SEXUAL PHARMACOLOGY

A NORTON PROFESSIONAL BOOK

SEXUAL PHARMACOLOGY

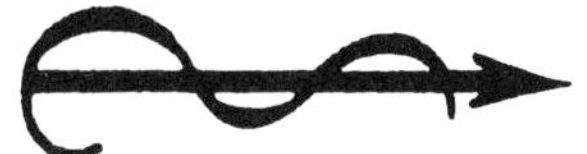

Drugs That Affect Sexual Functioning

Theresa L. Crenshaw, M.D.

James P. Goldberg, Ph.D.

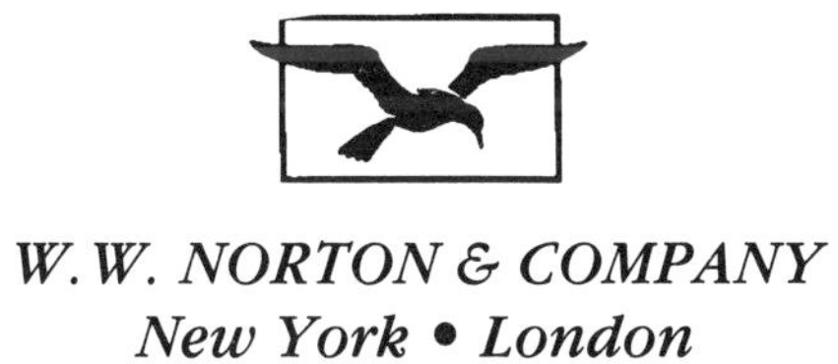

W. W. NORTON & COMPANY
New York • London

Copyright © 1996 by Crenshaw Writing Company

NOTICE

We have made every attempt to summarize accurately and concisely a multitude of references. However, the reader is reminded that times and medical knowledge change, transcription or understanding error is always possible, and crucial details are omitted whenever such a comprehensive review as this is attempted. We cannot, therefore, guarantee that every bit of information is absolutely accurate or complete. The reader should affirm that cited recommendations are still appropriate by reading the original articles and checking other sources including local consultants and recent literature.

DRUG DOSAGE

The authors and publisher have exerted every effort to ensure that drug selection and dosage set forth in this text are in accord with current recommendations and practice at the time of publication. However, in view of ongoing research, changes in government regulations, and the constant flow of information relating to drug therapy and drug reactions, the reader is urged to check the package insert for each drug for any change in indications and dosage and for added warnings and precautions. This is particularly important when the recommended agent is a new and/or infrequently used drug.

All rights reserved

Printed in the United States of America

First Edition

For information about permission to reproduce selections from this book,
write to Permissions, W. W. Norton & Company, Inc.
500 Fifth Avenue, New York, NY 10110

Library of Congress Cataloging-in-Publication Data
Crenshaw, Theresa Larsen.
Sexual pharmacology : drugs that affect sexual functioning /
Theresa L. Crenshaw, James P. Goldberg.
p. cm.
"A Norton professional book"—Ser. t.p.
Includes bibliographical references and index.
ISBN 0-393-70144-1
1. Generative organs—Effect of drugs on. 2. Drugs and sex.
3. Drugs—Side effects. 4. Sexual disorders—Chemotherapy.
I. Goldberg, James P. II. Title.
[DNLM: 1. Sex Disorders—chemically induced. 2. Sex Disorders—
therapy. 3. Sex Behavior—drug effects. 4. Drugs—adverse
effects. WM 611 C915s 1996]
RM380.C74 1996
615′.766—dc20
DNLM/DLC
for Library of Congress 95-42109 CIP

ISBN 0-393-70144-1

W. W. Norton & Company, Inc., 500 Fifth Avenue, New York, N.Y. 10110
W. W. Norton & Company, Ltd., 10 Coptic Street, London WC1A 1PU

1 2 3 4 5 6 7 8 9 0

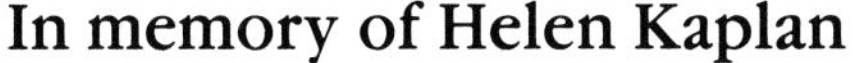

In memory of Helen Kaplan

Contents

Acknowledgments

Any author will tell you that a manuscript, as it goes to press, has acquired a life of its own that is more than just the sum of its parts—much like the strong identity of a giant fingerprint left by many people.

I am deeply grateful to all who have contributed to this project, especially my editor, Susan Barrows Munro, for her careful advice, patient counsel, and gracious deadline extensions; Linda Chester and Elizabeth Zongker, my agents, and their central support system, Laurie Fox, who did all they could to make sure that this book, the end result of years of patient research and compiling, found its respected niche; and Margaret O. Ryan, who sensitively cut the manuscript down to size and edited it for clarity.

To write a book of this magnitude is an ordeal. The sheer enormity of work involved can numb one's vision, blur all feelings, and overwhelm that sense of purpose so crucial to a successful project. The glue that held it together and made it all worthwhile was the spirit, determination, and cooperation of dedicated professionals who worked together in the face of formidable challenges. Dr. James Goldberg performed the majority of the literature research, conducted clinical research at the Crenshaw Clinic on my behalf, and contributed insights and new concepts to this venture. His tireless persistence and meticulous attention to detail were invaluable, his vision inspiring. With his help and support, I have been able to correlate, synthesize, and present as a comprehensive whole the result of my work of over 20 years of clinical and research experience.

With all our commitment and determination, Dr. Goldberg and I could not have completed the manuscript without a superb support staff, led by Allison Booth, including a tireless word processing crew, proofreaders, and an office staff who kept the logistics running smoothly and endured the fickle nature of our computer system with endless patience.

As final deadlines loomed time stood still for several weeks. Television was a distant memory and newspapers accumulated, unread. Somewhere in Florida there was a hurricane—we didn't know it. Among ourselves we shared a calm and utter sense of focus. We lived in the eye of our own hurricane, unruffled by events around us. As if on cue, we voluntarily diminished our world. We had a sense of mission.

For days on end, it was nothing but post-it notes and plastic flags; black, aromatic coffee; sinfully fattening pizza and delicious deli sandwiches; long bitter nights spent wrestling with uncooperative chapters; small, private moments on the balcony to drink in the charm of the San Diego Bay; hushed voices when somebody fell asleep in a beam of California sunshine or on the floor where they sat, manuscript in hand. Underneath it all ran a current of goodwill that must be rare among players as diverse as the cast that pulled together the finale. One might say that our molecules meshed.

This project drafted family and friends, who pitched in as needed and offered support whenever necessary:

- Ulrika Ehrenborg, a mother any daughter would be proud of, made of pure Dresden porcelain, aristocrat from head to toe and fingernail to perfect fingernail. Some years ago, she stepped out of another time and place into America. That perished world of hers—a world of kings and courts and noblemen—is still in every gesture.
- Brant Crenshaw, her American grandchild, my tousled puppy only yesterday. This was Brant's time. This project helped mature him. He quietly moved out of my lap to stand beside me as a man. He pitched in and pulled his weight. Between us, there was always love. Now there is respect and admiration.
- Allison Booth, a teenager *par excellence* who kept the book on track—without whom this project would not have been completed. This 19-year-old *wunderkind* chirps like a bird, moves like an Indian scout, smiles like 10,000 tiny suns, and marshals the troops (including me) as though she were Napoleon. That one has flawless timing, superb organizational skills. She has gold in her heart and steel in her eyes. We know she will always travel the distance.
- Lenny Thompson, who kept our world orderly throughout.
- Bob Morey, lifelong friend and valued critic, who put a rubber band around his pony tail and dug his Irish nose into assorted reference books to sharpen the text.
- My typing trio—Sue Daigle, Lillian Murphy, and Tiffany Booth—who threw themselves into ferocious battles with endless manuscript revisions—their fingers flew faster than words. Those three did all they could to keep computer glitches from defeating us, and performed a complicated waltz with discs of a nonmusical sort, without networks, and with a minimum of confusion. Christi Albouy typed the manuscript after final revisions.
- Toward the end, others were needed to meet the demand and the deadline: Gena Sproul, Arnold Crowson, Heidi Demer, Susan Sullivan, Cheryl Cerasoli, Kathy Herzog, and many others gave of their energy and time.
- Tim Swezey, who came on a moment's notice to sweet-talk our computers into cooperating during the numerous times they went on sudden strike.
- Larry Ritter, my neighborhood pharmacist, who located obscure and elusive information for me on short notice, and chuckled at my jokes.
- Peter Karlen, who helped me with legal aspects and made a fine "Dutch Uncle."
- To William H. Masters, M.D., Virginia Johnson, Robert Kolodney, M.D.,

Julian Davidson, Ph.D., Taylor Seagraves, M.D., John Buffum, Pharm.D., Alvaro Morales, M.D., and many others who courageously and persistently laid the groundwork for the field of sexual pharmacology through their research.

- To all my friends and colleagues who waded through this sometimes unintelligible, big, heavy, ugly manuscript during the awkward stages: Joseph Graedon, Ph.D., Joseph Pursch, M.D., Francis de Marneffe, M.D., William Stull, Paul Grant, Walter Bortz, M.D., Ralph Earle, Ph.D., Purvis Martin, M.D., Lennart Vetterberg, M.D., Bert McBride, M.D., Helen Kaplan, M.D., Elliott Richelson, M.D., Marty Weisberg, M.D., to name just a few.
- And especially to Ingrid Rimland, who arrived like a mix of the cavalry and the Salvation Army. Her editing talent and organizational sense took a massive task and made it manageable. Her stamina and determination rounded out the team and, briefly, we shared magic.

All of us appreciate the staff at the Crest Deli, who fed us, and the soft music by Enya, who soothed us. Annharriet Buck McLeod, through the charm and seclusion of the Golden Door, provided essential retreat and refreshment.

I owe special appreciation to my husband, William Gregoricus, who graciously altered our plans to make completion of this manuscript our top priority. Bill doesn't count time, he makes time count. He managed our schedule relentlessly, to best advantage, and streamlined my staff to peak efficiency. In response to his counsel, I hired Pamela Tipton as my executive assistant. She does the work of dozens. Although she entered the project toward the end, she made the home stretch smooth.

I have heard that books are never finished—they are abandoned. I thought that I would have the same uneasy feeling when it came to parting with this manuscript. Somehow, though, I am content—not because the book is finished or in any sense complete, but because it doesn't need to be. It is a good beginning, and as such, doesn't really need an ending. The ending should be written by others who continue this work by adding their contributions to the changing field of sexual pharmacology.

Introduction

Theresa L. Crenshaw

Sexual Pharmacology: Drugs That Affect Sexual Function is a comprehensive reference source on the sexual side effects of drugs, both positive and negative. Hundreds of commonly prescribed medications cause sexual problems; a smaller but growing group of drugs has the potential to improve sexual dysfunction.

Most physicians receive little or no training in human sexuality and even less information on the sexual side effects of drugs. When I was in medical school in the 1960s, the only information I was given about sex was delivered with a snicker: "Dyspareunia is better than apareunia." That is, painful intercourse is better than no intercourse—or, painful intercourse for the woman is better than no intercourse at all for the man!

Today the one-liner is, "Medications can cause sexual problems." End of subject. While even this minimal acknowledgment is a measurable improvement, the topic demands deeper exploration. *Sexual Pharmacology* addresses this void by serving as a resource for those who did not receive adequate training in human sexuality in medical or graduate school. It is also an essential reference for nonphysicians who evaluate and treat sexual problems.

A physician's treatment plan cannot be effective unless the patient follows instructions. It is well-known that patients frequently sabotage their own health care by abandoning certain medications prescribed for them without telling their doctors. Anything that threatens to interfere with this health strategy must be taken seriously and addressed accordingly. One of the greatest treatment obstacles is the adverse sexual side effects of commonly prescribed drugs. A physician's lack of information about the sexual side effects of drugs not only jeopardizes a patient's health but can actually be life threatening. Blood pressure medication that is not taken may cause a heart attack or a stroke; ulcer medication left on the shelf can result in gastrointestinal hemorrhage. This text will enable medical students, physicians, and others to make more appropriate diagnoses regarding medically and chemically induced dysfunction while enabling them to make better decisions regarding the medication they prescribe or recommend.

NEED FOR TEAMWORK

Sexual problems that result from prescribed drugs can lead to depression, divorce, and even suicide. It is ultimately the responsibility of the physician or therapist to be aware of the sexual consequences of prescription medications and to select the least sexually toxic option whenever possible. When a sexually toxic medication is unavoidable, the physician must know how to handle the situation with patients in an appropriate manner that promotes compliance and understanding.

Although nonphysicians need to be informed about the types of medications that can interfere with psychotherapy and sex therapy, numerous obstacles typically have blocked this seemingly simple mandate. First of all, until now a comprehensive text and reference has not been available on the subject. Moreover, new drugs are continually added to the marketplace. During research and development, drugs are not routinely evaluated for their sexual side effects, so neither researchers nor doctors are aware of the possible consequences before the drugs are made available for patient care. To further complicate matters, both patients and physicians often have difficulty discussing sexual issues. Even more insidious is the fact that many physicians are unaware of their own ignorance in this area. However, recognition of problems with noncompliance caused by the sexual consequences of drugs is becoming increasingly widespread in medicine. Armed with specific information about the sexual properties of drugs and general information on the mechanisms of action most likely to cause sexual problems, physicians can bridge the gap between recognizing this problem and solving it. *Sexual Pharmacology* provides the necessary information. In addition, since it is not possible to list all medications, and new ones are introduced each month, *Sexual Pharmacology* provides guidelines for evaluating the sexual properties of virtually any drug. These guidelines will enable physicians as well as nonphysicians to determine the probable effect of any particular drug or class of drugs on sexual functioning.

Even professionals who do not prescribe medications—psychologists, marriage and family therapists, social workers, pastoral counselors, nurses—need to know about sexual pharmacology. Without such information, they may misdiagnose as psychological, sexual problems that are actually chemical and easily treatable with drug substitution. In such cases even the finest therapy will fail to elicit the desired results, frustrating patient and therapist alike. Clearly, professionals who treat sexual problems cannot arrive at competent differential diagnoses without knowing how medications could be affecting their patients. An understanding of the medical conditions and medications that can cause sexual problems is extremely helpful in making appropriate referrals to physicians and evaluating the adequacy of the consults.

For the sake of simplicity, we will use the terms *doctor*, *physician*, and *therapist* interchangeably; the term *patient* includes the psychotherapeutic concept of *client*. To make the text readable for all professionals, we have made every effort to use generic language that is multidisciplinary. Complex material is presented in clear, simple terms without being simplistic (the necessary exceptions being the names of drugs and their mechanisms of action, which are unavoidably complex). Even patients will be able to use *Sexual Pharmacology* as a reference when necessary.

THE EVOLUTION OF AN IDEA

Ironically, this text on drugs began with my efforts to eliminate or at least minimize drug use. Throughout almost 20 years of clinical practice, prescription drugs have been my adversary. Numerous patients who were referred to me for sex therapy were taking medications for heart disease, depression, or other conditions; these drugs made it chemically difficult or impossible for them to function sexually. In order to treat them effectively, I had to find alternative medications to control their health problems without eliminating their sexual responsiveness. Whenever possible, I tried to eliminate medication altogether by utilizing nonchemical methods of improving their health, such as diet, exercise, stress management, cognitive therapy for depression and anxiety. If these strategies were not sufficient, and if no satisfactory substitute medication could be found, I attempted to reduce dosages.

When I began this process of examining cause-effect relationships between medications and symptoms, little information was available on the sexual effects of drugs. Anecdotal reports were rare and there were almost no pertinent research studies. Even *rumors* were scarce. In addition, patients were considerably more reluctant to discuss sex than they are today. My treatment strategy involved minimizing medication and maximizing other resources by improving diet and fitness, promoting exercise, eliminating drinking and smoking, and reducing stress. This comprehensive approach, when aggressively pursued, facilitated the reduction of dosage and in some cases even eliminated the need for medication.

At first there were few alternative medications from which to choose and most of those available had varying degrees of sexual toxicity. Drug substitution was mostly accomplished by trial and error. Over the years, better drugs have been developed in almost all categories, making drug substitution easier and more successful. While the first angle of attack in attempting to reduce or eliminate medication still should be to utilize nondrug therapies, drug substitution is often necessary. Psychotherapy can be successful with this strategy and most drug-induced sexual problems can be corrected or minimized. While there is still some trial and error involved in finding the best solution, the information presented in *Sexual Pharmacology* can make the effort much easier.

In the course of treating thousands of patients with prescription-related sexual problems, I have developed profiles of the medications that commonly cause problems and those that do not. Combining these findings with anecdotal reports in the literature, research studies, and networking among physicians, I accumulated a body of data that ultimately led to the writing of this book. Dr. John Feighner referred Warren Stern, Ph.D., to me after Dr. Stern expressed an interest in studying the sexual properties of bupropion. His vision and competence enabled him to convince a major pharmaceutical company to fund a properly controlled trial of drug treatment of sexual dysfunction. As a result, we had the opportunity to perform one of the first large-scale studies intended to investigate a drug for its positive sexual activity. Then, in 1983, Dr. James Goldberg, a research psychopharmacologist, joined my staff as chief of research at the Crenshaw Clinic in San Diego. Our mutual interest in drug-related sexual problems fueled my momentum in the collection and development of data in this area, eventually making this text possible.

OBJECTIVES OF *SEXUAL PHARMACOLOGY*

To integrate medical, pharmacological, and psychological arenas. One objective of this text is to increase understanding of the complex interaction of psychology, disease, and medication. In the past, medicine has taken a somewhat simplistic approach to distinguishing between physical and psychological causes. Norman Cousins expressed it best when he said that "emotions have biological consequences." This statement is especially true in the area of human sexuality. The emotion—sexual desire—typically results in predictable physical responses of erection and lubrication. However, certain chemicals (dopamine is one) can induce emotions that stimulate sexual desire. Appropriately, the differentiation between medical and psychological conditions is becoming increasingly blurred. In fact, the "psychological" is often physiological on a molecular level.

Throughout the history of medicine, diseases that could not be explained or cured were often diagnosed as psychological until medicine advanced to a more sophisticated level. Trichomonas was once considered a psychological disease, and publications in the psychiatric literature claimed to cure trichomonal vaginitis through psychoanalysis. These theories abruptly disappeared when metronidazole (Flagyl) was discovered and the condition could be corrected with a pill. I shudder to think of the numerous cases of drug-induced sexual dysfunction that have been misdiagnosed as psychological and treated with weeks, months, even years of psychotherapy, when a simple drug substitution in a timely fashion could have solved the problem.

To acknowledge pharmacological implications of gender differences. Men and women are different chemically, biologically, physiologically, anatomically, and emotionally. Although this statement may seem obvious, traditionally medicine has treated women as modified men, prescribing the same medications typically at the same dosages. Most drug research is usually performed on men by men under the questionable assumption that men and women are medically alike.

Physiological, psychological, hormonal, and anatomical differences between men and women are most clear and least debatable when it comes to sexual function and reproduction. Indeed, other aspects of physiology, psychology, and medicine are sex-linked as well, but have not yet received adequate attention or recognition. *Sexual Pharmacology* seeks to identify those aspects of gender that directly or indirectly interact with particular drugs.

To inspire further research. It is our hope that, through presenting this material and focusing attention on this new field, we will encourage pharmaceutical companies, the Federal Drug Administration (FDA), and researchers to assess the sexual properties of medication *prior to* its release for patient use. Until that time, the main method of discovering these adverse sexual side effects—prescribing them to the general population as an inadvertent sexual experiment—will continue to spawn considerable human suffering.

DRUGS THAT IMPROVE SEX

In the course of investigating adverse sexual side effects, we became curious about the possibility of *positive effects*. Through an appreciation of sexual pharmacology, beginning with the numerous mechanisms by which medicine and chemicals can interfere with sexual function, we concluded that chemicals had the potential to affect sex in the opposite direction. It is, therefore, no surprise that we are beginning to recognize and document a few medications that influence sexual function in a favorable way.

Does this mean we are on the threshold of discovering a true aphrodisiac? No. There is no *one* substance that solves all sexual problems. However, there are numerous medications currently available that can improve sexual function in one way or another. The term aphrodisiac is conventionally used to refer to virtually any substance that is believed to improve sex. There is an important distinction to be made, however, between substances that resolve sexual dysfunction, thus "normalizing" sex, and those that promote "supersex." The quest for medications that provide otherwise sexually normal people with "superhuman sexual prowess" is quite another concept, and is what many people think about when they hear the term *aphrodisiac*. This text will concentrate on the medications that can be used to correct sexual problems, thereby helping an individual return to normal sexual functioning, while acknowledging and identifying medications with the potential to induce hypersexuality.

COMPREHENSIVE THERAPY

A central theme of *Sexual Pharmacology* is the importance of psychotherapy. Tremendous benefit can be derived from medications that treat or cure sexual problems. They are valuable *supplements*; nevertheless, it is critical that these substances not be misused as *substitutes* for therapy. If treatment does not also address the emotional issues that are present, medication alone could actually aggravate a problem rather than resolve it. Chemicals should not be used to depersonalize sex or to transform it into a mechanically successful event that disregards the emotional context of the individual and his or her relationship. Neither should the sexual consequences of medical conditions and related drug regimens be overlooked or attributed to relationship problems. The prevalence of relationship distress can tempt both physician and patient to assume sexual symptoms are the consequence of an impending divorce or other emotional trauma, without appreciating the influence of a sexually toxic drug. Confounding the situation is the subtlety of sex drive disorders, which are difficult to measure. While low sex drive is the most common symptom to manifest as an effect of medications, sex drive is also most susceptible to the influence of many other stresses. Sorting out the variables can be a challenge.

ETHICAL CONSIDERATIONS

The medications available today that can improve various aspects of sexual function will become increasingly common and new ones will be discovered. The ethics of the use and misuse of these drugs needs to be addressed in view of the unusual nature of human sexuality. The potential for abuse of substances that stimulate sexual desire, correct impotence, and promote orgasm is substantial, particularly considering the fact that the appeal of most street drugs can be attributed partially to their sexual properties—be they real or imagined.

Even traditional medicine is not above misusing these drugs. Any tool can be used as a weapon. Most good medications (including penicillin) were overused until their potency and limitations were better understood. Also, all drugs can have dangerous side effects. Prescription drugs that affect sexual function must be placed in proper perspective and in a therapeutic context, which this book proposes to do.

SEXUAL CHEMISTRY AND "THE MOLECULES OF LOVE"

Today, the term *sexual chemistry* means more than the attraction between two people. We are actually beginning to define the molecules and chemical pathways responsible for desire, arousal, passion, lust, and sexual responsiveness. There is even reason to believe that the emotions, love and limerance, have a chemical basis—either as a catalyst or a consequence. A new understanding of the biological basis of human connection—what could be called "the molecules of love and lust"—is entering the mainstream of medicine and opening doors to exciting new possibilities.

Sexual pharmacology is a young, rapidly developing field that has a distinct contribution to make to other medical disciplines. Scientific interest in human sexuality is accelerating. Although it will probably be another decade before sexual functioning becomes a routine category of general medicine, such an inclusion is inevitable.

Twenty years ago, approximately 80% of sexual problems were considered to be psychological in origin. Today, these figures are almost the reverse. We have discovered increasing numbers of medical conditions and pharmacological agents that can cause or contribute to sexual disorders. As the etiology of sexual problems shifts from the psychological arena into the realm of concrete medical practice, physicians will be more inclined to acknowledge these conditions as their responsibility. If, in addition to defining the problem, it is within their power to solve it, their role becomes even more vital. Advances in medicine and chemistry have enabled us to cure some sexual problems; the future promises more.

THE INFLUENCE OF AIDS

Another force compelling physicians to address sexual issues is the AIDS epidemic. Physicians who did not address sex in general—much less homosexuality or anal intercourse—have been compelled to take sexual histories and ask questions that they would not have considered before. The pressure to ask personal and probing questions about sex will eventually help to integrate human sexuality into mainstream medicine. The continuing need to face sexual issues will gradually engender a sense of comfort and ease that will benefit patients and physicians alike.

The import of AIDS is also a consideration when exploring topics of sexually toxic and sexually effective drugs. Disrupting an otherwise stable relationship with sexually toxic drugs is not a desirable side effect of treatment at any time. In this age of AIDS, preserving a couple's sexual function in committed relationships is a noncontroversial and effective form of AIDS prevention. Unrecognized drug-induced sexual dysfunction can inspire affairs and destroy relationships, exposing more persons to the dating pool—and thereby increasing the risk of AIDS. Regarding drugs that facilitate sexual functioning, some might contend that the last thing society needs is drugs that cause more interest in more sex. However, any medication that improves sex within a committed relationship is a welcome resource for couples today.

"CONSUMER-DRIVEN" MEDICINE

The impact of sexual pharmacology will increase each decade. With the "graying" of America, before too long the elderly will comprise the majority of a doctor's practice. The shifting emphasis from disease management to wellness, longevity, and quality of life will bring sexual concerns into central focus. As people live longer, they will expect to retain, with the help of modern medicine, all their faculties—and they will not relinquish the pleasure of sexual functioning as willingly as they have in the past. The mature medical consumer will insist that the physician be sensitive and alert to these issues.

MAXIMIZING *SEXUAL PHARMACOLOGY*

There are two main ways to use this book: as a text to be studied and as a quick clinical reference source. As a text, *Sexual Pharmacology* is designed for use in medical schools, nursing programs, and graduate programs and is specifically intended to supplement courses in psychology, physiology, pharmacology, psychiatry, neurology, cardiology, gastroenterology, urology, and gynecology. Graduate school and training programs that would benefit from the information in *Sexual Pharmacology* include psychology, marriage and family therapy, sex therapy, pastoral counseling, social work, and pharmacology. In addition, as a reference *Sexual Pharmacology* is applicable to all areas of clinical medicine involving treatment with prescription drugs in which noncompliance is a concern. There is increasing awareness among physicians that sexual considerations are a central concern of their patients rather than an elective issue in patient management.

The first three chapters of the book discuss the development of fundamental skills: learning to elicit pertinent sexual histories; establishing baseline sexual histories efficiently and comfortably; differentiating between medical, pharmacological, and psychological factors in sexual dysfunction; and developing strategies for treatment. These chapters also provide a step-by-step procedure for evaluating the sexual properties of any drug, whether it is specifically included in this text or not.

After reviewing these chapters, clinicians can depend heavily on the index to locate information about individual drugs as needed. When a drug is not listed, refer back to Chapter 1 and follow the guidelines for evaluating the sexual properties of unlisted drugs.

The medical consumer—patients, clients, laypersons—can also use *Sexual Pharmacology* to learn about drugs they are taking, in order to be well informed when they address this issue with their physicians or therapists.

Part I

BASIC PRINCIPLES OF SEXUAL PHARMACOLOGY

1

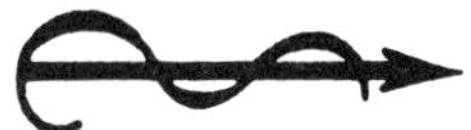

Understanding the Sexual Properties of Drugs

OBJECTIVES

- To provide clinically useful information on the sexual side effects of commonly prescribed drugs
- To identify categories of drugs that affect sex through a common mechanism of action
- To provide a method for evaluating drugs not specifically included in this book and/ or future drugs not yet developed

Many commonly prescribed drugs can cause a wide range of sexual problems. Since sexual problems were not taken into consideration during the developmental phases of drug research, this aspect of pharmacology was unappreciated for many decades. Physicians prescribed medications without considering the sexual implications or asking about sexual side effects.

As anecdotal information accumulated and insight developed into the sexual disturbances caused by medication, physicians developed a general understanding that adverse sexual side effects could develop. The prevailing view, however, was that the benefit of correcting a serious medical problem far outweighed the majority of side effects, including that of impaired sexual functioning. In addition, the absence of better pharmacological alternatives made it almost impossible for physicians to select drugs based on the presence or absence of sexual impact.

During the 1970s, the importance of pharmacological side effects gained increasing attention. The original premise that any medication offering a cure or symptom relief was automatically beneficial regardless of the price—in cost or in side effects—underwent a major revision. The battle against cancer with chemotherapy, surgery, and radiation raised questions about whether the cure was, in some cases, worse than the disease. Emphasis shifted somewhat from maximizing the duration of life to preserving its quality.

In the course of these general medical trends, new drugs were developed that could target specific systems more precisely, thereby affecting fewer physiological mechanisms. Once specific physiological functions could be pharmacologically modulated independently, patients could be maintained in relative health rather than simply rescued from debilitating disease—a dramatic departure from earlier medical practices. The continuing problem, however, remained the interference of adverse drug side effects.

Initially, side effects were tolerated as a necessary price of preserving health. Eventually, with more drugs from which to choose, treatment also involved minimizing side effects that interfered with quality of life: weight changes, sedation, depression, fatigue, allergies, cognitive debilities, emotional dyscontrol, and more recently, sexual dysfunction. These common complications of prescription medications have become medical concerns as well as the focus of pharmacological marketing.

Previously, sexual dysfunction was considered resolved once obvious symptoms (such as lack of erection or ejaculation) were eliminated. The priority remained, appropriately, the treatment of disease. Those drugs which were relatively free of major sexual side effects were readily accepted. However, when higher drug doses were needed to prevent sickness and debilitating sexual consequences ensued, physicians concluded that decreased sexuality was a small price to pay for the prevention of disease. Both doctor and patient settled for the adage that "sex was not particularly relevant if you were dead."

Most patients, regardless of the intensity of their concern, are embarrassed and confused by sexual changes brought on by drugs. They are often uncomfortable discussing these drug-induced sexual problems with anyone—their spouses, their doctors, even their therapists. As a result, most physicians remain unaware of the sexual complications of the drugs they prescribe. Indeed, physicians are confronted with two distinct lacunae in relation to the effects of the drugs they prescribe on sexual functioning: the first lacuna occurs with their patients (who do not tell them) and the second occurs in the literature (which is incomplete). Under these circumstances, it has been almost impossible for physicians to become aware of the sexual properties of drugs.

The material presented in the following chapters is the product of years of clinical experience, anecdotal reports, and an exhaustive search of the literature. Not infrequently, the information in the literature is contradictory. Studies vary tremendously in quality of design and content of research. Some researchers investigate sexual side effects through the use of questionnaires and/or interviews. More typically, the publications are based on information spontaneously volunteered by patients. Unfortunately, patients volunteer very little, if any, information about sex when they are not specifically invited to do so.

Information on the sexual side effects of drugs is spotty and incomplete. To complicate matters, there is no single compilation of the research. In fact, data are scattered throughout the literature, often in obscure journals, monographs, and doctoral dissertations. Surprisingly little can be found in publications that specifically address sexuality. Instead, relevant papers are spread across fields—in journals on pharmacology, psychiatry, obstetrics-gynecology, general medicine, cardiology, and various other specialties. A considerable number of pertinent reports can be found only in the animal literature.

SIDE EFFECTS AND SEXUAL FUNCTION

A prerequisite to understanding the sexual properties of drugs is a clear picture of the types of sexual problems drugs can induce. Most published information reports only male-related problems associated with erection or ejaculation. The term *impotence* is commonly misused to refer to all types of sexual dysfunction in males, whether involving libido, erection, or ejaculation. Meanwhile, women's dysfunctional sexual responses become invisible or appear nonexistent. Since the word *frigidity* (happily) has been eliminated from medical terminology, no comprehensive term has been conceived. For example, decrease in lubrication may be noted only when it becomes especially severe, and even then may be buried in the term *dyspareunia* (painful coitus). The influence of drugs on sex drive is even less frequently addressed, because it is a subtle symptom, difficult to measure objectively, and often dependent on interpersonal dynamics.

Anorgasmia is almost never described in side effect inventories. Apparently, female patients are not asked about changes in orgasm, even though this symptom is of as much concern to women as impotence is to men. Although recently rare case studies have reported the absence of female orgasm, historically there has been no systematic inquiry into the effects of medications on women's orgasmic responsiveness. Despite the "sexual revolution," women's sexual well-being is still seen as synonymous with reproductive health in most medical quarters. This limitation is even characteristic of specialties one would expect to be more sophisticated, such as obstetrics-gynecology, urology, and psychiatry. Anorgasmia, sex drive disorders, and even dyspareunia are considered so common in women that some doctors treat them as normal and routine.

In spite of all the limitations, inhibitions, and inadequate terminology, the literature is rich with reports on sexual side effects. Sometimes references are obscure and hard to find; more commonly, they are abundant and difficult to interpret. Nonetheless, the evidence, when compiled and properly analyzed, paints a compelling and surprisingly clear picture of the sexual side effects of commonly prescribed drugs.*

The detection of sexual side effects is not a mysterious or elusive task. When evaluating medications (whether listed in this chapter or not), depend heavily on your common sense. While sifting through the literature is a challenge, much can be accomplished by some simple detective work.

Based on our current understanding of the biochemical mechanisms that affect sexual function, medications can influence sexual function in a variety of ways. There are *direct* sexual side effects, which include chemical mechanisms of the drug that influence any or all aspects of sexual desire or activity. Drugs can also have *indirect* sexual side effects which result not from the chemical property of the drug but from some other drug effect such as sedation, changes in mood and energy levels, weight loss or gain, body image, etc. These indirect effects make a person too sleepy, too unhappy, too tired, or too confused for sex to be appealing or possible.

*In gathering the information presented here, we have consulted various texts and references. Original articles have been used as references whenever possible. General texts consulted include the *Physicians Desk Reference* (*PDR*, 1991a), the *PDR* Drug Interactions and Side Effects Index (*PDR*, 1991b), *American Medical Association Drug Evaluations* (AMA, 1991), *Meyler's Side Effects of Drugs* (Dukes, 1988), *Remington's Pharmaceutical Sciences* (Gennaro, 1990), *Goodman and Gilman's Pharmacological Basis of Therapeutics* (Gilman, Rall, Nies, & Taylor, 1990). Popular drug guides for the layperson include *Fifty Plus: The Graedon's People's Pharmacy for Older Adults* (1985), *Graedon's Best Medicine* (Graedon & Graedon, 1991), and *What You Need to Know About Psychiatric Drugs* (Yudofsky, Hales, & Ferguson, 1991).

As mentioned, the sexual effects drugs have on women may be the same or different from those they have on men.

Some medications that are best known for their adverse sexual side effects may, under some circumstances or at certain dosages, have positive sexual effects. In fact, paradoxical side effects of this nature are not uncommon. The most typical example of a paradoxical side effect is a drug that has one effect at a low dose and the exact opposite effect at a higher dose. Some drugs have adverse sexual side effects in some patients regardless of dose and positive effects in others at the same dosages.

Direct Side Effects

The most common sexually related consequence of medication is diminished desire, which applies fairly equally to both sexes. However, this symptom is seldom reported. Decrease in sex drive is often attributed to other causes, such as relationship discord, fatigue, job stress, and so forth. With so many feasible explanations, patients frequently do not associate the reduced drive with medication. For this reason, patients do not mention their symptoms to physicians, and physicians rarely ask. Because alterations in sex drive are less obvious than impairment of erection or ejaculation difficulties, changes are more readily missed by patients and physicians alike.

The next most frequent sexual side effect of prescription drugs is erectile difficulties, followed by orgasmic difficulties in both males and females. The most common orgasmic dysfunction for women is delayed orgasm. Most women find this delay particularly distressing, because even without adverse drug effects many women already feel under pressure to respond more quickly in order to keep pace with their partners. Additional delay is undesirable. Symptoms of gynecomastia, lactation, priapism, dyspareunia, and hypogonadism are less frequent but nonetheless disturbing when they occur.

Certain drugs can induce states of psychoses, which may initially manifest as hypersexuality. It is therefore particularly important to be vigilant for early signs of hypersexuality, regardless of the cause. The implications can be serious (as in psychosis) or readily correctable (as in a drug effect).

Symptoms of impending psychosis/hypersexuality may include:

- unusually vivid dreaming or nightmares;
- hallucinations and daydreaming;
- paranoid thoughts;
- driven, unusual repetitive behavior;
- excessive, unrealistic demands on the partner;
- frequent irritability or arguments;
- fascination and overindulgence in multiple "miracle cure" schemes;
- extreme withdrawal or obsessive intimacy;
- relentless overactivity.

Tables 1.1 and 1.2 list the direct sexual side effects that can be pharmacologically related. In order of frequency of side effects, these side effects include:

Sex drive disorders. Sex drive can be increased (hypersexuality) or decreased (inhibited) by certain chemicals. Hyposexuality refers to a lower than normal baseline interest. Inhibited sexual desire refers to a decrease from a higher baseline. Sexual aversion represents an avoidance of sexual activity. Symptoms can be mild and subtle, or frankly phobic. Sexual panic/phobia appears to be a distinct disorder involving avoidance of sex or intense symptoms of fear and nervousness before and/or during sexual activity. Obsessive-compulsive tendencies may manifest as either restriction of sex to a rigid routine or peculiar thoughts or behaviors connected to sexual stimulation and activity, often including excessive masturbation or need for excessive cleanliness.

Erection disorders. In the literature, penile erection often has been treated simplistically as an all-or-none phenomenon, but there are actually degrees of dysfunction that should be appreciated. Difficulty in achieving or maintaining an erection can be most distressing. The man who used to become erect as a result of a sexual thought or touch who now finds he is unable to develop an erection without vigorous manual stimulation has experienced a marked change in his sexual functioning. The inability to maintain an erection during intercourse usually results in distressing interruptions. The inability to achieve a full erection may not prevent inter-

Table 1.1 *Direct Sexual Side Effects Related to Drugs and Medications: Female*

Alterations in Desire	*Dyspareunia*
Hyposexuality	Pain during intercourse
Inhibition of desire	Pain after intercourse
Aversion	Painful orgasm
Hypersexuality	*Menstrual Disorders*
Panic/phobia	Dysmenorrhea
Obsessive-compulsive	Menorrhagia
Lubrication Disorders	Amenorrhea
Orgasmic Disorders	*Clitoral Hypertrophy*
Orgasmic inhibition	*Infertility*
Anorgasmia	Decreased frequency of ovulation
Diminished number of orgasms	Decreased quality of egg
Altered perception	Hypofertility
Anesthetic orgasm	*Breast Disorders*
Spontaneous orgasm	Galactorrhea
	Gynecomastia
	Pain/tenderness
	Paraphilia

Table 1.2 *Direct Sexual Side Effects Related to Drugs and Medications: Male*

Alterations in Desire	*Orgasm/Ejaculation Disorders*
Hyposexuality	Ejaculatory incompetence (inability)
Inhibition of desire	Ejaculatory inhibition (delay)
Aversion	Ejaculation without orgasm
Hypersexuality	Orgasm without ejaculation
Panic/phobia	Retrograde ejaculation
Obsessive-compulsive	Decreased ejaculatory volume
Erection Abnormalities	Anesthetic ejaculation
Inability/difficulty obtaining erection	Spontaneous orgasm
Inability/difficulty maintaining erection	Painful ejaculation
Decreased firmness of erection	Premature ejaculation
Ejaculation through flaccid or semi-erect penis	*Dyspareunia*
Painful erection	Pain during intercourse
Peyronie's disease	Pain after intercourse
Priapism	Painful ejaculation
Decreased or absent nocturnal/morning erections	*Breasts*
Infertility	Galactorrhea
Decreased or malformed spermatogenesis	Gynecomastia
Decreased sperm motility	Breast pain/tenderness
Hypogonadism	*Paraphilia*
Testicular atrophy	

course, but it will be worrisome to both partners. Partial erections that are insufficient for intercourse indicate some function but make penetration impossible. Many men are able to be orgasmic and ejaculate through a flaccid or semi-flaccid penis; thus orgasmic function can remain intact even when erections are diminished or absent. Not uncommonly these various alterations are due to the side effects of prescription drugs.

Lubrication disorders. The most common effect of medication on lubrication is to decrease it. This symptom can be easily corrected with a suitable artificial lubricant. However, it is remarkable to note how rarely women address the problem. Instead, they suffer discomfort, which results in local irritation, often severe enough to cause chronic infections and/or dyspareunia.

An *increase* in lubrication is usually perceived as sexually advantageous, but in some cases it causes lack of friction for the male, who may lose his erection due to lack of sensation. Herbs used as aphrodisiacs by many African women make the vagina hot and dry to better stimulate their male partner.

Alteration of odor caused by changes in vaginal pH or flora due to antibiotics and other medications can influence sexual receptivity, comfort, and practices.

Orgasm/ejaculation disorders. Conventional thinking does not distinguish between male ejaculation and orgasm, yet they occur via separate, albeit related, mechanisms. Complicating matters is the fact that many of these dysfunctions can be situational, meaning that the man who cannot ejaculate or sustain an erection during intercourse may be able to get a fine erection with masturbation or be able to have an orgasm with masturbation, oral sex, or manual manipulation by partner but not with intercourse or vice versa.

Ejaculation disorders include premature ejaculation, which is often subjectively defined; inhibited ejaculation, which involves difficulty in ejaculating when psychologically ready or motivated and in some cases leads to total inability to ejaculate (ejaculatory incompetence). Retrorograde ejaculation involves a rerouting of the ejaculate during orgasm. Instead of traveling out the urethra, the ejaculate travels the opposite direction into the bladder. At orgasm, there is no evidence of ejaculation, although it has occurred. The first time a man urinates after sex, however, the urine is cloudy due to the ejaculate. Retrograde ejaculation usually occurs as a result of a damaged internal bladder sphincter (i.e., due to prostate surgery) or as a consequence of some medications that relax the muscles of that sphincter. Other ejaculation disorders include painful ejaculation, ejaculation without orgasm, orgasm without ejaculation ("dry" orgasm), anesthetic ejaculation, decreased volume of ejaculate, and spontaneous orgasm. A man may be orgasmic without ejaculating and in some cases ejaculate without orgasm (emission alone). If ejaculation occurs without the sensation of orgasm, or with significantly decreased intensity of feeling, it is called anesthetic orgasm. Spontaneous orgasms are typically unexpected and unrelated to traditional sexual stimulation. They may occur for no apparent reason or be associated with an unusual event, such as yawning or walking.

Peyronie's disease. A condition resulting in the development of curvature of the penis, which, when severe, can cause pain with erection and/or penetration. It is also referred to as "penile fibromatosis," and results from the formation of plaques or strands of dense fibrous tissue surrounding the corpus cavernosum. It can be localized or diffused and is usually of adult onset. In most cases, the underling cause is not known. Frequent penile injections can cause or aggravate the condition.

Priapism. An involuntary erection lasting for hours or sometimes days, and often associated with pain. Priapism can lead to irreversible impotence if not treated promptly.

Orgasmic disorders. Orgasmic disorders in women can be universal or situational and include delayed, inhibited, or retarded orgasm (all synonymous), anorgasmia, anesthetic orgasm, spontaneous orgasm, and diminished number of orgasms. Anesthetic orgasms in women refer only to significant decrease in intensity. If orgasmic sensation is completely absent, orgasm is difficult, usually impossible, to identify. A more precise term to identify the phenomenon is "altered perception."

Altered perceptions of orgasm and arousal. Medications can intensify or diminish the perception and experience of sexual desire and responsiveness. If the effects are subtle, there may be little impact on the relationship unless the individual or couple was already marginally dysfunctional. Sometimes the effects can be quite pronounced. Unfortunately, however, patients rarely suspect medication as the cause.

Dyspareunia. This is a term originally used to describe female disorders, but is currently also used when males experience this category of symptoms (pain during intercourse with erection and penetration, pain with orgasm, and pain after orgasm).

Gynecomastia. If it occurs in a woman, this symptom usually goes largely unnoticed because it is masked by the size of a woman's breasts. Gynecomastia in the man is quite obvious and often associated with tenderness. Both women and men can experience tenderness or pain.

Lactation (galactorrhea). This symptom can occur in both sexes, but it is more frequent in women.

Breast tenderness. Certain medications can cause noticeable tenderness in the breast for both sexes. In the majority of cases this symptom is not a major concern, but on occasion it can severely inhibit sexual activity. Breasts become so tender that the touching, sucking, or pressing of foreplay and intercourse become uncomfortable or impossible. Although hypersensitivity is the more common problem, hyposensitivity can also cause significant distress.

Menstrual disorders. Any disruption of the menstrual cycle has the potential to interfere with sexual appetite, function, and frequency. Menstrual disorders include dysmenorrhea (painful menstruation), menorrhagia (excessively prolonged or profuse bleeding), and amenorrhea (the absence of menstruation). In addition, irregular and unpredictable bleeding, occurring in women of all ages but especially bothersome during the transition to menopause, can be particularly disruptive to sexual activity for couples who consider sex during menstruation unacceptable.

Clitoral hypertrophy. Hypertrophy refers to

a general enlargement of a part or an organ not caused by tumor formation. In response to certain medications, the clitoris may increase in size, with or without an increase in sensitivity.

Paraphilias (male and female). The dictionary definition of paraphilia is "sexual deviation." The term refers to a variety of aberrant sexual behaviors, e.g., necrophilia (sexual attraction to cadavers), pedophilia (sexual attraction to children), and numerous other sexual behaviors most societies consider abnormal. In general, paraphilias are considerably more common among men than women.

Infertility/sterility. These conditions comprise another area that typically has been viewed inappropriately in terms of extremes—the complete absence of viable sperm or the absence of ovulation versus the presence of normal reproductive facilities. In fact, more commonly at issue is the "gray zone" of decreased sperm motility, decreased frequency of ovulation, decreased quality of egg and sperm.

Hypogonadism. A variety of causes can induce this symptom in males, which results in subnormal gonadal function usually indicated by subnormal testosterone levels (less than 300 ng/dl) and/or impaired sperm production. In adult males, the most typical cause is testicular atrophy, which can be induced by various medications; in the developing male, arrested development (inadequate hypothalamic-pituitary function) can produce hypogonadism. Various substances (e.g., prolactin) and neurotransmitters (e.g., opioids) can block androgenic receptors necessary for testosterone production. When hypogonadism is due to lack of appropriate gonadotropin secretion from the brain, it is called "hypogonadotropic hypogonadism."

Hypofertility. Hypofertility is a new term intended to designate the relatively fertile individual whose baseline potency has been compromised to some degree.

Indirect Side Effects

It is important for physicians to be aware of the fact that medications which cause general physical and/or psychological side effects, making an individual feel ill or unwell, will also diminish sexual interest and responsiveness. Conversely, when a painful chronic condition is relieved (such as low back pain or migraine headache), sexual interest may revive as a result of the absence of pain, as long as the medication does not cause undue somnolence or absence of sensation. Similarly, medication that increases mobility (through pain relief or anti-inflammatory effects), such as the effective treatment of arthritis, can cause a major improvement in sexual participation. Decreased sensation, which may be a consequence of decreasing pain with medication, may allow sexual function but diminish sensation and enjoyment.

Common drug side effects that are not specifically sexual but can nonetheless affect sexual relations indirectly are listed in Table 1.3.

A "common sense" approach is required in order to appreciate the significance of these indirect sexual side effects to sexual well-being. It is important to recognize that indirect side effects can be as sexually disabling as direct ones.

Body image. An increase or decrease in weight can affect body image and self-esteem in a favorable or unfavorable fashion, resulting in an increase or decrease in sexual initiative and receptivity. Someone who gains or loses excessive weight may not wish to be seen nude and will be reluctant to participate in sex for fear of exposing real or perceived defects.

Halitosis and altered taste. Many medications (particularly the anticholinergics) cause bad breath by drying out the mouth. According to dental reports, anticholinergics can predispose individuals to caries and gingivitis, which are additional causes of halitosis. Although understandably overlooked as a sexual side effect, drug-induced halitosis can have an impact on sexual behavior. Taste may also be altered by many drugs. Kissing and hugging are often the first overture of sexual intimacy. If that simple bridge is broken, sexual opportunity may vanish altogether.

Comfort. Any drug side effect that makes an individual physically uncomfortable, such as nausea, bloatedness, or dizziness, can encroach on a sense of well-being sufficiently to interfere with the enjoyment of sex.

Endocrinological side effects. Endocrinolog-

Table 1.3 *Indirect Sexual Side Effects Related to Drugs and Medications*

Side Effects Influencing Body Image	*Endocrinological Side Effects*
Edema	Alterations in insulin metabolism, thyroid function, etc.
Halitosis	*Side Effects Influencing Mental States and Perception of Pleasure*
Weight loss/gain	Aggression
Side Effects Influencing Physical Levels of Comfort	Anhedonia
Constipation	Anxiety
Dryness (skin, mouth, mucous membranes)	Depression
Edema	Detachment
Hypothermia	Irritability
Indigestion	Mania
Nausea	Nervousness
Pain	Psychoses
Rash	*Side Effects Influencing Stamina/Movement*
Urinary problems (retention, incontinence, nocturia, cystitis)	Angina
Neurological Side Effects	Exercise intolerance
Analgesia	Shortness of breath
Cognitive deficits	*Vascular Side Effects*
Dizziness	Arrhythmias
Fatigue	Claudication
Headaches	Headaches
Movement disorder	Vasoconstriction
Neuropathy	Vasodilation
Pain	
Paresthesia	
Perceptual disortions and/or deficits	
Sedation	
Sleep disturbances	
Sensory loss	
Tremors	
Weakness	

ical influences on sexual function can be extensive. Whether a patient has disorders associated with diabetes, thyroid function, growth hormone, or more direct sexual endocrinopathies such as abnormal testosterone or estrogen levels, the influence of major hormone systems on sex must be factored into the equation.

Mood and mental states. Depression typically diminishes sexual interest. Manic states have been associated with hypersexuality or personality changes which are disturbing to one's partner. Anxiety can lead to sexual avoidance or compulsive sexual activity (e.g., repetitive masturbation prior to a major exam or other stressful situations). Premature ejaculation in men and retarded orgasm in women are often caused by or aggravated by anxiety. Aggressive behavior can disturb or promote sex, depending on the situation and circumstances. Also, aggressive behavior in one sexual partner can be perceived as offensive by the other. Some pharmaceuticals can diminish the perception of pleasure or the ability to appreciate pleasurable physical and/or emotional sensations, in which case sexual responsiveness becomes incidental. If the patient is experiencing an active psychotic episode, normal sexual expression cannot be anticipated until psychotic symptoms come under therapeutic control.

Neurological side effects. Medications that have a sedating effect usually affect sexual drive. The need for sleep impairs concentration and preempts the desire for sex under most circumstances. Medication can also impair motor coordination. The sexual response involves physical exertion and strategic maneuvering, both of which require coordinated movement. Any deficits in these physical requirements can make intercourse awkward, uncomfortable, difficult, or even impossible. Sex also involves a delicate interplay of visual, oral, olfactory, and tactile cues. Perception of these factors is vital to satisfying sex. Mental and psychological side effects of medications that diminish perceptual acuity have the potential to affect sexual function, sometimes dramatically. Finally, cognitive abilities play a role, facilitating communication, novelty, and concentration, all of which contribute to sexual satisfaction. When any of these factors is compromised, sex suffers.

Stamina. Medications that diminish energy and/or stamina affect sex accordingly.

Vascular side effects. Clearly, any medication (or disease) that affects the blood supply to the genitals will influence erection, lubrication, and perhaps responsiveness.

GUIDELINES FOR IDENTIFYING PHARMACOLOGICAL PROPERTIES THAT AFFECT FUNCTION

One of the most important objectives of *Sexual Pharmacology* is to teach the reader a *system* for understanding the sexual properties of drugs: learning how to analyze any drug for its sexual properties by applying existing knowledge together with common sense in a logical sequence of steps that leads to appropriate conclusions. This text was not intended to describe the sexual properties of each and every drug. There are too many drugs available, both nationally and internationally, for complete coverage to be practical. Most drugs have not been specifically studied for their sexual side effects; therefore, little relevant information is available. Often drug labeling (description in the *PDR* or package insert) is not changed after the drug's approval for clinical use, despite clear-cut side effects noted in clinical practice or further research (Woosley & Flockhart, 1994).

In the chapters that follow, many drugs are described in detail to serve as examples of the process. These summaries are meant as helpful references for the most commonly used drugs known to possess adverse sexual properties. They could also serve as a model for needed subsequent research on other widely used drugs.

The following steps should be used to evaluate the sexual properties of any drug not specifically described in *Sexual Pharmacology*:

- *Step 1* Find the drug in the *Physicians Desk Reference* (*PDR*). All drugs available in the United States are listed in this book. Similar references exist for each country around the world.
- *Step 2* Scan the list of adverse reactions for *indirect* sexual side effects—those symptoms that make a patient feel unwell, depress the central nervous system, stimulate mood disorders, or any other conditions listed in Table 1.3.
- *Step 3* Look for any specific sexual side effects noted, but bear in mind that if none are noted, it is not safe to assume that therefore none exist. Look for a table or other indication of how often a sexual or mood side effect occurs, since a sexual effect such as impotence may be listed but occurs so rarely as to be irrelevant.
- *Step 4* To further evaluate direct sexual side effects, review the mechanisms of action listed for the drug in the *PDR* and compare them to mechanisms of action listed in Tables 4.1 and 4.2 in Chapter 4. If the drug in question has any of these mechanisms of action, it could influence sexual responsiveness.
- *Step 5* Refer to the explanation of mechanisms of action in Chapter 3 to determine whether the drug in question has positive or negative effects on sex and which sexual function(s) is likely to be affected. Be sure to note if there are any gender-related differences.
- *Step 6* Look for the class of drug in *Sexual Pharmacology* that the drug in question resembles. For example, if the drug is a new beta-blocker, approved subsequent to the publication of this book, turn to beta-blockers and review the material on this class of drug. While some details may vary, the categorical attributes will provide a general sense of the sexual properties probably associated with this drug. If there is no matching class of drug, depend instead

on the mechanisms of action listed; also try to find the most similar drug and seek a probable analogical relation.

If you are simply looking for information about a drug that interests you, the next steps are not relevant. However, if you are pursuing this information to help a patient (or yourself) who is experiencing sexual dysfunction, proceed to the following steps:

- *Step 7* Review pertinent sections of Chapter 2 and follow the differential diagnosis protocol in order to determine, to the best extent possible, whether your patient is experiencing sexual side effects caused or aggravated by medication. Simply determining the potential of the drug in question to cause sexual problems by following steps one through six is not sufficient. Keep in mind that even the most sexually toxic drugs do not cause sexual problems for all patients.
- *Step 8* Consider performing nocturnal penile tumescence monitoring, Doppler studies, and laboratory tests to distinguish between physiological and psychological aspects of the sexual dysfunction.
- *Step 9* If the patient does not have adequate recollection of time sequences and medication dosages, speak with his or her sexual partner when possible. The spouse may have better recollection of when the problem developed in relation to initiating medication as well as insight into medical conditions or other events of potential significance.
- *Step 10* Ask patients for their opinions of the cause of the sexual problem. Often, patients are surprisingly "on target," but hesitate to express their conclusions to physicians or therapists without being asked.
- *Step 11* If the diagnosis is still not clear, it may be necessary to substitute another drug to see if the dysfunction resolves. If resolution occurs, the drug probably was responsible. If the dysfunction does not resolve, it *does not* indicate that the original drug was free from sexual side effects (see Chapter 2 for further information on this subject).

It is important to recognize that just because a drug is listed in an adverse category does not mean that it causes sexual problems in all cases. Indeed, there are no known cases of a drug causing sexual complications 100% of the time—although few medications are completely "innocent." Commonly, the adverse sexual side effects are dose-related, but not always. Some of the drugs mentioned cause sexual problems a significant percentage of the time; some recommended as alternatives may also cause sexual problems, but only rarely compared to the others. Some drugs, like analgesics, which usually have adverse side effects on sexual function, may also have indirect positive effects simply as a result of relieving pain. Various other drugs used to treat pain, such as opiates, evidently decrease sexual sensation, feeling, and vitality; however, failure to satisfactorily treat pain can cause equal or greater sexual dysfunction and reduction of sexual activity. Similarly, some diseases (e.g., epilepsy) are correlated with a high prevalence of sexual dysfunction regardless of drug treatment. Although the drug may intensify the dysfunction, the untreated disease is so severe that the compromise is necessary. Unnecessary "compromise" also occurs: Several sexually negative drugs are prescribed excessively or inappropriately, particularly for the elderly (Willcox, Himmelstein, & Woolhandler, 1994).

In many instances drugs are positively evaluated with regard to sexual side effects only because they do not cause certain symptoms that are assumed to result in sexual dysfunction. When fluoxetine (Prozac) was introduced, for example, it was believed by many to be a safe choice for preserving sexual function because it appeared to lack various symptomatic consequences considered to be detrimental to sex (weight gain, sedation, and anticholinergic effects). The *PDR* also initially noted Prozac as having few sexual side effects. Through extensive clinical experience, however, it has been discovered that Prozac may have more pronounced sexual side effects than many other antidepressants. Antidepressants similar to Prozac, such as paroxetine (Paxil) or sertraline (Zoloft), may have even more severe sexual side effects. Common sense (Prozac derives its therapeutic effects from serotonin, a known sexual suppressant) and attention to animal sex research would have resulted in a firm warning of such specifically sexual side effects.

For some conditions drugs with side effects that are sexually negative may nevertheless be preferred by patients. Sexual function alone cannot be the definitive criterion of a desirable state-of-being. Consider Prozac, again, which heightens serotonin activity but may directly reduce sexual desire and responsiveness. Nonetheless, if it permits sexual activity through relief of depression, anxiety, phobia, or aggression, it has sexually redeeming value that outweighs its sexual drawbacks. Antianxiety drugs are eagerly sought by many patients who would rather be free from debilitating panic than engage in sex—at least in the short term. A decrease in secretions, alertness, blood flow, sensation, movement, or intensity may seem negative in relation to sexual expression, but it is positive when compared to the overwhelming disability of panic disorder. The primary problem must receive priority. Then, with successful treatment of the primary problem, symptoms that interfere with sexual function may become of greater concern, shifting the focus of decision-making to whether the medication should be discontinued.

A FINAL NOTE

In considering medication for patients, quality-of-life issues are of paramount importance and need to be integrated into health-care deliberations. Discrimination and common sense must be optimally employed in weighing the multiple factors at play. An individual taking medication that diminishes memory, mental alertness, or level of energy is predictably less enthusiastic about life in general and activities such as sex in particular. Treatment plans that best suit patients, while also preserving or even improving their sex lives, *are* possible. In most cases, a caring attitude together with knowledge of the sexual side effects of drugs will foster healthier, happier, more appreciative patients.

2

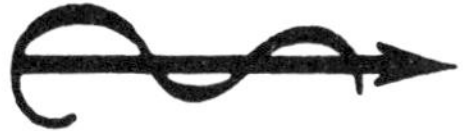

Differential Diagnosis of Sexual Dysfunction

OBJECTIVES

- To become aware of the compounding interplay of disease, drugs, and psychological factors
- To develop a system for differential diagnosis of sexual dysfunction that incorporates medical, pharmacological, and psychological evaluation

This chapter is intended to serve as a quick clinical tool for distinguishing medical, pharmacological, and psychological causes of sexual dysfunction. These three key factors play individual or combined roles in the differential diagnosis of sexual dysfunction. In exploring the relationship between disease, drugs, and sexuality, it is reasonable to attempt to distinguish between the organic and psychogenic factors. While there is a certain value in this approach, the complete etiological picture of sexual dysfunction is usually not black or white. More typically, multiple factors interact simultaneously. Consider the patient with arteriosclerotic heart disease who has diminished blood flow to the penis, who is placed on medication that interferes with the neurotransmitters mediating penile erection. Because of diminishing firmness of erection, he develops anxiety over his performance. Chances are high that he will consult his doctor about medication and his therapist about his mood, and both will work separately from one another.

The compounding interplay of disease, drugs, and psychological factors should not be underestimated. Almost any time there is an organic basis for sexual dysfunction, there are contributing psychological variables. A woman who has pain with intercourse for physical reasons also develops all of the emotional symptoms associated with the psychological inability to have intercourse with her mate. If medications are prescribed, additional complications can follow. A man who becomes organically impotent usually does not know that the cause of his dysfunction is physical—indeed, he might have been relieved, had he known. Yet it may be years before the correct diagnosis is made. In the meantime, he is subject to all the fears of performance and associated interpersonal anxieties that plague a man whose sexual problem is purely psychological.

If a man complains of a decrease in flaccid penis size, physicians may be tempted to dismiss the symptom ("Don't worry, it doesn't mean anything") when, in fact, it is a clue to several conditions, only one of which is drug-induced (any drug that causes peripheral vasoconstriction can precipitate the symptom). If a patient has peripheral vascular disease typical of arteriosclerosis, diabetes, Raynaud's syndrome, or if he smokes, one hallmark may be a decrease in flaccid penis size.

Other symptoms suggestive of arteriosclerosis extending to the penile vessels are delayed development of erection and difficulty maintaining an erection. If a patient reports that he used to get erect quickly, within seconds or minutes, and now it takes five to 10 minutes, it may be more difficult for the blood flow to contend with the narrowed channels. This mechanical vascular obstruction can also result in a less firm erection.

Other examples of the complex interplay of disease, drug, and psychology include symptoms such as: *dangling tip* (only half an erection, with the distal end hanging limp and useless), which may be caused by Peyronie's disease or by an old or recent sexual trauma with clot formation and fibrous tissue scarring; *orgasmic cramps* (if a man complains of cramping during orgasm, focus on pathology of the prostate; in a female patient, consider endometriosis or endometritis); *burning on penetration* (the woman who complains of burning on penile penetration in the absence of physical findings is describing a symptom pathognomonic of vaginismus); *orgasmic headaches* (if a woman complains of severe headaches at the moment of orgasm, consider the cerebrovascular system—in particular, an underlying Berry aneurysm [dilated blood vessel in the brain] or an impending stroke).

Clinically, it is essential to be aware of the disease-drug-psychology interplay. A physician who successfully treats the organic aspect of a sexual problem may be mystified that the problem does not resolve. A therapist working with the psychological components might wonder the same. In fact, even though the dysfunction has been corrected medically or chemically, the residual problem is typically perpetuated by the untreated psychological factors originally precipitated by the disease or the drug.

MEDICAL DIAGNOSIS OF SEXUAL DYSFUNCTION

Disease and illness can cause sexual problems by affecting desire, arousal, and/or function either directly or indirectly. Narrowed arteries due to arteriosclerosis can directly impair blood flow to the penis, preventing erection. A herpetic lesion at the introitus, or generalized endometriosis, can cause pain upon penetration. Certain neurological diseases also can directly interfere with erection and orgasm. In addition, any illness or disease that causes chronic pain, weakness, or unpleasant physical symptoms can indirectly affect sexual function in an adverse manner. For example, arthritis can render movement during sexual intercourse too painful; asthma can make breathing laborious and even exhausting. Table 2.1 lists common medical conditions that directly or indirectly result in a variety of sexual dysfunctions.

PHARMACOLOGICAL DIAGNOSIS OF SEXUAL DYSFUNCTION

Prior to evaluating a patient's prescription drug use, it is essential to ascertain the use of alcohol, nicotine, illegal drugs, and cigarettes—issues that are addressed in detail in Part III. This feature is one of the most commonly overlooked aspects of the pharmacological evaluation.

Dose, Latency, and Duration

In general, the higher the dosage of the medication, the more likely the sexual side effect. However, in some cases, sexual symptoms are independent of dosage and do not abate when the dosage of the drug is reduced. Typically, adverse side effects of medication are prominent and obvious at the beginning of treatment. However, the sexual side effects are often an exception. With certain medications—in particular, those that influence state of mind, mood, or hormones—sexual side effects may take weeks, months, and sometimes years to manifest. For example, the effect of certain antidepressants does not occur for two to four weeks. Sexual symptoms associated with these drugs may not be fully developed until such time. (On the other hand, as already noted, the successful treatment of depression may improve sexual desire and function if the sexually toxic aspects of the drug are not too severe.) There may be an initial sexual improvement the first four weeks due to relief from depression, but the negative sexual side effects of the drug become evident during longtime use.

Table 2.1 *Medical Conditions and Diseases Associated with Sexual Dysfunction*

Endocrine	*Gastrointestinal*	*Gynecological*	*Immunological*	*Neurological*	*Urological*	*Vascular*
Acromegaly	Constipation	Dysfunctional bleeding	AIDS/HIV	Alzheimer's disease	Chronic kidney disease	Arteriosclerosis
Adrenal dysfunction	Diarrhea	Dyspareunia	Arthritis & other bone/joint disorders	Brain lesions	Cystitis (acute, chronic & postcoital)	Fistula
Diabetes mellitus	Irritable bowel syndrome	Endometriosis	Cancer	Dementia	Epididymitis	Hypertension
Hyperprolactinemia	Ulcerative colitis	Genital warts	Chronic fatigue syndrome	Diabetic neuropathy	Peyronie's disease	Ischemia
Hypogonadism		Infertility/pregnancy	Respiratory diseases	Epilepsy	Priapism	Myocardial infarction
Thyroid dysfunction		Menopause		Multiple sclerosis	Prostatitis	Stroke
		Menstrual cycle disorders		Parkinson's disease	Renal failure	Transient ischemic attacks (TIAs)
		PMS		Spinal injury or tumors	Urethrocele/cystocele	Venous insufficiency
		Vaginismus		Stroke	Urinary incontinence	
		Vaginitis (bacterial, fungal, trichomonal, viral)				

The duration of the sexual side effect is dependent on numerous variables: whether the medication is taken occasionally, frequently, or regularly; how effectively the underlying disease is controlled; whether it is progressive; and/or the nature of the psychological forces contributing to or aggravating the problem, including relationship issues. For some medications, adaptation and tolerance to sexual side effects will eventually occur, along with tolerance of other side effects such as sleepiness. Another consideration is the therapeutic effect of the drug.

It is also important to consider the interaction of multiple drugs and the relationship to the treated disease over time. One of my patients, for example, successfully treated for impotence, began ejaculating only intermittently: Every third or fourth sexual experience, he had an orgasm but no ejaculate. Sometimes the volume was just reduced, and other times it was normal. I thought perhaps therapy had triggered some form of symptom substitution. These inconstant symptoms were a diagnostic puzzle until I learned that, a few weeks previously, another physician had placed him on thioridazine (Mellaril), a drug known to inhibit ejaculation. Because the patient took the medication on some days but forgot on others, this staccato pattern of ejaculation resulted.

Typically, the *physiologic* cause of adverse sexual effects will disappear shortly after the medication is discontinued (unless permanent damage has occurred to tissue, endocrine system, or neuronal circuits), but the psychological aftermath may be far more persistent. This is especially true if the drug was not recognized as the cause of the sexual dysfunction.

Consider a patient rendered impotent from propranolol (a "sex offender" drug), having taken this medication for 10 years or more. By the time the medication is discontinued or changed, dysfunctional sexual and psychological patterns have been well established. Often these patterns cannot be corrected without the help of sex therapy, even though the only reason the problem developed was chemical. Most patients and physicians mistakenly assume that if the cause of the problem is chemical, removing the chemical or replacing it with another is enough. However, this is usually not the case; therapy is generally required.

The Crossover Effect of Drug and Disease

Another important consideration is the nature and severity of the underlying disease. A drug with relatively mild sexual side effects can have a devastating impact under certain circumstances. For example, a man with generalized arteriosclerosis, whose penile arteries are narrowed but not occluded, may still be able to achieve a relatively full erection and function sexually, although it may take longer for erection to develop. Should he be placed on a blood pressure medication that has relatively mild negative effects on erection, however, the medication, though mild, may nonetheless "tilt the scales" from adequate functioning to complete impotence. Thus, the drug-disease interplay may have crossover effects that amplify sexual problems.

One must also consider temporal contributions to the crossover effect of the disease and the medication. A patient may be doing well on a particular drug regimen – for example, one of the beta-blockers. Blood pressure is satisfactorily controlled and, for a period of time, there are no sexual side effects associated with treatment. As this patient's disease progresses over five, 10, and 15 years, however, his penile arteries will gradually narrow, giving rise to sexual symptoms: difficulty achieving and maintaining an erection, and so on. Although the sexual symptoms may be due mostly to the natural progression of the disease and not the medication, a complicating factor may be the beta-blocker. As the patient becomes increasingly debilitated by the arteriosclerosis, he also becomes more vulnerable to the toxic sexual effects of the drug that accumulate over time. The combination ultimately may produce sexual dysfunction.

The temporal effects of the drug-disease interplay require monitoring and consideration. Obviously, it is worthwhile to avoid sexually toxic drugs from the beginning of treatment, or, if prescribed, to change to a relatively innocent drug as soon as the patient's medical condition allows *even when sexual symptoms are not present.*

Chronic or Acute Medical Conditions

How sexual functioning is affected will vary depending upon whether the medical condition is chronic or acute. With chronic conditions, some patients have accommodated sufficiently to their disease or distress that they are able to function sexually under adverse physical circumstances that would make it impossible for most people. Patients with diabetes, arthritis, or back pain may be able to tolerate thresholds of pain or discomfort that others cannot. Other alternatives involve changing positions (e.g., woman on top), communicating better about when pain is better or worse, and selecting times for sex when pain is reduced. Acute conditions are often so compelling that, with or without medication, the patient has no interest or ability to function sexually. After the acute episode has passed, medication may no longer be necessary; and, if the incident was brief, return of sexual function will occur naturally. Patients experiencing some types of acute conditions requiring only a week or two of treatment (such as the flu, a cold, a seasonal allergic response, an injury) can tolerate short-term treatment with drugs highly toxic to sexual function without suffering from any long-term consequences, as long as they are informed and prepared in advance. If an acute condition moves into a chronic state, the situation would require reevaluation: for example, if a patient who uses antihistamines only occasionally relocates to a place with long allergy seasons and has to take them for months at a time.

A basic if informal guideline for determining the drug-disease interplay might be: Consider how much pain, discomfort, and psychological distress debilitating to sexual function already exists without the added complication of medication. Then factor in the probable impact of the medication, including the length of treatment anticipated, whether a week or a lifetime. If the symptoms of the medical condition are so severe that the patient is unable to engage in sex or becomes disinterested in participating, then medication to relieve pain may be the best course of action even if it depresses sex drive and responsiveness to some extent. It is a balance that must be achieved by communicating clearly and specifically with the patient, then applying sound medical judgment and common sense.

Table 2.2 lists the classes of drugs associated with sexual dysfunction. Clearly, most classes include sexually toxic drugs, not just blood pressure medicines and psychotropics, as formerly believed.

PSYCHOLOGICAL DIAGNOSIS OF SEXUAL DYSFUNCTION

Although most psychological disorders have the potential to affect sexual functioning to varying degrees, they do not inevitably do so. Individual assessment is essential.

It is strongly recommended that possible psychological factors of sexual dysfunction be evaluated after all medical and pharmacological causes have been considered. Whether or not medical and pharmacological factors have been identified, there are usually secondary psychological factors. Avoid the common mistake of reversing the roles of cause and effect: Too often, physicians and therapists assume that if psychological factors such as relationship stress or impending divorce are present that they are responsible for the sexual problem, when, in fact, they may instead be an indirect consequence of a drug-induced sexual dysfunction.

We do not yet know all there is to know. Psychological diagnosis should not be based on an "elimination philosophy," a particularly offensive orientation common in medicine. When no medical or pharmacological cause can be substantiated by process of elimination, the sexual problem is attributed to a psychological cause. Back pain, migraine headaches, and depression are but a few psychosomatic conditions that have all been "written off" as having psychological origins simply because symptoms are

Table 2.2 *Drugs Associated with Sexual Dysfunction*

Antiandrogens	*Illicit and non-prescription drugs*
Antiarrhythmics	Alcohol
Anticancer agents	Amphetamines
Anticholinergics	Cocaine
Antihistamines	Heroin
Antihypertensives	Marijuana
Diuretics	Nicotine
Hormones	*Opiates*
Corticosteroids	Demerol
Progestins	Methadone
	Psychotropics
	Antianxiety
	Anticonvulsants
	Antidepressants
	Antipsychotics
	Sedatives/hypnotics
	Stimulants

common and it can be difficult or impossible to prove an underlying physical cause. Even AIDS symptoms first appeared to be psychologically based, until the virus underlying weight loss, fatigue, diarrhea, etc. (symptoms that were not taken seriously) was identified. Sexual problems are often psychologically contagious. They can spread to a person's sexual partner, and frequently do. This transmission of sexual dysfunction is particularly probable if the sexual problem lasts for a long time. The sexual problem of one person precipitates coping mechanisms in the other that frequently lead to dysfunction. A composite example might be the following:

A woman cannot have orgasms with intercourse. Her partner feels responsible, even though she has never had an orgasm during intercourse with any man. Nevertheless, he becomes anxious and determined to bring her to orgasm. He may even come to see her orgasm as a personal project, which he works persistently to bring to fruition. In the process, the sexual act loses its appeal; it has become a chore, and he grows increasingly frustrated, distracted, and impatient. After it is over he is disappointed and feels like a failure. Not surprisingly, as much as he used to enjoy sex, he begins to avoid it—at first in subtle ways and later more directly. Sexual frequency diminishes. When sex does occur, the quality is considerably inferior to diminishing memories of better times. During sex, he is so busy trying to make his partner respond that he loses his own responsiveness, and with it, his erection. This experience is so traumatic that he avoids sex even more.

Another composite scenario: A comparable situation to the above example occurs in the sexually healthy women mated to a man who is experiencing premature ejaculation or impotence. With this premature ejaculator, she becomes so angry, impatient, and disgusted that she would rather not have sex at all than be left without her orgasm. With the impotent man, she is more inclined to be sympathetic and behaves much like the man in the above example. She works diligently to fix his problem, turns sex into a chore, and loses enthusiasm for the whole experience.

Suffice it to say that, if a sexual problem persists in one partner for any length of time, a complete diagnosis requires that the therapist work with the other partner as well. It is probable that a secondary sexual dysfunction has developed and, unless it is defined, it will be difficult to correct the original problem.

A multitude of psychological factors can influence a patient's sexual behavior. If a patient has an altered body image unfavorable to a sense of sexual attractiveness, this alone can be enough to damage intimacy. For example, a woman who believes that her breasts are too small, even if her partner adores them, is unlikely to feel appealing. She may continue to feel defective and self-conscious sexually, believing that his reassurances are just a kindness.

A man who has (or who perceives he has) a small penis is in a similar position. Convinced that he does not "measure up," he may actually feel deformed and undesirable. His confidence, manner, personality, and sexual function will be altered accordingly.

Other real or perceived body flaws can seriously inhibit sexual comfort. Stretch marks, big hips, fat thighs, beer bellies, and hairiness are just a few of the obstacles that can inhibit sexual pleasure for women and men.

Sometimes the problem is fear that sex could precipitate illness or a fatal event. The sexual partner or spouse of someone who has had a stroke, transient ischemic attack, myocardial infarction, or other vascular episode, may fear killing a lover with sex. Both the patient and the sexual partner may find that their sex life has been brought to an abrupt halt by the cloud of fear in the bedroom.

3

Interpersonal Techniques and Treatment Strategies

OBJECTIVES

- To facilitate comfort in patients as well as health practitioners
- To establish a baseline sexual history
- To provide interview techniques for physicians
- To provide interview techniques for therapists
- To demonstrate design of treatment strategies

Physicians typically find it difficult to discuss the sex lives of their patients comfortably and professionally because most have received inadequate training in human sexuality. It was not until the 1960s that the first course on human sexuality was offered in any medical school in the nation and several decades passed before most medical schools addressed the subject.

Today the majority of medical schools offer at least one course on human sexuality, but few are *required* courses. Many offer human sexuality as an elective, meaning that *physicians can still graduate from medical school without any training whatsoever in this subject*. Of those schools that require courses in human sexuality, the time devoted is minimal, averaging eight to 13 hours of course work. Of this time, less than an hour is allotted to examining the sexual side effects of prescription drugs—sometimes no more than a sentence or a phrase is offered. Other graduate programs are no exception. Human sexuality courses are usually electives even for psychologists.

With this unpromising background it is no surprise that physicians frequently do not ask their patients about sexual subjects. They have not been taught how to ask appropriate questions and consequently feel awkward inquiring about sex. Patients, usually inhibited by embarrassment, rarely volunteer information in this area, incorrectly assuming that the physician would ask if it were important. This inadvertent conspiracy of silence leads many physicians to believe that their patients have no sexual problems. No one mentions them; therefore, they do not exist.

Some physicians are afraid that raising sexual issues will open "Pandora's Box," eliciting questions they will be unable to answer and taking extensive consultation time they do not have scheduled. Many physicians still assign sexual function low priority compared to the medical condition at hand. Some physicians are afraid of offending certain patients just by mentioning the subject; others are concerned that raising sexual issues could be misunderstood by patients, thus increasing their liability exposure should a patient misconstrue their intent. The opposite effect is more likely. With increasing recognition of the relationship between drugs and sexual impairments, patients may sue because a sexual problem occurred that could have been avoided.

A common reservation among physicians is their fear of "the inverse placebo effect": If the information is not presented properly, telling a patient that a drug *might* have sexual consequences could precipitate a self-fulfilling prophecy, causing a sexual problem that would otherwise not occur. For example, if a physician tells a patient, "This drug causes impotence," that patient may, in fact, develop impotence from the power of suggestion alone. Although it is true that suggestion is particularly strong in the area of sex, if the physician expresses the information in the correct way, iatrogenically induced sexual dysfunction is unlikely.

Financial considerations are a practical but insidious factor contributing to the reluctance of many physicians to suggest sex therapy for pharmacologically related sexual dysfunction. While many types of sexual dysfunction are not covered by medical insurance, sexual dysfunction that is the result of medical problems or the side effect of medical treatment is covered. If the underlying cause of a sexual problem is a medical condition (i.e., arteriosclerosis, diabetes), and the insurance company is billed properly, coverage will usually be at 80% (or whatever the patient's medical coverage ordinarily provides), *even when there is no specific psychological or sexual coverage noted in the policy, and even when sexual problems are specifically excluded.* The same is true if the sexual dysfunction results from medical treatment (i.e., prescription drugs). It should be noted that occasionally it is necessary for an attorney to write a brief letter to an insurance company, pointing out their legal areas of responsibility.

ESTABLISHING A BASELINE SEXUAL HISTORY

One of the clinical objectives for physicians and therapists should be to *establish a baseline sexual history before prescribing medication or beginning therapy. Determining what is normal for a patient prior to prescribing any medications or designing a treatment plan minimizes the risk of noncompliance.*

When physicians do not establish and record these baselines, it is very difficult retrospectively to distinguish those problems precipitated by medication from those that were pre-existing.

Patients may be unable to recall whether their sexual problem developed before or after instituting medication – especially if the medication was first prescribed many years previously. Therefore, it is important to determine whether any problems existed prior to the prescription of new medication.

Determining a sexual baseline can play a strategic role in selecting the best drug and/or therapeutic approach for a patient. If one of several medications would be suitable, one that tends to inhibit ejaculation might be preferable if the patient historically experiences premature ejaculation. Conversely, it would be best to avoid drugs with these characteristics if inhibited ejaculation is a pre-existing condition. If a female patient complains of headaches during orgasm, labetalol, an antiadrenergic antihypertensive, might be indicated (see Chapter 15). In this way, the sexual side effect profile of a drug, in combination with an accurate baseline history, can enable physicians to prescribe medication from a considerably more inclusive perspective. During intake therapy, a baseline sexual history also could help determine if individual or joint counseling would be worthwhile for a couple at the onset of the medication or after a few weeks.

Probably the most important reason for taking a baseline sexual history is to prevent patient noncompliance. The best treatment plan will fail if a patient does not follow it. Sometimes the consequences of noncompliance can be fatal. More commonly, the patient stops taking the drug and changes doctors. A therapist could help maintain continuity by giving feedback to the physician if sexual changes develop after a new drug is prescribed. Professional feedback, of course, works both ways.

Another important function of the baseline sexual history is simply to prevent gross misunderstandings and miscommunication that lead to unnecessary sexual dysfunction, as the following case demonstrates. A couple who had been in psychotherapy elsewhere for some time arrived for treatment. The presenting complaint was that the wife, who could only be orgasmic with oral sex, had been informed by her husband that he would no longer participate. She was devastated; he was adamant. She had never asked him the reason for his unexpected refusal, he had never volunteered the information, and the therapist they were seeing had not inquired.

During their individual intake interviews, I asked the woman if she had any idea why he had refused oral sex. Although she had been puzzled and hurt, she reiterated that she had never inquired. When I asked her husband, he was not at all reluctant to explain. He informed me that he had a serious sinus condition and, when he was under the covers performing oral sex, he could not breathe easily through his nose. As she became aroused, she would clamp his head with her legs, making breathing all the more difficult. Each time, he felt as though he were suffocating, and after many years, simply could not take it anymore.

The solution was straightforward. Once the wife heard her husband's reasons, her anger dissolved. She was sympathetic and dismayed, indicating that it would be no problem to stop gripping him with her legs. I suggested they throw the covers off and he make arrangements to breathe as necessary.

Unfortunately, because they were at the threshold of divorce due to the anger and misunderstandings that had flourished in this tense and unhappy atmosphere, several months of therapy were necessary before their situation was stable again. If, years earlier, their physician or therapist had taken a competent baseline history, appropriate advice could have been offered and relationship therapy would not have been necessary.

INTERVIEW TECHNIQUES FOR PHYSICIANS

The central concerns to be aware of when in discussing sexual issues with patients are facilitating comfort, establishing context, and clarifying appropriateness of topic. Consideration must be given to ages of patients, individual value systems, and overall comfort level. The office nurse or other personnel can expedite matters in some cases by administering sexual/relationship questionnaires, or by being trained to take a brief sexual history.

Comfort

Your level of comfort, or lack thereof, is communicated to your patients. Knowledge and practice will bring increasing comfort in this area, enabling you to help make your patients more at ease with the subject. Remember back to the times you struggled to maintain your dignity while asking a patient, "Do your stools float?" The first prerequisite is to use awkward or potentially embarrassing sexual phrases frequently enough to feel familiar and at ease with the words. Eventually the objective is to develop comfort with the concept behind them. Developing comfort with sexual questions involves practice and persistence. If you are not comfortable discussing sexual issues, you might admit it. Tell your patients that, although you find it somewhat intrusive to inquire into their sex lives, the information is important for their health and well-being, and you hope they will help you out by volunteering any information they think could be important. Acknowledge that you may not have all the answers, but if there is a problem, you will certainly help them find a solution or refer them to someone who can help them. A candid approach, at this point, can be quite successful.

Context

Do not ask sexual questions "out of the blue." Put them into a clear context. For example: "I am planning to prescribe some medications for you and want to be sure that I don't give you something that could adversely affect your sex life or your relationship. Let me find out a little about what is typical for you before I make my decision. Have you ever, or are you now, experiencing any sexual difficulties?" Another approach: "As I am taking your medical history,

I am also going to ask you a few questions about your sex life. It is not my intent to intrude on your privacy, but sometimes symptoms show up in the sexual area that provide important clues about your general health."

Discussing sexual issues is appropriate any time medications are being considered or changed, during a review of systems, and typically whenever the patient's chief complaint concerns the urogenital/gynecological tract. It is also appropriate to take an interval sexual history during periodic health updates, when you are routinely checking other aspects of a patient's health and well-being.

In view of the AIDS epidemic, a history of sexual practices as well as sexual orientation and drug use—both IV and non-IV—has become more than appropriate—it has become essential. It is important to know how many sexual partners your patient currently has, particularly if diagnosing any sexually transmitted diseases (including candidiasis, chlamydia, and hemophilus), so that the partners can be treated as well. Otherwise, your patient will become reinfected. Physicians often assume that, if a patient is married, the sexual relationship is monogamous, while statistics and common sense suggest otherwise.

The best way to broach sexual issues with new patients is to integrate the discussion into the review of systems during the initial evaluation. Both male and female patients appreciate being interviewed prior to disrobing, particularly if it is their first appointment with a new physician. Patients commonly complain that their first introduction to a physician is in the examining room, where they are naked, chilly, uncomfortable, and usually irritated by being kept waiting. Women, in particular, feel at a tremendous disadvantage under these circumstances. Do not broach sexual topics for the first time with a patient in this condition. Although men do not complain as frequently about being naked on the first meeting with a physician, questioning usually reveals a discomfort with it.

If a check list is utilized for a patient's review of systems, add a section on sexual function between the urological and gynecological categories. If the patient responds positively to any questions about sexuality, three courses of action are possible:

1. Tell the patient that you would like to pursue the discussion of sexual issues at a later appointment when adequate time can be scheduled.
2. Tell the patient that, because you need to know more about the sexual issues, for your next meeting you would like the patient to fill out a more detailed sexual questionnaire to facilitate the discussion. (Such a questionnaire can be developed from the tables available in this chapter.)
3. Pursue the review of sexual systems in detail at that time, if you have the comfort and the knowledge to proceed, as you would with any other section of the review of systems.

For example, if a female patient complains of pain during intercourse, the questions in Table 3.1 can be asked. Parallel questions for a male patient are given in Table 3.2.

Masturbation history is also important if the complaint is Peyronie's disease or pain with intercourse. You want to know whether the pain occurs only with intercourse or if the same pain occurs with masturbation. For Peyronie's disease, you want a description of the curvature of the penis when erect. It is useful to ask the patient to take a photograph of the penis erect from several different angles so you can clearly evaluate the degree of deformity. If a man complains of difficulty in achieving or sustaining an erection, ascertaining how well the man functions with masturbation determines whether his problem is predominantly psychological or physical. Many physicians are uncomfortable inquiring about masturbation. Explore the subject during the review of systems, *not* while you are examining the patient. The questions in Table 3.3 can be asked.

As a general rule, do not ask patients *if* they masturbate, which requires that they either admit or deny engaging in the activity. Ask instead, "*How often* do you masturbate?" Patients can always answer, "I never do," or "I never have."

Table 3.1 *Painful Intercourse* (*Female*)

1. When did you first notice discomfort during intercourse?
2. Does your partner do anything that causes you physical discomfort?
3. Does the pain occur each time you have intercourse or only sometimes?
4. Is the pain constant or intermittent? Does it worsen or lessen as intercourse continues?
5. Where does it hurt? Is it deep or shallow?
6. What does the pain feel like? Is it sharp, dull, burning?
7. On a scale of 0 to 10, how intense is the pain?
8. Does changing position change the pain in any way?
9. Does using artifical lubrication improve or change the degree of pain?
10. Is there a discharge or an odor?
11. Does the pain cease when intercourse ends or does it persist?
12. What contraceptive method are you using?
13. What have you tried to do to relieve or diminish the pain?
14. (If a patient has more than one sexual partner, ask:) Is the pain equally intense with all partners?

However, the question has been posed in a manner that implicitly assumes that most people masturbate; the phrasing in itself makes it easier for patients to respond openly and honestly.

A particularly sensitive subject for male physicians involves inquiring about the orgasms and masturbatory patterns of female patients (see Table 3.4). The best method of approaching this area of inquiry is first to screen for painful intercourse, followed by the natural segue of "Do you have the same type of pain during masturbation?" Additional questions about masturbation can follow: "Do you have any difficulty being orgasmic with masturbation?" "Do you have orgasms as easily with your partner as you do by masturbating?" The answer to this question is typically no. Female patients are usually more efficient and effective sexually by themselves. However, the difference between self-stimulated orgasms and those with partners should not be too great. Ask, "How much of a time difference exists?"

Your next question will depend upon whether the answer is five minutes or an hour. If the difference is five to 20 minutes, there is no problem as long as the patient is not unhappy about it. Ask her if she worries that her partner is getting tired or if she feels she takes too long.

It is also important to know by what means the patient is orgasmic when she is with her partner: by oral manipulation, by manual manipulation, and/or intercourse. In addition, ask whether any mechanical devices or vibrators are used, either with a partner or when alone.

If a woman can masturbate to orgasm without difficulty, it is likely that her physiological and hormonal connections are intact, and that her difficulty responding with a partner has to do with her lack of comfort, reluctance to communicate, and/or her partner's techniques.

If the patient is orgasmic with partner manual manipulation but not with thrusting, ask whether or not either of them provides additional manual stimulation during thrusting. If the answer is no, including this extra dimension can be suggested.

It is important for physicians and therapists to avoid the common error of suggesting that women

Table 3.2 *Painful Intercourse* (*Male*)

1. When did the pain begin?
2. How frequently do you experience it?
3. What does the pain feel like?
4. Do you have pain with masturbation as well? If so, is the nature of the pain the same?
5. When during sex does it occur?
6. On a scale of 0 to 10, how intense is the pain?
7. Does the pain persist after intercourse?
8. Is there any pain in your testicles or rectum?
9. Is the pain associated with erection or ejaculation or both?
10. Do you have any curvature of your penis?
11. Has the degree of curvature changed in the last year or two?
12. Is the curvature associated with the pain?
13. Do you have this pain at any other times?
14. What have you tried to do to relieve or diminish the pain?
15. Does changing position relieve or aggravate the pain in any way?

Table 3.3 *Impotence*

1. Is the problem with your partner intermittent or constant?
2. Is there a predictable time when you lose your erection?
3. Grade your erections on a scale of 0 to 10. 0 is a completely flaccid (or limp) penis. 10 is a completely erect penis. Half an erection would be graded a 5.
   a. morning erections
   b. night time erections
   c. erections with masturbation
   d. erections with partner stimulation (manual)
   e. erections with partner stimulation (oral)
      (i) with her mouth on your genitals
      (ii) with your mouth on her genitals
   f. erections with fantasy only
   g. erections with intercourse
   h. erections with extramarital sex
   i. erections with prostitute experience
   j. other
4. How frequently do you masturbate?
5. Do you fantasize during masturbation? During intercourse?
6. When was the very first time in your life that you can remember losing an erection, or not getting one, at a time that you thought was inappropriate? Include those times you were drunk or tired.
7. When was the very next time that you lost an erection after gaining one, or could not get an erection at all?
8. When did the loss of erections equal the number of successful intercourse opportunities?
9. When was the last time you had intercourse?
10. How frequently now are you attempting intercourse?
11. How frequently do you succeed?
12. How frequently do you think about intercourse?
13. Have you ever ejaculated through a flaccid penis?
14. What was the best grade erection you have had under any circumstances during recent months? What were the circumstances?

who are not orgasmic with intercourse are inherently deficient or abnormal. They feel this way already. Instead, help them understand that, according to the available statistics, it is common to *not* achieve orgasm with intercourse alone. Depending upon which references are consulted, approximately 40% of women are routinely orgasmic with intercourse (Kelly, Strassbert, & Kircher, 1990). The majority of women who can be orgasmic with intercourse are not orgasmic with intercourse every time. Many women (approximately 60%) who enjoy sex thoroughly and are orgasmic in a variety of other ways do not have orgasms with thrusting alone.

In men you will want to know about any ejaculatory or orgasmic disturbances (see Table 3.5). These valuable symptoms can guide you in your differential diagnosis. Although ejaculation and orgasm normally occur simultaneously in males, medical conditions and pharmacological interference can separate them. A man can be orgasmic without ejaculating if he has had a certain type of prostatectomy, or he may be orgasmic but experience retrograde ejaculation if he has had a transurethral prostatectomy that damaged his internal urinary sphincter. He may ejaculate without the sensation of orgasm as a result of a genito-urinary anesthetic effect of medication, or he may ejaculate through a semi-erect or flaccid penis. Orgasm and ejaculation ordinarily occur together, but sometimes ejaculation occurs in the absence of orgasm.

Also determine subjective and objective time frames for ejaculation. Ask the patient if he thinks he ejaculates too quickly or takes too long. Then ask him to estimate the span of time between the development of the erection and the moment of ejaculation (in thrusts, seconds, or minutes). Some men ejaculate prior to penetration. Make no assumptions, and use care in phrasing your question. Asking a man how many minutes he lasts during thrusting will be awkward if it is only a few seconds. You want to make it easy for him to volunteer the circumstances, without making him feel embarrassed or inadequate.

It could also be valuable to know whether the patient's ejaculate has decreased in volume (possible anticholinergic effect) or changed in color, odor, or taste, suggesting infection and/or diet concentrations (e.g., garlic). In one case, a woman mentioned that her husband's ejaculate tasted sweet. As it turned out, laboratory studies confirmed the presence of diabetes, which their general practitioner had not yet identified. Problems in the area of sexual desire can be the most complex of all sexual dysfunctions to evaluate *and* the most commonly overlooked.

The key elements of physical sensation and pleasure are not well conveyed by any of the terms used to describe sex: *libido, desire, arousal, response.* The relation between sexual arousal and desire, imagination, attention, motivation, appetite, and drive is often identified as *libido.* For convenience, we usually use *desire* and *libido* interchangeably to cover all anticipatory/motivational/maintenance aspects of sexual behavior, excluding physical arousal and response. However, neither *drive* nor *libido* includes the essential interpersonal, perceptual, and reinforcement aspects of sexual behavior.

Perhaps the most important aspect of desire

Table 3.4 *Orgasms (Female)*

1. Do you have difficulty having orgasms?
2. Do you have orgasms less than half the time you desire them?
3. Do you ever fake orgasm or exaggerate your sexual response?
4. Have you experienced orgasms in any of the following ways: in dreams, through masturbation, through partner manual stimulation, through partner oral stimulation, through intercourse, with a vibrator?
5. What method do you use for masturbation: manual stimulation, vibrator, other?
6. Have you ever experienced more than one orgasm at a time through any method?
7. Do you have orgasms as easily with your partner as you do by masturbating? (If the answer is no, ask:) How much of a time difference exists? Are you concerned about it?

Table 3.5 *Orgasms/Ejaculation (Male)*

1. How long do you last—from the moment of penetration to the moment of ejaculation (in seconds, thrusts, or minutes)?
2. Do you ever ejaculate prior to penetration without meaning to?
3. Have you ever ejaculated without direct physical stimulation of the penis:
   a. under emotional stress, such as during an examination?
   b. under physical stress, like rope climbing?
   c. while fully clothed, from kissing or petting?
4. Do you try to think nonsexual thoughts to distract yourself so that you are able to last longer?
5. Do you skip foreplay hoping to last longer during intercourse?
6. Have you ever tried numbing ointments or other home remedies for premature ejaculation?
7. Do you ejaculate twice (starting intercourse again immediately after your first orgasm) hoping to last longer the second time?
8. How long do you think your partner wants you to last?
9. Do you ejaculate more quickly when you are on top or on the bottom?
10. Have you always ejaculated rapidly? If not, when did it begin?
11. Are there some circumstances under which you can last longer:
    a. if you drink alcohol, smoke marijuana, or consume other drugs?
    b. with some women and not others?
12. Do you sometimes lose erections or have difficulty obtaining one?
13. Is your partner hostile and angry with you for ejaculating too soon?

disorders—the one most difficult to understand—is that sexual responsiveness can exist independent of sexual desire. A woman who has no sexual desire, or who admits she detests sex, can be orgasmic and physically responsive once she agrees to participate. Even though she has been orgasmic, she usually avoids participating unless her partner pressures her.

It is easier to comprehend lack of desire leading to lack of responsiveness. This situation is more often true for men: those with reduced or little interest in sex typically do not pursue it and consequently do not function unless pressured into it by their partners. Physiologically normal men can then respond with manual stimulation, even when psychological interest is minimal. It is also easy to understand that some women who have no sexual desire do not respond sexually. The point is that it is not uncommon for both women and men to be normally responsive sexually, even though they are experiencing a desire disorder, if someone persuades them to participate.

Sexual aversion manifests as a desire disorder, but it has phobic components. This sexual aversion may be mild or clearly phobic. Again, as with other disorders of desire, the aversive individual may function well and even enjoy the experience, but maneuvers to avoid sex in-between episodes. A patient who is mildly aversive may cringe at a touch or caress for fear that it might lead to sex. Severely aversive behavior with phobic components may manifest as hysteria, suicidal threats, panic reactions or physical responses (i.e., nausea, vomiting, dizziness, at the thought of sex or at a suggestive touch). By contrast, a non-aversive patient with low sexual desire may not respond receptively to touch or sexual overtures, and may decline to participate due to lack of interest, but without the anxious, avoidance component. Panic may be eased or avoided by initiating discussion and non-sexual touching, and letting the fearful partner decide whether sexual activity will occur on any given occasion. Also, the partner should be assured that he or she can discontinue sexual activity if physical symptoms of panic appear. See Table 3.6 for questions to evaluate levels of desire.

Table 3.6 *Levels of Desire*

1. As a rule, do you desire sex more or less often than your partner?
2. How often did you have sex this past year?
3. Have you experienced any decrease in frequency?
4. Would you like to have sex more often than you do?
5. Do you enjoy having sex?
6. When exactly did you last have intercourse?*
7. Do you have sex when you would rather not?
8. Do you have any difficulty lubricating/becoming erect?
9. Are you easily distracted during sex?
10. Grade your relationship/marriage on a scale of 0 to 10.

*This may be the only time you find out that a couple has a 20-year unconsummated marriage; that your patient has not had intercourse for several years due to pain; or that your patient is having an affair and has intercourse frequently but not with his or her mate.

Issues with Long-Term Patients

Introducing sexual subjects to patients you have treated for many years can be distinctly awkward. There are several ways to approach this situation. Address the subject during the next scheduled history and physical examination and health review. Begin by linking the discussion to new medications or a change in current medications. When prescribing a new medication, preface your remarks by noting how numerous medications can adversely affect sexual functioning in a percentage of patients. However, even drugs that are known to cause sexual problems do not do so in all patients, and drugs that do not have a reputation for causing these problems *can* do so in *certain* patients. In other words, there are no hard-and fast rules. Therefore, you would like your patient to inform you of any sexual changes, should they occur, as well as any other side effects that he or she suspects are associated with the new medication. A sample introduction to a 60-year-old patient of 20 years follows: "When you first became my patient, discussing sexual issues was not a common medical practice. However, times have changed and we have a little catching up to do. I would like to make sure that we have not overlooked anything important to your health and well-being, so let me ask you just a few questions. Are you experiencing any sexual problems at this time? Have you experienced sexual problems in the past? If so, how were they resolved? Is your mate/partner/spouse experiencing any sexual problems? Have you had any pain associated with sexual activity?"

By integrating the subject of sexual side effects whenever general side effects of drugs are discussed, the topic ceases to stand out as sensitive or delicate and becomes merely one more item on the list. By understanding why sexual information is needed and how to elicit it comfortably from patients, the sexual review of systems can be covered as efficiently as the urological or gynecological reviews.

Ideally, medical knowledge should be used as an adjunct to sex therapy, and vice versa. With both new and long-term patients, your most valuable asset in addressing the sexual problems patients bring to your attention is a list of dependable sex therapists similar to those you use for surgery, neurology, psychiatry, etc. Until you have developed a dependable referral list of your own, solicit suggestions from your colleagues. Be sure to ask patients whom you refer to a sex therapist to let you know how they felt about their care. In addition, find out if the patients made use of the therapist's suggestions. The ability to engage patients in treatment programs and motivate follow-through is a necessary therapeutic skill. If most of the patients you refer to a particular therapist go for one visit and never return, it would be advisable to find another referral.

INTERVIEW TECHNIQUES FOR THERAPISTS

The clinical intake procedures conducted by therapists follow similar lines of inquiry, with more emphasis on psychological dimensions. A certain number of medical questions must be asked in order to ascertain whether sexual difficulties have a physiological or pharmacological basis, as can easily happen when a patient comes for therapy while taking sex-offender drugs (be they legal or illegal). Therapists should first determine if a referral or a phone call to a physician is indicated. Sharing a patient's intake with a physician saves time for both professionals. A written evaluation of the therapist's intake interview should be sent to the physician for inclusion in the patient's chart. A partial intake could be similar to the medical form patients fill out in physicians' offices when they first seek help for a physical complaint.

It is important to explain to patients that physicians and therapists serve two complementary functions. The main reason for teamwork is that each discipline can fill in part of the "sexual puzzle." Communication about a potential treatment strategy might include a succinct summary of how best to take advantage of professional expertise. Therapists, who usually see patients on a weekly or biweekly basis, can be particularly helpful to both patients and physicians, if they are alert for noncompliance with health-care recommendations. They can also contribute by communicating interdisciplinary information that addresses the medical, pharmacological, and psychological issues in an integrated fashion, and by reinforcing dietary limitations, stop-smoking protocols, and alcohol recovery programs. It is also comforting for therapists to know that they can consult with physicians on problems in "gray areas."

Physicians typically do not take full advantage of clinical therapy as a resource. They are even less inclined to refer to for sexual conditions. Even when they do refer, only one in four patients is willing to pursue treatment—although these statistics can be improved with follow-through. A partnership between physicians and other therapists is therefore essential. Sex therapists are the best source of information regarding sex drive and levels of response; clinical therapists are the best source for psychological evaluations of responses to medications; and physicians are the best source of information about the physiological side effects of prescription drugs. Unfortunately, physicians and therapists rarely benefit from one another's experience and expertise. A physician may prescribe a drug but fail to alert the therapist regarding its side effects. Usually the therapist does not realize that these effects are due to the drug. Both physicians and therapists could consult on these side effects to mutual advantage.

DESIGNING TREATMENT STRATEGIES

Designing a treatment strategy intended to avoid or manage the sexual side effects of drugs is a very straightforward task that can be clearly delineated (see Table 3.7).

- *Step 1* Investigate alcohol and illegal drug abuse and cigarette smoking, as appropriate.
- *Step 2* Be assertive about helping your patients utilize the resources that self-discipline, diet, exercise, and habit control can provide. Explore and implement all non-drug strategies that could enhance the patient's condition, such as weight loss; special diet regimens for blood pressure, ulcer, and diabetes; exercise; stress reduction techniques; and any other strategies beneficial to the physical problem and/or to sexual health. Suggestions to patients about changes in lifestyle generally net no tangible results without the follow-up discussion of Step 3.
- *Step 3* Establish realistic goals (weight loss, exercise, quitting smoking, etc.) through discussion with the patient and determine what avenues of implementation are most suitable. For example, if weight loss is the goal, will the patient be helped more by a twelve-step-type program, by working with a nutritionist, by physician supervision, etc. Regarding smoking, examine the best approach for your patient individually—smokenders, nicorettes, the nicotine patches, etc. Establish short-term and long-term goals: e.g., weight loss perhaps in five-pound increments, a minimum satisfactory health weight, and an ideal weight. If alcohol, smoking, weight, diet and exercise are all important elements, decide on priorities, sequence, and strategy. Be sure to refer your patient to suitable programs as appropriate. Advising a patient to stop drinking is an important first step, but not sufficient in most cases. Some patients will need to be helped to understand that they require an aggressive inpatient program. Others may respond well to outpatient treatment.
- *Step 4* Set specific deadlines. Ask the patient by what date he or she thinks the particular objective can be reached. Solicit a commitment that, if the goal is not achieved, the patient will pursue whatever form of therapy is appropriate to achieve it. For example, if your patient decides to stop smoking, set a date for stopping (within two weeks to a month, for example) and together set a date to evaluate the success of the program three to six months in the future.
- *Step 5* Ask the patient what alternative program ("phase 2") would be acceptable if "phase 1" is ineffective. The first impact of this two-phase commitment is to increase the likelihood that phase 1 (achieving the goal) will occur. The second impact is to minimize the damage of failure if phase 1 does not work. The patient has made an agreement to proceed to phase 2, to which you, as the physician, can influence and facilitate compliance.
- *Step 6* Schedule the next appointment before your patient leaves the office.

After exploring all relevant and meaningful non-prescription health strategies, evaluate the following questions:

Table 3.7 *Strategy and Goal Setting*

1. Investigate alcohol/illegal drug abuse and smoking.
2. Discuss all non-drug strategies/lifestyle changes.
3. Establish realistic goals and means of implementation.
4. Set a specific date for achieving the goals.
5. Define a phase-2 strategy in case phase 1 is not successful.
6. Schedule a return appointment before patient leaves the office.

1. If medication is still necessary, which drug is most suitable and has the fewest sexual side effects?
2. Does the patient have a persisting sexual condition that might make one drug preferable to another (e.g., if the patient suffers from premature ejaculation, is there a relevant drug with a side effect that inhibits ejaculation)?
3. If your patient is already on medication that is adversely affecting sexual functioning can the dosage of the drug be reduced without negatively affecting the patient's health?
4. Can the drug be discontinued for a month or two without unacceptable risk in order to determine whether the sexual dysfunction is relieved by removal of the drug?
5. If your patient cannot tolerate the absence of medication or reduction of dosage, or if reduction of dosage is ineffective, is there a suitable alternative drug with less potential for adverse sexual side effects?

If the original drug has been reduced or terminated, or if a substitute drug has been prescribed and no sexual improvement is clinically evident, do not assume that the original drug was not the problem; it may have precipitated sexual problems that persist long after the drug is discontinued. The medication caused the sexual problem, but the sexual problem usually causes psychological reactions that reinforce the dysfunction. Fears of performance develop, for example, that can persist long after the drug is withdrawn, and that perpetuate a sexual disorder on a psychological basis that was originally triggered by a drug effect. *Do not* dismiss chronic sexual dysfunction with comments like, "It comes with age." At this point, refer the patient to a skilled sex therapist; short-term sex therapy can usually correct any long-term adverse psychological effects of sexually toxic drugs. In some cases the severity of the disease and/or the need for multiple drugs make it difficult or impossible to find a satisfactory therapeutic alternative that does not compromise sexual function. A patient's condition can be so unique that it can only be managed medically by one of the most sexually hazardous medications. Even under these circumstances, however, do not tell your patient to "learn to live without sex." More positive options are available, such as further medical evaluation and intervention; therapy to help the patient to enjoy a somewhat limited sexual repertoire; surgery (penile implant); supplemental lubricants/dilation procedures; and the addition of sexually effective medications to counteract the adverse effects of necessary drugs.

The differential diagnosis of drug-induced sexual dysfunction is essential to developing an appropriate treatment strategy. While the forces that influence human sexual response are complex, a systematic diagnostic approach can usually distinguish between the medical, psychological, and pharmacological etiologies. Since they are typically all present to some degree, it is particularly important to have a comprehensive clinical picture of the role each plays.

Part II introduces gender differences and hormonal therapies. The distinctions between men and women are more obvious sexually than in any other respect. Even so, these marked sex-linked patterns have not been fully appreciated by modern medicine. While Part I provided general principles and strategies for dealing with drug-related sexual problems, Part II develops the foundation for understanding why men and women must be evaluated and treated separately with regard to drugs and sex. It will become clear that the same drug often affects men and women in distinctly different ways sexually. But in order to fully appreciate the scope of these differences, a thorough grasp of the neuroendocrine gender gap is essential.

Part II

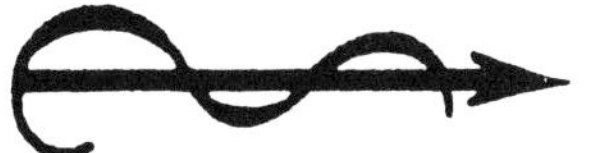

SEX DIFFERENCES AND HORMONAL THERAPIES

4

Sexual Aspects of Neurochemistry

OBJECTIVES

- To identify and clarify the neuroendocrinological mechanisms of action that influence sex
- To provide quick reference summaries of each known sexual mechanism of action
- To identify gender-based differences in pharmacological side effects
- To provide a description of the various neurotransmitter hormones and structures involved in the sexual aspects of neuroendocrinology

Much of our information about human sexuality comes from animal studies which have obvious limitations. Very few researchers have observed and measured human sexual activity. (Masters and Johnson [1966] are an exemplary but unfortunately rare research team who have provided objective sexual data in this fashion.) Most recently, valuable information about living subjects has been obtained through therapeutic penile injections, which have enabled us to add to our knowledge of neurotransmitter effects on male sexual functioning (see Chapter 31). When various vasodilators have been injected directly into the penis, in an effort to produce an erection, the clinical response varies according to the underlying disease causing the impotence. Other data about human sexual functioning have been charted from the sexual consequences of naturally occurring diseases, such as cerebrovascular accidents (strokes), neurological (spinal cord injuries, multiple sclerosis), and endocrine diseases (diabetes, hyperprolactinemia). As we identify sexual changes associated with these diseases, we can analyze retrospectively and indirectly the mechanisms involved. Some speculative aspect remains, however, because living humans are obviously not available for dissection and laboratory documentation; cadavers can only facilitate our investigations of the anatomical and neurological structures implicated in human sexuality.

Even though our data base and resources are restricted by these realities, research conducted throughout the last decade has netted a wealth of discoveries. Ten years ago, scientists considered testosterone and estrogen to be the basic hormones involved in sexual drive and response. Over 30 mechanisms that influence sex directly or indirectly are identified in this text. In addition, the neurotransmitters that interact with specific brain structures are also becoming more clearly understood. However, this mapping process is still very much in its infancy. Here especially, animal research is insufficient. In this chapter, we summarize what is known to date and speculate upon possibilities that will be better defined in the future.

In the 1940s the endocrine system was conceptualized as existing outside the blood-brain barrier and therefore not controlled by the brain. The pituitary, situated below the barrier, was known to signal various glands throughout the body. During the 1950s research revealed direct endocrine influence from the hypothalamus; and, finally, in the 1960s, peptide hormone-releasing factors were identified in the hypothalamus. For example, the newly identified hypothalamic luteinizing hormone releasing hormone (LHRH) peptide was recognized as regulating the luteinizing hormone (LH) pituitary-gonadal feedback circuit. Several such hypothalamic-releasing peptides were identified, establishing the still-expanding field of peptide neurotransmission.

The synthesis and secretion of pituitary peptide hormones, luteinizing hormone (LH), and follicle-stimulating hormone (FSH) are regulated by a hypothalamic releasing factor or hormone (designated alternatively as gonadotropin-releasing hormone [GnRH], LHRH, or luteinizing hormone releasing factor [LRF]). Although this releasing hormone is chiefly localized in the median eminence of the hypothalamus, its activity involves anterior hypothalamic (AH), medial preoptic (MPO), and ventromedial (VMH) control which, in turn, is sensitive to activation of neurotransmitter (DA, NA, 5-HT) and sex hormone (androgen and estrogen) receptors that are abundant in these areas. While LHRH regulates both LH and FSH, differences in the nature of LH and FSH secretion indicate that a separate FSH releasing factor may be operating. Our increasing understanding of this complex and fascinating puzzle points to the inevitable conclusion that the biochemistry of sex is inextricably linked with our emotions and thoughts, and therefore mediated through the higher structures of our brain, in synchrony with a concert of hormones and chemicals circulating throughout our bodies.

This neurochemical identification of interactive mind-body circuits has been vital to the development of sexual pharmacology (as well as to other neurochemical areas of study such as immunology). In fact, currently the brain is being redefined as an endocrine organ because it not only controls distant endocrine functions, but also produces certain hormones itself called neurosteroids (Baulieu, Robel, Vatier, Haug, Le Goascogne, & Bourreau, 1987). Neurotransmission by dopamine and serotonin involves less than one percent of human nervous system activity. The excitatory amino acid system, including glutamate transmission, a separate neurotransmitter system, is currently the focus of advances in molecular pharmacology.

Various studies have indicated positive effects on the nucleus accumbens brain reinforcement center by dopaminergic agents, marijuana, odors, brain stimulation, and other processes that have also been shown to affect sex positively (see Chapter 26). Testosterone potentiates the sexual effects of dopamine through synergistic action in brain sex centers, such as the medial preoptic nucleus. Conversely, the nucleus accumbens is inhibited by agents that negatively affect sex, such as serotonin, GABA, and opiates. Specific activation of the nucleus accumbens by sexual stimuli and sexual activity also has been demonstrated. The connection between sexual activity and activation of the brain reward center is important because it assures reproduction by making sex rewarding.

Of particular interest in research is identifying the distinctions between the male and female brain anatomically and histologically. A central premise of sexual pharmacology is that men and women are sexually more different than alike—from their anatomy to their hormones, emotions, and needs—and that these differences will affect sexual responses to various pharmacological agents. Biochemical and hormonal differences between men and women are clear. While both sexes have all the mechanisms of action we will be describing, each has dramatically different concentrations of these substances and they behave differently in males and females. Behavioral and psychological differences, while often clear, are far less standardized. It generally appears that men and women process sexual data differently and respond differently. For example, typically, the male must concentrate in order to delay orgasm; by contrast, the female must concentrate in order to have an orgasm. Men are usually mono-orgasmic; women commonly have the capacity to be multi-orgasmic. Men usually detumesce abruptly after sex, while women prefer to bask in the afterglow and continue cuddling.

The age-old debate about whether nature or nurture is responsible for certain differences between the sexes undoubtedly will continue indefinitely into the future. We do not intend to end this debate—only to point out demonstrable biological, physiological, neurochemical, anatomical, and hormonal differences and whatever behavioral implications will shed light on these important gender distinctions.

MECHANISMS OF ACTION AFFECTING SEXUALITY

In order to appreciate the sexual properties of a drug, it is important to understand which mechanisms of action have been identified that can affect sex. All drugs work through one or more mechanisms of action. For example, aspirin is an anticoagulant that prevents strokes by interfering with platelet aggregation. Interfering with platelet aggregation is one of the general mechanisms of action of aspirin. It is also specifically beneficial sexually because, via the same mechanism, the patency of the fine vessels to the penis is also protected, promoting erections in men who might otherwise be obstructed. Consequently, interfering with platelet aggregation qualifies as a sexual mechanism of action. It is not necessary to have a degree in pharmacology or to understand all dimensions of the particular mechanism of action, but it is important to grasp the basic principles. We need to ask: When a particular mechanism of action is affected in one direction, does it activate or inhibit any aspect of sexual response? What sexual emotion or function is influenced? Is the effect similar or different in men and women? When the mechanism is affected in the opposite direction, are sexual changes also associated? Or is there no effect?

Our first insights into sexual mechanisms of action involved hormones. With the identification of numerous neurotransmitters, additional sexual mechanisms of action were identified. Both hormones and neurotransmitters are variously mediated by the brain. The mechanisms described in Tables 4.1 and 4.2, therefore, consist primarily of hormones and neurotransmitters (as well as a few other recognized sexual mechanisms of action) and reflect our current understanding of the neuroendocrinology of sex. As our knowledge and sophistication increase, sexual mechanisms of action will expand further, just as they grew beyond the scope of endocrinology alone.

Understanding the sexual influence of each mechanism of action not limited to the endocrine system is the basis for understanding the sexual properties of drugs. One way to evaluate these mechanisms is to consider them in related groups based upon an axis of effect ranging from excitatory to inhibitory. The excitement/inhibition axis is directly related to sexual function and dysfunction. Sexual desire and response are associated with excitement. Consequently, as long as excitement is not excessive or disrup-

Table 4.1 *Mechanisms of Action Affecting Sexual Response*

NATURALLY OCCURRING ENDOGENOUS SUBSTANCES WITH GENERALLY EXCITATORY SEXUAL ACTIONS (Increase in dose or activity favorable to sex; decrease in dose or activity unfavorable to sex.)
Adrenergic (Alpha$_1$) Activity
Adrenergic (Beta$_2$) Activity
Calcitonin-Gene-Related-Peptide (CGRP)
Cholinergic Activity
Dehydroepiandosterone (DHEA/DHEAS)
Dopamine (DA)
Endothelium-derived Relaxing Factor (EDRF)
Estrogen (female only)
Excitatory Peptides
Growth Hormone (GH)
Histamine
Luteinizing Hormone Releasing Hormone (LHRH)
Nitric Oxide (NO)
Oxytocin
Prostaglandins
Substance P (SP)
Testosterone
Vasoactive Intestinal Peptide (VIP)
Vasopressin
Zinc (replacement value only)

tive, drugs which increase excitement generally enhance various aspects of sex while drugs with inhibitory effects generally decrease desire and/or responsiveness.

However, sexually activating features are not universally desirable. In keeping with this spectrum, excessive excitement can trigger hypersexuality and other aberrant sexual patterns. Excitatory substances include: epinephrine, acetylcholine, dopamine, histamine; androgens such as DHEA/DHEAS and testosterone; and various peptides including oxytocin, vasopressin, LHRH, prostaglandins, Substance P, CGRP, and VIP. Inhibitory substances include: GABA, cortisol, melatonin, MAO, opioids, progesterone, prolactin, and serotonin.

Specific side effects can also be associated with sexual repercussions along an excitatory/inhibitory axis. Sedation, decreased sensation, inactivity, lack of initiative, depression, weakness, and fatigue are consistent with the inhibitory pole; activation, movement, attention, increased sensation, and intensity correlate with the excitatory pole. It should be noted that some drugs which are capable of promoting sexual desire and response may also be potentially problematical and pathological. For example, activation and intensity are also associated with anger, aggressiveness, poor impulse control, and psychosis. Tables 4.1 and Table 4.2 list the various mechanisms of action that influence human sexuality according to whether they generally improve or detract from sexual responsiveness.

Table 4.2 *Mechanisms of Action Inhibiting Sexual Response*

NATURALLY OCCURRING ENDOGENOUS SUBSTANCES WITH GENERALLY INHIBITING SEXUAL ACTIONS (Increase in dose or activity unfavorable to sex; decrease in dose or activity favorable to sex.)
Adrenergic ($Alpha_2$) Activity
Angiotensin II (Ang II)
Cortisol
Estrogen (male only)
Melatonin
Monoamine Oxidase (MAO)
Neuropeptide Y (NPY)
Opioids
Progesterone
Prolactin
Serotonin (5-HT)
Thyroid Hormone*
Vasoconstrictive Peptides (Ang II and NPY)

*Both increase and decrease in thyroid activity unfavorable to sex.

Adrenergic ($Alpha_1$) Activity

(*Primarily excitatory*)

- enhances desire and arousal
- facilitates the action of dopamine, testosterone, acetylcholine, vasopressin, and prostaglandins
- promotes peripheral vasoconstriction
- can cause impotence and trigger ejaculation

$Alpha_1$ adrenergic receptors increase adrenergic (sympathetic) stimulation by mediating norepinephrine and epinephrine release. Norepinephrine (NE) release is the key agent in general physical and mental arousal, not just sexual arousal. In the brain, norepinephrine is released from the locus coeruleus (LC), which is involved in activation, arousal, and attention. Norepinephrine can specifically modulate sexual reactions by stimulating LHRH secretion.

$Alpha_1$ adrenergic stimulation also facilitates other excitatory substances, including dopamine, testosterone, acetylcholine, vasopressin, and prostaglandins. Of the two major catecholamines – norepinephrine and dopamine – norepinephrine is more nonspecific for sexuality and pleasure than dopamine. Even so, norepinephrine is an essential prerequisite; it functions much like a battery current that must be activated in order for the rest of the sexual apparatus to ignite and operate. However, norepinephrine also can have a paradoxical effect: Excessive sympathetic stimulation can cause enough anxiety to short-circuit sexual function. Excess $alpha_1$ activity can cause sexual problems via two different mechanisms: centrally, through CNS activation of anxiety which can inhibit erection or trigger ejaculation; peripherally, through vasoconstriction that can prevent or abort erection.

Adrenergic (Alpha$_2$) Activity

(*Primarily inhibitory*)

- decreases desire and arousal
- prompts peripheral vasoconstriction
- antagonizes alpha$_1$ activity
- can decrease anxiety-related premature ejaculation

Alpha$_2$ adrenergic receptors essentially have the opposite effects of alpha$_1$ adrenergic receptors: They *decrease* adrenergic (sympathetic) stimulation. Located pre-synaptically to alpha$_1$ receptors, many but not all alpha$_2$ receptors indirectly inhibit alpha$_1$ receptor firing by reducing the release of NE. Thus, alpha$_2$ receptors reduce adrenergic activity by inhibiting alpha$_1$ stimulation. Alpha$_2$ receptor agonists (stimulators) have the same effect. The function of post-synaptic alpha$_2$ adrenergic receptors has not yet been adequately studied.

One property that alpha$_1$ and alpha$_2$ agonists have in common is peripheral vasoconstriction, particularly in surface tissue like the genitals. Consequently, both agonists have the potential to affect erection adversely. Alpha$_2$ agonists such as clonidine, used to treat hypertension, decrease sexual desire and response in males, while alpha$_2$ antagonists such as yohimbine can increase male sexual desire and response. The sexual effects of these drugs appear to be caused by actions in the brain rather than the penis. The only sexual advantage of alpha$_2$ agonists may be to decrease sexual anxiety and perhaps anxiety-related premature ejaculation.

The sexual effects of alpha$_2$ agonists in female animals and in women are unclear, but until proven differently, it would be logical to assume that sexual arousal and orgasm would be decreased. When possible, avoid this potential problem by selecting an alternative.

Beta$_2$ (β_2) Adrenergic Activity

(*Primarily excitatory*)

- vasodilator
- promotes nervousness, "stage fright"

Beta$_2$ adrenergic stimulation has strong smooth muscle relaxing properties that can be used to treat bronchoconstrictive disorders, disorders of peripheral vasoconstriction, as well as erectile disorders (particularly arteriosclerosis, which reduces blood flow to the extremities). Beta$_2$ agonists also can cause peripheral nervous reaction such as tremor and shakiness, which is why beta-blockers have been useful in treating the symptoms of "stage fright." Although the excitatory effect of beta-agonists appears to enhance sexual arousal, the nervous reactions can contribute to anxiety.

GABA

(*Primarily inhibitory*)

- sedating
- disinhibiting paradoxical effects
- reduces anxiety, panic
- diminishes active sexual response in both sexes
- promotes receptive sexual response in females

The inhibitory action of GABA activity (best represented pharmaceutically by benzodiazepines) occurs chiefly in the limbic system, which modulates sexual attention, arousal, cognition, and personal reaction to others. Partners of patients treated with benzodiazepines may feel that the drug detracts from interpersonal and emotional reactions so that sexual interactions are less satisfying by muting responses due to CNS depression. Inhibition and sedation due to benzodiazepines may cause disorientation and disrupt sexual interest and rhythms indirectly. In addition, the dynamic range of sexual responses and reactions may be decreased directly. It is often difficult to differentiate deficits in general arousal (sedation) from specific sexual effects. Results of animal studies indicate that benzodiazepines seem to have different effects on males and females. In both sexes they may diminish "active" sexual responses; in females, however, they may increase selectively "receptive" sexual responses, such as lordosis.

Because of a reduction in anxiety, aversive or fearful sexual attitudes may be blocked by benzodiazepines, decreasing sexual avoidance, phobia, and panic. However, without concomitant psychotherapy, the negative sexual reactions will return once the medication is discontinued. Thus in the short term, sexual activity may be facilitated by the reduction in anxiety and avoidance patterns, in the long term, however, the most predominant effect of benzodiazepine/GABA medications is to lower sexual arousal and responsiveness.

Calcitonin-Gene-Related-Peptide (CGRP)

This peptide appears to be involved in peripheral vasodilation and perception of genital sensation. In animals, CGRP appears to be a cofactor in sexual arousal. As yet, little is known of its neural and peripheral actions.

Cholinergic Activity

(*Primarily excitatory*)

- once considered to be solely responsible for erection and lubrication mediated by parasympathetic nerves
- generates theta rhythms
- involved in both seizure and orgasm

Cholinergic activity was once credited as the neurotransmitter responsible for the parasympathetic stimulation necessary for erection and lubrication. Currently, it is believed only to facilitate other noncholinergic factors, which in turn are directly responsible for these sexual reactions. Cholinergic activity, by its involvement in limbic system arousal and excitement, mediates all types of sexual thoughts, attitudes, and memories (REM dream sleep is a cholinergic-driven process). Cholinergic activity in limbic structures (septum, hippocampus) is characterized by theta rhythms. EEG theta rhythms that accompany sexual arousal and orgasm indicate the participation of cholinergic activation. (Interestingly, neural hyperexcitation generated during cholinergic activity is involved in both seizure and orgasm.)

Peripheral cholinergic activity also promotes various secretory processes associated with nonsexual genital function (urination, defecation), as well as tissue secretion essential to sexual activity (e.g., cholinergic inhibition causes dry mouth, which can interfere with taste and kissing and may also diminish vaginal lubrication).

Cortisol

(*Acutely excitatory, chronically inhibitory*)

- paradoxical patterns
- long-term depressant effect on sex

Cortisol is a steroid secreted by the adrenal gland along with progesterone and DHEA. Cortisol release is triggered from the brain by neural peptides—directly by ACTH from the pituitary and indirectly by corticotropin releasing factor (CRF) and vasopressin from the hypothalamus. While the involvement of these neural peptides with cortisol is not yet completely clear, ACTH and vasopressin apparently mediate the "emergency reaction" property of cortisol when it is experienced on an acute basis. However, the long-term consequence of cortisol seems to be suppression, depression, and exhaustion. While this suppressive action is beneficial in reducing rash and other troublesome immune reactions, tissue (whether it be brain or bone cells) degenerates during prolonged cortisol exposure.

The emotional effects of cortisol are also paradoxical. Psychoses, derangement, and aggression can be promoted by cortisol-like steroids such as prednisone and anabolic steroids. Excessive cortisol levels can have either a depressant or destabilizing effect, ranging from decreased sex drive to perverse behavior in psychotics.

Dehydroepiandosterone (DHEA/DHEAS)

(*Primarily excitatory*)

- most abundant androgen
- associated with sex drive, especially in women

DHEA/DHEAS are androgens produced in the adrenal gland. While they are the most abundant androgens in humans, they have only about 3% of the androgenic potency of testosterone. They are thought to be a precursor substance for testosterone, peripheral androgens, and other sex hormones including estrogen. They have been of clinical interest mainly for their contribution to hirsutism and acne.

DHEA/DHEAS have received little scientific attention until their recent association with longevity research; their sexual profile is just beginning to emerge. A few years before puberty (adrenarche), DHEA/DHEAS levels begin to increase and reach a peak in the third decade of life, declining steadily thereafter. Some researchers have associated the drop of DHEA/DHEAS below a critical level as a factor in aging and as a male climacteric analogue (adrenopause) of menopause. DHEA/DHEAS may stimulate sex drive in both men and women, but less potently than testosterone. In addition, DHEA/DHEAS appear to have an excitatory impact in the limbic arousal system of both women and men, in contrast to the suppressive actions of cortisol and progesterone that typically have negative sexual effects (see Chapter 9).

Dopamine

(Primarily excitatory)

- mediates pleasures
- increases sex drive
- promotes orgasm

Dopamine is perhaps the most important neurotransmitter for experiences of pleasure, reinforcement, reward, movement, attraction, and various other processes intrinsic to sexual attraction, desire, arousal, response, orgasm, and satisfaction. It is so closely intertwined with sex that it is unclear whether dopamine promotes sex or sex promotes dopamine. However, its excitatory properties can cause or contribute to psychoses as well as sexual compulsion, addiction, and some perversions.

In men, dopamine may promote premature ejaculation; in women, it may facilitate orgasm. In both sexes, it appears to increase sex drive. Its action appears to be potentiated by sexual stimulants such as testosterone and estrogen and inhibited by sexual depressants such as serotonin. The sexual properties of dopamine and dopaminergic drugs are discussed in detail in Chapters 26 and 27.

Estrogens

(Excitatory and inhibitory in women; inhibitory in men)

- contributes to sexual desire and responsiveness in females
- promotes lubrication
- facilitates action of serotonin, opioids, prolactin, and oxytocin

Estradiol and other estrogens, which are produced in the ovaries and through metabolism from other body steroids, can promote all aspects of female sexuality including desire, attraction, lubrication, orgasm, and satisfaction. Estrogens are essentially female hormones, although men have small amounts in their systems. Female cycles and secondary sex characteristics are dependent upon estrogen activity.

In women, estradiol is sexually and mentally activating; it may also have an antidepressant effect in women through inhibiting monoamine oxidase. Beneficial moisturizing and lubricating actions on skin and body tissues have been identified. The relative sexual potency of estradiol in women compared to testosterone in men is under debate. The sexual role of estrogen in men is unclear, except for a feminizing influence on secondary sex characteristics (i.e., gynecomastia, hair patterns).

On both physical and mental levels, estrogens in women serve to attract males. As female sex steroids, estrogens facilitate the actions of serotonin, opioids, prolactin, and oxytocin. Their activating effect on sensation is exemplified by the superior sense of smell in women compared to men. (See Chapter 5 for a detailed discussion of the relation between estrogens and pharmacological agents.)

Growth Hormone (GH)

Growth hormone supports the growth of body tissue and appears to generate a feeling of calm and confidence which promotes satisfying sex.

Histamine

(*Primarily excitatory*)

- antagonism causes sedation through CNS depression

Histamine has arousal, sensitizing, and blood flow facilitating properties similar to excitatory peptides, particularly substance P. Its inhibition causes sedation, increased appetite, and reduction of cutaneous sensitivity and secretions.

Luteinizing Hormone Releasing Hormone (LHRH or GnRH)

This peptide hormone is released from the hypothalamus and triggers release of luteinizing hormone (LH) from the pituitary. It simulates gonadal testosterone production and regulates the menstrual cycle and other estrogen-related activities. LHRH may also act as a neurotransmitter in the brain directly stimulating libido. It appears to be the primary neural releasing substance initiating sexual attraction and approach. Through its triggering action on testosterone production, it mediates communication of sexual impulses from the brain to the body. LHRH not only triggers hypothalamic-pituitary function essential to sex, but also appears to be secreted in the brain during sexual encounters, facilitating sexual attraction.

Melatonin

(*Primarily inhibitory*)

- involved in diurnal and seasonal cycles
- central to understanding the relationship of light and sex

Melatonin is a serotonin-like substance inhibited by light and promoted by sleep (and hibernation in animals). It is produced and secreted by the pineal gland. In animals its secretion causes gonadal recession which accompanies the shortening days during winter, often preparing animals for a period of sexual quiescence. With the recent therapeutic success of light therapy for winter depression, we may be able to determine if melatonin has sexual effects in humans similar to those in animals.

Monoamine Oxidase (MAO)

(*Primarily inhibitory*)

- may cause depression
- MAO-A decreases norepinephrine, serotonin, dopamine
- MAO-B is more specific for dopamine and excitatory phenylethylamines (PEA) and can decrease sex drive and responsiveness

MAO is the enzyme that breaks down monoamines and degrades NE, E, 5-HT, and DA. It is speculated that increased activity is associated with depression, but one cannot yet state definitively that it causes depression. Generally, MAO activity is thought to cause depression by decreasing these monoamines. There is evidence that people who tend to seek out excitement and sensation of all kinds are deficient in MAO.

MAO inhibitors block the action of these MAO enzymes, resulting in increased levels of norepinephrine, serotonin, and dopamine. MAO-A enzyme inhibition may decrease feelings of depression, phobia, and panic, but may also increase serotonin production, leading to decreased orgasm and lowered sexual sensitivity.

By contrast, MAO-B enzymes are specific for dopamine and phenylethylamine, which are endogenous adrenergic-like stimulating chemicals. Consequently, their inhibition by drugs such as deprenyl (Eldepryl) can lead to heightened levels of these stimulating adrenergic chemicals and consequently to increased sexual desire, arousal, response, orgasm, and ejaculation.

Nitric Oxide (NO) or Endothelium-derived Relaxing Factor (EDRF)

(*Primarily excitatory*)

- vasodilators

Drugs that promote endothelium-derived relaxing factor (EDRF) activity will facilitate blood flow necessary for sexual response in general and erection in particular. The chemical identity of EDRF is not known, but it appears identical or similar to nitric oxide. Nitric oxide is generated by nerves in minute amounts to signal the cells of the endothelial lining of blood vessels to relax, allowing the vasodilation particularly important to erections.

Opioids

(*Primarily inhibitory*)

- inhibit orgasm/ejaculation
- diminish sex drive in both sexes
- disinhibitory at low doses
- facilitated by serotonin, estrogens, and progesterone

Opioids are perhaps the most powerful inhibitory neurotransmitters/peptides in the body. Despite the association of endorphins and romance, opiate drugs or endogenous opioids (endorphins, enkephalins = endogenous opioids) reliably decrease all aspects of sexual desire and response in animals. While feeling no pain and being tranquilized may be soothing, it is obvious that opiates/opioids are sexually inhibitory.

Male drug addicts may initially attribute sexual properties to opiates because they can delay orgasm/ejaculation. Similarly, female opiate users may benefit initially by reduction of anxiety and the inhibition of physical pain. Addictive opiates may also decrease sexual repression and psychological aversion to sex. Sooner or later, though, the essentially inhibitory effect of opiates/opioids will decrease sexual desire and response. Withdrawal from opiate addiction in men is characterized by spontaneous erections and orgasm/ejaculation. The sexual effects of endogenous opioids are presumably integrated into body chemistry so as not to be disruptive to sexual expression, but research into the sexual effects of endogenous opioids is just beginning. Opioid action is facilitated by serotonin, estrogens, and progesterone.

Oxytocin

Oxytocin facilitates attraction and touch sensation. It is a key substance known to spike during orgasm. It is integrally involved in bonding both as a cause and as an effect. Oxytocin levels increase secondary to touch. Once a touching pattern has been established, oxytocin levels increase with anticipation of touching. Its multifaceted role in attraction, touch, mating, sex, orgasm, bonding, labor, parenting, nursing—to name only a few—makes it a complex chemical with influence on human biology and emotion only marginally understood.

Progesterone

(*Primarily inhibitory*)

- sexual depressant independent of testosterone
- can also lower testosterone
- can cause depression, irritability

Progesterone is an inhibitory hormone that can reduce sensation, neural excitation, and irritative skin reactions in both women and men. Its role seems to be more to protect than to attract. In females, progesterone plays a dominant role in protection and nourishment of the fetus and may limit sexual and social interaction with males, because attention to men can interfere with care for offspring. In women, progesterone may be involved in defensive aggression. However, in female animals progesterone has a short-term effect in association with estrogen.

Progesterone seems to be an *anti*aphrodisiac, reducing sexual attraction generated by smells and other reflexive pheromonal stimulus cues. Its inhibitory function is analogous to the inhibitory effects of serotonin, opioids, melatonin, and cortisol. It often operates in opposition to testosterone and is more prevalent in females than males. By increasing monoamine oxidase (in contrast to estrogen and testosterone, which inhibit monoamine oxidase), progesterone has a depressant effect on monoamines, thus decreasing erotic desire and sexual sensitivity in both men and women.

Prolactin

(*Primarily inhibitory*)

- decreases sex drive/orgasm
- can cause impotence
- involved in sperm production

Prolactin is secreted by the pituitary. Elevated levels of prolactin seem to depress sensation and alertness in general, and may be associated with mild depression and fatigue. Chronically elevated prolactin levels can reduce sex drive in both men and women and can also cause impotence.

Prolactin normally increases in nursing mothers; excess secretion of prolactin can cause gynecomastia and galactorrhea in both men and women. An abnormally high level of prolactin can also decrease testosterone to subnormal levels. Therefore, it inhibits sex drive in a manner characteristic of low testosterone levels in both sexes. Whether the diminished sex drive secondary to prolactin is due to a direct mechanism of the drug or indirectly due to its reduction of testosterone is unclear.

Prolactin levels spike during copulation and orgasm, but quickly return to normal levels. The implications of this finding have not yet been fully explored. Prolactin also surges during stressful experiences such as nausea, vomiting, or fainting.

Involved in sperm production and the "maintenance" of genital tissue, prolactin may function as a precursor substance, nutrient, or lubricant. The sexual effects of low prolactin levels have not been studied.

Prostaglandins

This group of peptide substances prominently localized in the stomach and genital tissue facilitate smooth-muscle vasodilation and tissue sensation. It appears to be a primary mediator of erection and lubrication. Prostaglandin E1 is currently used as a vasodilator for penile injection-erection therapy.

Serotonin (5-HT)

(*Primarily inhibitory*)

- inhibits arousal and orgasm in both sexes
- decreases anxiety and aggressiveness
- symbiotic with estrogen
- facilitates opioids and progesterone

Serotonin appears to restrain excessive excitation, blunting impulsive pleasurable arousal and, in some cases, inhibiting orgasm completely. It appears to fall on the inhibitory pole of a dopamine-serotonin sexual axis. On the other hand, serotonin decreases excessive anxiety and aggressiveness that can make sex unpleasant and facilitates the warm sociability that is necessary for continued intimacy short of sexual peaks. It can prevent premature ejaculation in men and exhibits a preferential relationship with estrogen in women similar to the DA-testosterone connection in men. Serotonin also seems to facilitate other chemicals such as opioids and progesterone that mute sexual excitation.

Substance P (SP)

This substance is one of a group of peptide chemicals prominently involved in local tissue reactions, including skin, muscle, and the gastrointestinal tract. It is intricately involved in peripheral sensation and blood flow. Although generally studied as a mediator of pain transmission, it modulates both sensations of pleasure and pain. It contributes to dilation of blood vessels involved in the response of the sexual organs and the skin to sexual stimuli and touch.

Testosterone

(*Primarily excitatory*)

- promotes sex drive, assertiveness, aggression in both sexes
- facilitates action of dopamine, epinephrine, and vasopressin
- inhibits actions of serotonin, opioids, and prolactin
- inhibits MAO

Testosterone is the archetypical male hormone. It promotes sex drive, assertiveness, and aggression in both sexes and sexual responsiveness in men (including orgasm and ejaculation); excessive levels can result in destructive aggression, psychotic reactions, and irritative skin reactions like rash and acne.

Most testosterone production occurs in the gonads, but it is also derived from adrenal androgens and skin steroids. Secondary physical sex characteristics are maintained by its metabolite dihydrotestosterone (DHT). As an anabolic steroid, testosterone promotes growth hormone secretion. It also facilitates activating neurotransmitters like dopamine and epinephrine and is inhibitory to muting or restful neurotransmitters and hormones like serotonin, opioids, and prolactin. The excitatory action of the peptide vasopressin appears to be linked to testosterone, furthering or contributing to its qualities of arousal, alertness, and attention. Testosterone weakly inhibits monoamine oxidase, an action which can raise monoamines and have an antidepressant effect.

Thyroid Hormone

(*Primarily inhibitory, may be excitatory*)

- both increases and decreases in thyroid hormone are toxic to sex
- may interfere with testosterone

Thyroid hormone is essential to normal body vitality and metabolism. A deficiency can result in fatigue, weakness, sexual disinterest, dry or coarse skin, weight gain, impaired attention, constipation, muscle aches, decreased muscle reflexes, polyneuropathies, and bradycardia. From 50 to 80% of hypothyroidal men and women experience decreased sex drive and insufficient sexual response. This sexual deficiency may be partly due to general anergia and lack of initiative. Fertility and testosterone production also may be impaired by hypothyroidism. Hyperthyroidism has a general toxic effect on tissue metabolism, which indirectly undermines normal sexual responses.

Vasoactive Intestinal Peptide (VIP)

This peptide is abundant in genital tissue and the lumbosacral spinal cord. It is co-localized with acetylcholine in parasympathetic nerves and mediates genital vascular and smooth muscle relaxation previously associated solely with cholinergic action.

Vasoconstrictive Peptides

(*Primarily inhibitory*)

- angiotensin II (Ang II)
- neuropeptide Y (NPY)

These vasoconstricting peptides are similar to adrenergic agonists: They can have a negative effect on sexual function due to powerful vasoconstricting actions. The specific nature of their relationship to sexual response has not been studied. NPY has a powerful hyperphagic promoting action that distracts from sexual feelings. When given to animals, NPY can quickly halt any sexual activity and cause a switch to voracious eating behavior. Both directly and indirectly, NPY seems to discourage sexual attraction and attractiveness. A clinically useful NPY antagonist could have facilitating effects on sexual activity and dieting, but as yet, none exists.

Vasopressin

(*Primarily excitatory*)

Vasopressin facilitates limbic activation, which allows sexual arousal to be focused. This peptide appears to modulate adrenergic sexual excitation. Its action is linked with testosterone, possibly modulating masculine sexual social behavior and pheromonal communication. In the brain, it appears to mediate activation of attention to and concentration on sexual stimuli. As a potentiator of limbic cholinergic activity, it facilitates cognitive activity essential to sexual interactions. More specifically, it is a key thermoregulator which limits "overheating" of brain areas involved in sexual activity. Also known as antidiuretic hormone (ADH), it prevents water and salt depletion by stimulating thirst and inhibiting urination.

Zinc

(*Primarily excitatory*)

- involved in spermatogenesis
- abnormally low levels associated with impotence and hyperprolactinemia
- reduces GABA and opioids

Zinc is an essential mineral associated with proteins involved in spermatogenesis. It may also sensitize Leydig cell testosterone production to LHRH-LH stimulation. Zinc levels are particularly high in prostatic secretions and men have higher overall zinc levels than women.

Zinc has excitatory effects on limbic and hypothalamic activity, apparently through reduction of GABA and opioid activity (Baraldi, Giberti, Caselgrandi, & Petraglia, 1986). Manifestations of this excitatory action in animals include seizure, the stretching-yawning-penile erection (SYE) syndrome, and hyperalgesia.

Reduced serum zinc levels are common in male and female geriatric patients (Bogden et al., 1990). Abnormally low zinc levels have been associated with impotence and hyperprolactemia (in kidney dialysis patients depleted of zinc), which can be reversed with zinc supplementation (Antoniou, Shalhoub, Sudhaka, & Smith, 1977). However, zinc supplements have not exhibited any sexual effects in men with normal zinc levels. Zinc is also involved in proper immune function (Bogden et al., 1990), tissue healing, and prostaglandin action. The best form of zinc supplementation is zinc acetate. Deficient zinc availability can decrease cognitive function.

MECHANISMS OF ACTION AND THE BRAIN

Over 30 mechanisms of action affecting sexual function have been identified to date. How these mechanisms of action affect the brain and how drugs interact with both is still frontier territory. The brain can be separated into five main regions, from top to bottom: cerebral cortex, limbic system, basal ganglia, hypothalamus, and pituitary. The higher regions primarily process sensory information, thoughts, learning, memory, and associated emotional reactions. The lower regions primarily mediate reflexive and vegetative functions and hormonal and neural peptide activity.

These five regions and their effects on sexual function are summarized in Table 4.3.

The limbic system and the hypothalamus play central roles in sexual function. Specific structures within these areas seem to have control of distinct aspects of sexual behavior. The anterior hypothalamic medial preoptic nucleus (MPO), for example, governs sexual approach and active

Table 4.3 *The Sexual Effects of Localized Brain Activity*

Focal Brain Area	*Presumed Sexual Effects*
Cerebral cortex	Processes sensory and cognitive information and stores learning essential to interpretation of sensations and cognition
Frontal cortex	Stores consolidated memories of past sexual encounters which guide sexual choices and biases; involved in relationships; learning involved in sexual strategies
Limbic system	
Entorhinal cortex	Routing and processing of sensory input (sight, sound, touch, smell, taste)
Hippocampus	Consolidation of learning and memory traces; sexual dreams
Septum	Reverberating pacemaker mediating activation of sexual emotions within the limbic system; sexual dreams
Amygdala	Processing social and relational learning and thought. Locus of sexual feelings involving social learning such as sexual aversion, aggression; locus of fight/flight response and phobic reactions
Basal ganglia	
Nucleus accumbens (NACC)	Stimulates initiative and pleasure; charging and potentiating of sexual feelings experienced prior to and during sexual responses
Striatum	Directs and facilitates active movement in pursuit of sexual attractions; turns intentions and desire into action
Hypothalamus	
Anterior hypothalamic medial preoptic nucleus (MPO)	Generates *active* sexual behavior; mediates "masculine sexual behavior"; functions prominently in testosterone/dopamine activation; mediates coordination of sexual response execution and accompanying vegetative states (e.g., temperature, digestion)
Ventromedial nucleus (VMN)	Generates *passive*, receptive sexual behavior; mediates "feminine" reactions; functions prominently in estrogen/serotonin activation; connection with spinal reactions (central gray) (e.g., thrusting, lordosis)
Pituitary gland	Distributes hormonal messages from the brain to the rest of the body; produces various hormones which regulate sex hormone metabolism. The sexual effect depends on which hormone(s) are being influenced in which direction.

execution of copulatory behavior. Its function is so powerful in animals that it is referred to as the "active sexual behavior center" of the brain. It contains a prominent sexually dimorphic area which is larger in males than in females (Gorski, 1987). By contrast, the posterior hypothalamic ventromedial nucleus (VMH) controls passive, receptive, sexual behavior (i.e., lordosis) characteristic of both animals and humans. Activation of one of these hypothalamic nuclei can inhibit the expression of the other (e.g., activation of VMH decreases active sexual behavior characteristic of medial preoptic nucleus activation [Whitney, 1986]).

Observations during direct electrode stimulation to the human brain have brought attention to the limbic septum, which is a focal center of cholinergic activity (Heath, 1964a, 1972). Electrode stimulation of the limbic septum in surgical patients has resulted in pleasurable sensation, including intense sexual arousal and orgasm. When Heath (1972) directly stimulated the areas of the septum in these patients, intense pleasurable responses were accompanied by ecstatic sexual arousal, including compulsion to masturbate as well as actual orgasm in both female and male patients. Stimulation of other regions of the brain, especially in the hypothalamus, produced pleasurable feelings, but did not induce these specifically sexual reactions.

Preorgasmic and orgasmic sensations in a man and a woman studied by Heath were associated with seizure-like discharges in the septum and the nucleus accumbens, particularly on the right side (Heath, 1972). This seizure-like activity was restricted to the limbic nucleus accumbens area so that an epileptic seizure did not occur. Painful emotions such as fear and rage were associated with heightened limbic activity centered in the amygdala. It is interesting that orgasm, seizure, and psychotic states were all associated with septal activation. While monitoring patients during free association, electrical activity was most noticeable in the amygdala during painful emotions of fear and anger and most noticeable in the septum during pleasurable and positive sexual thoughts (Heath, 1972).

Animal research has indicated that, while animals usually avoid direct electrical stimulation to the amygdala, they will press for electrical stimulation of the septum. It is quite likely that the septum modulates and stimulates dreams, since dreams occur during REM sleep when the EEG theta rhythm characteristic of the septum is active. Indeed, the theta rhythm generated from the limbic area is specifically associated with both orgasm and REM sleep (Cohen, Rosen, & Goldstein, 1976; Kling, Steklis, & Deutsch, 1979). For this reason, it is possible to speculate that orgasms occurring during dreams in both sexes are somehow associated with the septum.

A study using normal volunteers treated with the dopaminergic antidepressant amineptine showed increased REM sleep and improved attention and concentration in the morning (Bramanti et al., 1985). Given the association of EEG theta rhythm with REM sleep and orgasm (Cohen et al., 1985), amineptine's sleep effects indicate a potential for sexual stimulation. Amineptine and other known dopaminergic sexual stimulants, including bupropion, apomorphine, and lisuride, all induce EEG theta in rabbits (Bo, Patrucco, & Savoldi, 1984). Theta rhythm is driven from the limbic hippocampus and septum, where cognitive and emotional stimuli are integrated, and is associated with cholinergic and dopamine D_1 receptor activation. The connections of dopamine to these sleep and theta phenomena have not been investigated. Dopamine appears to have special stimulant properties for women, suggesting that it could facilitate female orgasm (see Chapters 26 and 27).

In Heath's brain stimulation studies (Heath, 1964a), stimulation of the limbic hippocampus, a center for cholinergic activity, was often accompanied by adverse emotional states ("I feel sick all over"). Apparently, sexual stimulation is not chiefly the result of cholinergic activity per se, but of activation within a circuit that includes the cholinergic-driven septum. In one female patient, rage, fear, and depression induced by hippocampal stimulation were replaced within minutes by intense sexual feelings, including spontaneous orgasm, when the septal region was subsequently stimulated.* Heath (1964a) noted that "this patient, now married to her third husband, had never experienced orgasm before she received electrical stimulation to the brain, but since then has consistently achieved climax during sexual relations." The area of the septum stimulated by Heath was adjacent to the nucleus accumbens, which is active during pleasurable behavior. It is possible that electrical current had spread to this area, thereby intensifying pleasurable sensations from septal stimulation.

Pleasurable sexual sensations may be generated by a circuit running from the septum to

*Open human brain stimulation such as practiced by Heath is generally prohibited and his findings have not had the opportunity to be replicated.

the nucleus accumbens and, from there, into the anterior hypothalamus and medial preoptic nucleus (MacLean, 1990; Sachs & Meisel, 1988). Without actual human experimental studies, such a pathway cannot be confirmed. When such studies are eventually performed, other human brain regions are expected to demonstrate prominent sexual reactions as well, but this circuit probably will remain central to pleasurable sexual responsiveness.

Comprehensive and interesting reviews of sex-related brain literature and detailed descriptions of specific brain activity can be found in MacLean's 1990 book, *The Triune Brain*, which focused on the limbic circuit as the most relevant to human sexual behavior. Sachs and Meisel (1988) and Pfaff and Schwartz-Giblin (1988) focused on sublimbic hypothalamic structures most relevant to animal sexual behavior. Ascending and descending neural connections allow evaluation and control of lower brain function (e.g., temperature, digestion) by higher brain areas, so that there is a continuum of cognitive, emotional, and somatic reactions. (Discussions of these brain areas in relation to particular neurotransmitters and drugs are included throughout this book. For example, fear and phobia modulated by limbic brain areas are discussed in Chapter 18 on GABA/benzodiazepines; initiative and pleasure modulated by the nucleus accumbens are discussed in Chapters 26 and 27 on dopamine/bupropion.)

The Adrenaline Reflex*

The fight/flight circuitry of the brain (the epinephrine reflex) seems to be centrally involved in an animal's response to the sexual approach of another. Briefly, there are three major structures hierarchically involved in the fight/flight response:

thought and emotion/limbic: amygdala (AMD)

hormone-driven brain: ventromedial hypothalamus (VMH)

peripheral output/brainstem/spinal: midbrain central gray (MCG)

The midbrain central gray includes the spinal structures involved in fight/flight responses to aversive stimuli, whether direct (pain) or indirect (threat). The fight/flight response of the midbrain central gray is normally kept in check (tonic inhibition) by the ventromedial hypothalamus. To the extent that the ventromedial nucleus is activated (for example, by food satiation), the fight/flight will not occur. However, amygdala activation can inhibit the ventromedial hypothalamus, releasing the midbrain central gray fight/flight response.

Amygdala output contains the learning and conditioning of social and emotional reactions. Essentially, the amygdala serves as a "watch out!" structure mediating negative arousal reactions in response to threat. Conditioned fear and anxiety "output" by the limbic system are concentrated in the amygdala. The epinephrine response" is mediated by the amygdala through the adrenal glands (epinephrine) and the locus coeruleus (norepinephrine). However, the locus coeruleus-norepinephrine is a general arousal factor that can amplify the response to positive as well as negative factors.

The "command center" where memory and thought are integrated with emotion and reaction is located within the limbic system. Positive attentional responses seem to be mediated through the septum, which is another limbic structure that links thought with emotion and action. The septum is more directly connected to the hippocampus (memory and thought processor) than is the amygdala. The septum works in tandem with the hippocampus, while amygdala output more often reaches the hippocampus through a circuitous route (perhaps up through the cortex for evaluation and back into the hippocampus via the entorhinal cortical input path). Though also a "stop-and-attend" structure like the amygdala, the septum is more tuned to positive responses, whether they determine approach, reflection, or simply return to "automatic pilot."

***Adrenaline* is synonymous with *epinephrine*. Adrenaline is the preferred term in England, while epinephrine is preferred in the United States. Use of the term *adrenaline* facilitates understanding for laypersons.

Oxytocin Release

The "burst-and-spurt" nature of oxytocin release (Chard, 1985) (such as occurs with suckling) represents another variable involved in sexual stimulation. Given that oxytocin reaches saturation levels rapidly, refractory intervals are a natural part of the rhythmic flow of highly intense sexual stimulation. (This same principle works for the pituitary regulation of sex through LHRH pulsatility.) However, It is difficult to relate oxytocin to differences in orgasmic potential, or to explain the different postcoital patterns of men and women.

Oxytocin may be involved in the postcoital inertia that typically follows orgasm in men. Oxytocin generates a characteristic EEG theta after-reaction in breastfeeding rabbits (Kawakami & Sawyer, 1959) that resembles this refractory state. This theta response occurs at orgasm in both men and women, though more so for men, and usually is associated with activation of the right hemisphere (Cohen et al., 1976). Although we do not know why men become so much more refractory than women, sedation during the postejaculatory period may be a refractory effect of the oxytocin orgasmic "flush."

Oxytocin increases both centrally and peripherally during and after coitus. Stoneham, Everitt, Hansen, Lightman, and Todd, (1985) have reported oxytocin release during coitus in male rabbits, most often occurring at ejaculation but sometimes occurring during preliminary pelvic thrusting or in anticipation before entry of the female. The same group of researchers (Hughes, Everitt, Lightman, & Todd, 1987) found cerebrospinal fluid oxytocin increments after ejaculation in male rats, but no change when males were put with sexually unreceptive females.

Vasopressin Suppression

Vasopressin suppression may be an indirect route by which benzodiazepines reduce responses of sexual aversion, avoidance, fear, panic, and phobia. However, contrary to the conceivable positive association of vasopressin with sexual fear and avoidance, Onaka and his colleagues (Onaka, Yagi, & Hamamura, 1982) have shown in rats that, although physical stress increases vasopressin, emotional stress generated by fearful conditioning suppresses vasopressin secretion.

Vasopressin and oxytocin excite hippocampal neurons, enhancing glutamate action (Van Den Hoof, & Urban, 1990; Mazurek, Beal, Bird, & Martin, 1987). Benzodiazepine sedative/hypnotics may suppress excessive glutamate/excitatory amino activity involved in seizure; they reduce vasopressin through GABA activation. As with many sedative/hypnotic effects, the disturbance of abnormal excitation also involves the disturbance of normal excitation. Specifically, benzodiazepine sedative/hypnotics and alcohol (which also activates GABA) can suppress theta rhythm activation (Ehlers, Chaplin, & Koob, 1990). Consequently, even when sexual receptivity is facilitated by benzodiazepine sedative/hypnotics, sexual drive and excitement may be lowered or lost due to suppression of vasopressin. Benzodiazepines can also inhibit other peptides which promote sex, including LHRH, ACTH, substance P, and oxytocin. On the other hand, inhibition of CRF and cortisol can eliminate the potent sexual inhibitory action of benzodiazepines.

ANATOMICAL, HISTOLOGICAL, AND BIOCHEMICAL DIFFERENCES BETWEEN MALE AND FEMALE BRAINS

Studies in rats and other animals have shown distinct "sexually dimorphic" differences between males and females in the size of certain brain structures, which appear to be determined prenatally by differences in sex hormone secretion (e.g., testosterone and estrogen) at strategic points of fetal development. Although Gorski (1985) and his research group at UCLA have reviewed these differences and reported on various male-female differences in brain structures in both animals and humans, the relevance of the gender-linked anatomical variations to sexual desire and sexual behavior remains unclear. Science and medicine have not (and perhaps will never) develop a method whereby modification of human brain structures for the purpose of experimental investigation and clinical observation is morally feasible.

Though sex differences exist throughout the brain, the most obvious sexually relevant difference is found in the medial preoptic nucleus-anterior hypothalamic area, which governs active masculine sexual behaviors (Hines & Gorski, 1985) and appears to be dependent upon prenatal testosterone secretion. This region has been labeled as the sexually dimorphic nucleus of the preoptic area. Typically, it is more than twice as large in male rats as in female rats. Size differences exist in other animal species as well as in humans.

The medial preoptic nucleus-anterior hypothalamus generates active "masculine" sexual behaviors (labeled *proceptive* when displayed by females). It appears to operate in a reciprocal balance with the ventromedial nucleus which mediates typical receptive "feminine" behaviors such as lordosis. Such a reciprocity means that an increase in medial preoptic nucleus-anterior hypothalamic activity may decrease the probability of ventromedial nucleus activity, and vice versa.

The activity of these complementary hypothalamic regions is influenced by specific neural transmitters such as dopamine, serotonin, and GABA. Evidence to date indicates that dopamine receptors are abundant in the medial preoptic nucleus, while serotonin receptor terminals are few (Gorski, 1987). Such a finding is consistent with research associating dopamine with active sexual behaviors and serotonin with decreased active sexual patterns and an increased tendency toward receptive sexual behaviors.

LeVay's (1991) discovery of a size difference in the hypothalmic structure between the brains of homosexual and heterosexual men within this "masculine-oriented" region has suggested that a physical, neurological factor may cause homosexual men to have a decreased sexual attraction to women and, perhaps, an increased attraction to men. In a small study of 41 male and female brains, LeVay found that the size of the interstitial nuclei of the anterior hypothalamus was smaller in the brains of women and in homosexual men than in heterosexual men. LeVay's findings and his speculations may encourage examination of the sexually dimorphic nucleus of the preoptic area for more complex sexual attributes (such as attraction and choice) that would expand the active-passive, "masculine-feminine" dichotomization of copulatory behaviors.

Another prominent sexually dimorphic feature of the human brain has been identified in the size of the corpus callosum, which connects the left and right hemispheres. Some researchers have proposed that the corpus callosum is up to seven times larger in the female brain. Durden-Smith and deSimone (1983) have described this finding and its ramifications for differences in left-right brain cognitive function between men and women. (Presumably, women have greater access to right-brain emotional processes and are better able to integrate left brain-right brain impulses than men.) However, strong disagreement remains regarding whether such a gender-specific size difference actually exists, and whether the difference would lead to the cognitive disparities proposed to exist between men and women (Allen, Richey, Chai, & Gorski, 1991). In any event, the contribution of drugs and neural transmitters to such left-right brain differences is at this time unknown.

There is no clear physical sexual response in the human female comparable to the characteristic lordosis response in animal females. The lordosis posture may indicate passivity or submission rather than active sexual desire. Animal studies indicate that, when the female can control the male's access to her by using an "escape door," a decrease in lordosis posturing occurs. Conversely, an increase in sexual behavior occurs when she cannot get away.

The extent to which impulse-limiting drugs (like those that increase serotonin levels) have different effects on men and women is unclear. However, in clinical practice we have noted that sexual dysfunction in men (lack of orgasm/ejaculation) due to use of the serotonergic antidepressant fluoxetine (Prozac) and other serotonin–specific antidepressants (SSRIs) can be contrasted to beneficial sexual relaxation in women with only minor deficits in orgasmic response.* The fact that certain chemical substances may have generally beneficial effects on female sexuality and generally adverse effects on male sexuality (and vice versa) complicates any simple statements on the direction and nature of pharmacologically-induced sexual side effects. Clear or hypothetical discrepancies between a drug's sexual effect on males and females will be discussed in the appropriate chapters.

GABA

- common denominator of alcohol, benzodiazepines, barbiturates
- facilitates lordosis
- diminish fight/flight reactions
- post-yawning elevation of GABA

GABA, an abundant transmitter present in approximately one-third of CNS synapses, has effects common to inhibitory neurotransmitters which promote sleep, such as serotonin, endogenous opiates, and progesterone neurosteroids. (Unfortunately, GABA as a neurotransmitter has not been as extensively studied as dopamine, serotonin, norepinephrine, and the opiates.) Benzodiazepines, barbiturates, and alcohol all produce sleep and lessen anxiety due to their influence on GABA transmission. Our focus here will be on the possible sexual effects of GABA as they relate to behavioral inhibition, hopefully resulting in a meaningful understanding of the sexual effects produced by benzodiazepine sedative/hypnotics and their associated antianxiety mechanisms.

*Specific female-male differences are discussed in various chapters in this book in relation to particular drugs or drug classes. The active-passive sexual dimension is examined in detail in Chapter 19 on sedative/hypnotics (for passive emphasis), Chapters 26–28 on dopaminergic stimulants and PCPA (for active emphasis), and extensively in this chapter. Chapters 26 and 27 discuss differences in drug sensitivity between women and men.

For the female, GABA mutes the fear/avoidance response and promotes sexual receptivity. As illustrated by animal research, sexual avoidance and sexual receptivity are opposite behaviors mediated by the same structures: the ventromedial hypothalamus, the amygdala, and the medial preoptic nucleus. GABA and other inhibitory transmitters can directly inhibit pain sensation from and to the spine and periphery at the midbrain central gray, thus facilitating lordosis by removing incompatible fight/flight actions. These neurotransmitters can also mute the midbrain central gray indirectly by potentiating inhibitory actions of the ventromedial hypothalamus or by suppressing excitatory actions of the amygdala. Conversely, sexual responding can be decreased by concurrent GABA medial preoptic nucleus hypothalamic suppression of the active masculine sex center. When benzodiazepines are injected systemically (reaching all areas of the brain), even lordosis is diminished. Proceeding further up the fight/flight circuit, GABA can inhibit amygdala activation and thus the fear, anger, and other avoidance reactions that are mediated by the amygdala. When amygdala activity is inhibited by GABA, lordosis may be facilitated through the prevention of incompatible avoidance and resistance behaviors.

A GABA inhibitory action can also be generated by sexual activity itself. After orgasm/ejaculation, male rats show a marked increase of GABA. This increase of GABA continues for a definite refractory period, during which time the rat cannot be roused to copulate. If orgasm/ejaculation does not occur during copulation, GABA elevation does not occur. The post-ejaculatory increase in GABA and refractory period also occur in female rats after the males have ejaculated. It is unknown whether GABA elevation would occur in female rats after ejaculation if the ejaculate was prevented from reaching the vagina and cervix. Whether GABA elevation occurs after orgasm in human males and females is unknown. Internal sleeping pills seem to be triggered in males after ejaculating. Whether or not this effect is transferred to or shared by women is yet to be determined.

GABA also reduces vasopressin, a peptide hormone linked to testosterone and released during sexual activity in men (Murphy, Seckl, Burton, Checkley, & Lightman, 1987), which reinforces the cholinergic mental processes of the limbic system that control attention to and evaluation of sexual cues involved in active sexual behaviors.

It is important to remember that the limbic area around the septum was once the "smell brain," where pheromone cues were received in lower animals. During evolution, sexual stimuli increasingly were routed through the cortex for evaluation and learning and then sent back into the limbic system. It appears that dopamine localizes in the lower brain (hypothalamus) where it influences sex drive, while the higher brain (limbic, cortex) controls sexual thoughts. In the transitional limbic structures, vasopressin appears to sensitize cholinergic and glutamate activity involved in sexual thoughts and learning, unless it is reduced by GABA activity.

Estrogen can increase GABA and benzodiazepine binding (Lasaga, Duvilanski, Seilicovich, Afione, & Debeljuk, 1988; Mansky, Mestres-Ventura, & Wuttke, 1982; Perez, Zucchi, & Maggi, 1988). Vasopressin can also inhibit female receptive lordosis, whereas destroying the cortex and limbic areas can facilitate it. Under certain circumstances, vasopressin may increase sex drive and attention to sexual cues. On the other hand, vasopressin may sustain sexual fear and avoidance which are learned behaviors (i.e., conditioned emotional response, CER).

Benzodiazepines inhibit brain centers that mediate attention, thought, and emotional reactions by suppressing activity in the limbic area where thought and emotion are integrated into cognitions and attitudes. Barbiturates have other neuronal inhibitory actions (possibly on glutamate excitatory amino acid transmission and strychnine-like processes), which can depress the nervous system beyond the limit of GABA modulation.

Serotonin

- inhibits sex drive
- inhibits orgasm
- most effective way to delay ejaculation is to increase serotonin
- paradoxical effects
- promotes contentment
- lower levels promote aggression, violence, and sexually aberrant behavior
- multiple receptors

Pharmacological modification of serotonin levels can cause distinctive changes in sexual functioning. Animal research indicates that serotonin has an inhibitory effect, while dopamine is generally excitatory. Sexual effects can occur as much through a shift in the dopamine-serotonin balance as through an increase or decrease of either one alone. Effects may alternate back and forth due to compensatory reactions involving changes in metabolism and sensitivity.

Excessive activity in a neurotransmitter can lead to a refractory period during which the characteristic effects of the transmitter are reversed. Because of its more active and erratic nature, dopamine activity is more subject to refractory or inverse reactions (either burn-out or reversal). Although serotonin neural activity is slower and more regular than that of dopamine, when it is disrupted the result can be more acute because it involves the loss of chemical and emotional stability.

The lowering of physical sexual responsivity with serotonin potentiators in monkeys has been shown to produce beneficial psychological and behavioral effects such as increased relaxation, huddling, grooming, and decreased defensiveness (Raleigh et al., 1983). The hostility, defensiveness, impulsivity, restlessness, and aggression that results from serotonin depletion also may be decreased by serotonin potentiators (see Chapter 21). Both excitement and relaxation can result in a positive change in sexual desire and/or behavior. The initial relaxation and decreased defensiveness with serotonergic drugs initially may improve sexual compliance, desire, and responsiveness. However, from what is known of the sexual symptoms generated by serotonin depletion, one must speculate that sexual excitement and response will decrease with long-term serotonin elevation. A decrease in serotonin may contribute to the paradoxical aggression often noted with benzodiazepines. For instance, lesions of the dorsal raphe (DR), which may be analogous to reduction of dorsal raphe serotonergic firing, facilitate muricide (mouse-killing in rats) and defensive aggression (Potegal, Antilla, & Glusman, 1988).

Buspirone appears to stimulate 5-HT_{1A} receptors on neurons. Stimulation of these receptors suppresses serotonin activity through an unexplained autoreceptor or negative feedback mechanism. When researchers first used 5-HT_{1A} agonist drugs on rats, they found (somewhat to their amazement) that these drugs caused large increases in sexual activity rather than the decreases found with other drugs that stimulate the serotonin system. Thus, it was a difference in sexual effects that led to the discovery of these paradoxical, but distinct receptor effects within the serotonin system. Subsequently, many other types of serotonin receptors have been found, each with its own particular behavioral effects; however, even the experts do not yet know the exact function of the different serotonin receptors.

Curiously, propranolol blocks 5-HT_{1A} receptors, which may have something to do with its ability to lower sexual desire. We have observed that, even when only orgasm/ejaculation is delayed by beta-blockers or other medications, with continued use erection and desire are eventually affected. In the end, the result is a weaker erection, decreased arousal, and diminished orgasmic sensation. Propranolol occasionally can help control ejaculation, not so much because it is a beta-blocker, but because it facilitates serotonin and possibly blocks excitatory amino acid transmission. However, the most effective way to delay ejaculation is by increasing serotonin levels (with serotonin uptake inhibitors), not with an adrenergic decrease.

Unexplained paradoxical effects of serotonergic drugs are relatively common. Recently, reports of suicidal ideation by patients being treated with fluoxetine for depression have conflicted with previous findings in which serotonin was found to decrease suicidal feelings (Teicher et al., 1990). Hypomania sometimes associated with hypersexuality may occur with extended SSRI treatment, often requiring drug withdrawal. Nonetheless, animal and human research on SSRIs, MAOIs, the serotonin precursor 5HTP, and the sexual effects of serotonin depletors such as PCPA indicates that serotonin is predominantly inhibitory to sex drive and response, particularly to active male sexuality.

Dopamine

Dopaminergic stimulants have an excitatory effect on the nucleus accumbens, a small brain area at the base of the limbic system adjacent to the basal ganglia and in front of the hypothalamus. Speculation on the contribution of nucleus accumbens activity to pleasure motivated behavior in general and to sexual stimulation in particular is a continuing source of interest for those interested in sexual pharmacology. Unfortunately, most of the experimental work on the nucleus accumbens has been done on rats. In higher animals, nucleus accumbens involvement may be more intricate or may be obscured by less direct expression of desire.

The nucleus accumbens appears to act as a nodal interface between dopaminergic incentive motivation drives and the actual behavior necessary to satisfy these drives. If there are areas in the brain that get a "charge" during vigorous and pleasurable activities, the nucleus accumbens is certainly one of them. Perhaps it is the most focused of such incentive-activity-charged centers because of its tangential location bordering to the reflex-driven "reptilian" brain and its functional connection to the nigrostriatal brain structures governing initiation, direction, and modulation of physical movement. This connection allows intentions, thoughts, habitual actions, and emotional reflexes to be translated into purposeful and routine activity. Thus, limbic and cortical learning and memory may be expressed with appropriate action, and the nucleus accumbens may function as a transformer, resonator, or charger within this circuit.

Because the nucleus accumbens is located next to the olfactory nucleus, even reflexive smell and touch stimuli are remembered through their cognitive associations. We remember that a particular person has a pleasant or unpleasant odor from our overall memory of that person. The additional brain area in the prefrontal cortex allows us to look forward to smelling and touching someone, even when he or she is not present. When the person is present or expected imminently, the nucleus accumbens receives a charge from memory structures to be on alert to move toward the person.

If these brain areas do not charge when appropriate, behavior is depressed and listless. Sexual overtures and initiatives from the partner will not be stimulating. A favorite desert or the chance to attend a much-admired play will also fail to arouse. When the person actually participates in sex, eats the dessert, or attends the play, he or she may enjoy the activity; but enjoyment does not occur until the person is directly engaged in the activity. Such a lack of anticipatory and/or subsequent pleasure may underlie bulimic and other addictive behaviors in which the addict is satisfied only while directly involved in the activity or substance. Patients who avoid sex but enjoy it once involved may be experiencing the same neuroendocrinological phenomena.

Although the evidence that the nucleus accumbens is a pleasure resonator is very strong, only a handful of researchers in behavioral psychopharmacology and neurology appreciate the fact that pleasure and reinforcement are central to brain activity of all kinds. The prevailing view concentrates on the role of pleasure and reinforcement in abuse and indulgence that corrodes or stops the system from performing normally. For example, positive sexual effects of increases in endorphins may occur due to opioid stimulation of dopamine in brain reinforcement centers, such as the nucleus accumbens, which also may partly account for opiate abuse and dependency. Negative and positive interactions of opioids with dopamine reinforcement activity must be further investigated to determine any sexual benefits of endorphins.

The nucleus accumbens is involved in directing attention and behavior in accord with available external cues. It facilitates the association of sensory "filtering" of the environment to incentive-directive-reward processes. The function of cognitive sex therapy is to promote optional interchange among these associations so that the nucleus accumbens remains charged and active. Much of this therapy is directed toward activation of associated brain areas through instructions for conscious attention to positive aspects of sex.

Dopaminergic drugs may have their stimulatory effect on sexual response through an oxytocinergic mechanism that applies to both erection and orgasm/ejaculation. Oxytocin and dopamine pace one another by mutual reinforcement. Oxytocin injection can elicit stretching-yawning/penile erection syndrome. In animals, like cats and monkeys, stretching associated with yawning and erection is a typical feature of sexual response. Oxytocin can stimulate this response directly, or dopaminergic drugs can generate the syndrome through stimulating oxytocin activity. Drugs that block dopamine will not block oxytocin-induced stretching-yawning/penile erection (Argiolas, 1989); but a drug that blocks oxytocin can prevent the syndrome when it is induced by dopaminergic drugs (Argiolas, Melis, Stancampiano, & Gessa, 1989). When dopamine or oxytocin was injected into various brain regions, stretching-yawning/penile erection was elicited, but only with injections into the paraventricular nucleus, which secretes oxytocin and vasopressin throughout the brain (Melis, Argiolas, & Gessa, 1986). Conversely, paraventricular nucleus lesions prevented yawning and erection induced by both apomorphine (dopamine) and oxytocin (Argiolas, Melis, Mauri, & Gessa, 1987). The paraventricular nucleus also contains magnocellular neurons that release oxytocin to the posterior pituitary, where it acts as a birth and lactation hormone.

The medial preoptic nucleus (MPO) active sex center functions synergistically with the paraventricular nucleus to stimulate sexual and parental behaviors. Additionally, progesterone and estrogen from the ventromedial nucleus receptive sex lordosis center activate female sexual initiation behavior in part by stimulating neighboring oxytocinergic neurons of the paraventricular nucleus and the dorsomedial nucleus

(Schumacher, Coirini, Pfaff, & McEwen, 1990). Thus the curious yawning-erection behavior reaction has enabled researchers to recognize crucial chemico-anatomical bases for sexual and reproductive activities, and the recent availability of potent oxytocin antagonists has led to further understanding. Dopamine-induced yawning, erection, and male copulatory behavior in rats have been shown to depend upon oxytocin, but these same behaviors were blocked by oxytocin antagonists (Argiolas, Collu, Gessa, Melis, & Serra, 1988; Argiolas, Melis, Vargiu, & Gessa 1987).

Oxytocin-induced yawning and erection can be blocked by the cholinergic antagonist atropine, indicating that oxytocin requires some cholinergic activity for its stimulation of this syndrome. However, cholinergic stimulation alone, such as with physostigmine, causes yawning but does not induce erections (Gower, Berendsen, Princen, & Broekkamp, 1984). Parvicellular oxytocin neurons of the paraventricular nucleus project to cholinergic areas of the limbic system (hippocampus, septum, and amygdala) and the spinal cord. Injection of apomorphine, a dopamine agonist, elevates oxytocin levels in the hippocampus while inducing yawning and erection (Melis, Argiolas, Stancampiano, & Gessa, 1990). Oxytocin can also elicit yawning and erection by direct injection into the hippocampus (Argiolas & Gessa, 1987). Oxytocin itself stimulates the release of luteinizing hormone releasing hormone (Johnston, Lopez, Samson, & Negro-Vilar, 1990). Potency studies of the oxytocin-induced stretching-yawning/penile erection syndrome show that the oxytocin receptors that stimulate erection are similar in intensity to those that stimulate uterine contraction and breast milk ejection (Melis, Argiolas, Stancampiano, & Gessa, 1988).

The data gathered from these stretching-yawning/penile erection syndrome experiments indicate that oxytocin apparently activates erection through a complex circuit involving the cholinergic limbic system through the dopaminergic hypothalamus to the pituitary and into the spinal cord. This effect is sensitized by testosterone, vasopressin, and possibly ACTH and epinephrine, and can be blocked by the anticholinergic antagonist atropine and by morphine (Argiolas & Gessa, 1987).

Adrenergic Stimulation

While the positive actions of dopamine on sexuality have attracted increasing attention, adrenergic arousal has been of less interest. Conventionally, adrenergic activity was believed to be more relevant to general levels of arousal than to sexual arousal; and, indeed, excessive adrenergic levels of arousal causes nervous energy and behavior that can interfere with or compete with sexual activity. At the level of the genitals, excess noradrenergic release constricts blood vessels, preventing vascular dilation essential to the sexual response, and may trigger the ejaculatory mechanism prematurely.

With the advent of penile injection erections, we now know that an increase in $alpha_1$ adrenergic action in the penile cavernosum causes vasoconstriction that either prevents erection or mediates detumescence. In fact, the adrenergic nerves in the cavernosum are chiefly $alpha_1$ and can be stimulated by both epinephrine and norepinephrine. Benard et al. (1989) reported that intravenous infusion of epinephrine into dogs completely aborted erections generated by stimulation of the cavernous nerve. However, capacity for erection recovered within 15 minutes. Crenshaw (1983) described how the "adrenaline reflex" reaction can cause loss of erection. Many urologists administering penile injections have observed that stress can prevent an adequate erection, even with direct intracavernous injection of erection-inducing drugs (Benard et al., 1989). To some extent phenylpropanolamine (often in cold and diet pills) will interfere with erection and cause stressful elevation of norepinephrine and epinephrine in the body. With many adrenergic stimulants, including phenylpropanolamine, there may be decreased "genital tone" in the resting penis, presumably due to tonic elevation in adrenergic/sympathetic activity. As yet, no research has been conducted to measure whether such increased vasoconstriction actually occurs. Supposedly, *Koro* (an Asian term describing penile shrivelling and "withdrawing into itself") is due to stress-related adrenergic hyperactivity.

Zorgniotti, Rossman, and Mitchell (1987) identified impotence induced by chronic use of phenylpropanolamine and other nasal decongestants in 16 patients. Few of these patients had other risk factors for impotence (e.g., diabetes, hypertension, smoking). The researchers suggested a parallel between nasal and penile vasodilation and observed that some men may experience nasal congestion during sexual excitation. However, the reverse may also be true: Men with rhinitis may experience alleviation of nasal congestion during sexual excitement and a return of congestion following ejaculation (Blumberg & Moltz, 1988).

Phenylpropanolamine is sometimes used successfully to treat urinary incontinence in women. Other adrenergic stimulants such as ephedrine and pseudoephedrine also have been used successfully. Alpha$_1$ adrenergic stimulation of the bladder neck and proximal urethra increases bladder outlet resistance, thus decreasing incontinence and, to some extent, reversing retrograde ejaculation in men.

Given the abundance of alpha$_1$ adrenergic receptors in the vagina, any action sufficient to decrease incontinence should also change genital responses, particularly orgasm, which is partly generated from adrenergically mediated pelvic musculature. However, anxiety generated from brain adrenergic centers (e.g., locus coeruleus) increases stress and urination. Consequently, although orgasm may be facilitated from a local adrenergic urethral action, anxiety transmitted through CNS action can block sexual response. Furthermore, general sympathetic arousal sustained by phenylpropanolamine can lead to muscle spasms, difficulty in concentrating, and inability to relax. Stimulants may provide adequate sympathomimetic tone for the bladder neck to close and facilitate the sympathetic actions of the posterior urethra, vas deferens, bulbocavernosus (BC) and ischiocavernosus (IC) muscles, prostatic musculature, and the seminal vesicles. Sympathetic arousal is normally phasic (rises and falls appropriate to the situation), but the arousal generated by phenylpropanolamine and other stimulants is tonic. To the extent that one is too active to eat due to an anorectic stimulant, one may also be too active to make love.

Epinephrine

While it is clear that nervousness can prevent erection by causing tension in the smooth muscle of the cavernosum, its effect on swelling, lubrication, and clitoral sensitivity is unknown. Increasing adrenergic stimulation through phenylpropanolamine and other stimulants could have either positive or negative effects on coital reflex circuitry. The bulbocavernosus-ischiocavernosus reflex (also called pudendo-pudendal reflex) is used to test neural function in the lumbosacral-genital area. In rats, male and female reflex responses were similar, although the musculature is much greater in males in order to sustain rigid erection. The external urethral sphincters and motorneurons are not sexually dimorphic. The bulbocavernosus reflex of the female rats is the same as for males but occurs with a greater delay after stimulation of the pudendal nerve.

Researchers (Chung, McVary, & McKenna, 1988; McKenna & Nadelhaft, 1989) have extended the study of pelvic muscle reflexes to what has been termed the "coitus reflex"—"rhythmic movements of skeletal and smooth muscles of the pelvis in males and females following (more or less) prolonged genital stimulation." The reflex is associated with ejaculation; it can be reliably generated solely by stimulation of the urethra in both male and female rats subsequent to spinal transection. In female rats, mechanical stimulation of the dorsal wall of the distal urethra elicited the same coital reflex as elicited by distension of the male urethral bulb. The reflex in females consisted of "regular, rhythmic bursts of activity in the pudendal efferents and the cavernous nerve and rhythmic movements of the vagina, leading to increases in vaginal pressure." Although these responses appear to be orgasmic in nature, there is no documentation to determine whether or not female rats have orgasms. Clonic contractions of striated perineal muscles and the vagina/urethra occur in females as they do in males, but there is no emission-ejaculatory mechanism, as determined by measuring EMG recordings of the bulbocavernosus and bulbospongiosus muscles. McKenna and Nadelhaft (1989) speculated that the reflex is generated from spinal circuitry because of the necessity for spinal transection. The reflex is not altered by castration or ovariectomy, even though castration decreases penile erection.

Marson and McKenna (1990b) have traced the innervation of the coital reflex up to the paragigantocillular reticular nucleus (PGi) in the brainstem rostral ventromedial medulla. PGi innervation apparently mediates the spinal sexual reflex circuitry for the coital reflex in tonic inhibition. Elicitation of the reflex by urethral stimulation requires spinal transection so that descending inhibitory control is removed. An isolated lesion of this small PGi area of the medulla removes inhibition to the same extent as spinal transection. Since pelvic pain sensations are routed along the same spinal-medulla circuit as the coital reflex, genital stimulation during sexual activity may block or modify pain sensations, causing pelvic analgesia. The PGi brainstem area regulates breathing, blood pressure, heart rate and sensory responses. Release from PGi inhibition may account for parallel changes in these functions characteristic of the sexual response and orgasm. Marson and McKenna (1990a) have further shown that serotonin injected into the spinal-genital region inhibited the coital reflex. Consequently, they proposed that serotonin may be a key neurotransmitter mediating tonic inhibition from the PGi to the spinal coital reflex generator.

The adrenergic locus coeruleus (LC) has an excitatory innervation from the brainstem PGi region mediating the spinal-genital coital reflex (Rasmussen & Aghajanian, 1989). Since LC activation (for example, during morphine withdrawal) causes urination, defecation, and erection, there is an obvious connection between the locus coeruleus and genital activity that apparently passes through the medulla PGi. Depending on the circumstances, this connection may be excitatory or inhibitory. Since the locus coeruleus facilitates sensory attention, the genital sexual response would be potentiated during sexual arousal but inhibited by an attentional shift away from the genitals during other excitatory states (such as fear). The negative effect of LC stimulation is involved in the "adrenaline response" that interferes with the sexual response. Bladder contraction and relaxation of the urethral sphincter may be elicited by activation of this circuit, producing urinary incontinence that may further interfere with relaxed attention to the genital sexual response action.

Overreaction to LC activation in susceptible individuals during sexual activity may result in panic and phobia, which either block or distort the coital reflex. If this is true, then repeated benign exposure to the sexual stimuli should eliminate the panic reaction, because the locus coerulus quickly becomes tolerant to repeated environmental stimulation. On the other hand, the locus coeruleus is stimulated by novel stimuli, so that lack of novelty in sexual stimulation may fail to produce the pleasant epinephrine flow and focus generated during sexual arousal from the locus coeruleus to the spine to the genitals.

Since the adrenergic increase due to stimulants is an internal, chemically triggered response regardless of the outer environmental situation, conditioning to sexual cues may be disturbed because the conditioned stimulus–unconditioned stimulus relationship (e.g., dog salivating to Pavlov's bell) is weakened (e.g., ringing the bell many times during the day when food is not expected or received). If a drug only potentiates natural adrenergic reactions to stimuli, it will have a positive effect on normal arousal; but if a drug itself induces adrenergic reactions, the phasic attention to sexually arousing events will suffer from lack of focus and a weakened conditioned response. To some extent, sex therapy sensate focus training involves conditioning the patient to changes in his or her threshold of physical sensitivity and arousal, so that these changes can enhance rather than inhibit sexual response. If the nervous system is sympathetically overcharged by phenylpropanolamine, such subtle changes may go undetected. Though the adrenergic effects of phenylpropanolamine probably influence genital sexual response in either a positive or negative direction depending on the circumstances, there is really no research to document an effect in either direction. Until we have more definitive data, men should be monitored for changes in penile tone and maintenance of erection; women should be monitored for changes in orgasmic intensity.

Lesion of ascending noradrenergic fibers to the hypothalamus increases active masculine and proceptive male sexual behavior in both male and female rats, but reduces receptive female lordosis behavior. Conversely, noradrenergic stimulation of these fibers increases receptive lordosis but decreases female proceptive and active masculine behavior (Everitt & Hansen, 1983; Sachs & Meisel, 1988; Pfaff & Schwartz-Giblin, 1988). Consequently, it is conceivable that the noradrenergic stimulation component of stimulants *decreases* active masculine and proceptive sexual behavior, while dopaminergic stimulation by stimulants *increases* such behavior.

Norepinephrine levels are higher in females than in males and estrogen treatment of female rats increases norepinephrine in the medial preoptic nucleus brain sex center (Pfaff & Schwartz-Giblin, 1988). Along with greater endogenous serotonin and less dopamine in females, the greater noradrenergic influence in females may inhibit active masculine and proceptive sexual behaviors but facilitate receptive ones.

It should be noted that epinephrine is lower in females than in males and may even inhibit norepinephrine activity. A relative deficiency of epinephrine in females in comparison to males may favor receptive sexual behavior and prevent more active and proceptive sexual behavior. With such counteractive influences operative between norepinephrine and dopamine, the effect of stimulant activation on sexual behavior is difficult to predict. When amphetamine is given to female rats with the dopamine component blocked by concurrent pimozide, lordosis is increased apparently through noradrenergic stimulation (Everitt, Fuxe, Hokfelt, & Jonsson, 1975).

The dynamic range of positive excitatory sexual response may be decreased due to a continuous sympathetic elevation by noradrenergic stimulants, which reduce the impact of specifically sexual phasic adrenergic increases occurring during sexual activity. Muscle contractions during orgasm are characterized by sharp rises and falls. With noradrenergic stimulants, the peak effect may be unchanged or increased, but the subsequent relaxation may be decreased. Essentially, a sharp fall back to a normal, low baseline is required so that a subsequent sharp increase can occur; otherwise, large changes will not occur or be noticed. With less extreme rises and falls, there may be a decrease in orgasm intensity. Rivas, Barradas, Montiel, and Bianco (1990) reported that women who regularly experienced orgasm during intercourse showed the lowest resting pubococcygeus muscle action by electromyogram (EMG); anorgasmic women, the highest resting EMG; and women who experienced orgasm only by direct clitoral stimulation fell in the middle. In contrast, the strength of intentional pubococcygeus muscle EMG flex was greatest in the women who experience orgasm through intercourse and least in the anorgasmic women. Expansion from normal rest to a climax peak may be optimal for orgasm, and lack of relaxation at rest may preclude or desensitize genital climax.

From the intricacies of the multiple mechanisms of action governing sexual function, we will now proceed to explore the specific characteristics of hormones in detail. Subsequent chapters on psychoactive and prescription drugs will return our attention to neurotransmitters and their interplay with various peptides and hormones.

5

Estrogens

OBJECTIVES

- To describe nature and function of naturally occurring estrogens
- To explore key psychological, physiological, and sexual consequences of estrogen replacement therapy (ERT)
- To present benefits of ERT in areas of heart disease and osteoporosis
- To consider cancer risks of ERT
- To give therapists an overview of the medical issues involved

Sex hormones have two functional modes: organizational and activating. During prenatal and neonatal life, they are chiefly organizational, directing selective physiological development into distinct male and female configurations. Central and peripheral structures and organs may be altered and various biochemical systems (including neurotransmitters, peptides, and metabolic enzymes) are modified by hormonal signals.

Later in life, hormonal function is predominantly activational in nature: Patterns of behavior and function characteristic of organizational predispositions are now activated. However, neither the organizational nor activating actions of sex hormones occurs in isolation. Rather, complex interactions with other body chemicals modify, amplify, facilitate, retard, or inhibit hormonal activity.

Treatment with estrogens is controversial. During a woman's reproductive years, she may decide to use estrogen for birth control; when she reaches menopause, she may decide to use estrogen replacement therapy (ERT). There is a continuing debate throughout the medical field about the safety of long-term treatment with estrogens and a noteworthy concern for the cancer risk associated with estrogen replacement therapy. Indeed, the debate concerning estrogens becomes a difficult dilemma for many women as they approach menopause. In an effort to make a wise decision about estrogen replacement therapy, women often discover that well-respected experts disagree. Because it may be one of the most important medical decisions a woman makes in her lifetime, it is crucial that she obtain enough information and guidance to make an intelligent choice.

Estrogen, progesterone, and testosterone are the chief hormones involved in cyclical female sexuality. Testosterone plays a minor role in the overall picture, but seems to have a major impact on sex drive and perhaps attitude. Dehydroepiandrosterone (DHEA) has a yet to be defined role, but appears to impact sex drive. The role of estrogen is complex. It is intricately involved in reproductive cycles and other rhythmic, sensitizing processes which affect sexuality. Although this hormone is one of the most studied, its sexual effects are probably the least clear.

The control circuit for reproductive hormones in general and estrogen in particular is mediated through the pituitary and the gonads. When circulating blood hormone levels are low, the pituitary signals the ovaries to produce more of these hormones through an auto-feedback mechanism. Altogether it is a well-balanced system that modern medicine has learned to manipulate for therapeutic purposes.

THE MENSTRUAL CYCLE AND SEX DRIVE

The word *estrogen* is derived from the words *estrus* (sexual excitement, receptivity, heat) and *generate*. In animals, sexual desire and receptivity is usually confined to specific periods of estrus, which is dependent upon estrogen stimulation. In humans, levels of estrogen and sexual desire do not seem to be correlated. In highly developed mammals, the capacity for sexual desire and receptivity has expanded beyond estrus periodicity. Only in human females, however, does this freedom from hormonal determination of sexual responsiveness seem to be relatively complete.

Curiosity about the role of female hormones in women's sexuality is relatively recent. During the 1930s, Therese Benedek conducted a series of intensive psychoanalytic investigations of sexual desire. She studied the changes in sexual desire that occurred in nine "neurotic women" over a period of 75 menstrual cycles (Benedek & Rubinstein, 1939a, 1939b). The nature of sexual desire was ascertained from an interpretation of the unconscious meaning of dreams at different phases of the cycle. Benedek estimated estrogen and progesterone activity by temperature changes and cytological examination of vaginal smears. She concluded that heterosexual desire and activity was stimulated by estrogen, while nurturant feelings were induced by progesterone.

In the late 1970s, a series of studies investigating the relation between hormone levels and mood and sexual changes failed to show significant correlations of sexual desire with differences in estradiol levels (Abplanalp, Rose, Donelly, & Livingston-Vaugh, 1979; Persky, Lief, Strauss, Miller, & O'Brien, 1978). Persky, Charney, Lief, O'Brien, Miller, and Strauss (1978) found positive correlations between sexual activity and testosterone. They suggested that ovulatory increases in sexual activity could be due to increased testosterone near ovulation, rather than to estradiol. A series of studies followed, demonstrating that sexual activity correlated with testosterone elevation, but not to estradiol levels. Since both testosterone and estradiol reach peak levels at ovulation, it is difficult to determine which hormone is responsible for sexual changes.

In women, follicle stimulating hormone (FSH) controls the growth and maturation of the ovarian follicle. Luteinizing hormone (LH) controls ovulation and the formation and maintenance of the corpus luteum by signal mechanisms involving estrogen and progesterone changes. The control of testosterone production in females has not been defined, nor has the relation among LH, estradiol, and testosterone.

Luteinizing hormone releasing hormone (LHRH) secretion is differentially influenced by various neurotransmitters, peptides, and hormones. Apparently, norepinephrine is chiefly stimulatory; dopamine and serotonin are both inhibitory and indirectly stimulatory; opiates are predominantly inhibitory; and some peptides, such as prostaglandins and angiotensin, are strongly activating.

Since sex hormones are involved in interactive feedback circuits with LHRH, they may be either stimulatory or inhibitory. Small amounts of estrogenic stimulation may be stimulatory to LHRH secretion, while elevated estrogen levels are inhibitory. However, outside of the hypothalamic feedback circuit, estrogens are predominantly stimulatory on LH in the pituitary. Testosterone, progesterone, and inhibin are chiefly inhibitory, each in its own particular fashion. Testosterone and progesterone inhibit LH, while inhibin appears to be the inhibitory control factor for FSH. Differences between activation of LHRH and LH directly are not clear.

The secretion of LH and FSH is relatively constant in males, but varies cyclically in females. Triggered by increasing levels of estrogen, the short secretory peak of LH/FSH at the mid-point of the menstrual cycle results in ovulation and the subsequent formation of the corpus luteum accompanied by the rise of progesterone. In nonfertilized cycles, estrogen and progesterone levels drop, which produces wasting of the corpus luteum during the bleeding period of the menstrual cycle.

Although the intricate relation between peptides and sex hormones is recognized and routinely manipulated in reproductive medicine, the interrelationship of sex hormones with peptides is seldom appreciated when sexual behavior is considered. Simplistic notions of "too little," "normal," or "too much" have dominated discussions of sex hormones. The enormous reproductive impact of minute levels of exogenous estrogen and progesterone in new sequential oral contraceptives indicates that sexual functioning is not simply increased or decreased by changing levels of sex hormones, but instead may depend upon a delicate balance of quantal changes and set-point deviations.*

The paucity of information relating reproductive endocrinology to sexual function is surprising and distressing. A comprehensive text on sexual arousal by Rosen and Beck (1988) hardly mentions estrogen. A more recent volume, *Reproductive Endocrinology*, by Yen and Jaffe (1991), with over 1,000 pages, has a great deal of information on estrogens but only a few paragraphs on sexual function. Despite the enormous amount of data available on estrogen hormones and sexual function, the relationship between the two remains largely unexplored in the traditional literature.

MENOPAUSE AND ESTROGEN REPLACEMENT THERAPY (ERT)

A variety of physiological, sexual, and psychological changes and symptoms occur throughout the perimenopausal and menopausal time period. Before the 1960s, women had no alternative but to go through surgical or natural menopause. Research performed during the 1950s resulted in the use of exogenous estrogens as treatment for the discomforts of menopause. Random controlled studies of estrogen replacement therapy are difficult and frustrating to conduct on treatment programs which extend over 30 years or more. Furthermore, any new medications or changes in care (e.g., transdermal or injected estrogen, synthetic analogues, or addition of progestogens) cannot be adequately evaluated for risks until they are used long enough for adverse effects or lack of benefits to become apparent. Consequently, patients may feel that they are "guinea pigs." Unfortunately, in this case, they *are*, because these effects cannot be evaluated in real guinea pigs or other animals. Wellness measures and "health-store pharmacology" for treatment of menopause-related symptoms are also experimental, with outcomes far less certain than when standard low-dose estrogen is included in such care.

Table 5.1 summarizes the signs and symptoms that have been associated with the diminishing estrogen levels that characterize menopause. Taken singly, the symptoms are manageable; taken collectively, they can result in depression, physical discomfort, and sexual dysfunction. Table 5.2 summarizes the therapeutic and adverse side effects of estrogen replacement.

Psychological Symptoms and ERT

Estrogens and progesterone cause mood and performance problems in some women, so that the decrease in these hormones with menopause may in some cases improve mood and performance. It can be expected that this change would be particularly true for women who have suffered from severe premenstrual syndrome.

However, the reverse is usually true. Mood, sexuality, and attitude usually diminish with hormone deprivation and improve with replacement. Estrogen replacement can provide relief for psychological problems associated with menopause and thus enhance sexual response directly and indirectly.

Because estrogens are weak monoamine oxidase inhibitors (Broverman, Klaiber, Vogel, &

*The menstrual cycle is described in greater detail in Chapter 7. Tables 7.2 and 7.3 illustrate the interactive patterns of several hormones (including testosterone and DHEAS) during the menstrual cycle, and clarify why it is difficult to correlate sex drive with specific hormones.

Table 5.1 *Signs and Symptoms of Estrogen Withdrawal*

Cognitive	Cognitive deficits Inability to concentrate Poor memory
General	Headaches Hot flashes/hot flushes Thinning skin, collagen Weight gain
Genitourinary	Stress incontinence Urinary frequency/nocturia
Psychological	Anxiety Fatigue Insomnia Irritability Lack of initiative Tenseness
Sexual	Decreased intensity of orgasm Decreased sex drive
Vaginal	Adhesions Atrophy Dyspareunia Lubrication decrease Senile vaginitis Tissue loss in vulva Tone decrease (elasticity, expansion, pliability) Vulvar leukoplakia

Table 5.2 *Therapeutic and Adverse Effects of Estrogen Replacement*

General (Adverse)	*Physiological (Therapeutic)*	*Psychological (Therapeutic)*	*Sexual (Therapeutic)*
Breast tenderness Cancer risks increased Depression Fatigue Irritability Malaise Nausea Taste and touch aversions	Decreases appetite Reduces heart disease risk Eliminates hot flushes Prevents osteoporosis Maintains skin tone and collagen Prevents stress incontinence and urethral, bladder, and uterine prolapse Improves taste and smell	Antidepressant Decreases anxiety, irritability Cognitive benefits, increases memory Mood improves, stabilizes Increases performance	Body odor remains attractive Improves senile vaginitis Promotes vaginal lubrication Preserves vaginal rugae Preserves vaginal, urethral, genital tissue

Kobayashi, 1974), it is conceivable that they could have antidepressant effects. Klaiber, Broverman, Vogel, Kobayashi, and Moriarty (1972) found that premenopausal depressed women have higher MAO activity than normal women. Although oral conjugated estrogen therapy can reduce MAO levels, it is unlikely that the degree of MAO inhibition achieved with estrogen replacement therapy would be sufficient for therapeutic effect.

Some studies have concluded that psychological improvement with estrogen replacement was due to improvement of vasomotor symptoms (Ballinger, 1975; Utian, 1972a, 1972b) while others (Regestein, Schiff, Tulchinsky, & Ryan, 1981; Thomson, 1976; Utian, 1975) have attributed therapeutic psychological benefits to a placebo effect. Other early research (Campbell & Whitehead, 1977; Lauritzen, 1973) noted substantial relief from a variety of physical and psychological symptoms, including hot flushes, depression, anxiety, and nocturnal sweating.

Improved quality of life, including sex life, has been reported in two European studies of transdermal estradiol patch therapy (Estraderm). In a 12-week double-blind placebo-controlled study of 223 postmenopausal women (mean age = 52.6) using Estraderm with no progestogen supplementation, quality of life improved on both estradiol and placebo, but improvements in health, climacteric symptoms, and sex were significantly greater on Estraderm (Nathorst-Böös, Wiklund, Mattsson, Sandin, & von Schoultz, 1993; Wiklund, Karlberg, & Mattsson, 1993). Sexual improvements appeared to be related to overall improved well-being, decrease in anxiety, and reduction of climacteric symptoms. There were no differences in orgasm frequency and sexual arousal scores between estradiol and placebo groups, but significant differences in favor of enjoyment, vaginal lubrication, and pain during intercourse. As is usually the case, in this study it is difficult to determine the extent to which psychological sexual benefits derived from relief of physical sexual problems such as decreased lubrication. Without a comparison to testosterone-estradiol combined, it is difficult to determine to what extent the psychological components of sexual drive, arousal, and orgasm are improved by estrogen hormone replacement therapy.

Similarly, a large six-month multi-site study (Limouzin-Lamothe, Mairon, Joyce, & Le Gal, 1994) with the Estraderm TTS patch supplemented with the progestogen chlormadinone on 499 postmenopausal women found significantly greater improvement in quality of life on estradiol compared to symptomatic treatment of hot flush vasomotor upset with veralipride (not available in the United States). Both treated groups improved on all measures, except for no increased rating of attractiveness in women treated with veralipride. On the Sexual Behavior Questionnaire, there were no significant differences between estradiol and veralipride. Though both of these estradiol patch studies showed sexual benefits for estrogen replacement, neither showed these benefits to be distinct from the relief of physical symptoms and other mood problems.

Ditkoff, Crary, Cristo, and Lobo, (1991) reported psychological benefits attributed to estrogen replacement (conjugated estrogens/Premarin) in healthy asymptomatic postmenopausal women, but no significant cognitive/memory benefits. They found few significant findings with meaningful measurements, despite great care in recruiting surgically menopausal patients free of confounding factors such as other medications, illnesses, or hot flushes. The contrast with earlier referenced pronounced psychological responses to ERT reflects the continuing controversy surrounding medical opinion on its value.

A well-performed study by Sherwin (1991) has shown positive sexual and mood benefits with estrogen replacement in naturally menopausal women. Women were treated with 0.625 or 1.25 conjugated estrogen (Premarin) for 12 months, with or without 5 mg medoxyprogesterone (MPA). In concurrence with Dennerstein's prior study (Dennerstein, Burrows, Wood, & Hyman, 1980), progesterone decreased the positive mood and sexual effects of estrogen (more so with the 0.625 dose of Premarin than the 1.25 dose).

Recently, with more careful and comprehensive evaluation, limited cognitive *benefits* of estrogen have been shown in postmenopausal women. Conversely, it now appears that, due to estrogen deficiency, small though significant cognitive/memory *deficits*, which can be corrected with conventional ERT, may be present in postmenopausal women. Sherwin and Phillips (1990) studied cognitive functioning in 12 women (mean age = 47) prior and subsequent to hysterectomy/oophorectomy. Post-operatively, women were placed on either monthly 10 mg estradiol injections or placebo. Measured at the end of the second month of treatment, the estradiol-treated women showed significantly higher scores on paired-association and paragraph recall tests than placebo-treated women.

As part of the extended longitudinal Rancho Bernardo health study conducted from 1972 to the present, Barrett-Connor and Kritz-Silverstein (1993) found that age-related cognitive declines occurred in their cohort of 800 women over age 65, regardless of whether or not they were on ERT. Only on one task (a short-term recall category task) out of a large battery of 12 cognitive tests was a difference found in favor of women on ERT for at least 20 years compared to women who had never used estrogen replacement.

Robinson, Friedman, Marcus, et al. (1994) tested 72 women (aged 55–93) on ERT (54 of 58 on Premarin; mean use duration, 13.4 years) and a control group of 72 women not on estrogen. Only two cognitive tasks were administered: a proper name recall test and a word recall test. There was no significant difference between groups on the word recall test, but on the proper name recall task, the ERT-treated group did significantly better than the control group. However, the difference was small: Out of a possible 12, the ERT group recalled 4.3 names versus 3.1 names recalled by the non-ERT group. The authors noted that prior memory research using word recall tasks had failed to show significant benefits of estrogen replacement therapy.

Kampen and Sherwin (1994) studied a sample of 71 healthy women over age 55 who were at least two years postmenopausal (28 women were on ERT, usually conjugated estrogens, and 43 were untreated; 9 of 28 ERT users had surgical menopause compared to 4 of 43 of the non-users). No differences were found on selective remembering or paired association tasks, but the ERT group did perform slightly better on the paragraph recall tasks (the difference was only marginally significant, since significance was improperly measured with one-tailed t-tests; on two-tailed tests, the significance would be less than a P of ≤ 0.05). In summary, convincing evidence of cognitive benefits distinct from improvement in mood and health has yet to be shown for extended use of estrogen replacement therapy.

Since estrogen increases or potentiates prolactin, serotonin (DeLisi, Dauphinais, & Hauser, 1989), opiates/endorphins (Nappi et al., 1990), GABA (Mansky et al., 1982), renin and angiotensin II (McCaffrey & Czaja, 1989), and corticosteroids (Lesniewska, Nowak, & Malendowicz, 1990), it is not surprising that some women feel relief when estrogen levels drop to postmenopausal levels, and may even experience increased well-being, confidence, and sexual desire.

Postmenopausal studies investigating the relation between estrogen replacement and sexual function generally have demonstrated only an indirect connection: improvement in overall well-being and decreases in uncomfortable symptoms, which promote the maintenance of sexual activity. Lorraine Dennerstein has been an influential proponent of estrogen replacement therapy. Her frequently cited study (Dennerstein et al., 1980) demonstrated beneficial effects on mood and sexual function. She performed a 12-month crossover double-blind trial comparing the effects of estradiol and/or progestogen treatment on 49 surgically menopausal women (hysterectomy and oophorectomy for benign symptoms). Women were evaluated for three months in each of four conditions: ethinyl estradiol (50 mg/day), levonorgestrel (a progestogen, 250 mg/day), Nordiol oral contraceptive (a combination of ethinyl estradiol and levonorgestrel), and a placebo.

If patients could not tolerate one condition, they could request an immediate switch to the next. Apparently due to hot flushes in the placebo condition, 12 women (24%) were prematurely switched. There was no wash-out period between conditions, so that carry-over effects (including estrogen withdrawal) were a compounding factor. Women who had been using hormonal preparations before the trial were requested to stop two weeks prior to the study. Consequently, some women would have been in a state of estrogen withdrawal upon entering the trial (hot flushes are an estrogen withdrawal symptom).

No significant differences were found between the four groups in frequency of intercourse or on any of 15 visual analogue scales for various aspects of sexual desire and response. The results of this study indicated that estrogen had no sexual benefits beyond resolving the general psychological and somatic difficulties of estrogen withdrawal. Increases in sexual desire were correlated with general feelings of well-being. Women on estradiol or estradiol-levonorgestrel showed slight but insignificant increases in sexual desire and enjoyment, lubrication, and orgasmic frequency. Progesterone-only treatment failed to provide any psychological benefits or complete relief of physical symptoms. The authors concluded that addition of the progestogen, levonorgestrel, clearly decreased the benefits of estradiol. With the lower estrogen dose, progesterone caused a considerable decrease in testosterone levels. Although there was no placebo control for estrogen, the positive effects diminished the week without hormone treatment each month. The positive sexual and mood benefits were enduring and stable over a twelve-month period.

Even if a woman later receives estrogen replacement, the decrease in the pleasure of sexual contact, in a woman's sexual attractiveness (estrogen generates attractive body odor and skin texture), in her ability to accommodate penile penetration and thrusting, and in her receptiveness to touch can aggravate physical problems occurring in men. Since men are also undergoing a decline in physical sexual response during their forties and fifties, perimenopause and menopause are times when sexual dysfunction commonly arises for couples and, unaddressed and untreated, continues for the rest of their lives, generating reticence, depression, frustration, anxiety, anger, and even aversion.

Although the physical difficulties triggered by estrogen withdrawal (hot flushes, sweating, loss of lubrication, dyspareunia) tend to cause problems in relationships, couples often wait until a crisis (such as an affair) provokes them into seeking help. By this time, "natural" approaches such as changes in nutrition, vitamin supplements, and increased exercise may be "too little and too late" to correct the physical changes which have undermined sexual attractiveness and responsivity. Bitter over their own sexual decline, men may blame their difficulties on their wives' "growing old and unattractive." Sleep problems, arthralgia, and irritability promote further tension in menopausal women (which may be avoided by estrogen replacement), and require evaluation of personal and environmental interventions. Sarrel (1982), for example, has reported that husbands of postmenopausal women with sexual symptoms developed fear of hurting their wives (as a result of postcoital bleeding resulting from vaginal atrophy) and feelings of insecurity, rejection, and anger due to their wives' sexual difficulties (vaginal dryness, vaginismus, tactile aversion).

Physiological Symptoms and ERT

The most immediate and noticeable effects of irregular secretion and decreased levels of estrogens are vasomotor alterations experienced as hot flushes and sweating. In 1977 Sam Yen labeled these thermoregulative disturbances as part of the "estrogen withdrawal syndrome." He pointed out that women who have never had normal estrogen levels (for example, due to gonadal dysgenesis) do not experience hot flushes during aging. If these women are treated with estrogen for several months and then treatment is withdrawn, however, classic hot flush symptoms are experienced for the first time. Hot flushes are preceded by hot flashes, which are the subjective feelings experienced just prior to the physiological flush. The flush is caused by sudden dilatation of cutaneous capillaries due to increased blood flow. Temperature increases by about 3 °C and lasts about 31 minutes (Notelovitz, 1986). Because of the high concentration of cutaneous blood vessels in the face and upper neck region, flashes and flushing are most often experienced in these areas.

These bothersome temperature changes affect about 75% of perimenopausal and postmenopausal women. Decreasing levels of estradiol may produce hot flushes even when the hormone is still within normal limits during the perimenopause (Notelovitz, 1986). Though symptoms are greatest near the end of the perimenopause and the first few postmenopausal years, 65% of women between the ages of 54 and 63 and 30% of women over 65 may still experience flushes (Notelovitz, 1986).

Flushes are usually accompanied by night sweats, abnormal perspiration, and palpitations, which often disturb sleep and cause irritability and anxiety. Estrogen replacement can resolve these thermoregulative symptoms. Though it is not clear what triggers hot flushes, estrogen seems to exert its effect in the hypothalamic thermoregulatory centers, which also regulate appetite and sexual behavior (Yen, 1977).

Estrogen also functions outside the genital zone to maintain health, lubrication, thickness of skin, and the secretion of attractive odors and sense of touch. Postmenopausal women may complain of thin, dry, flaky skin and easy bruising. Researchers (Brincat & Studd, 1988; Moniz, Savvas, Brincat, & Studd, 1989) have shown that skin collagen content decreases during the postmenopausal period by about 2% per year. This decrease is greater during the initial years (as much as 30% during the first five years after menopause) and levels off over several years. Interestingly, the postmenopausal decline of collagen content and skin thickness is significantly correlated with loss of bone mass and degree of osteoporosis (Nordin, Crilly, & Smith, 1984). Castelo-Branco et al. (1994) analyzed 76 nulliparous women from 20 to 60 years old and found that collagen decreased significantly after age 40 and after menopause, and changes in bone mass were closely related to changes in collagen. Basically, the fullness and resiliency of skin and maintenance of a sexually attractive body fragrance is facilitated by estrogen.

Decreased collagen synthesis has been shown in urinary stress-incontinent postmenopausal women compared to continent postmenopausal women (Falconer, Ekman, Malmström, & Ulmsten, 1994). An analysis of skin fibroblast cultures showed that stress-incontinent women accumulated 30% less collagen than continent women. A questionnaire survey of 355 premenopausal women and 858 postmenopausal women showed 25.1% urinary incontinence reported by premenopausal women. However, more than twice as many (7.1% vs. 3.1%) postmenopausal as premenopausal women experienced incontinence on a daily basis (Rekers, Drogendijk, Valkenburg, & Riphagen, 1992). Urgency nocturia and dyspareunia, which could be due to degeneration of urogenital tissue, were more prevalent in postmenopausal women; vaginal itching and discharge were more prevalent in premenopausal women. The prevalence of incontinence was higher after surgical than natural menopause. Among premenopausal women, 86.8% were sexually active, compared to 50.7% of postmenopausal women. Estrogen replacement therapy or vaginal estrogen cream has been shown to decrease urinary incontinence (see Elia & Bergman, 1993, for a comprehensive review).

Estrogen replacement can prevent collagen loss and even restore collagen toward normal levels in older postmenopausal women in less than two years (Brincat et al., 1987). Punnonen, Vilska, and Rauramo (1984) have shown that long-term (six years) estrogen-treated postmenopausal women have significantly greater skin thickness (21–39%) than nontreated controls. Other physiological actions of estrogen replacement on skin include (Brincat & Studd, 1988; Moniz et al., 1989): increased vascularization of skin, increased dermal moisture content, increased number of capillaries, less fragmentation of collagenous fibrils, reduced adhesion of collagen fibers in connective tissue, and decreased thinning action of corticosteroids.

Quite a few women experience dysphoric effects from estrogen replacement therapy that indirectly inhibit or discourage sexual responsiveness: Nausea, malaise, breast tenderness, and peculiar taste aversions are common complaints (Gustavson, Gustavson, Young, Pumariega, & Nicholas, 1989). Estrogens may also disturb tryptophan metabolism, causing a vitamin B_6 deficiency which can manifest as depression, fatigue, and irritability (correctable by vitamin B_6 supplements [Haspels, Bennink, van Keep, & Schreurs, 1975]). When these estrogen-induced symptoms are not correctly associated with replacement therapy, women may be treated with potentially toxic and unnecessary drugs such as tricyclic antidepressants, benzodiazepines, and neuroleptics.

As the number of women who receive estrogen progressively increases, a postmenopausal estrogen syndrome (PES) may soon emerge. In fact, with the current cancer-preventative recommendation of a 10–13-day progesterone addition to estrogen replacement therapy each month, we are already facing an outbreak of iatrogenic postmenopausal PMS as well.

Sexual Symptoms and ERT

A study from Julian Davidson's Stanford laboratory (Morrell, Dixen, Carter, & Davidson, 1984) showed that postmenopausal women have 16% lower vaginal pulse amplitude (a measure of physical sexual response) than premenopausal women, but no difference in subjective sexual arousal. Although healthy, sexually active untreated postmenopausal women may show some decline in vaginal response, it does not seem to be enough to significantly lessen subjective sexual arousal.

A later study (Myers & Morokoff, 1986) in Davidson's lab revealed that both untreated and treated postmenopausal women had similar vaginal pulse amplitudes when sexually stimulated by visual erotic stimuli. Lubrication in the untreated group was self-reported at a lower level than in the other groups and time to achieve maximal arousal was nonsignificantly increased. However, sexual arousal by self-report appeared similar in both groups of women. Beneficial increases in vaginal response to sexual stimulation with estrogen replacement may only be obvious when there is a marked deficiency or when vaginal atrophy causes discomfort.

A study by Myers, Dixen, Morrissette, Carmichael, and Davidson in 1990 evaluated the sexual responsiveness of 40 healthy naturally menopausal women using a double-blind prospective trial of four conditions: 0.625 mg/day conjugated estrogen (Premarin); 0.625 Premarin with 5 mg/day medroxyprogesterone (Provera); 0.625 Premarin with 5 mg/day methyltestosterone; and placebo. No significant group differences were found except that pleasure from masturbation was significantly greater for the estrogen-testosterone group. Use of oral testosterone instead of testosterone injection or implant probably resulted in a smaller advantage to the testosterone-added group. No group differences were noted for laboratory vaginal responses (lubrication, blood volume, or vaginal pulse amplitude). The researchers concluded that differences in sexual activity and response due to hormone replacement or supplementation may be less evident in asymptomatic naturally menopausal women than in those experiencing surgical menopause.

Greenblatt (1987) and Studd and Magos (1987) have shown that the full benefits of hormone replacement in relation to sexual desire are reliably achieved only with addition of testosterone. Smaller and less reliable sexual benefits and resolution of dysphoric mood and somatic/vaginal discomfort are achieved with estrogens alone. A study by Dow, Hart, and Forrest (1983) shows equal sexual benefits for estradiol and estradiol-testosterone combinations, demonstrating that estrogen replacement alone can be sufficient to maintain sexual desire.

Double-blind studies by Utian (1972a) and Campbell (1976) did not find significant sexual benefits for estrogen. An often-cited study by Fedor-Freyburgh (1977) showed that estrogen was beneficial to sex drive in open trials, but the sexual improvement was not statistically significant in the double-blind condition. There was, however, considerable improvement in depression, emotional dysphoria, and performance reaction, and a decrease in somatic symptoms such as hot flushes and vaginal dryness.

Some studies have shown no significant correlations between estrogen levels and sexual interest in perimenopausal (Ballinger, Browning, & Smith, 1987) or postmenopausal women (Bachmann et al., 1985). Cutler, Garcia, and McCoy (1987) found no significant relationship between estrogen levels and sexual desire, thoughts, response, or satisfaction in perimenopausal women. However, estrogen replacement therapy during perimenopause has been shown to delay the onset of menopause. Increased sexual activity during perimenopause may be responsible for higher estradiol levels, rather than the reverse. Frequent intercourse has been associated with fewer aberrant menstrual cycles, luteal phase defects, and perimenopausal hot flushes (Cutler, Garcia, & Krieger, 1979; McCoy, Cutler, & Davidson, 1985). In Cutler's study, frequency of intercourse decreased in women with estradiol levels lower than 35 mg/pl.

Animal researchers (Michael, Zumpe, & Bonsall, 1982) have shown that estrogen alone is sufficient to maintain normal sexual behavior in ovarectomized female monkeys. They induced menstrual cycles pharmacologically with daily injections of estradiol, progesterone, and testosterone. Results indicated that estradiol increased the females' sexual attractiveness to the males in the group and also increased female behaviors of aggressive soliciting and competitive sexual responses, which assure dominance over other females (Michael & Zumpe, 1990). Testosterone was not necessary for these distinctive effects of estradiol to occur. Submissive females may become more sexually attractive to males when estradiol peaks at midcycle. No significant sexual deficits were observed in the absence of testosterone injections.

There has been surprisingly little investigation of surgically or naturally postmenopausal primates, and most existing research has been compounded by the unnatural restraints of captivity, isolation, or special "model" groups. Research on captive postmenopausal rhesus monkeys has shown decreased active (proceptive) and passive (receptive) sexual behaviors unless females receive estrogen replacement (Young, 1961). In most cases, female primates available for study do not even reach the age of postmenopause due to declining health.

Our review of the research investigating the relation between estrogen and sex drive indicates that either estradiol does not specifically maintain sexual desire and activity or its sexual effects are less potent than those of testosterone. Nonetheless, estrogen replacement therapy is often sufficient to maintain a normal sense of well-being, including continuing sexual desire and activity. However, if sexual dysfunction becomes severe, estrogen replacement may not be adequate treatment. Estradiol does not seem to be the sole or even primary "libido" hormone and may not stimulate the degree of sexual desire necessary for normal sexual functioning.

Sex drive is also affected by the physiological changes that occur in the sexual organs during menopause. Estrogen replacement therapy has been found to have generally beneficial effect on many of these changes.

Vaginal Symptoms Vaginal changes occur soon after estrogen withdrawal. The earliest change is usually a reduction in lubrication and transudation; dryness and atrophy are commonly signaled by dyspareunia. The combination of reduced lubrication, friable tissue, and mechanical friction from intercourse predisposes postmenopausal women to vaginal infections that can become chronic and difficult to eliminate. Artificial lubrication can serve as a substitute, preventing many undesirable consequences (irritation, pain); however, women may view the need to use artificial lubrication as a mark of sexual inadequacy. For women who are unable to use estrogens, one approach that is more effective than most artificial lubricants currently available is the use of vitamin E capsules (punctured) or cream intravaginally; it serves as an excellent lubricant and as a daily supplement simultaneously.

Semmens, Tsai, Semmens, and Loadholt (1985) provided quantitative documentation of increased vaginal health with estrogen replacement therapy. They evaluated vaginal physiology in 23 postmenopausal women before and after treatment with 0.3–1.25 mg/day conjugated estrogen treatment (Premarin). Laboratory vaginal blood flow measurements using thermosensors and fluid measurements with tampons were included in each evaluation. Treatment resulted in vaginal improvement in several areas which continued over 24 months (pH levels decreased; vaginal fluids and blood flow increased).

This study demonstrated that frequent sexual activity alone, without estrogen replacement, will not suffice to maintain normal sexual function. No correlations between vaginal parameters and frequency of sexual activity were found other than pH.

Vaginal atrophy includes narrowing, shortening, and shrinkage of the vaginal barrel; in more severe cases, vaginal adhesions may develop. If a woman has been estrogen-deprived and sexually inactive for years at a time, intercourse should be approached with caution. Once vaginal atrophy and adhesions have become well-established, penetration can cause pain, rips, and tears. This physical condition can be reversed rapidly (within weeks) and effectively with estrogen replacement therapy—ideally, before renewing sexual relations.

Leiblum, Bachmann, Kemmann, Colburn, and Swartzman (1983) showed that weekly intercourse decreased vaginal atrophy without estrogen replacement in 52 women approximately seven years postmenopausal. Sexually active women (intercourse three or more times monthly) were compared with sexually inactive women (intercourse less than 10 times per year), whose decreased sexual frequency was the result of their partners' disinterest. Although sexual activity had decreased in the sexually active group during postmenopause, masturbation had increased. The vaginal atrophy index used showed a small but significant superiority in the sexually active group, chiefly in the condition of the pubic hair, labia and introitus. Estrogen levels did not differ between the two groups, but androgens were significantly higher in the sexually active group. It could be concluded that vaginal atrophy can be reduced by regular sexual activity and that androgens play some role in vaginal maintenance, possibly by facilitating increased sexual activity, including masturbation.

Glycogen levels also decline during menopause with the general reduction of moistness; hemorrhagic submucosal laceration and excoriation of the vaginal wall may occur. While trichomonas vaginalis thrives in the estrogen-deficient alkaline state, candida albicans is inhibited. A rise in vaginal pH from acid to alkaline, a decrease in Doderlein's bacilli, and thinning of vaginal and bladder epithelium all increase the risk of vaginal infection and lesions. Estrogen replacement returns pH levels toward normal and increases lubrication and blood flow.*

A decrease in pheromonal secretions dependent upon estrogen may accompany a decline in lubrication. Although the presence of these vaginal pheromones and their estrogenic nature has only been confirmed in female primates, it is likely that they do occur in women during sexual activity and probably throughout the day and during sleep as well.

The vagina may show decreases in elasticity, expansion, capacity, resilience, and pliability. A loss of vaginal tone can affect relaxation of the tissue around an inserted penis. The decrease in lubrication and lack of vaginal tone can make intercourse more difficult and less enjoyable for the male. The vaginal walls are composed of mucous membrane covered with squamous epithelium. The membrane occurs in a wave of transverse folds called *rugae*. Without estrogen support, the rugae recede and the vaginal wall becomes smooth and pale due to vascular atrophy. These rugae help to grip the penis, causing gentle drag and traction pleasurable to both partners.

Studies have shown that estrogens usually are effective in resolving sexual dysfunction due primarily to dyspareunia and secondarily to vaginal dryness (Sarrel, 1988). Lubrication occurs during REM episodes similar to sleep erections in men. Estrogens promote REM sleep, during which time secretions may "irrigate" the vagina. However, progestogen supplementation may impede or prohibit this estrogenic facilitation of sleep lubrication.

---

*Since the vagina and vulva may remain somewhat more alkaline even with estrogen replacement, postmenopausal women should avoid soaps with detergent or Ivory soap, which is alkaline, using instead baby and nondetergent soaps.

Topical estrogen-based vaginal creams are easily absorbed and usually reverse most of these symptoms within a week of treatment; tissue begins to thicken and nonspecific itching usually disappears (Byyny & Speroff, 1990). Treatment should be applied daily for the first week or two, followed by a weekly maintenance dose. Blood levels should be monitored to determine dosage. Since estrogen cream is systemically absorbed through the vagina, this method of estrogen replacement can also provide adequate therapeutic blood levels.

Vulvar Symptoms The chief vulvar structures are the *labia majora*, which contain sebaceous and apocrine glands embedded in fat and fibrous tissue, and *labia minora*, which are composed of flat connective tissue relatively free of fat. They are more prominent prior to the onset of puberty and may become more noticeable again postmenopausally as the labia majora atrophies. Vulvar skin is composed of dermis and epidermis in continuous interaction. Estrogen loss has little effect on the epidermis itself, but causes fibrosis and loss of fat and moisture in the dermal tissue. Small blood capillaries below the surface, *telangiectasia*, may become exposed and painful. Even hot baths can precipitate trauma; bleeding from telangiectasia can triggered by penile thrusting or even by the friction of towel drying.

Vulvar cutaneous changes due to hormone deficiency usually occur later than vaginal changes and are more difficult to differentiate from normal aging than the associated vaginal symptoms. Although less noticeable than vaginal changes, they are also less reversible. Given that the vulva is homologous to the male scrotum, it may be as dependent on androgen maintenance as on estrogen replacement.

External itching and burning due to vulvar dystrophy is indicated by whitish skin lesions or white patches (leukoplakia [Byyny & Speroff, 1990]).* A severe form of vulvar dystrophy, called *lichen sclerosis*, is characterized by a thin, parched, dry, whitish epithelium. Itching causes scratching, which in turn leads to ulceration and further pathology of the primary lesions. The minor labia may develop adhesions to the adjoining major labia. Scarring may develop around the clitoris, which may become recessed behind the whitish tissue. Corticosteroid-based ointments or creams usually cause further drying and thinning of the skin. However, topical testosterone cream, or a mixture of testosterone and cortisone, can be helpful.

The vulva of female primates is often called a "sex skin" due to the obvious and sometimes colorful changes that occur during sexual heat (estrus). In women, there is a more subtle "sex skin" reaction to sexual arousal, with engorgement and flushing of the vulva. This local reaction typically decreases during postmenopause, probably due to a combination of estrogen deficiency and aging. In one study, estrogen replacement treatment resulted in a fourfold blood flow increase in the labia minora and clitoris (Sarrell, 1986).

Cervix and Uterus The uterus may shrink and the cervix may flatten after menopause. Uterovaginal prolapse may also occur due to thinning, weak tissue. Abnormal endometrial proliferation may occur with unopposed estrogen, so that cyclic progesterone treatment may be necessary even in women who do not take estrogen replacement therapy (for example, in obese women who continue postmenopausally to produce large amounts of estrogen from fatty tissue). The normal endometrial proliferation due to estrogen replacement is beneficial for maintaining the smooth and soft texture of the uterus and for preventing cystic hyperplasia.

Urogenital Urogenital atrophy commonly occurs as a result of estrogen deficiency. In the majority of women, the atrophy can be corrected or substantially reduced with estrogen replacement. However, the drying and thinning of skin, which comprises the largest sexual organ in the body, may decrease both sexual attractiveness and the pleasure of touching. Philip Sarrel (1988, 1990) has eloquently described these postmenopausal sexual deficits in touching and sensation, which he attributes to decreased estro-

*These patches were believed to be premalignant or malignant until research established their benign nature.

gen, and which in large part can be reversed by continuing estrogen supplementation. Accompanying feelings may include hyper-irritability or a vague sense of numbness. Negative touch symptoms correlate with loss of sexual desire, hot flushes, and insomnia.

Sarrel (1987) also cited evidence for shrinkage of touch zones along the pudendal nerve after ovary removal in rats and estrogen enhancement of sensory perception, vibration sensitivity, taste, and smell. He concluded that neural transmission is slowed as when there is a state of peripheral neuropathy and that retarded peripheral neurotransmission can be corrected by estrogen replacement.

Urethral pressure is correlated with estradiol levels. Atrophic urethritis and voiding problems are therefore common: About 30–40% of postmenopausal women suffer from these disturbances. The function of the urinary sphincter of postmenopausal women may be improved by estrogen treatment (Hilton & Stanton, 1983; Rud, 1980). In a sample of 75 women, 35% complained of nocturia and 40% of urinary frequency (Wren, 1985). Within four months of estrogen treatment, these urinary symptoms were resolved in all but 3–4% of the women. Versi and Cardoza (1988) found that three months of estradiol implant therapy reduced urinary frequency, nocturia, and incontinence in postmenopausal women from 32–54% to 12–24%. However, they pointed out that comparative studies before and after menopause have been few and may not show significant differences; placebo-controlled studies of estrogen-induced improvement in urinary function are also rare.

Unfortunately, many women do not seek medical treatment for urinary incontinence or sexual dysfunction until their symptoms become intolerable. In a sample of middle-aged women (ages 42–50), Burgio, Matthews, and Engel (1991) found that 58% had experienced urine loss on occasion and 30% reported incontinence that occurred at least once a month. Only 25.5% of women with chronic incontinence had sought medical treatment. Even among women with daily incontinence or large-volume urine loss accidents, only 54–60% sought medical treatment.

Rekers et al. (1992) found that only 26.1% of postmenopausal incontinent women had consulted their doctors about it, compared to 38.2% of incontinent premenopausal women. Urinary incontinence was found to be much more frequent in the surgical menopausal subgroup (n = 242) compared to the natural menopausal subgroup (36.0% vs. 21.5%). Additionally, other urogenital symptoms (e.g., vaginal pain, dysuria) showed much greater prevalence in the surgical menopausal group compared to the natural menopausal group.

Urinary incontinence can be particularly frequent during sexual intercourse. Walters, Taylor, and Schoenfeld (1990) reported urine leakage during coitus or orgasm in 60–65% of the incontinent women sampled. From a statistical perspective, incontinence symptoms can adversely affect sexual relations in as much as 43% of incontinent patients (Vereecken, 1989). Decrease or abstinence from intercourse among incontinent women may be due to dyspareunia, decreased sex drive, embarrassment, and/or depression.

Estrogen loss is primarily responsible for irritable and thin urethral mucosa. The thinning of the urethral mucosa contributes to dysuria, tenderness, burning sensations, and decreased urethral resistance. Burning can be due to urine contact with the thinned mucosa, or to inflamed tissue resulting from infection caused by the rise of pH from acid to alkaline, which increases susceptibility of tissue to bacterial invasion.

Atrophy of the bladder and urethral walls is similar to atrophy of the vaginal mucosa. The pathology of the urethra also parallels postmenopausal vaginal pathology. Atrophic distal urethritis can result in partial bladder outlet blockage. Nonbacterial urethritis will not respond to antibiotic or sulfa drugs; corticosteroid creams will thin tissue even further. Topical estrogen creams and/or estrogen replacement can resolve many of these urinary problems (Elia & Bergman, 1993). However, failure to treat promptly with estrogen can result in chronic susceptibility to infection and irritation.

Inability to empty the bladder completely may be due partly to estrogen loss and partly due to peripheral neuropathy associated with aging. Because the urethra and bladder trigone have high concentrations of estrogen receptors, these areas are very sensitive to decreases in estrogen levels. Chronic interstitial cystitis (trigonitis) can be aggravated by estrogen withdrawal. Often a weakness of the paraurethral musculature develops and an ectropion of mucous membrane tissue is formed.

Neuropathy associated with decreased alpha-1 adrenergic tone can be reversed by estradiol (Hamlet, Rorie, & Tyce, 1980; Schreiter, Fuchs, & Stockamp, 1976; Wein, 1991). The findings of numerous animal studies have supported this adrenergic-estrogenic synergism. Hodgson, Dumas, Boling, and Heesch (1978) have shown that castration-induced decreases in alpha adrenergic sensitivity in female rabbits were reversed by low-dose estrogen treatment. Larsson, Andersson, Batra, Mattiasson, and Sjogren (1984) also found that urethral tension was improved in female rabbits by estrogen treatment. An increased sensitivity to norepinephrine and an increase in adrenergic receptors appeared to be responsible. Estrogenic facilitation of adrenergic tone in women can also be expected to improve orgasmic capacity, given the improvement in muscle contraction and excitatory receptor sensitivity.

Wein (1991) has promoted the combination of the alpha adrenergic stimulant phenylpropanolamine (PPA) (the generic ingredient of most over-the-counter diet pills) and estrogen to treat urinary incontinence. Beisland, Fossberg, Moer, and Sanders (1984) have shown that, while PPA alone was not sufficient to resolve postmenopausal urethral sphincteric insufficiency, combinations of PPA with estriol vaginal suppositories resulted in total continence or great improvement in 17 of 18 incontinent women. Coopland (1989) reported the success of treating postmenopausal stress incontinence with 25 mg vaginal estrogen cream three times a week, PPA three times a day, and Kegel exercises.

Urinary sphincter incompetence is rarely caused by estrogen deficiency alone unless there is tissue weakness due to aging (Karram, Yeko, Sauer, & Bhatia, 1989). However, estrogen alone is sufficient treatment for many postmenopausal women with stress incontinence. The first report of estrogen treatment of postmenopausal dysuria and incontinence was by Salmon, Walter, and Geist (1941), the same authors who first recommended the use of testosterone to treat decreased sexual desire in females. Onuora, Ardoin, Dunnihoo, and Otterson (1991) reviewed the clinical records of 43 postmenopausal women with stress incontinence, who were treated over a period of four years with alternating amounts of intravaginal estrogen cream. Seventy percent of the women were cured and 21% improved. (On the average, improvement occurred within four weeks.) Treatment with oral estrogen alone may also be helpful (Rud, Andersson, Boye, & Ulmsten, 1980), but resolution of symptoms is more likely with vaginal cream.

A general increase in urogenital blood flow (Batra, Bjellin, Sjogen, Iosif, & Widmark, 1986), more pliable and less irritable genital mucosa and skin, and a softening and thickening effect due to estrogen treatment can improve objective and subjective urinary health. All these improvements in the urinary tract and urinary symptoms with estrogen treatment suggest the probability of improved genital sexual responses with estrogen replacement. Untreated urinary symptoms, however, can only be exacerbated by frequent intercourse, which furthermore adds to the likelihood of infection, inflammation, and chronic pelvic and genital pain.

NON-MENOPAUSAL BENEFITS OF ESTROGEN REPLACEMENT THERAPY

Heart Disease

After menopause, death from heart disease in women may increase by as much as 18 times (Rosenberg et al., 1981); it is by far the greatest health risk and cause of death in aging women. Estrogen replacement therapy appears to reduce heart disease risk by 30–70%. Henderson, Ross, Paganini-Hill, and Mack (1986) estimated that, with a standard (0.625 mg) dose of conjugated estrogen, women between the ages of 50 and 75 would show a reduction of 25-year death risk for ischemic heart disease of 5,250 per 100,000 women compared to a death risk of 63 per 100,000 for endometrial cancer (reduction of

5,250 deaths versus increase of 63 deaths). Since few women die of endometrial cancer, relatively few additional deaths can increase the statistical risk several fold. By contrast, death in women from heart disease is frequent and the reduced risk effected by ERT can prevent a significant number of early deaths. Gorsky, Koplan, Peterson, and Thacker (1994) reviewed past ERT risk data with a standard-size hypothetical cohort of 10,000 postmenopausal women aged 50 to 75. Estrogen use for 25 years would decrease fatal heart attack by 48% (567 cases), decrease deaths from hip fracture by 49% (75), increase deaths from breast cancer by 21% (39), and increase deaths from endometrial cancers by 207% (29 excess deaths).

Barrett-Connor and Bush (1991) have reviewed 18 studies of estrogen impact on cardiovascular disease risk. Reduced risks of at least 20% were reported in 12 of the studies, with 50% reduction reported in seven. Of the four studies that showed increased risk, three were unreliably small or used confounded variables. The much-criticized Framingham study (Wilson, Garrison, & Castelli, 1985) was the only published study suggesting an increase in cardiovascular risk with estrogen. However, a later re-analysis of the study data by some of the authors showed that estrogen use reduced cardiovascular deaths in women in their fifties and caused no difference in women in their sixties (Eaker & Castelli, 1987).

Postmenopausal estrogen supplementation prevents or reverses negative cholesterol/lipid changes which occur after menopause, when cardiovascular risks in women sharply increase to approximate levels in men (Barrett-Connor & Bush, 1991). In one study, oral conjugated estrogen usage resulted in about a 10–14% increase in HDL cholesterol and a 4–8% decrease in LDL cholesterol (Henderson, Paganini-Hill, & Ross, 1991). Maintenance of HDL cholesterol levels and increased levels of apolipoprotein A-1 are typical findings with postmenopausal estrogen supplementation (Lindheim et al., 1994; Mathews et al., 1989; Tepper, Goldberger, May, Luz, & Beyth, 1992). A comprehensive review that supported the beneficial cardiovascular effects of estrogen on cholesterol-lipid formation has been presented by Barrett-Connor and Bush (1991). They concluded that 25–50% of estrogen reduction of cardiovascular risk was due to changes in HDL and LDL cholesterol, noting that 50–75% of the reduction remained inexplicable.

In addition to the favorable effect on cholesterol, the protective benefit of estrogen replacement therapy on survival of women with preexisting angiographically identified blood vessel stenosis disease has been shown to be particularly strong, indicating a direct antiatherosclerotic effect (Sullivan et al., 1990). Other studies of subjects with angiographically-defined coronary disease have also shown significant risk reductions of approximately 50% (Gruchow, Anderson, Barborick, & Sobocinski, 1988; McFarland, Boniface, Hornung, Earnhardt, & Humphries, 1989).

Osteoporosis

After menopause, the incidence of hip fracture increases steeply, about ten-fold (from 0.6 to 6.0%, Nordin et al., 1984). Over 100,000 hip fractures and 250,000 femoral neck fractures occur yearly in the U.S., costing over seven billion dollars for medical care (Libanati, Schulz, Shook, Bock, & Baylink, 1992). Approximately 20% of patients with these fractures die within three months of complications due to fracture (Christiansen & Riis, 1989). Among survivors of hip fracture, there may be a 50% rate of incapacitation requiring nursing home care (Thorneycroft, 1989); most experience subsequent chronic pain which can destroy quality of life.

Bone loss after menopause is universal. During the first 20 years postmenopause (until about 65 to 70 years old), approximately 75% of bone loss can be attributed to estrogen deficiency rather than to aging itself (Byyny & Speroff, 1990). Though particularly great within the first few years after menopause, bone decay continues relentlessly, increasing the risk of disabling fractures.

There is a sharp acceleration in fracture incidence after the age of 60 (Christiansen & Riis, 1989), and by 80 years of age (the average life expectancy of women in the United States), bone mass in untreated postmenopausal women shows an average loss of almost 50% in trabecular bone and 35% in cortical bone (Doren & Schneider, 1989). Estrogen replacement therapy is remarkably effective in preventing and inhibiting bone loss and consequent osteoporosis in more than 90% of patients for as long as 10 to 15 years (Lindsay, 1986a, 1986b). Structural skeletal damage and associated atrophy of muscle and skin are also largely prevented. Although major fractures may not occur for 10 to 20 years, deterioration in bone, muscle, and skin may progressively compromise quality of life, including a possible decrease in enjoyment from exercise and the physical rough-and-tumble of sexual intercourse. Onset of chronic pain from deterioration of spinal architecture and brittle bone almost certainly discourages sexual activity, and pain relief medication may further decrease sexual sensitivity. Preservation of bone density by estrogen can prevent minor fractures which make movement uncomfortable or painful. Cauley, Cummings, Black, Mascioli, and Seeley (1990) found that ERT users participated in significantly more physical exercise per week than women never treated with ERT. Zhang, Feldblum, and Fortney (1992) examined 352 perimenopausal women aged 40 to 54 for both energy expenditure during physical exercise and bone density at various body locations. Women who by history and three-day metabolic monitoring showed moderate energy expenditure physical exercise and increased bone density at all sites were compared to women with low energy expenditure physical activity.

When estrogen is not started at menopause and osteoporosis is not identified until later, prophylactic estrogen treatment may be ineffective in preventing gross osteoporosis. Consequently, for prevention or optimum reduction of osteoporosis, estrogen replacement therapy should be started immediately at menopause and continued indefinitely. Osteoporotic bone loss has also been shown during the perimenopause in women with longer menstrual cycles (Gambacciani et al., 1994), indicating that women should be monitored during the perimenopause and prescribed ERT, even though menopause has not yet occurred. It should also be noted that, when osteoporosis is clearly identified, calcium supplementation is unlikely to retard further bone loss, except when given in conjunction with estrogen (Ettinger, 1987).

Calcitonin, a peptide hormone secreted by C-cells of the thyroid gland, reduces bone resorption by inhibiting osteoclasts and reducing calcium efflux from bone surfaces (Ravn, Rosenberg, & Bostofte, 1994). Since it has no contraindications, calcitonin is an obvious alternative when estrogen is inadvisable. It should be noted that, while there is no doubt that calcitonin reduces excessive bone resorption, its efficacy in long-term prevention of bone loss and treatment of osteoporosis has not been demonstrated to any degree comparable to estrogen replacement therapy.

For this reason, nasal calcitonin (Miacalcin) is not yet approved by the Federal Drug Administration for marketing in the United States, even though it is available and widely used in more than 20 other countries. Approval is expected after efficacy trials are completed (possibly 1996). Some believe that estrogen prevention of bone loss occurs through stimulation of calcitonin secretion (Stevenson et al., 1981; Whitehead, et al., 1982). In fact, estrogen has been found to increase calcitonin both in the test-tube and in postmenopausal women (Greenberg et al., 1986). However, studies have not consistently shown reduced calcitonin in postmenopausal osteoporotic women (Aloia, 1985).

Calcitonin also stimulates the uptake of tryptophan and the synthesis of serotonin in the brain (Nakhla, 1987). It has been shown to be an effective analgesic in various bone diseases that may involve inhibition of sensory processing through stimulation of endorphin and serotonergic activity (Pietrowsky, Dentler, Born, & Fehm, 1990; Wisneski, 1992).

An anorectic effect of calcitonin has also been related to its activation of hypothalamic serotonergic activity. Since both calcitonin and serotonin are co-localized in human genital paraneurons (Cecio & Vittoria, 1989), calcitonin may decrease genital sensitivity and inhibit orgasm. Consequently, women (and men) should be closely monitored for decreased sexual response when treated with calcitonin. Conversely, nasal calcitonin should be investigated as a treatment for premature ejaculation or for pelvic pain.

The best alternatives to estrogen replacement therapy in the prevention of osteoporosis are calcitonin and diphosphonates. Various androgens such as DHEA are also promising, particularly as antagonists to bone destroying glucocorticoids. These alternate androgen treatments may avoid the cancer risks of estrogen and virilization of conventional testosterone use.

CANCER RISKS AND ESTROGEN REPLACEMENT THERAPY

Many physicians are reluctant to prescribe prophylactic estrogen replacement therapy despite its benefits for heart disease and osteoporosis, because of their concern about the relationship between estrogen and cancer. However, the weight of the evidence indicates that standard doses (0.625 mg) of conjugated estrogens, with or without adjunctive progestogen, do not increase risk of breast cancer and may even reduce the overall cancer mortality rate (Colditz, Egan, & Stampfer, 1993; Dupont & Page, 1991; Grady et al., 1992; Henderson, Paganini-Hill, & Ross, 1991; Nachtigall, Smilen, Nachtigall, Nachtigall, & Nachtigall, 1992; Ravn et al., 1994). The only form of cancer definitely increased by estrogen replacement therapy is endometrial cancer, which occurs far less frequently and has lower mortality rates. This risk can be virtually eliminated with the addition of progestogen or with hysterectomy.

This decreased risk of death from cancer may partially be due to the fact the women at less risk are put on estrogen replacement therapy. However, the death rate due to cancer is less in ERT users than in nonusers, both for endometrial cancer (Fitgerald, Elstein, & Mansel, 1993) and breast cancer (Strickland, Gambrell, Butzin, & Strickland, 1992) indicating that ERT may be a health and longevity factor (Gambrell, 1989; Henderson et al., 1991).

Estrogen replacement therapy users may show an elevated incidence of breast cancer but a lowered rate of breast cancer mortality (Hunt, Vessey, McPherson, & Coleman, 1987). Other studies have also found higher breast cancer risks with estradiol than typically found with conjugated estrogens (e.g., Premarin).

While European studies have shown significantly increased breast cancer with estrogen replacement therapy, this increased risk is usually due to the use of synthetic forms of estradiol rather than the conjugated estrogens contained in Premarin (Bergkvist, Adami, Persson, Hoover, & Schairer, 1989; Hiatt, Bawol, Friedman, & Hoover, 1984; Hulka, Chambless, Deubner, & Wilkinson, 1982; Hunt et al., 1987). Dupont and Page (1991) pointed out that the highly publicized 1989 Bergkvist study in the *New England Journal of Medicine*, which showed an increased breast cancer risk, found a small overall risk 10% (1.1 risk) increase in ERT users; the risk increased to 20% in estradiol ERT uses and increased with duration of exposure. The risk for women on conjugated estrogens (Premarin) or estriol was not significantly increased and did not increase with duration of exposure. A recent update of their study (Persson, Yuen, Bergkvist et al., 1992) shows that there is no increased risk for breast cancer among estradiol or conjugated estrogen users (relative risk = 1.0) and a slightly higher risk for users of the estrogen-progestogen combined therapy (relative risk = 1.3).

Conjugated estrogens (Premarin) contain estrone, a form of estrogen that is less tissue active. While circulating estrogen levels are low after menopause, estrogen levels in breast tissue decline only slightly. Estradiol rather than estrone is the chief estrogen within the breast (Miller & Anderson, 1988). Differences in breast cancer risk between estrone-containing ERT and estradiol ERT taken orally (e.g., Estrace, ethinyl estradiol) or by injection, pellet implant, or transdermal skin patch have scarcely been investigated.

Therefore, while estradiol replacement is perhaps more beneficial psychologically and sexually, it may result in greater breast cancer risk. Breast cancer risk does appear to increase to about 30% (risk of 1.3) after 15 years of estrogen use (Steinberg et al., 1991). However, studies of such extended ERT use inevitably include women who have used higher than currently recommended doses. Moreover, death rate in long-term ERT users is radically decreased (30% lower) rather than increased due to other health and longevity benefits (Henderson et al., 1991).

Some researchers have proposed that inadequate progesterone or lack of progesterone opposition to estrogens is the cause of increased breast cancer risk (Gambrell, 1989; Korenman, 1980; Miller & Anderson, 1988). Inadequate progesterone may occur with anovulatory cycles in infertile women or during late perimenopause. An elevated risk of breast cancer continues throughout the postmenopause when estrogen levels are lower but present, and progesterone production is usually all but absent. Breast cells are not shed cyclically by progesterone as in the endometrium, so any progesterone breast-protective effect must operate through cellular or enzymatic processes as yet unknown.

Gambrell (1989) contended that, in addition to eliminating the risk of ERT-induced endometrial cancer, progestogen addition to estrogen replacement therapy (though not progestogen use alone) also protected against breast cancer in estrogen-progestogen users. Two other studies (Lauritzen & Meier, 1984; Nachtigal, Nachtigal, Nachtigal, & Beckman, 1979) found a decreased breast cancer risk in estrogen-progesterone users. By contrast, European studies (Bergkvist et al., 1989; Ewertz, 1988) have found a higher risk of breast cancer in estrogen-progesterone users, possibly indicating that addition of progestogens to estradiol rather than to conjugated estrogens will not lower and may raise breast cancer risk.

Overall, weighted risk of breast cancer from estrogen-progesterone use in the few studies reported is 0.99 (Sillero-Arenas, Delgado-Rodriguez, Rodigues-Canteras, Bueno-Cavanilli, & Galvez-Vagas, 1992). The latest meta-analysis of breast cancer risks with conjugated estrogens (Premarin), regardless of duration or dose, shows an 8% increase (Sillero-Arenas et al., 1992). The most thorough meta-analysis of risk due to conjugated estrogens has been conducted by Dupont and Page (1991), who also found a nonsignificant 8% increase for the recommended dose of 0.625 mg or less. The overall risk with a 1.25 mg dose was not significantly different from that with 0.625 mg. However, separate large studies have occasionally shown a significantly increased risk for breast cancer of over 50% (Colditz et al., 1990), while others (Kaufman et al., 1984) have shown significantly reduced breast cancer risk, particularly in surgically menopausal women.

The relative risk of breast cancer does not appear to be significantly increased by estrogen replacement therapy in women with a history of benign breast disease (Dupont & Page, 1991). However, ERT is contraindicated where epithelial hyperplasia has been identified and when there is a history of breast cancer.

In summary, ERT treatment with estradiol appears to increase breast cancer risk significantly (30% overall and about 60% with extended use over many years) (Dupont & Page, 1991; Sillero-Arenas et al., 1992; Steinberg et al., 1991). (It has not yet been determined if there is an increase in deaths due to breast cancer even when there is an increase in incidence of breast cancer.) However, ERT treatment with conjugated estrogens or other nonestradiol estrogens appears to carry an overall cancer risk of 0–10%, which may increase with long-term use (over 10 years) and current use to 28–50%. This increased risk may reflect a true increase or merely increased surveillance and detection.

CONCLUSIONS

The role of estrogen in female sexuality is both direct and indirect. The most direct and obvious genital symptom that occurs as a result of estrogen withdrawal—lack of lubrication—can be corrected artificially. However, the indirect effects of estrogen depletion on sex are more global, since positive states of mind and mood, as well as an overall sense of well-being, are facilitated by this hormone. To help ensure that sexual symptoms related to estrogen withdrawal are not overlooked, complete and comprehensive information on possible menopause-induced problems should be given to women and the possible benefits and risks of estrogen treatment should be routinely explained and discussed.

Changes in sexual organ function are usually an early indication of the degeneration occurring throughout the body during menopause. Urogenital atrophy and resultant tissue injury and pain are clear harbingers of the progressive degeneration of less visible tissue such as vertebral bone and muscle mass. To treat urogenital symptoms in isolation (such as with estrogen vaginal creams) ignores the probability that similar pathology is occurring in other skin, muscle blood vessel (arteriosclerosis), and bone (osteoporosis) tissue. This additional pathology, which is less evident and bothersome, can become severely disabling in the long term if it is not adequately treated by estrogen. When treatment is not initiated at the beginning of menopause, estrogen replacement at any time will be valuable and can begin to prevent the progression of osteoporosis, heart disease, and other symptoms.

Estrogens can also preserve attractiveness by keeping hair soft and full-bodied and by reducing appetite so that weight is kept within normal limits. The absence of hot flashes/flushes, sweating, and dizziness with estrogen replacement also contributes to comfort and sexual receptivity.

Obviously, the benefits of ERT must be balanced against the risk of breast and endometrial cancers. Breast cancer is unfortunately increasing in both users and nonusers of estrogen. It is important to note that breast cancer is more highly correlated with the use of estradiol than with conjugated estrogen (Premarin). (However, the sexual and psychological effects of conjugated estrogens may not be as intense as with estradiol.) While some studies have shown increased cancer risk with long-term use of conjugated estrogens (Sillero-Arenas et al., 1992), the majority have not shown a significantly increased risk with long-term use.

The concern regarding uterine cancer can be largely resolved by the use of supplemental progesterone, which has not only reduced the risk of endometrial cancer for estrogen users, but may even reduce it below what is normal for non-estrogen users (Gambrell, 1992). With the combination of estrogen and lower dose progesterone replacement therapy, many women can have "the best of both worlds" while being carefully monitored for any signs of breast abnormalities.

If a woman has had both her uterus and ovaries removed, it is important that she consider testosterone replacement therapy in addition to estrogen, if she wishes to maintain certain qualities of her character including assertiveness, energetic sexual libido and bright mood. There is no medical rationale for adding progestogens to ERT when the uterus has been removed. This aspect of hormone replacement therapy will be discussed in depth in the chapter on testosterone.

For comprehensive care, prophylactic estrogen treatment is as efficient and considerably less dangerous than the combination of drugs that are usually used to treat the consequences of estrogen withdrawal. These drugs include antihypertensives (including calcium blockers which may promote Parkinson-like changes) and methyldopa (which can cause loss of memory and other cognitive impairment), cholesterol and lipid-lowering drugs, weight-reducing drugs, and a variety of pain relievers ranging from nonsteroidal anti-inflammatories (which decrease tissue prostaglandins) to opiates (which have an evident adverse effect on sexuality). A bewildering array of prescription alternatives is currently available for mood disorders associated with menopause. As a result, menopausal symptoms may be treated with psychotropic drugs including benzodiazepines for insomnia and anxiety, tricyclic antidepressants for depression, beta blockers for hypertension and nervousness, and SSRIs (e.g., fluoxetine/Prozac) for almost any other emotional condition ranging from phobia to obesity. Combinations of these drugs can lead to complete sexual and emotional anesthesia.

Sexual intimacy between partners in their late forties and early fifties is sometimes the only bond that enables a couple to bridge the gap that midlife changes have brought to bear on their relationship. When sexual continuity is broken due to lack of adjustment to or therapy for menopausal changes, depression, anxiety, anger, frustration, and sexual aversion can take an irreversible toll on the relationship. Although sexual therapy may correct the major psychological consequences of menopausal sexual problems, consulting a sex therapist is still relatively infrequent in our society and tends to be precipitated by a crisis of separation or divorce. This emotional upheaval is a painful and expensive way to deal with symptoms that may have been prevented in the first place.

We do not mean to imply that estrogen is a panacea. Estrogen therapy is not without complications. However, it is our opinion at this time that the complications of estrogen deprivation are considerably more severe. The extent to which estrogen replacement therapy is a viable solution to postmenopausal changes must be judged in the light of continuing, comprehensive research—which, furthermore, should include intensive clinical monitoring of postmenopausal women. The addition of alternatives such as DHEAS, testosterone, and dopamine stimulants, and other forms of currently used medications, such as nasal spray calcitonin and adjunct micronized progesterone in place of progestogens, holds enormous promise for improved sexual functioning throughout menopause in the near future.

6

Progesterone

OBJECTIVES

- To describe the nature and function of naturally occurring progesterone
- To distinguish between the effects of natural and synthetic progesterones
- To describe the sexual impact of progesterone in oral contraceptives and estrogen replacement therapy
- To discuss therapeutic applications as treatment for prostate cancer and criminal sex offenders

Progesterone is a female hormone that functions as an intracellular/receptor like other natural hormones such as estrogen and various steroids. Secreted by the ovaries, corpus luteum, and adrenal glands, it is synthesized from the cholesterol metabolite pregnenolone. As indicated by its name, progesterone promotes gestation by protection of the corpus luteum and reduction of myometrial activity. Although it works in concert with estrogens, in many circumstances it has an effect opposite to estrogens. For example, progesterone increases MAO activity, while estrogen decreases it (consequently, progesterone has the potential to cause depression). It also inhibits orgasm through mechanisms not yet clearly defined. Progesterone may also potentiate estrogenic action, but the behavioral interaction of progesterone and estrogen involves cyclic differences, so that an initial stimulatory effect becomes inhibitory a short time later—a process that may involve protein and RNA modifications, which require time to occur (24 hours in some cases).

Therapeutic actions of progestational agents include:

- preservation of corpus luteum when natural luteal phase progesterone secretion is inadequate
- contraception
- postmenopausal hormone supplementation
- suppression of endometrial hyperplasia and anovulatory bleeding
- use as antiandrogen for treatment of acne and for inhibition of prostate growth
- treatment of sex offenders

Many of the side effects of progesterone documented by Glick and Bennett (1981) and listed in Table 6.1 have the potential to affect sexual function either directly or indirectly.

SYNTHETIC VERSUS NATURAL PROGESTERONES

Synthetic progesterones (progestogens or progestins) are progesterone derivatives (e.g., medroxyprogesterone) or testosterone derivatives which have chiefly progestational and antiandrogen actions (e.g., norethindrone and norgestrel).

Progestogens derived from testosterone are more virilizing, may reduce high-density-lipoprotein cholesterol (HDL) and may eliminate the beneficial rise in HDL from estrogen replacement therapy. These negative cholesterol

Table 6.1 *Side Effects of Progesterone That Negatively Affect Sexual Function*

General Physiology	*Sexual Physiology*	*Psychobiological*
Sedative in moderate doses and anesthetic at high doses	Potential to inhibit orgasm	Decreased sex drive
Depression of neuronal arousal	Decreased sex drive	Potential to cause depression
Potential to reduce physical sensitivity	Decreased sensitivity of hypothalamic neurons to reflex stimuli from genital area	Negative body image
Potential to reduce physical activity	Decreased LHRH reactivity	
Increased MAO activity	Blocked endometrial growth and change of proliferative estrogen pattern to secretory state	
Thermogenic effect of raising hypothalamic set-point for body temperature	Decreased uterine contractile activity	
Stimulation of respiration	Stimulation of breast alveolar development	
Weight gain and water retention	Irregular vaginal bleeding	
Overall discomfort		

effects are not found with natural micronized oral progesterone (Fahraeus, Larsson-Cohn, & Wallentin, 1983; Hirvonen, Malkonen, & Manninen, 1981).

There are important differences between synthetic and natural progesterones in regard to side effects and how they influence mind and body. Farquhar et al. (1989) found that medroxyprogesterone (Provera) caused a five-pound weight gain in 38 of 45 (84%) women treated over four months for pelvic pain, compared to 14 of 40 (35%) women who gained weight on a placebo.

Table 6.2 provides a comprehensive listing of natural and synthetic progestational agents currently available.

Studies of sexual receptivity throughout the human menstrual cycle have not shown a clear lowering of sexual desire or response during the luteal phase when progesterone levels are substantially elevated. In fact, complicating the picture, various clinical studies have reported *increased* sexual desire during the premenstrum, when progesterone levels are changing rapidly. Other studies have indicated the potential of progesterone or progestogens to impact sexual desire negatively (Dennerstein et al., 1980; Holst, Backstrom, Hammerback, & von Shoultz, 1989; Magos et al., 1986; Sherwin, 1991). The negative sexual effects of progesterone and progestogens could be due to biochemical changes in other neurotransmitters and peptides that effect sexual mood, as well as: reduction of dopamine (Lofstrom, 1979); increase in brain opioid levels (Genazzani et al., 1989); and antagonism of oxytocin (Luck, 1989). The ability of progesterone to diminish sex drive is partially due to its reduction of testosterone (Gottesman & Schubert, 1993). However, since progesterone can reduce sex drive in men even when testosterone levels are not decreased, other factors appear to be involved.

Primate and rabbit studies have indicated that progesterone or progestogens may decrease positive pheromonal cues or increase negative pheromonal cues, making females less sexually attractive to males, despite no change in the females' sexual receptivity (Hudson, Gonzalez-Mariscal, & Beyer, 1990; Linn & Stecklis, 1990). This aspect of progestational activity has not been investigated in humans.

Although progesterone appeared to facilitate lordotic passive sexual behavior in female rats, after initial facilitation the sexual response was reduced (Gorski, 1976; Nadler, 1970). In ovariectomized female rats, administration of progesterone added sequentially to estrogen induced both lordosis and active proceptive sexual behavior (i.e., brought the female rats into estrus). The extent to which progesterone acts as a complement to estrogenic sexual stimulation in human females is unknown. In female rats, progesterone promoted estrogenic sexual stimulation only over a short period (about 24 hours), after which the rats became refractory to further sexual stimulation (Gorski, 1976).

Research has indicated that facilitation of female rat sexual behavior is generally dependent on the presence of estrogen (Beach, 1976). The combination of progesterone and estrogen noticeably increases active proceptive (female-initiated) sexual behavior toward males (Fadem, Barfield, & Whalen, 1979). However, further increases or inhibition of progesterone-induced proceptive behavior with progesterone administered over many days has not been investigated systematically, nor have we learned much from research involving drugs with opposite effects. Administration of the progesterone antagonist RU 486 (mifepristone, also known as "the abor-

Table 6.2 *Available Natural and Synthetic Progestational Agents*

Natural	
Progesterone	Micronized for oral use (50, 100 mg); vaginal suppository (25, 50, 100, 400 mg); injectable in oil (25, 50, 100 mg/Ml)
Synthetic	
Levonorgestrel	Norplant contraceptive (subdermal implant)
Medroxyprogesterone acetate	Provera (2.5, 5, 10 mg); Depo-Provera (100 or 400 mg/Ml); Amen, Curretab, Cyorin (10 mg)
Megestrol acetate	Megace (sex offender drug) (20, 40 mg)
Norethindrone	Norlutin (5 mg)
	Micronor, Nor-Q D (the minipill) (0.35 mg)
Norethindrone acetate	Norlutate, Aygestin (5 mg)
Norgestrel	Ovrette (the minipill) (0.75 mg)
Progesterone-estrogen oral contraceptive combinations:	
Norethindrone (NE) combinations with ethinyl estradiol (EE)	
Norethin 1/35 E	1.0 mg NE and 35 mcg EE
Norinyl 1 + 35	1.0 mg NE and 35 mcg EE
Ortho Novum 1/35	1.0 mg NE and 35 mcg EE
Brevicon	0.5 mg NE and 35 mcg EE
Modicon	0.5 mg NE and 35 mcg EE
Ovcon 35	0.4 mg NE and 35 mcg EE
Loestrin 1/20	1.0 mg NE (acetate form) and 20 mcg EE
Ortho Novum 10/11	0.5/1.0 mg NE biphasic and 35 mcg EE
Ortho Novum 7/7/7	0.5/1.0 mg NE triphasic and 35 mcg EE
Tri-Norinyl	0.5/1.0 mg NE triphasic and 35 mcg EE
Norgestrel/levonorgestrel (NG/LNG) combinations with ethinyl estradiol (EE)	
Lo/Ovral	0.3 mg NG and 30 mcg EE
Levlen	0.15 mg LNG and 30 mcg EE
Nordette	0.15 mg LNG and 30 mcg EE
Tri-Levlen	0.05–0.125 mg LNG triphasic and 30–40 mcg EE
Triphasil	0.05–1.25 mg LNG and 30–40 mcg EE
Ethynodid diacetate (ED) combinations with ethinyl estradiol (EE)	
Demulen 1/35	1.0 mg ED and 35 mcg EE

tion pill") to female rats has not yet been shown to have clear effects on their sexual behavior (van der Schoot & Baumgarten, 1992).

Shively, Manuck, Kaplan, and Koritnik (1990) studied social and sexual interactions among 30 adult female cynomolgus monkeys (*Macaco fascicularis*) treated for eight months with either Ovral (0.05 mg ethinyl estradiol/0.5 mg norgestrel), Demulen (0.05 ethinyl estradiol/1.0 mg ethynodiol diacetate), or no treatment (control). Ten monkeys were in each treatment group and all monkeys lived in social groups of five females each. Once a week a vasectomized male monkey was placed in each social group for 50 minutes. Generally, interfemale social behavior and time spent alone were influenced by hierarchy/status factors but not by oral contraceptive treatment. However, time spent in affiliative passive body contact was reduced by Ovral (containing norgestrel). In reaction to the presence of the male monkey, dominant females aggressively interfered with sexual approach attempts by subordinate females among controls, but this aggressive sexual competitive behavior was apparently suppressed in oral contraceptive-treated females. Oral contraceptive treatment did not affect frequency of sexual intercourse with males, but males ejaculated less with Ovral (norgestrel)-treated monkeys (mean rate of 1 per 50-minute test) than with controls (mean rate of 3.7) or with Demulen-treated females (mean rate of 4.3). Oral contraceptive treatment did not affect rate of male sexual approach, copulation initiatives, or rate of female receptivity. The doses of norgestrel used in this study were comparable (adjusted for each monkey's weight) to those used by Dennerstein et al. (1980), who also noted a negative sexual effect of norgestrel added to ethinyl estradiol. The progestogen in Demulen (ethynodiol diacetate) is less androgenic and more estrogenic than norgestrel.

PROGESTERONES IN CONTRACEPTION

Oral contraceptives prevent ovulation by eliminating peak secretions from the hypothalamus and pituitary, which normally trigger ovulation. Oral contraceptive research began in the United States about 1950, when Gregory Pincus, supported by Margaret Sanger, began experiments on the inhibition of ovulation by progesterone derivatives (a concise history of the development of contraceptive steroids can be found in Henzl, 1993). Oral progesterone itself was tested in female volunteers in 1953 by Pincus and Boston gynecologist John Rock. However, progesterone was associated with excessive breakthrough bleeding, so that stronger synthetic progestogens were needed. A derivative of testosterone, with little androgenic activity due to the removal of a methyl side chain, 19-nor-testosterone was developed by Carl Djerassi's group during 1951. A potent progestational agent, 19-nor-progesterone, and another, 19-nor-testosterone derivative, were synthesized, and to this day, progestogens are either norethindrone or norgestrel products.

The first estrogen-progestogen combination oral contraceptive was marketed in the United States in 1960. Addition of the synthetic estrogens (either ethinyl estradiol or mestranol) reinforced pituitary inhibition by progestogens, allowing reductions in dose for safety without loss of efficacy (Goldzieher, 1993). All oral contraceptives, except the progestogen-only minipill, contain either ethinyl estradiol or mestranol. Physiological estrogen, estradiol-17-beta, does not have a sufficiently potent pituitary inhibiting effect. Note that physiological estradiol and the conjugated estrogens used for menopausal estrogen replacement are not sufficiently potent for use in oral contraceptives, and the synthetic estrogen, ethinyl estradiol, is probably too potent for use as estrogen replacement.

Progestogens are widely used as female oral contraceptives because they reliably and safely suppress the mid-cycle gonadotrophin peaks that trigger ovulation. Progestogens chiefly inhibit luteinizing hormone secretion, while estrogens more potently suppress follicle-stimulating hormone. Progestogens, which can be used alone (without estrogen) as an oral contraceptive (i.e., the "minipill"), may lower DHEA/DHEAS in addition to lowering testosterone. Medroxyprogesterone is far less potent than norethindrone or norgestrel, which are used for contraception at doses of 1 mg or less. Klove, Roy, and Lobo (1984) found decreased DHEAS in normal women after four to five months of treatment with oral contraceptives containing norethindrone (Ortho-Novum, Ovcon), but not from an oral contraceptive containing levonorgestrel (Nordette), or the levonorgestrel implant, Norplant. Vermeulen and Thiery (1982) and Gaspard, Dubois, Gillain, Franchimont, and Duvivier (1984) found only nonsignificant reductions of DHEAS after six months treatment with levonorgestrel triphasic oral contraceptives. Injectable medroxyprogesterone (Depo-Provera) used as an oral contraceptive was found to lower DHEAS levels by Trienekens, Schmidt, and Thijssen (1986).

Our clinical impression is that norgestrel progestogens in oral contraceptives such as Triphasil cause androgenic side effects (such as acne) that are not caused by oral contraceptives containing norethindrone. Agitation and tension (suggestive of androgenic stimulation) also seem more frequent with oral contraceptives containing norgestrel than with those containing norethindrone. The sexual consequences of this apparent androgenic effect of norgestrel are unknown.

There is no doubt that most oral contraceptives, including current low-dose versions, more or less reduce both total and free testosterone by about 16–60% (the decrease in free testosterone is usually, but not always, greater than in total testosterone [Bancroft et al., 1980; Bancroft & Sartorius, 1990; Jung-Hoffman & Kuhl, 1987; Kuhl, Gahn, Romberg, März, & Taubert, 1985; Kuhnz, Sostarek, Gansau, Louton, & Mahler, 1991]). However, it is unclear to what extent the reduction of testosterone in pill users affects sexual desire and activity. Differences in frequency of intercourse and masturbation and in levels of sexual motivation and enjoyment are rarely found between oral contraceptive pill-user groups and non-user groups (Bancroft & Sartorius, 1990). Differences in sexual behavior between pill users and non-users are confounded by the fact that pill users are more likely to have intercourse, given that they use the pill for contraception during, or in anticipation of, intercourse. However, differences are also not found (or are found in favor of pill-user groups) when only sexually active non-users and pill users are compared (Bancroft, Sherwin, Alexander, Davidson, & Walker, 1991). Bancroft et al. (1980) compared 20 women complaining of sexual problems due to oral contraceptives to 20 pill users without sexual problems. While there were clear differences in sexual desire and behavior, androgens were abnormally low in both pill-user groups, with and without sexual problems. Furthermore, sexual difficulties were not improved when users with sexual problems were given androgen supplements.

In the early days of birth control pills, the progestogen dosages used were sufficiently high to interfere markedly with women's sexual response. Today it appears that the levels of progestogen used in birth control pill combinations (as well as for postmenopausal estrogen replacement therapy) are sufficiently low to minimize, if not eliminate, these adverse sexual properties. At this time, there is no reliable evidence that moderate doses of progestogens suppress sexual desire or response, despite lowering testosterone levels and often lowering general mood. However, further controlled research is clearly needed. In the meantime, if a patient complains of decreased sex drive when given progestogens, the lowered sexuality should be assumed to be a true effect of progestogen treatment until controlled research trials indicate that such a negative sexual effect does not exist. When a patient experiences unpleasant symptoms from one form of progestogen (e.g., norgestrel), whether on oral contraceptives or postmenopausal cyclic progestogen therapy, another form of progestogen (e.g., norethindrone) may be more comfortable.

Studies up to 1970 on the sexual and mood effects of oral contraceptives indicated a greater incidence of loss of libido and depression in women taking contraceptives with higher progestogen content (Cullberg, 1972; Grant & Pryse-Davies, 1968). Unfortunately, many physicians are more aware of the conclusions of this 30-year-old research than they are of more current work. However, with the lower estrogen and progestogen content of current oral contraceptives, sexual and mood effects appear far less frequently and are milder when they do occur (Kay, 1984). Lowered sexual desire with these low-dose contraceptives may be due to either the progestogen component or to the synthetic ethinyl estradiol suppression of natural estradiol and LHRH activity.

Despite the frequent report of adverse sexual effects of oral contraceptives high in estrogen and progestogen content, Glick and Bennett (1981) have shown that most studies during the 1960s showed a far greater incidence of increased sex drive on oral contraceptives (18–54% increased) than decreased sex drive (0–13% decreased). Such positive effects of oral contraceptives containing progestogens are apparently due to the practical benefits of reliable contraception, which may far outweigh less evident changes in sexual desire and mood. Perhaps the most powerful test of progestogens' negative sexual potential would be to give them to very assertive, easily orgasmic women (e.g., Meshorer & Meshorer, 1986), who may be most aware of and bothered by inhibitory effects.

A further confounding variable in ascertaining the impact of oral contraceptives on sexual function has been the discovery that oral contraceptives may cause vitamin B_6 (pyridoxine) deficiency, which may lead to depression if not corrected by vitamin B_6 supplementation (Parry & Rush, 1979). Oral contraceptives may also suppress endogenous levels of progesterone (Dalton, 1990), thereby increasing feelings of anxiety that can interfere with sexual desire and activity.

In essence, the research pertaining to the sexual side effects of contraceptives is deceiving because early studies were performed on much higher dosages than those in use today, and various psychological features compete with biochemical effects. Relief from fear of pregnancy may outweigh the sexual depressant effect of progesterone, such that the net result is improved interest and responsiveness. However, if all other psychological and physiological variables remain constant, the addition of progesterone can be expected to diminish sexual desire and responsiveness.

Depot medoxyprogesterone supplementation with testosterone enanthate has also been clinically tested as a reversible male contraceptive (Wu & Aitken, 1989), but its use in men at doses necessary for contraception seems unlikely, given the complications of testosterone supplementation and excessive side effects in men.

Norplant

Norplant is a system of subdermal levonorgestrel capsules set for minimal release so that contraception occurs for two to five years after the rods are inserted (Shoupe & Mishell, 1989). Its mechanisms of action include suppression of ovulation at least 50% of the time, conversion of the cervical mucus to a "thick and scanty" state so that sperm cannot penetrate the cervix to the uterus/ova, and suppression of endometrial growth due to continuous exposure to low levels of progestogen (Shoupe & Mishell, 1989). Since it is implanted, there can be no failures as a result of user noncompliance, a particularly important feature for adolescents and women who may not follow instructions rigorously. The most common side effect is irregular menstrual bleeding, which lasts from three to six months to a year (Shoupe & Mishell, 1989). Since levonorgestrel has some residual androgenic potency (it is a testosterone derivative) about 5–20% of women may experience acne and, we expect, as yet unexplored psychological effects. Five percent of users also experience weight gain (Shoupe & Mishell, 1989).

Norplant was first marketed in the United States in February, 1991. Surveillance at Johns Hopkins Medical Clinic in Baltimore since May of 1991 produced the following response information (van Amerongen, 1994): Through the first 14 months, 1,074 systems were implanted and 22 removed (after counseling). Removal occurred in seven (31.8%) cases due to irregular bleeding, four (18.1%) due to headache, three (13.6%) due to hair loss, and three due to nausea, fatigue, and lethargy (van Amerongen, 1994). Seventeen of 22 removals occurred at six months or less and none occurred after 12 months. Twelve of 21 women switched to oral contraceptives and five of the 21 became pregnant within six months of Norplant removal.

While there has been recent media reports of

frequent problems with Norplant side effects and difficulty in removal, there is as yet insufficient documentation of these problems in the literature. A particularly interesting case in our clinical practice was that of an 18-year-old young woman suffering from panic attacks and agoraphobia. Upon removal of Norplant after about two years of use, the woman experienced an extreme chronic exacerbation of her panic symptoms, which required treatment with an SSRI antidepressant. This case should serve as a reminder that progestogens have tranquilizer, anticonvulsant, sedative, and anesthetic properties (MacDonald, Dombroski, & Casey, 1991), so that chronic continuous treatment with even very low doses may result in severe withdrawal/rebound anxiety in susceptible individuals.

Mifepristone (RU 486)

Mifepristone (RU 486) is the new antiprogesterone steroid that has gained medical acceptance as a method of non-surgical abortion in France, Sweden, and Great Britain (despite enormous controversy that centers on its "abortion pill" repercussions). It is approved to be used in conjunction with a uterine contractive prostaglandin (usually oral misoprostol, approved as an anti-ulcer drug in the United States). By itself, mifepristone causes about an 80% rate of abortion, but when combined with prostaglandin, its success rate is about 96% (Ulmann, Teutsch, and Philibert, 1990, give an excellent review of its early clinical testing). Ulmann et al. (1992) report a 95.3% success rate in 15,709 women treated at 300 medical centers in France after its introduction in 1990.

Mifepristone is given as a 600 mg oral dose after counseling at a clinic, followed by clinic administration of the prostaglandin two days later (Thong & Baird, 1992; Ulmann et al., 1992). After prostaglandin administration for abortion, the patient is kept at the clinic for a few hours to monitor for adverse effects such as bleeding, nausea, vomiting, abdominal pain, diarrhea, fainting, and cramping (many of the gastrointestinal symptoms are due to the prostaglandin, not to mifepristone). Bleeding and residual gastrointestinal and pelvic upset may continue for many days for some women. Ulmann et al. (1992) report a median duration of bleeding of 8 days, and 12 days or less in 90% of cases. Continued bleeding required vacuum aspiration or dilatation and curettage in 0.8% of the 15,709 cases reviewed. If pregnancy termination is not achieved with mifepristone/prostaglandin, surgical abortion is usually performed.

Due to rare but possible cardiovascular complications, mifepristone/prostaglandin pregnancy termination is prohibited in France for women over 35, regular smokers, or women with any indication of cardiovascular pathology (Ulmann et al., 1992). For the first 60,000 mifepristone abortions performed in France up to 1992, there were three heart attacks, one fatal (Ulmann et al., 1992). Mifepristone may be used for abortion from six to nine weeks of pregnancy (49 to 63 days from the first day of the last menstrual period) (Thong & Baird, 1992; Ulmann et al., 1992). The rate of severe complications is considerably less than surgical abortion, particularly in regard to the risk of infection.

Grow and Wiczyk (1994) give a comprehensive review of the possible clinical applications of mifepristone and other antiprogestogens and the recent research and testing for these applications, which include postcoital contraception, treatment of endometriosis, gynecological tumors (leimyomata), breast cancer, labor induction, and even brain tumors (meningioma). Mifepristone also has strong antiglucocorticoid effects, which may be used to treat glaucoma or hypercortisolism due to Cushing's syndrome (Grow & Wiczyk, 1994). Mifepristone is the most promising contraceptive since, by antagonism of progesterone, which is required for fetal growth and protection, it provides a natural way to prevent fetal development.

Contraceptive Vaccines

Contraceptive vaccines are still in an early stage of development and clinical testing (Aldhous, 1994). Vaccines to keep the egg and sperm apart, or to suppress or disable sperm, have only reached the testing stage in primates. The two vaccines in current human efficacy testing work by producing antibodies (immunity) against human chorionic gonadotropin (hCG), the hormone from the fertilized egg, which is measured to indicate pregnancy in blood and urine tests. This hormone is necessary for the fertilized egg to implant itself in the uterus, and is produced by the developing embryo prior to implantation. Though this vaccine appears to be quite reversible (frequent booster shots are currently required to keep it going), its efficacy is still considerably below oral contraceptives and there is concern that it may adversely produce antibodies to other pituitary gland secretions.

PROGESTERONE AND PREMENSTRUAL SYNDROME

Progesterone is implicated as both cause and cure for premenstrual syndrome. It is thought that natural progesterone is responsible for some PMS symptoms, since the drug is known to cause irritability and a certain type of protective (maternal) aggressiveness. Women with prior histories of premenstrual irritability seem to show increased disturbance when started on oral contraceptives high in synthetic estradiol, while women without pre-existing premenstrual irritability seem to become depressed more frequently when taking contraceptives with higher progestogen content (Cullberg, 1972).

While Katharina Dalton (1990) has used natural progesterone injections or suppositories to treat PMS symptoms, placebo-controlled trials generally have not shown significant benefits (Freeman, Rickels, Sondheimer, & Polansky, 1990; Maddocks, Hahn, Moller, & Reid, 1986; Rausch & Parry, 1987). Furthermore, even Dalton has insisted that synthetic progestational agents do not have any beneficial effect on PMS and, in contrast to natural progesterone, may even exacerbate these symptoms (Dalton, 1990). Dennerstein et al. (1985) found marginally significant improvements in stress, anxiety, and tissue swelling in 23 PMS women treated for two months with 300 mg oral micronized natural progesterone compared to a two-month period on placebo, but drowsiness was a bothersome side effect. Studies of postmenopausal women treated with cyclic progestogens added to estrogen replacement therapy have shown that the progestogens can produce negative moods and physical symptoms similar to those experienced in PMS (Backstrom, Bixo, & Hammarback, 1985; Holst et al., 1989; Magos et al., 1986).

Chan, Mortola, Wood, and Yen (1994) note that there are no consistent findings that relate luteal phase levels of endogenous progesterone to PMS, and the majority of studies find no differences. Consequently, they hypothesize that it could be progesterone receptor disturbances rather than progesterone per se that is responsible for PMS. To test this hypothesis, they treated seven women who had PMS with low doses (5 mg) of the progesterone antagonist RU 486 (mifepristone) or placebo for three months during the luteal phase of the menstrual cycle. Improvement occurred with both placebo and RU 486, and there were no differences between the two groups. A prior study that used higher dose RU 486 also failed to show significant amelioration of PMS symptoms (Schmidt et al., 1991). If PMS were caused by aberrant or insufficient action of progesterone receptors or insufficient levels of progesterone, use of RU 486 could be expected to worsen the symptoms compared to placebo; instead RU 486 and placebo produced equivalent improvement.

POSTMENOPAUSAL PROGESTERONE SUPPLEMENTS

Progesterone supplements are needed to prevent endometrial hyperplasia (cancer) by regularly "bleeding the uterus" as an adjunct to estrogen supplementation in naturally postmenopausal women who are predisposed toward endometrial cancer. (Progestogens are often routinely given to hysterectomized women, who may receive no medical benefit from them and many of the negative side effects.) In the early 1970s, progestogens were given cyclically for five to seven days each month, which was often insufficient to reverse endometrial hyperplasia. Even ten days of cyclic progestogen each month may leave an occurrence of endometrial hyperplasia 1.6% of the time; consequently, 12-to-14-day usage is currently recommended (Gambrell,

1992). Typically, 5–10 mg/day of medroxyprogesterone (Provera) or norethindrone is prescribed. However, with the use of 12-to-14-day cycles, lower doses may be sufficient (2.5 mg/day medroxyprogesterone or 1–2.5 mg/day norethindrone).

Cyclic progestogen treatment is rejected by many women due to the inconvenience of resumed menstrual bleeding. A recent alternative has become increasingly popular, which consists of continuous combined treatment of low-dose estrogen and progestogen. During the initial four to 12 months of continuous treatment, there may be unpredictable breakthrough bleeding, which some women find intolerable. However, within a year the endometrium typically becomes atrophic and bleeding stops altogether. The continuous use of lower progestogen doses (2.5 mg medroxyprogesterone or 1 mg or less of norethindrone) avoids some progestational side effects, and the avoidance of regular bleeding makes adjunct progestogen use acceptable to more women.

According to current literature, sexual side effects of this treatment approach appear to be minimal to non-existent. An investigation by Sherwin (1991) of naturally menopausal women ages 47 to 57 treated with conjugated estrogen (Premarin) combined with either 11-day cyclic medroxyprogesterone (Provera) or placebo for one year showed decreased testosterone with 0.625 mg conjugated estrogen and 5 mg medroxyprogesterone but no difference in sexual desire, and only nonsignificantly less sexual arousal with 0.625 estrogen (Premarin) and 5 mg medroxyprogesterone compared to 0.625 estrogen and placebo. However, women given 0.625 estrogen and 5 mg medroxyprogesterone showed more overall dysphoric mood than those on 0.625 estrogen alone, or placebo.

In a double-blind crossover study of 49 hysterectomized-ovariectomized women given (1) estradiol, (2) the progestogen levonorgestrel, (3) estradiol and levonorgestrel, or (4) placebo, there were some positive sexual effects of estradiol alone when compared to placebo and a slight inhibitory effect with levonorgestrel alone (Dennerstein et al., 1980). The Dennerstein study intentionally gave different hormonal combinations to test their mood effects, not to treat hysterectomized women in general clinical practice.

CHEMICAL CASTRATION

Understanding of the sexual properties of progestogens may come from continued study of their administration for sex offenders (Berlin, 1981). For the past 30 years, medroxyprogesterone has been used in Europe and the United States to suppress deviant male sexual behaviors, including rape, exhibitionism, voyeurism, and other paraphilias (Cooper, 1986). While medroxyprogesterone also has been used to treat non-sexual aggressive behaviors (Blumer & Migeon, 1975), it may be insufficient to treat violent sex offenders effectively (Walker, Meyer, Emory, & Rubin, 1984). In Europe, the progesterone derivative cyproterone acetate (CPA) has received more attention than medroxyprogesterone (Bradford, 1988; Bradford & Pawlak, 1993).

In the United States, medroxyprogesterone treatment of sexual offenders began in the 1960s at John Hopkins Sexual Disorders Clinic, which remains a major treatment center for paraphilias (Money, 1987). Medroxyprogesterone is used in its injectable form, Depo-Provera. Treatment begins with weekly doses of 300–500 mg (note that these doses are far higher than those used in women for hormone replacement or contraception). Maintenance doses of 150–800 mg per week are titrated individually. Gottesman and Schubert (1993) treated seven male patients showing noncontact paraphilias with low-dose 60 mg/day oral medroxyprogesterone acetate for an average of 15 months. Six of the seven patients were successfully treated (no paraphilic behaviors and fewer paraphilic fantasies).

The sexually inhibitory effect of medroxyprogesterone has been attributed to its reduction of testosterone activity, but decreased sexual arousal has been noted even when measured testosterone levels do not change (Berlin & Shaerf, 1985). Within one month of medroxyprogesterone treatment, testosterone levels may decrease by more than 90%; however, deviant sexual activities have been observed to remain suppressed even when testosterone levels return toward normal, suggesting a combination of sexually depressant effects (Cooper, 1988). The decrease in testosterone is generally attributed to inhibition of the luteinizing hormone signal necessary for testosterone production (Cordoba & Chapel, 1983; Money, 1987). Medroxyprogesterone also reduces testosterone by accelerating metabolic clearance through induction of liver testosterone-A-reductase (Bradford, 1988).

At low to moderate doses, Depo-Provera has been observed (Money, 1987) to be sexually "calming or tranquilizing." Money attributed the Depo-Provera-induced decrease in sex drive, erection, and ejaculation to depression of testosterone levels and contended that these sexual changes are reversible within weeks of discontinuing the medication—a reversible form of "chemical castration." The chief non-sexual side effects are drowsiness and weight gain.

Given the criminal nature of sexual offenses, long-term placebo-controlled studies of sexual offenders are considered unethical. Wincze, Bansal, and Malamud (1986) have conducted one of the few extended placebo-controlled laboratory evaluations of the sexual effects of medroxyprogesterone. They studied three chronic pedophiliac offenders treated with medroxyprogesterone over a period of at least three months. Reductions in sexual urges and fantasies occurred on both medroxyprogesterone and placebo, indicating that either the drug effect has a strong placebo component or that patient reports were unreliable. Erections measured in the laboratory during arousal from visual erotic stimuli declined only slightly during medroxyprogesterone treatment and remained depressed during the subsequent placebo crossover. Nocturnal penile tumescence (NPT) erections decreased during medroxyprogesterone treatment, compared to no change on placebo.

Despite the inconclusive findings in their laboratory study, the authors reported that, in their clinical experience, medroxyprogesterone usually reduced pedophiliac urges and that these urges returned after discontinuing the drug. Their study indicated that the capacity for erection is not strongly reduced during medroxyprogesterone treatment, but that brain mechanisms involved in generating NPT are inhibited. Reductions in sexual urges are more difficult to determine and to some extent may involve strong placebo effects. It should be noted that chronic treatment with depot medroxyprogesterone may induce or exacerbate osteoporosis in both men and women (Cundy et al., 1991), though such negative effects on bone density is not seen with natural progesterone (Dalton & Dalton, 1991).

PROSTATE CANCER

Progestogens, typically megestrol (Megace), are also used to treat men with prostate cancer (Geller, Nelson, Albert, & Pratt, 1979). As a progestational antiandrogen, megestrol blocks DHT receptors and inhibits 5-alpha reductase. Since megestrol potently reduces DHEA/DHEAS and powerfully inhibits male sexual desire, it may be that a decrease in DHEA/DHEAS is an additional cause of the drug's negative sexual effect in the majority of prostate patients (marked loss of libido occurs in 50–70% [Donkervoort et al., 1975; Geller et al., 1979]).

A promising alternative to megestrol for treatment of benign prostatic hypertrophy (BPH) and prostate cancer is the 5-alpha-reductase inhibitor finasteride (Proscar) (MK-906), which was approved for marketing in the United States in 1992 (Stoner, 1994). Finasteride blocks the enzymatic conversion of androgens to peripheral testosterone (DHT). At this early stage of clinical use over the past three years, the sexual side effects reported include impotence (5%), decreased libido (4.8%), and ejaculation disorders (3.5%), and are the most prevalent side effects of this drug (Stoner, 1994). Otherwise, finasteride shows impressive efficacy and safety and deserves widespread use for symptomatic treatment of BPH. Finasteride does not appear to decrease non-peripheral circulating testosterone and does not decrease DHEA/DHEAS levels (Rittmaster, Antonian, New, & Stoner, 1994). Currently, finasteride is chiefly prescribed for BPH (Stoner, 1994). Since male-pattern baldness is peripheral testosterone DHT-dependent, finasteride topical treatment of baldness is currently being tested and appears very promising (Dallob et al., 1994).

Gonadotrophin Hormone-Releasing Agonist: Alternative to Progestogens

A safer and more reliable form of chemical castration to treat paraphilias may be the use of a synthetic, potent, long-acting gonadotrophin hormone-releasing agonist (GnRHa) given by injection daily or even monthly. Thibaut, Cordier, and Kuhn (1993) used such an agent (triptorelin 3.75 mg per month injection) to treat six men with severe paraphilia. Deviant sexual behavior was fully suppressed in five men within a month and suppression continued during follow-ups that varied from seven months to three years. One patient stopped treatment at the end of one year and relapsed within 10 weeks. Sexual fantasies and activities were also markedly decreased. Clinical improvement paralleled the gradual decrease of plasma testosterone levels to castration levels during the first month of treatment.

Rousseau, Couture, Dupont, Labrie, and Couture (1990) reported a single case of a severe exhibitionist who had openly masturbated in public libraries over 2,000 times (three to six times per week). Within a month of being treated with daily GnRH agonist injections, supplemented daily with the oral antiandrogen flutamide, excess and exhibitionist masturbation had ceased, and the patient was able to continue normal sexual activity (coitus, masturbation in private, and occasional sexual fantasies). However, cessation of treatment after 26 weeks resulted in rebound elevation of testosterone and greater than baseline masturbatory activity. Disturbances upon withdrawal of treatment could be an unpredictable and dangerous complication of extended GnRHa therapy for paraphilia.

Many GnRH agonists (e.g., leuprolide/Lupron, goserelin/Zoladex, nafarelin/Synarel) are currently marketed in the United States or are in clinical testing. Given the abundance, promotion, and putative safety of GnRH agonists, and knowledge gained during their extensive clinical testing as a male contraceptive (e.g., Doelle et al., 1983) and in prostate cancer treatment (DeBruyne et al., 1988; Denis et al., 1993; Parmar, Edwards, Phillips, Allen, & Lightman, 1987; Smith, Jr., 1987), depot GnRH agonists may soon become the treatment of choice for testosterone-related paraphilias (Richer & Crisman, 1993). However, there is some evidence that gonadal suppression by long-term GnRH agonist treatment of humans may not be completely reversible (Decensi et al., 1989; Rolandi et al., 1988; Smith, Jr., & Urry, 1985). GnRHa treatment for male contraception is often combined with supplemental testosterone for maintenance of libido (Doelle et al., 1993). Consequently, evaluation of the efficacy and side effects of these agents should prove to be an extended, convoluted process over the next 10 years. Additionally, direct GnRH antagonists can be expected to be developed as alternatives to present GnRH agonists.

GnRH agonists also have varied treatment applications in women, including menstrual cycle manipulation in preparation for in vitro fertilization, female contraception, treatment of endometriosis, fibroids, uterine leimyomata, hirsutism, and menstrual cycle disorders (Andreyko, Marshall, Dumesic, & Jaffe, 1987). Side effects typical of estrogen withdrawal, such as hot flushes, can be expected with such use. Testosterone is also decreased, which could cause reduced sexual drive.

7

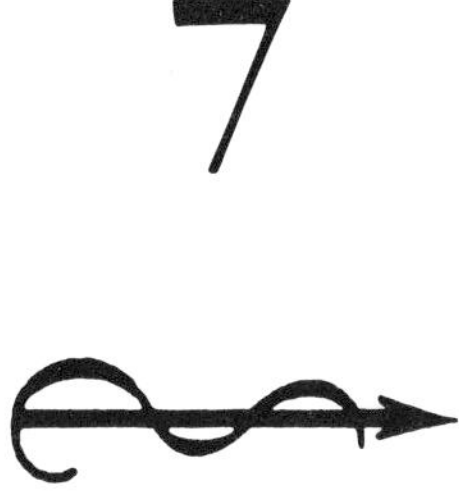

Testosterone in Women

OBJECTIVES

- To illustrate the dynamic role of testosterone in women
- To examine the effects of testosterone treatment for sexual dysfunction in women
- To define significant differences in testosterone activity between surgically-induced and natural menopause
- To evaluate the role of testosterone replacements and supplements

Historically, testosterone has been considered "the male sex hormone" because there is over 10 to 20 times more testosterone in men than in women. However, as we have become more sophisticated in our understanding of this hormone, we have learned that it plays a pronounced role in women, particularly in regard to sex drive.

The female sex drive is more complex than that of the male and, consequently, more difficult to study. Men, as far as we know, have one basic sex drive pattern, which is predominantly governed by testosterone. Women have several sex drive patterns, which are governed by a multitude of cycling hormones. These patterns change from day to day, depending upon the particular combination of sex hormones circulating through the female system.

The two most prominent sex drives in the human female are the *receptive* sex drive and the active, *aggressive* sex drive. The receptive sex drive is governed primarily by estrogen; it is responsible for a woman's desire for penetration and motivates her to have sex with a partner rather than masturbate. The aggressive sex drive, by contrast, is governed by testosterone, and promotes a woman's interest in genital sex, including her drive for orgasm. It also promotes masturbation more than coitus. Progesterone, which fluctuates naturally throughout a woman's cycle, is a formidable sexual deterrent, eliminating lust, desire, and receptivity (diminishing her sex drive) and making her more nurturant, more interested in cuddling and holding, and less desirous of genital stimulation. Progesterone has essentially the same effect in both sexes. When prescribed for men, it eliminates sex drive quite efficiently.

While testosterone appears to be a significant determinant in a woman's active sex drive, along with DHEA and other hormones perhaps yet to be identified, there are still other substances, such as progesterone and estrogen, that compete with or complement testosterone's effect, depending on their relative concentrations in the bloodstream.

What mixture of these sexually influential hormones is present at any given time in a woman's menstrual cycle or life cycle will determine her sexual impulses. Whether and how she acts on them are influenced by other forces, such as the relationship, her values, etc. Her testosterone levels are also subject to environmental influences, which are often difficult to measure.

In the female, testosterone is produced by the ovaries; additional testosterone can be derived from adrenal steroids. The metabolism of testosterone is discussed in Chapter 8, "Testosterone in Men," because the majority of the research in this area has been limited to the male.

In addition to sex, testosterone influences other aspects of behavior, including competitiveness, irritability, assertiveness, and aggressiveness. It also appears to have some antidepressant qualities.

The relatively recent discovery of the fact that testosterone exists in both free and bound forms has confounded much of the data gathered in this area of research. Prior to the discovery of an active form of testosterone (Vermeulen & Verdonck, 1972), only total testosterone was measured, which actually included protein-bound testosterone as well as free circulating testosterone. Consequently, studies attempting to correlate total testosterone levels with sex drive or function could not identify any relationship whatsoever, because only total testosterone was measured, rather than biologically active free testosterone.

However, if the roles of free and bound testosterone are viewed as analogous to the roles of free and bound thyroid, it is easy to understand that minute amounts of free hormone are metabolically active and cannot be related to symptoms or behavior unless measured separately. Now we have the capacity to conduct separate measurements and recent studies have taken full advantage of this additional ability (Free testosterone can be approximately measured through simple salivary tests.)

Nonetheless, it is important to appreciate the fact that the bulk of research on testosterone in relation to sexual function was performed with only total testosterone as an available measure. Because total testosterone correlated either negligibly or very poorly with any sexual parameter, further studies in these directions were not considered worthwhile.

As we understand more about the properties of testosterone, the functions it performs in female physiology will become clearer. At this point in time, we know that testosterone, in concert with other hormones, promotes sex drive, affects mood, and contributes to an overall sense of well-being.

TESTOSTERONE AND THE MENSTRUAL CYCLE

In women with normal menstrual cycling, blood testosterone levels range between 20–60 ng/dl, with a progressive increase during the follicular period to a peak near ovulation, followed by a decrease as menstruation approaches (Soules, Cohen, Clifton, Brenner, & Steiner, 1987). This mild rise and fall is paralleled by free testosterone and salivary testosterone levels (Dabbs & de la Rue, 1991).

However, the circadian rhythm of testosterone shows variation far greater than changes up and down during menstrual cycle phases. Salivary testosterone levels were measured in 22 cycling women (mean age = 32) during the morning and evening across menstrual phases (Dabbs & de la Rue, 1991). Menstrual phase samples were taken at menses, a week later, at ovulation (detected with a urine LH kit) and every three days subsequent to ovulation. A similar circadian rhythm, with highest levels in the morning, was shown regardless of cycle phase. Circadian variations were much greater during each day than between menstrual cycle phases: Levels were 80% greater in the morning than in the evening, but only 12% greater in the highest week of the menstrual cycle compared to the lowest week. Menstrual cycle differences were also far less than individual differences in salivary testosterone levels. As expected, testosterone levels increased to a peak at ovulation and decreased during the luteal phase.

The relation of endogenous testosterone levels to sexual drive and behavior, even disregarding menstrual phase, is inconsistently related to positive sexual measures (Sherwin, 1988b).

Some studies have identified a high correlation of testosterone with masturbation but not with interpersonal sexuality (Myers, Dixen, Morrissette, Carmichael, & Davidson, 1990; Sanders & Bancroft, 1982), raising the possibility that testosterone chiefly enhances self-directed and self-controlled behaviors. Sanders and Bancroft (1982) found that women with higher testosterone levels had a higher masturbatory frequency. Among women who had never masturbated, however, high testosterone levels were associated with decreased sexual feelings and less sexual activity with their partners. Monti, Brown, and Corriveau (1977) also reported that the only sexual activity found to be positively correlated with testosterone levels was masturbation.

There does not appear to be as precipitous a surge in testosterone as occurs in the LH burst which signals ovulation. Since almost 50% of blood testosterone and androstenedione comes from adrenal gland precursors rather than the ovaries (Abraham, 1974), actual ovarian testosterone secretion intrinsic to the menstrual cycle may show a sharper rise and fall than is noted when overall levels are measured. The adrenal androgen DHEAS, which is chiefly (over 90%) secreted by the adrenal gland, does not show concentration changes over the menstrual cycle.

Ovulation is marked by a drop (nadir) and subsequent rise in basal body temperature. A peak level of estrogen triggers the LH surge at ovulation. The total period around ovulation, called "periovulation," normally consists of the three to four mid-cycle days during which ovulation occurs. Although many studies have shown increased sexual activity around ovulation, which is attributed to peak testosterone levels, positive sexual effects at ovulation may be due to peak estrogen levels and the potent sexual effects of peak LHRH/LH (see Part VII on Sexually Effective Drugs), which can increase sexual desire independently of testosterone. Even the expectation that sexual desire should be greatest at ovulation could cause a positive placebo effect. Testosterone increases during the follicular period (prior to ovulation), generally following the rise in estradiol. During the luteal phase there is a smaller secondary rise and fall of estradiol, while testosterone slowly drops to initial levels (Genazzani et al., 1978). Table 7.1 charts the patterns of four hormones—progesterone, estradiol, luteinizing hormone, and follicle stimulating hormone—over the course of the menstrual cycle. Testosterone is typically not included in these kinds of measurements—another reflection of the degree to which its role in female physiology is overlooked. Table 7.2 summarizes the hormonal changes involved in the normal menstrual cycle, including the androgens, testosterone, and DHEAS.

Generally, reproductive researchers have assumed that sexual interest in human females will be greatest at ovulation when estrogen and testosterone levels peak and progesterone is still very low. Some researchers have affirmed this assumption. For example, Adams, Gold, and Burt (1978) found that women not on oral contraceptives showed peak autosexual activity (masturbation, fantasies, dreams, arousal from books and films) and female-initiated heterosexual activity at ovulation (reverse cycle days 13–15). In contrast, women on oral contraceptives did not show any increase in sexual activity at this time. For an intrusive nonpill group (e.g., using diaphragm for birth control), masturbation increased during ovulation and male sexual initiations decreased. The authors suggested that ovulatory sexual peaks may be best evaluated by female-determined measures such as autosexual activity and female-initiated heterosexual activity, rather than overall intercourse frequency. Premenstrual sexual increases consistently occurred in all groups, but were considerably smaller than at ovulation.

Persky, O'Brien, and Kahn (1976) found that peak mid-cycle testosterone levels were significantly correlated with overall intercourse frequency, whereas average or baseline testosterone levels were not correlated with intercourse frequency. Persky also found that young women with more frequent sexual activity had higher ovulatory testosterone levels than less active women (Persky et al., 1976). In a subsequent study, Persky and his associates (Persky, Lief, et al., 1978) found that sexual activity correlated significantly with ovulatory testosterone levels, but not with mean testosterone levels.

Morris, Udry, Khan-Dawood, and Dawood (1987) replicated Persky's finding that periovulatory total testosterone levels significantly correlated with young couples' intercourse frequency (Persky, Lief, et al., 1978). In addition, they found a similar significant correlation between periovulatory free testosterone and intercourse. However, because the women in this study appeared to be sexually "conservative"

Table 7.1 *The Normal Menstrual Cycle*

The hormonal, ovarian, endometrial, and basal body temperature changes and relationship throughout the normal menstrual cycle.

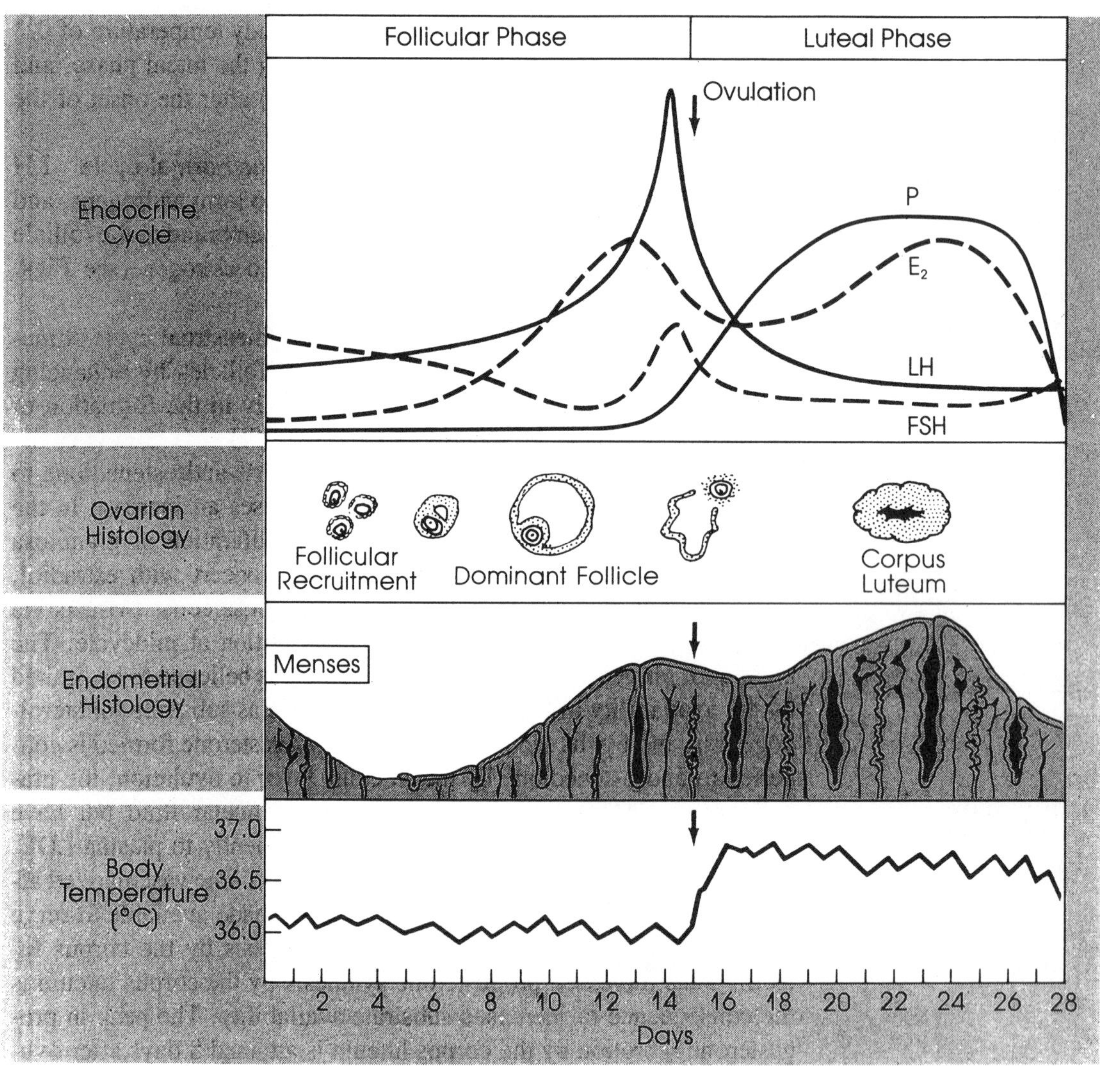

P = progesterone
E_2 = estradiol
LH = luteinizing hormone
FSH = follicle stimulating hormone

Reprinted with permission from *Harrison's Principles of Internal Medicine (11th Edition)*. Braunwald, E., et al. (Eds.). Copyright 1987 McGraw-Hill Book Company.

Table 7.2 *Hormonal Changes During Menstrual Cycle Phases*

Phase	*Hormonal Changes*
Menstruation	Minimum/low levels of estradiol and progesterone
Early follicular	Slow daily increase in estradiol Low levels of progesterone Little change in testosterone/DHEAS
Late follicular	Large daily increase in estradiol to peak level at end Low levels of progesterone Small gradual increase in testosterone No change in DHEAS
Ovulation	Large 24 hour LH surge Smaller 24 hour FSH surge Slight decrease in estradiol Increase in progesterone level begins Small increase in testosterone to peak level No change in DHEAS
Early luteal	Decrease in estradiol Large increase in progesterone Return of LH and FSH to low levels Gradual decrease of testosterone from peak level No change in DHEAS
Late luteal	Increase in estradiol to second peak (lower than follicular peak) Peak level of progesterone Gradual decrease of testosterone from peak No change in DHEAS
Premenstruum (last three days)	Precipitous drop in estradiol Precipitous drop in progesterone No change in testosterone No change in DHEAS

(only 35% initiated intercourse within the 100-day study span and only 32% reported masturbation), it was not possible to determine to what extent intercourse was determined by female choice. Males' sexual initiations did not significantly correlate with their wives' periovulatory testosterone levels.

However, other studies have reported peak sexuality at various stages of the menstrual cycle, including the mid-follicular period (days 6–9), ovulation (days 13–15), and late luteal premenstrual (days 25–28). For example, Genazzani et al. (1978) found self-reported peaks in sexual desire and activity during the early and middle follicular phases, the ovulatory phase, and the premenstruum. These times correspond hormonally to the initial rise in testosterone levels (follicular), the peak in testosterone levels (periovulatory), and the precipitous decline in progesterone (premenstruum).

In one study that measured intercourse frequency throughout the menstrual cycle, Hedricks, Piccinino, Udry, and Chimbira (1987) found that the highest rate of intercourse occurred on the day of the luteinizing hormone (LH) surge, when estradiol, and possibly testosterone, have reached peak levels. The increased coital rate may have occurred due to increased female sex drive and attention, increased initiative and assertiveness, or increased attractiveness to the male partner, who may even have coerced the women to have sex.

Dennerstein et al. (1994) conducted a remarkably comprehensive study of sexual and mood changes in relation to the menstrual cycle. Patients formed three groups: (1) a *premenstrual syndrome group* (n = 65) with negative symptoms limited to the late luteal/premenstrual period; (2) a *menstrual distress group* (n = 51) with persistent negative symptoms throughout the cycle that are exacerbated premenstrually; and (3) a *no change group* (n = 34) without significant negative mood or distress. Daily 24-hour urine samples were collected for hormone analysis and to confirm menstrual phase changes. Though it is difficult to tell from the article, the premenstrual period apparently consisted of about the last six days of the cycle prior to menses. Rated sex interest increased during the follicular phase, with a nonsignificant peak at ovulation; it significantly decreased during the luteal and premenstrual phases, with somewhat lower-rated sexual interest during the premenstrual phase compared to the luteal phase in both the premenstrual syndrome and menstrual distress groups. Well-being ratings showed changes in the sex interest ratings. Urinary estrogens and pregnanediol levels showed no significant correlations with either sex interest or well-being. Unfortunately, measurements of testosterone levels and sexual activity were not reported in this article.

In a 1981 review of studies reporting sexual peaks during the menstrual cycle, several sexual peaks were found: Eight studies showed peaks at ovulation, 17 studies showed peaks premenstrually, 18 showed follicular peaks, four identified peaks during menstruation, others showed no peaks at all, some studies concluded that women do not have sexual cycles (Schreiner-Engel, Schiavi, Smith, & Shite, 1981). In the discussion section of this review article, the authors presented an extended examination of the studies that reported no sexual response changes during the ovulatory phase despite significantly higher testosterone levels.

Despite confusion over how many days constitute the premenstrual period (we believe sexual urge may increase for just the three days prior to menses), it appears from past and recent studies that sexual measures reach a low during the luteal phase and menses, while there may be a slight peak around ovulation, perhaps due to testosterone. This peak may also be due to peak estradiol at ovulation. We can be more sure that sexual interest and activity typically decrease during the luteal phase elevation of progesterone. Three subsequent laboratory studies of subjective and vaginal response arousal to erotic stimuli have reported no differences between menstrual phases (Hoon, Bruce, & Kinchloe, 1982; Meuwissen & Over, 1992; Morrell et al., 1984). Thus there is some evidence against the commonly held view that women are normally more physically responsive during sex occurring around ovulation. Sensitivity to genital sensations and reactions to possible pheromonal cues may also vary throughout the menstrual cycle, as a result of complex chemical interactions we have not yet defined.

Phillips and Sherwin (1992) comprehensively reviewed the literature on cognitive changes throughout the menstrual cycle and, in their own study, measured memory, mood, and hormone levels in 25 women during the menstrual and luteal menstrual phases. Menstrual phase measurements were conducted on days 3–5 of menses (days 1–2 were avoided, due to possible distraction from physical symptoms), and luteal phase measurements were conducted on days 19–24 of the cycle (at least five days before the start of the menses). Appropriately, progesterone and estradiol were far higher during the luteal phase compared to the menstrual phase, but free testosterone levels were not significantly different between phases. There were no significant correlations between mood measures and memory task performance. Though differences between phases were small and insignificant on most tasks between phases, there was a significant decrement on a visual retention-recall task during the menstrual phase. Though this study did not include the follicular and ovulation phases, other studies reviewed by Phillips and Sherwin (1992) have generally failed to find consistent differences on various cognitive tasks that may be required during academic or work performance.

During the luteal phase when progesterone levels are high, a woman may feel a need to be "nurturant" and have a desire for touching and cuddling rather than genital sex. When progesterone drops precipitously three days prior to menstruation, there is a rather sudden reversal in the testosterone-progesterone ratio which could cause a rebound, testosterone-driven sexual increase. Though testosterone levels do not actually increase, progesterone no longer blocks testosterone receptors. However, women also may become sexually hostile and irritable in response to a rise in testosterone or dysphoric due to withdrawal from the tranquilizing effects of progesterone.

The increased sexual desire and activity experienced during the three premenstruum days may even be unrelated to testosterone and different in kind from the increase which occurs around ovulation. Certainly, it does not seem to include the general positive feelings of active well-being and assertiveness associated with the ovulatory peak. Rather, it seems associated with physical sensations and a need for genital stimulation. Unfortunately, both the characteristics of testosterone-induced sex drive in women and the increase in sex drive experienced by some women premenstrually are yet to be adequately described. Indeed, Sanders, Warner, Backstrom, and Bancroft (1983) have shown that increased sexual desire may occur despite the effects of severe, concurrent PMS symptomatology. Bancroft, Sanders, Davidson, and Warner (1983) found a peak of sexual activity during the mid-follicular and the premenstruum phases. Their sample, which included women with PMS, reported a premenstruum rise in sexuality despite a decrease in well-being. Furthermore, they found a clear mid-cycle peak of testosterone and androstenedione, which was strongly correlated with masturbatory frequency among women who masturbated, but was negatively correlated with sexual feelings and intercourse frequency in women who did not masturbate. Harvey (1987) found significant increases in orgasmic response and self-ratings of sexual pleasure and arousal during the three-day premenstruum, but female-initiated heterosexual activities and increased receptivity to male advances occurred more commonly at ovulation. On a retrospective questionnaire, 20.9% of the women reported feeling more sexual during the three-day premenstruum versus 14.9% who said they felt more sexual during ovulation, and 28.3% who noticed no differences over the course of the menstrual cycle.

The restriction of this sexual peak to the three-day premenstruum period could be explained in terms of progesterone withdrawal, which triggers dispersal of the corpus luteum, releasing blood saturated with sensory peptides (such as oxytocin) that trigger prostaglandin secretion. This "spicy" blood may cause pain and genital dysphoria or cramping, but may also mimic genital and uterine feelings of sexual stimulation during the crescendo of response toward orgasm. Whether due to premenstrual syndrome or sexual arousal, the uterus responds by becoming engorged with blood. The pelvic congestion may trigger impulses to the limbic system that are interpreted as sexual. In fact, orgasm (with its expulsive uterine contractions) relieves cramping and pelvic discomfort for some women. In any event, whether the uterine signals are mixed sexual messages or a reflexive physiological response to relieve premenstrual and menstrual symptoms, a considerable percentage of women find that their highest sexual interest occurs at this time.

Other factors contributing to this three-day period of sexual peaking may be a combination of opioid and estrogen withdrawal, which occurs even more abruptly than progesterone withdrawal and, in fact, potentiates any hypersensitivity that may occur due to progesterone withdrawal. Endorphins evidently rise during the luteal phase and then subside abruptly, premenstrually. (See Chapter 12 for information on spontaneous orgasms due to opioid withdrawal.) A secondary estradiol rise-and-fall occurs during the luteal phase (much smaller than during the follicular stage), which apparently reinforces progesterone receptor activity.

The relative increase in testosterone activity freed from progesterone inhibition in conjunction with chemical mechanisms of sexual facilitation (which typically potentiate one another) may provide another explanation for premenstrual sexual peaks. The sexually activating peptides (oxytocin, vasopressin, substance P, calcitonin gene-related peptide, LHRH) and neurotransmitters (dopamine, epinephrine), which may be stimulated by decreases in inhibitory substances such as opioids/endorphins, GABA, serotonin, estradiol, and progesterone, are mutually reinforcing with testosterone.

PSYCHOSEXUAL EFFECTS OF ENDOGENOUS TESTOSTERONE

Persky, Lief, et al. (1978) found that women with higher testosterone levels reported less depression, experienced more sexual gratification with their husbands, and showed a "greater capacity to form good interpersonal relationships." The women's testosterone levels were significantly correlated with both their husbands' and their own Locke-Wallace Marital Adjustment Scale scores. This finding indicated either that successful marital and sexual adjustment leads to high-normal testosterone levels, or that high-normal testosterone levels lead to optimum marital and sexual adjustments. Persky et al. (1982) proposed that higher testosterone levels in women will lead to better marital and sexual adjustment (what he termed "pair bonding"). His controversial position has been contradicted in other studies. Note that these authors are referring to testosterone levels in *women* as the determinant of optimal marital adjustment; male testosterone levels were not correlated with the Locke-Wallace Scale or a separate marital support measure (Persky et al., 1982).

Persky et al. (1982) added a group of 19 sexually normal postmenopausal married women (mean age = 54) to their 1978 sample of 11 normally cycling young married women (mean age = 24), and analyzed the psychosexual effects of all four androgens (testosterone, dihydrotestosterone, androstenedione, and DHEA). Beneficial effects of high normal testosterone on sexual drive and activity were shown for all circulating androgens (overall androgen levels were used instead of specific periovulatory measures). Levels of testosterone, dihydrotestosterone, and androstenedione in postmenopausal women (who apparently were not receiving any hormonal replacement supplementation) were 50–63% lower than in younger women, presumably due to reduction of ovarian secretion; DHEA was 86% lower, due to increased age and reduced ovarian secretion.

In spite of their reduced androgen levels, these postmenopausal women showed only minor and nonsignificantly reduced levels of sexual desire, arousal, initiation, and responsivity. However, intercourse frequency and Persky's sexual gratification measure showed significant 40% reductions in the postmenopausal group compared with the premenopausal group.

Sexual activity and adjustment were significantly and positively associated with higher normal androgen levels in both groups. Androgen correlations were calculated for both groups combined, because it was assumed, perhaps inappropriately, that sexual desire and activity were not significantly different between the two groups. Given the reduced variance due to the vastly increased data, even intercourse frequency was now significantly correlated with overall mean testosterone levels. This finding contrasted with the 1978 study (Persky, Lief, et al., 1978), in which only periovulatory testosterone level correlations were sufficiently large and consistent to yield a significant correlation.

Intercourse frequency and sexual gratification were significantly correlated with blood levels of all four androgens. Sexual initiation, sexual responsivity, and lack of sexual avoidance were significantly correlated only with testosterone, though other androgens showed smaller nonsignificant correlations with these measures. Orgasmic frequency was not significantly correlated with any androgen.

General mood scales, which included measures of depression, anxiety, and hostility, did not show any significant correlations with androgen levels. More surprisingly, special sexual interaction scales, including LoPiccolo and Steger's Interaction Inventory, also failed to show any significant correlations with androgen levels, indicating insignificant effects on specific sexual initiation-responsivity interactions. In contrast, Locke-Wallace Marital Adjustment Scales administered to the postmenopausal women showed both wife and husband scores to be positively and significantly correlated to each of the female androgen levels.

There is a possibility that peak periovulatory testosterone levels sensitize the sexual "system" for many weeks or show optimal capacity for brain-gonadal (hypothalamus/pituitary/gonad) functioning (Schon & Sutherland, 1960; Sopchak, 1957). Autosexual behavior and female sexual desire ratings, however, seem to correlate well with levels of testosterone (Adams et al., 1978; Persky et al., 1976).

Evidence suggesting negative effects of testosterone on sexual activity also has been reported. The Schreiner-Engel et al. 1981 study showed a decreased sexual response during the periovulatory stage. A further analysis of low and high testosterone subjects showed that, despite higher vaginal and self-reported sexual arousal during laboratory testing, high-testosterone women reported less frequent intercourse, lower sexual desire, less sexual responsiveness and satisfaction, less positive attitude toward sex, less physical exercise, poorer body-image, and more premenstrual and menstrual discomfort (Schreiner-Engel, Schiavi, Smith, & White, 1982). Some of these adverse effects can be explained by testosterone's selective impact on masturbatory behavior as opposed to sex with a partner.

Bancroft et al. (1983), however, did find a positive association of female testosterone levels with frequency of masturbation, while other measures such as sexual feelings, intercourse frequency, and subjective quality of orgasm showed insignificant negative associations. Many of the women in this study complained of PMS, which may have interfered with sexual receptivity. Also, positive correlations between testosterone levels and sexual interest/activity may only be found among women free of affective, marital, or sexual dysfunction (Bancroft et al., 1980).

TESTOSTERONE TREATMENT OF SEXUAL DYSFUNCTION IN PREMENOPAUSAL WOMEN

The physiological effects of testosterone (and other steroids such as androstenedione, DHEA, estrogen, progesterone, glucocorticoids, and mineralocorticoids) are not adequately researched at this time. Consequently, their influences on sexual function, immune function, and aging are poorly understood and replacement/supplementation is inevitably controversial. A balanced perspective based on a comprehensive overview of existing research is the physician's and therapist's most important asset in this area of pharmacology.

The first evidence from a controlled trial of a therapeutic effect of testosterone supplementation on female sexual dysfunction in premenopausal women was reported by Carney, Bancroft, and Mathews (1978), who found that sexually aversive women showed significantly more improvement with 10 mg/day sublingual testosterone (Testoral) combined with sex therapy than with 10 mg/day diazepam (Valium) combined with sex therapy. Since there was no placebo group, this finding could mean either that testosterone increased sexual function or that diazepam decreased it.

Subsequently, when testosterone was tested against placebo in a similar design, it not only failed to facilitate sex therapy, but appeared to decrease improvement compared to placebo and sex therapy groups (Mathews, 1983; Mathews, Whitehead, & Kellet, 1983). At a six-month follow-up evaluation after testosterone-placebo treatment had stopped, women who had been treated for three months with testosterone were rated as having a significantly worse sexual relationship than those treated with placebo.

The sublingual testosterone (Testoral) used in both of Mathews' studies may lack sufficient hormonal potency. The failure to confirm a beneficial effect of sublingual testosterone should not discourage further trials for treatment of female sexual dysfunction with other forms of testosterone.

Bancroft et al. (1980) found that the testosterone levels of oral contraceptive users complaining of sexual dysfunction were no different from testosterone levels in oral contraceptive users without sexual complaints (oral contraceptives lowered testosterone in both groups of women regardless of sexual function). Since treatment of sexually dysfunctional oral contraceptive users with the exogenous androgen androstenedione caused no sexual improvement, sexual dysfunction could not be attributed to an absolute androgen deficiency.

Schreiner-Engel, Schiavi, White, and Ghizzani (1989) reported normal testosterone levels in women with rigorously defined *DSM-III-R* hypoactive sexual desire, who were compared to 13 matched controls free of any sexual dysfunction and who had sexual activity weekly. Careful blood sampling throughout the menstrual cycle showed no significant differences in hormone levels between sexually hypoactive women and the control group. In fact, the peak ovulatory testosterone levels and follicular free testosterone levels of sexually hypoactive women were slightly but nonsignificantly higher than in control women. Lower testosterone levels did not appear even in a subset of the most extreme sexually hypoactive patients. (DHEA levels were not measured.)

Given the general failure to show testosterone deficits in healthy premenopausal sexually dysfunctional women, successful testosterone treatment would not be explained as correcting a deficiency; rather it would function as a pharmacological supplement. In the future, more specific measures of testosterone activity (not just gross overall levels) may show in what ways and in what circumstances female sexual desire is dependent on testosterone.

In view of the apparent reluctance to treat menopausal women with testosterone to correct menopausal physiological deficiencies, the use of testosterone supplements for "sexually sluggish" younger women is likely to be highly controversial, even if these supplements were shown to be efficacious in treating female sexual dysfunction. Robert Greenblatt's apparently routine treatment of female low sexual desire (Greenblatt, 1987), even in women with normal testosterone levels, is not sufficient to warrant wider use of testosterone supplements in premenopausal women at this time.

Increased prolactin with no evident cause occurs more often in premenopausal women than in men. While bromocriptine is normally used to treat this condition in both women and men, hyperprolactemic women with low sex drive or orgasm difficulty may be given a course of oral small-dose methyltestosterone. Although hyperprolactemia often disappears without any treatment, its occurrence in women nonetheless may signal abnormal activity of neurotransmitters such as serotonin or opioids, which can raise prolactin and lower testosterone and/or sexual responsivity. If sexual drive continues to wane after hyperprolactemia spontaneously regresses, testosterone given over two to four months may correct the problem directly or indirectly (by antagonizing serotonin, opioids, or prolactin).

As may be gleaned from this review, the data gathered in these hormonal studies can be bewildering, contradictory, and susceptible to selective attention, emphasis, and bias. Identification of consistencies between the findings of different research groups, different patient samples, different measures, and different statistical tests is difficult. However, there is sufficiently compelling correlational data to suggest that androgens (particularly testosterone) have positive effects on levels of sexual desire in women, which have not been adequately investigated.

Helen Singer Kaplan and Trude Owett (1993) have labeled states of low sexual desire as the "female androgen deficiency syndrome," characterized by markedly decreased sexual desire and fantasy, decreased orgasm, global sexual symptoms, and low circulating testosterone (plasma testosterone levels of 10 ng/ml or less compared to the normal range of 20–60 ng/ml). Kapan studied a sample of 41 women who had histories of treatment (for carcinomas and other medical conditions) with cytoxic drugs or of removal of their ovaries. Of these 41 women, 11 were grouped as "low testosterone," with plasma testosterone levels of 10 ng/ml or less; a "normal testosterone" group of 11 women had testosterone levels above 30 ng/ml. All women were currently sexually active and had been satisfied with their sex life prior to medical treatment. Significant differences in sexual dysfunction between these groups were shown for decreased orgasm and global sexual dysfunction: 100% of the low testosterone group reported these sexual complaints compared to 45% of the normal testosterone group. Other sexual symptoms, such as decreased desire and sexual avoidance, showed a nonsignificant greater prevalence in the low testosterone group. The chief sexual complaint of all the low testosterone women was "a complete loss of their spontaneously occurring feelings of sexual desire and a loss or significant decrease in the ability to become aroused in response to sexual stimulation."

Given the evidence that female sexual desire is dependent in some part on testosterone, what can explain the general reluctance to use testosterone supplementation clinically for menopausal women who have lowered testosterone levels and lowered sexual desire? Perhaps there is an underlying concern that, in addition to inducing secondary sex characteristics (increased weight in the wrong places, low voice, hirsutism, small breasts, enlarged clitoris, and acne), testosterone supplementation in women may also induce unpleasant qualities associated with male sexual expression (such as aggressiveness, surliness, raunchiness, genital overemphasis), which could distort the nature of female sexual behavior and adversely affect male/female interaction, creating a reverse of the improved "pair bonding" claimed by Persky, Lief, et al. (1978) for high-normal testosterone levels. While research in this area indicates that such an undesirable alteration of female sexuality would not be inevitable or even frequent, it could occur in some patients. It is conceivable that sexual crimes such as rape and molestation as well as crimes of assault committed by testosterone-treated women could be attributed to the treatment (or mistreatment). Ehlers, Rickler, and Hovey (1980) have reported relatively high testosterone levels (73 ng/dl) in violent female outpatients compared to nonviolent patient controls who had testosterone levels similar to normal healthy women (46.7 ng/dl vs 49 ng/dl). Among elderly women, testosterone could exacerbate harmful behavior brought on by dementia, leading to increasingly destructive behavior.

TESTOSTERONE TREATMENT OF SEXUAL DYSFUNCTION IN NATURALLY MENOPAUSAL WOMEN

Although the appearance of male secondary sex characteristics may be relatively frequent with oral supplements such as Halotestin (fluoxymesterone), liver toxicity and other major side effects are mostly avoided by testosterone injections, implants, and sublinguals. At this time, testosterone supplements (tested for use with surgical and normal menopausal women) produce higher than normal testosterone levels. Sherwin (1988b) currently is working with half-dose testosterone supplements which produce normal range testosterone levels but may have inconsistent or non-existent sexual benefits. However, Burger, Hailes, and Nelson (1987) have shown reliable resolution of low sexual desire in postmenopausal women with smaller doses (50 mg instead of 100 mg), which yield testosterone blood levels about 20% above normal.

With the advent of estrogen replacement therapy, it was assumed that estrogen supplementation alone could correct menopausal decreases in sexual desire. As noted in Chapter 5, research on estradiol during the 1970s failed to verify the anticipated effects on sexual function. During the 1980s, controlled comparisons of testosterone and estradiol supplementation generally showed the definite superiority of testosterone (with or without estradiol) in maintaining or correcting menopausal sexual desire. At this time, however, there is still minimal professional discussion of testosterone supplementation in women because, in addition to concerns about distorting female sexual function, positive comprehensive controlled trial evidence for the effect of testosterone on menopausal sexuality is relatively new.

A number of pharmacological options are in the process of being developed. Testosterone supplements delivered directly to the brain by carrier molecules (thus avoiding most adverse side effects) are theoretically possible, although such high-tech pharmacology probably will be too expensive for general use. Testosterone esters, which supply normal levels of testosterone over months with a single injection, are being developed for birth control in men by a World Health Organization task force (Nieschlag, Waites, Paulsen, & Handelsman, 1990) and may soon be available for women as an alternative to pellet implants. Transdermal patches should be available even sooner. Currently, the cost of monthly or bimonthly injections of generic testosterone enanthate or testosterone enanthate/estradiol (150 mg) is modest, making this method affordable as well as safer and more effective than available oral supplements.

Along with dopaminergic stimulants, testosterone is a possible treatment for sexual dysfunction in women with normal testosterone levels. However, given the tendency to avoid hormonal treatment other than to replace deficiencies, we expect that nonhormonal drugs such as bupropion or deprenyl, as well as specific serotonergic modification, will become more readily accepted treatment modalities. When nonhormonal treatments are not sufficiently effective, the addition of testosterone by injection or implant is a logical alternative, since dopamine and other pharmacological sexual stimulants have consistently been shown in animals to work synergistically with testosterone. Though as yet untested for treatment of low sexual desire in women, DHEA/DHEAS oral androgen supplementation may prove to be the optimal treatment, either alone or in combination with other nonhormonal sex stimulants (see Chapter 9).

TESTOSTERONE TREATMENT OF SEXUAL DYSFUNCTION IN SURGICALLY MENOPAUSAL WOMEN

Much of what we currently know about testosterone we have learned from studying surgically menopausal women who are abruptly deprived of testosterone. There is a greater incidence of depression with surgical menopause than with natural menopause. Because abrupt loss of testosterone and estrogens (from ovarian removal) seems to cause much more depression than natural withdrawal from estrogens, which does not ordinarily diminish testosterone, we wish to emphasize the hormonal consequences of hysterectomy. Typically, these consequences are minimized and described as the premature experience of natural menopause. In actuality, surgically induced menopause does *not* emulate natural menopause; it is far more abrupt and the symptoms more severe. Furthermore, since we do not yet fully appreciate all the physiological and psychological ramifications, caution is all the more in order. Yet the performance of unnecessary hysterectomies remains a disturbingly common occurrence (Ryan, Dennerstein, & Pepperell, 1989).

It has been our observation that most physicians are considerably more reluctant to remove the testicles of a man for malignant disease than to remove the uterus and/or ovaries of a woman for benign conditions. Considering that the hormonal consequences of surgical menopause are usually more severe than natural menopause, even when the ovaries are not removed, surgical remedies should be approached more conservatively. In addition, it would be appropriate to provide a woman with comprehensive information about the post-surgical consequences. In California, there is a state law requiring physicians to provide informed consent and present the alternative therapies prior to this procedure.

Richards (1974) has described a posthysterectomy syndrome that includes depressed mood, hot flushes, urinary problems, fatigue, headache, insomnia, and dizziness. For such symptoms, estrogen and testosterone replacement offers a healthier pharmacologic alternative than a combination of pain pills, benzodiazepines, or antidepressants. With estrogen, other benefits (e.g., decrease in osteoporosis, in vaginal atrophy, in cardiac morbidity) are also realized. However, the true psychological benefits of estrogen and testosterone replacement for women with somatization disorder have not yet been determined.

After menopause the ovary is still a functional endocrine organ, even though it supplies very little estrogen by direct production (Adashi, 1994). Most menopausal ovarian estrogen comes from aromatization of the androgen androstenedione. However, the menopausal ovary remains an androgen-secreting organ: It produces about 20% of total daily androstenedione (compared to 50% prior to menopause) and 40% of total daily testosterone (up from 25% prior to menopause), but this increased contribution is predominantly due to decreased testosterone from the adrenal gland. The ovary also remains responsive to gonadotropin stimulation, though far less than before menopause (Adashi, 1994).

While testosterone has long been considered a libido hormone in men and more recently in women, its sex-enhancing properties had not been convincingly identified until a series of impressive studies on hormone replacement were conducted in the 1980s by Barbara Sherwin, Morrie Gelfand, and their McGill University colleagues in Canada (Sherwin, 1988a, 1988b; Sherwin & Gelfand, 1985a, 1985b; Sherwin, Gelfand, & Brender, 1985). The initial studies reported in 1985 were performed on surgically menopausal women within a prospective, double-blind, crossover design. In all subjects, hysterectomy and bilateral oophorectomy had been performed for reasons other than malignant disease (e.g., benign uterine fibroids). The women had been in stable relationships for at least two years, had no prior history of psychological illness requiring treatment, and were in good general health.

Study 1: Sherwin and Gelfand (1985a)

This seven-month study included one month of establishing preoperative baseline values and two three-month treatment phases separated by an intervening placebo month. Each three-month phase consisted of a different treatment, which was given by injection every 28 days:

1. estradiol-testosterone combination—Climacteron (150 mg testosterone enanthate with 8.5 mg estradiol) (n = 12)
2. estradiol-alone—Delestrogen (10 mg estradiol valerate) (n = 11)
3. testosterone—Delatestryl (200 mg testosterone enanthate) (n = 10)
4. placebo—hysterectomy and oophorectomy-sesame oil injection (n = 10)
5. hysterectomy control—intact ovaries–no treatment (n = 10)

There were two control groups: Number 4 controlled for ovary removal and hormone replacement, while number 5 controlled for effects of surgery without treatment.

Subjects were evaluated on two scales: the Daily Menopausal Rating Scale (DMRS) and the Menopausal Index.

Results indicated that the control hysterectomy group with intact ovaries either showed no changes or improved. The testosterone-estradiol and testosterone-alone groups did not differ from the hysterectomy control in the menopausal index factors and were the same or somewhat better on daily energy, well-being, and appetite scales. During the placebo month, testosterone and testosterone-estradiol groups showed symptomatic worsening, while the hysterectomy control remained unchanged. During the seven months of study, the placebo group deteriorated on most measures, as did the estradiol-only group (though somewhat less than placebo). Deterioration was worst for placebo and estradiol groups during the first month of postsurgery. Interestingly, testosterone groups improved despite inadequate relief from hot flashes.

The authors commented that the relative lack of difference between estradiol replacement and placebo groups on the index of well-being was consistent with other controlled studies of hormonal replacement in surgical menopause women, suggesting a facilitative role for testosterone. They also stated that no adverse side effects of exogenous testosterone were observed or reported during the three-month treatment periods.

Study 2: Sherwin and Gelfand (1985b)

This study reported the psycho-emotional data gathered during the first study from two mood scales, which were self-administered four times during the study: the Multiple Adjective Affect Checklist (MAACL), measuring anxiety, depression, and hostility and the "Today Form" measuring current affective dimensions.

Depression scores on the MAACL increased only in the placebo group, remaining unchanged in the hysterectomy control. Depression scores in the hormonal supplement groups were unchanged or lower than at pre-surgery baseline, but increased during the placebo month prior to crossover. The androgen-treated group had the lowest depression scores and the highest hostility scores. Hostility scores in other groups did not change, except for a slight rise in the estradiol-testosterone group during the second treatment stage.

The results of this study indicated that, while estradiol was sufficient to prevent depression in subjects, the combination of testosterone and estradiol was more effective. Also, estradiol alone was not sufficient to prevent a decrease in energy and well-being.

Study 3: Sherwin, Gelfand, and Brender (1985)

This study reported the sexual data gathered during the first study* from two items on the daily DMRS scale:

1. "Indicate the degree of your sexual desire during the past 24 hours" on a scale from 0 to 7 (0 = low sexual desire; 7 = high sexual desire).
2. "Rate the level of arousal experienced during sexual activity during the past 24 hours" on a scale from 0 to 7.

Additionally, each day subjects noted the number of sexual thoughts or fantasies, number of sexual encounters with partner, and number of times orgasm had occurred during these encounters.

The hysterectomy control, testosterone, and estradiol-testosterone groups showed unchanged or increased sexual desire, arousal, and number of sexual thoughts/fantasies; the estradiol and placebo groups showed decreases in all the above. The frequency of coitus and orgasm did not differ among the five groups: It was reduced during the three months following surgery for all groups, but recovered during months five through seven. Unfortunately, the lack of measurable change in sexual activity was invalidated by failure to measure masturbation activity. In a two-year follow-up, the testosterone-treated groups still showed greater sexual desire and sexual activity than the estradiol group.

Study 4: Sherwin (1988c)

This study also reported data gathered from cognitive tests measuring short-term memory, long-term memory, and logical reasoning. Hormone-treated groups did not differ from the hysterectomy-alone control, but the placebo-treated group showed decrements on all tests. Furthermore, the cognitive performance of all hormone-treated groups decreased when they were treated with placebo during month four.

Study 5: Sherwin (1988b)

This study of surgically menopausal women (hysterectomy and oophorectomy for benign fibroids) was conducted subsequent to the research reported in Sherwin's 1985 articles (studies 1, 2, 3, 4) and examined mood benefits of hormonal treatment in well-adjusted and healthy surgically menopausal women two or more years after surgery for a period of 3.8 to 4.9 years. There were three groups: One was treated with 10 mg estradiol valerate injections (Delestrogen) each month; another with 150 mg testosterone

*It should be emphasized that data from studies 1, 2, 3, and 4 were gathered simultaneously from the same 53 women but reported separately in the three separate articles.

enanthate and 8.5 mg estradiol (Climacteron) each month; the third was left untreated. The normally scheduled monthly injection for hormonally-treated patients was initially withheld so that all women were without hormone treatment for one month. During the non-hormone month, baseline moods were recorded. The hormone-treated patients were given their hormone shot at the beginning of the next month; the untreated controls continued as before. During hormone treatment, patients were given psychological tests on days 2, 4, 8, 15, 21, and 28, along with blood sampling.

At baseline, hormone-treated patients had nonsignificant but slightly better mood scores than untreated patients, even after a month without hormone treatment. Estradiol patients had higher estradiol levels even without their prior month's shot, and the testosterone-estradiol group had much higher testosterone-estradiol levels. With reinitiation of hormonal injections, estradiol increased ten-fold in the estradiol group and four-fold in the testosterone-estradiol group. Hormone levels peaked within a week of injections and thereafter declined to baseline. Correlating with the rise in hormone levels, the testosterone-estradiol patients were less depressed, less anxious, less hostile, less tired, more clear-headed, more confident, and more energetic than untreated controls. These positive changes decreased toward baseline toward the end of the month. Similar mood improvements appeared in the estradiol group, but were approximately half that of the testosterone-estradiol group. Although this study was not placebo-controlled, it suggested that psychological/mood benefits of hormone supplementation persist many years after surgical menopause.

SIDE EFFECTS OF TESTOSTERONE TREATMENT SUPPLEMENTATION

The toxic side effects of oral testosterone treatments usually exceed the benefits in postmenopausal women. The efficacy, safety, and cost-effectiveness of monthly or bimonthly testosterone enanthate injections is not yet fully appreciated, and testosterone pellet implants have not been approved for use in this country. There is currently no medical momentum in this direction making change unlikely in the near future.* The virilizing and metabolic side effects of testosterone continue to be of concern, even though these side effects have been found to be infrequent and minor when injection and implants are administered (Greenblatt, 1987; Sherwin, 1988b). In menopausal women, hypoandrogenic states are not yet recognized as pathological and the concept of prophylactic testosterone replacement therapy is not yet widely accepted in medicine. More studies will be necessary and perhaps new forms of testosterone administration (i.e., brain delivery) before testosterone use for female menopausal sexual dysfunction becomes routine medical practice.

Sherwin (1988b) found that side effects with monthly 150 mg testosterone enanthate or testosterone-estradiol injection treatment for surgically menopausal women were minor. Of more than 1,000 women, only 15–20% experienced mild facial hirsutism, which was reversible. There were no other signs of virilization and no effect on lipoprotein lipids or liver function. Benign clitoral hypertrophy was rarely noted. Sherwin has correlated significant psychological and sexual benefits with testosterone supplementation in surgically menopausal women for up to five years.

The combination of estrogen and testosterone withdrawal after surgical menopause has considerable impact on female genitals. To some degree, the cutaneous health of human female genital structures such as the vulva is dependent on testosterone. Deslypere and Vermeulen (1985) have shown that, despite large differences elsewhere, androgen concentrations in genital tissue are nearly as great in women (labia majora and clitoris) as in men (scrotum and prostate). Skin thickness and collagen concentration in pubic structures are dependent on androgens in both sexes; androgen concentrations in female genital

*Reflecting the lack of attention to this subject, an otherwise superb handbook on gynecological care of woman's health, *Gynecology: Well-Woman Care*, edited and written by women, does not even include the word *testosterone* or *androgen* in the index (Lichtman & Papera, 1990).

tissues decrease with age much more than in men (Deslypere & Vermeulen, 1985). In addition, surgical menopause is accompanied by cutaneous blood vessel and nerve tissue atrophy (Punnonen, 1973), that are estrogen dependent. In the United States, the only approved testosterone treatment for female genital androgen deficiency problems (lichen sclerotic vulval dystrophy) is a 2% topical testosterone ointment (Sideri, Origoni, Spinaci, & Ferrari, 1994). However, various states of undiagnosed pubic dystrophy and atrophy may be due to androgen deficiency, which testosterone injections and implants could correct (Nishida et al., 1989).

Testosterone rather than estrogen is needed for reinvigoration of normal vulvar tissue growth and blood flow. It may be applied as an ointment or by injections. Testosterone is particularly effective in resolving local burning sensations unrelated to infection. The relative contribution of estrogen and testosterone to dry and sparse pubic hair is unclear, but the dryness and vaginitis resulting from estrogen loss is probably harmful to hair growth and maintenance. Treatment with androgens other than testosterone, such as DHEAS, has not been evaluated.

For many years Robert Greenblatt in the United States (an endocrinologist) and John Studd in England (a gynecologist) have been strong proponents of testosterone supplementation for sexual enhancement in surgically and naturally menopausal women. However, their recommendations for testosterone use have not been widely accepted, probably because physicians are concerned about the potential virilizing side effects and metabolic abnormalities.

Some physicians argue that testosterone supplementation benefits are due to the fact that testosterone is metabolized to estrogen so that estrogen supplementation should be sufficient for whatever benefits hormone supplementation may provide. As previously noted, however, Sherwin's extensive work has documented definite benefits from testosterone, separate from and not provided by estrogen.

In the United States, Greenblatt, Mortara, and Torpin (1942) and Salmon (1941) first proposed use of androgens to treat sexual disorders in women, regardless of hormonal status and including both pre- and postmenopausal women. Implantation of testosterone pellets (75–225 mg) reversed libido deficiency in several hundred women (Greenblatt, 1943). Even women suffering weakness and cachexia due to terminal cancer experienced increases in sex drive with testosterone supplements (Greenblatt, Jungck, & Blum, 1972).

Greenblatt contended that, although testosterone increases "susceptibility to sexual excitement," it does not affect sexual behavior itself. Salmon observed that testosterone injection could induce receptivity to mental and physical sexual stimulation, increase sensitivity of the clitoris, and facilitate more intense sexual gratification (Salmon & Geist, 1943). The researchers dispensed testosterone as a drug to treat sexual problems, without discriminating among groups of women.

In one double-blind study, Greenblatt, Barfield, Garner, Calk, and Harrod (1950) treated postmenopausal women with one of the following: (1) oral formulations of 5 mg/day of methyltestosterone (MT); (2) 0.25 mg/day, diethylstilbestrol (DES) synthetic estrogen; (3) a MT-DES combination; or (4) placebo. Hot flashes were relieved in 97% of diethylstilbestrol patients, 90% of methyltestosterone-diethylstilbestrol patients, 76% of methyltestosterone patients, and 16% of placebo patients. Sex drive was increased in 42% of methyltestosterone patients, 23.5% of methyltestosterone-diethylstilbestrol patients, 12.3% of diethylstilbestrol patients, and 1.8% of placebo patients.

In another study, Greenblatt (1987) found decreased depression and improved sex drive in depressed, postmenopausal patients with low sexual desire when treated with 50 mg estradiol pellet implantation. He found even greater benefit when testosterone pellets were added. It was not clear from this study whether improved sexual desire was due directly to hormonal supplementation or indirectly due to decreased depression.

For over 40 years, Greenblatt has treated low sexual desire in menopausal and nonmenopausal women with various testosterone formulations, including daily oral methyltestosterone, monthly testosterone propionate injections, testosterone pellet implantation every three months, and testosterone-estrogen combinations. When compared to these testosterone supplements, progesterone or placebo have shown no consistent benefits. In older women, Greenblatt notes that testosterone supplementation counteracts many of the catabolic actions of aging caused by glucocorticoids—the thinning skin, bruising, loss of muscle mass, bone loss, and impaired carbohydrate metabolism. Oral methyltestosterone adversely affects lipoprotein metabolism, but testosterone by injection or cell implantation has no such effect (Greenblatt, 1987). Greenblatt has contended that most of testosterone's side effects can be managed by dosage adjustment. Without further monitoring, however, Greenblatt's argument for testosterone treatment of low sexual desire as part of routine clinical practice is difficult to evaluate.

Currently, pellet implants are being administered outside the United States, especially in England, where John Studd has promoted their use. Studd et al. (1977) treated sexual dysfunction in 76 postmenopausal women with one of the following: (1) pellet implants of 50 mg estradiol, (2) a combination implant of 100 mg testosterone and 50 mg estradiol, or (3) placebo. Only the testosterone-estradiol group showed improvement in sexual response and coital frequency.

Another study by Studd's group (Montgomery et al., 1987) of perimenopausal and postmenopausal women being treated for psychiatric problems (depression, anxiety, irritability) reported mixed results. Testosterone-estradiol and estradiol implant supplements produced significant improvement in perimenopausal patients, but differences in the postmenopausal treatments were not significant due to a high placebo response rate. Testosterone-estradiol implant treatment showed the greatest improvement in symptoms for both perimenopausal and postmenopausal patients.

An influential study by Dow et al. (1983) convinced most experts that estradiol-only replacement was sufficient to resolve sexual desire deficits for both surgically and normally menopausal women. However, the study was flawed by the lack of a placebo control, the mixture of natural menopausal and surgically menopausal women, and treatment of all patients with a seven-day monthly cycle of progestogen.

Dow treated 40 postmenopausal women experiencing decreased sexual desire with either 50 mg estradiol pellet implants or 50 mg estradiol-100 mg testosterone pellet implants. There was no significant difference between the treatment groups. Both treatments reduced the psychological and physical symptoms of menopause and increased sexual interest, responsiveness, and orgasm. Marital dissatisfaction was not improved.

At the time, Dow was a psychologist working with gynecologists in Glasgow, Scotland on a series of hormonal replacement studies, which were reported in his doctoral dissertation (Dow, 1983). His failure to find special sexual benefits for testosterone in women seems to have reinforced similar findings by Andrew Mathews, a London psychologist (Mathews, 1983; Mathews et al., 1983), and those of a major Edinburgh sex researcher, John Bancroft (Bancroft et al., 1986). This series of studies, which effectively discouraged the use of testosterone supplements, set the standard for menopausal replacement therapy for many years to come.

By contrast, a later study confirmed the benefits of testosterone supplementation. Henry Burger, an Australian endocrinologist, showed that loss of sexual desire in postmenopausal women could be treated effectively with combinations of 40 mg estradiol and 100 mg testosterone implants. Estradiol, alone, was ineffective (Burger et al., 1984).

In response to Dow's negative findings, Burger further investigated the sexual benefits of testosterone added to estradiol supplementation (Burger et al., 1987). He treated 20 women (mean age = 45), who complained of severe loss of sexual desire despite adequate relief of physical symptoms by oral estrogen/progesterone supplementation. Nearly all (19 of 20) had hysterectomies and a third had oophorectomies. For six weeks, they were randomly assigned (a 40 mg estradiol pellet implant or a combined implant of 40 mg estradiol and 50 mg testosterone). The study was single-blind. At each six-week evaluation, both groups were prescribed 2.5 mg per day norethisterone progestogen for 10 days. After six weeks, there was no change in the estradiol implant group. At this point two women in the estradiol group dropped out of the study and the remaining eight chose to switch to the combined estradiol-testosterone implant. Subsequently, all 18 women on combined estradiol-testosterone noted relief of sexual desire deficiency for 18 weeks, despite mean testosterone levels only 20% above the normal range upper limit. Furthermore, no significant changes were noted in cholesterol or triglycerides.

Burger's study replicated the work of Studd et al. (1977), who had reported that conjugated equine estrogen treatment improved sexual symptoms in women with dyspareunia due to atrophic vaginitis discomfort. However, only combined pellet implants of 50 mg estradiol and 100 mg testosterone improved sexual desire in 80% of libido-deficient postmenopausal women without primary dyspareunia.

Burger has shown that estradiol/testosterone implants do not raise cholesterol or triglycerides over two to three years of use and may even allow the beneficial decrease of LDL cholesterol achieved with estradiol alone. The implants are effective for three to six months and require replacement as symptoms return (Brincat et al., 1984). For hysterectomized women, progestogen interval supplements are not needed.

Barlow et al. (1986) randomly allocated postmenopausal women (mean age = 44) to either 50 mg estradiol or 50 mg estradiol-100 mg testosterone implants, re-inserted every six months for three years. About 80% of women in each group was menopausal due to hysterectomy and oophorectomy. Sexual symptoms were not measured. (As a point of interest, this study was run by the Glasgow Menopause Clinic that had earlier conducted Dow's study.) A few more women (12 of 48) dropped out of the estradiol-only group than in the estradiol-testosterone group (9 of 48). Vasomotor symptoms were reduced equally well in both groups. Estradiol levels accumulated in both groups from about 400 pmol/L at six months to over 600 pmol/L at 36 months. Weight, blood pressure, and liver enzymes did not change significantly over three years in either group. Bone density did not change significantly in the estradiol group and even rose significantly but slightly in the estradiol-testosterone group (+2.5%). Testosterone levels did not change in the estradiol-only group, but rose 20–70% above normal levels in the estradiol-testosterone group within the first few months after each six-month implant, returning to the normal range by the end of six months. Given the high testosterone levels maintained, it was surprising that no patients complained of excess hair growth.

CONCLUSIONS

The extensive research by independent investigators Sherwin and Greenblatt has demonstrated sexual and psychological benefits of testosterone treatment for sexual deficiencies which occur during surgical or natural menopause. However, the amount of testosterone administered always resulted in greater than normal physiological levels. Therefore, testosterone treatment, technically, became supplementation rather than replacement.

Barbara Sherwin's comprehensive and thorough monitoring has contributed greatly to our understanding of postmenopausal endocrinology. Her findings have verified that testosterone replacement maintains sexual desire and arousal after ovary removal in contrast to estradiol alone or placebo. Testosterone but not estradiol alone can maintain or improve well-being and energy. Both testosterone and estradiol can prevent depression and decline in cognitive performance after ovary removal.

Although testosterone supplements have been shown to increase sexual desire in women with below normal testosterone levels, research has not yet determined whether there is a positive effect for those in the normal range.

In the Sherwin studies, testosterone levels by injection reached 120–250 ng/dl (above the female normal range of 20–100 ng/dl). However, Burger et al. (1987) showed resolution of postmenopausal loss of sexual desire with a considerably lower dose—50 mg testosterone pellet implants, which resulted in testosterone levels only about 20% above the normal range. The sexual benefits persisted for three to six months, even though testosterone levels fell back into the normal range toward the end.

Sherwin (1988a) reviewed the rise and fall of testosterone and estrogen levels with injections and pellet implants. She noted that regular changes in hormone levels may be as important as absolute levels for normal function, particularly since sexual deficits and hot flashes may return even when testosterone and estradiol remain at supranormal or normal levels.

Although estradiol supplementation alone seems to be sufficient treatment for many postmenopausal sexual problems, some women get little or no effect without testosterone supplementation. For women who have negative sexual and psychological reactions to estrogen therapy, testosterone alone may be an appropriate alternative. Injection or pellet implantation delivers enough testosterone so that some of it can be sequestered, aromatized, and released as estradiol, potentially preventing osteoporosis and some cutaneous menopausal symptoms. Neither testosterone pellets nor the oral form, testosterone undecanoate, has been approved for use in the United States.

In contrast to definite evidence of beneficial effects of testosterone supplements on female sexual drive, the contribution of endogenous testosterone to female sexual desire is yet to be specified. While testosterone does not necessarily influence the frequency of intercourse, some studies have indicated that it does increase masturbation. It is not clear whether testosterone causes increased sexual desire and activity. Conversely, decreased sexual desire and activity or mildly depressed states may decrease testosterone levels.

In many animal studies, testosterone has been shown to rise in animals victorious in combat. In humans, it can be increased by "top of the hill" states of mind which include confidence, self-esteem, optimal coping, and well-being as well as positive sexual desire. As part of our clinical sex therapy program, we often "prescribe" David Burns' (1980) excellent cognitive therapy book, *Feeling Good.* Ultimately, frequent and satisfying sex and an overall positive state of mind are mutually reinforcing and enhancing.

8

Testosterone in Men

OBJECTIVES

- To describe the brain-body pathways of testosterone production and function
- To define the influence of testosterone on male sexuality
- To examine the influence of testosterone on aggressive male behavior
- To determine suitability of testosterone replacement therapy in men
- To evaluate the various methods of testosterone supplementation

Testosterone is the chief testicular steroid, produced predominantly from Leydig cells residing in the interstitial tissue of the testes. Leydig cells occupy about 5–12% of human testicular volume. At maturity, human testes contain about 700 million Leydig cells. Within the Leydig cells, cholesterol is converted by mitochondrial enzymes to pregnenolone and then to testosterone, similar to androgen production in the inner regions of the adrenal gland. Testosterone levels in blood may not reflect Leydig cell concentrations, because blood levels reflect other processes such as metabolic degradation and excretion.

Additional testosterone is derived as a product of metabolism from adrenal steroids (e.g., DHEAS, androstenedione). Peripheral tissue effects are due to metabolism of testosterone to dihydrotestosterone. In lower animals such as rats, testosterone can be metabolized (aromatized) to estrogens, producing many of its effects on sexual behavior. The influence of aromatization on human sexual desire and behavior appears to be relatively minor, although there is some research to the contrary.

Secondary sex characteristics of the male (e.g., hair patterns, distribution of muscle and body fat) are governed by testosterone. Specific tissues controlled by testosterone include accessory sex organs as well as production and maintenance of sperm. Testosterone is the hormone which differentiates males from females. It controls fetal and neonatal brain development and organization by appropriate coding and direction of growth processes. It does not simply cause "more" masculine tissue activity; it prescribes the way in which organs and tissue will act and react. Much of the organizational/directive function of testosterone is complete after peaks in activity during the fetal or neonatal period. Subsequently, its level declines for many years until reactivated by the onset of hypothalamic/pituitary rhythmic function during puberty. During and after puberty, its chief role is to stimulate brain and body function and tissue which was organized and developed during the fetal/neonatal period. (Though it is assumed that the organizational functions of testosterone are mainly confined to the fetal/neonatal period, there may be additional, not-yet-discovered functions that occur later in life.) The sexual role of testosterone is primarily preparatory and directional; in other words, it influences sex drive and promotes masculine characteristic behaviors.

Testosterone levels are flexible: relatively constant basal levels will fluctuate considerably in response to environmental events, attractions, and repulsions. Testosterone levels are also subject to diurnal fluctuations (highest in the morning) and seasonal cycles (highest in the fall). Even basal testosterone levels fluctuate widely due to changes in episodic secretion over 15–20-minute periods, caused by frequency and amplitude fluctuations in LHRH secretion. Consequently, for reliable testosterone level determination, blood samples every 20 minutes over at least an hour should be taken. Otherwise, levels may represent nadirs or peaks in secretion.

Testosterone production is modulated by luteinizing hormone (LH) within a feedback loop involving the gonads, the hypothalamus, and the pituitary. Production of testosterone in Leydig cells is regulated by pituitary luteinizing hormone (gonadotrophin), which is in turn regulated by luteinizing hormone-releasing hormone (LHRH) or gonadotrophin-releasing hormone (GnRH) from the hypothalamic arcuate nucleus. The anterior pituitary secretes LH and FSH to maintain normal steroidal balance. In the testes, LH triggers production and secretion of testosterone and dihydrotestosterone in the Leydig cells, which maintain male genital and accessory sex organ tissues as well as male sex behavior. Small amounts of estradiol are also secreted from the testes. While the function of testicular estradiol is unclear, too much can act as a negative signal to the hypothalamic-pituitary feedback loop, as if it was testosterone, and decrease LH secretion. Increases in estradiol can confound the testosterone-LH feedback set points, just as exogenous testosterone inhibits normal LH activity.

Any significant decrease in circulating testosterone is communicated to the hypothalamus, which triggers the LHRH/LH mechanism that signals the gonads to produce more testosterone. Conversely, when testosterone levels reach an acceptable level, a signal is sent back to the hypothalamus to decrease LHRH/LH secretion. Female LHRH/LH secretion is integrated into a menstrual cycle with a peak at ovulation. Male LHRH/LH secretion seems to lack such cyclic organization; rather, it appears to operate on a continuous feedback principle, so that the male will "always be ready" to take advantage of sexual opportunity.

The LHRH/LH mechanism can be shut down by administration of exogenous testosterone, which signals a reduction in secretion, even though testosterone levels in the Leydig cells are decreasing. Fluoxymesterone (Halotestin) and other synthetic androgens cause a decrease in LHRH pulse frequency with little change in amplitude. Administration of potent and long-lasting LHRH supplements down-regulates the LHRH/LH mechanisms. These manipulations can result in reduction of testosterone and sperm to castrate levels without actually blocking androgen receptors. The system essentially shuts itself off.

Seminiferous tubules are maintained by androgens and FSH, which is secreted with LH from the anterior pituitary (pars distalis) and participates in stimulation of Leydig cell testosterone production. FSH controls sperm production by stimulating Sertoli cells which store and maintain sperm. FSH provides a more extended signal than LH because it is less altered by hypothalamic releasing hormone fluctuations. A separate testicular substance called *inhibin* may regulate FSH secretion separately from LH, but its role has not been fully explained. Increased inhibin will decrease FSH.

Prolactin is also involved in the stimulation of Leydig cells, which contain prolactin receptors. Testosterone levels transiently increase in human males injected with the dopamine antagonist haloperidol, which increases prolactin. However, prolactin stimulation soon down-regulates Leydig-cell functions, and elevated prolactin over an extended period of time (hyperprolactemia) results in lowered Leydig-cell testosterone production. A given amount of prolactin at proper times will increase testosterone, but higher or lower amounts, or improper timing, will desensitize and down-regulate Leydig-cell production.

Estrogen, on the other hand, can decrease testosterone production because it operates like testosterone in the feedback loop to the LHRH-LH mechanisms. If estrogen levels rise, LHRH/LH secretion decreases so that less testosterone is produced in the Leydig cells. Essentially, estrogen substitutes for testosterone. However, instead of the robust LH pulsatile spikes generated by testosterone, there are smaller and smoother pulses characteristic of female LH secretion. There are estrogen receptors in Leydig cells and estrogen may be produced in the interstitial tissue. Thus, testosterone and gonadal activity can be undermined by interference of competing steroids as well as by disregulation of testosterone loop function caused by excessive or insufficient levels of normal chemicals within the loop.

As testosterone levels decline, or when levels are chronically low, there is no compensatory rise in LHRH-LH secretion signaling the gonads to produce more testosterone. Failure of chronic supplemental LHRH administration to raise testosterone is due to the fact that LHRH requires an optimum rhythm of pulsatile secretion in order to stimulate the gonads. Too much or too little, or inappropriately timed secretion, eliminates LHRH effects. Hypogonadotrophic hypogonadism is the result.

When LHRH is secreted continuously, a progressive desensitization of pituitary reactivity occurs. In fact, when highly potent synthetic LHRH superagonists with continuous extended action are ingested, testosterone declines toward castrate levels. Consequently, synthetic LHRH analogues can be used to achieve a reversible "chemical castration" to treat prostate cancer. However, there is evidence that such extended treatment for prostate cancer in elderly men may irreversibly decrease testicular Leydig cell response (Decensi et al., 1989).

Synthetic LHRH agonists have been tested clinically as male contraceptives due to their power to shut down the production of sperm (Doelle et al., 1983). However, when the body's testosterone production drops to low levels, sex drive is frequently lost along with sperm production. Pharmacological investigations suggest that the primary effect of lowered testosterone is to reduce sex drive rather than sexual potency (Creed, 1989; Johnson & Jarow, 1992). Investigators are currently attempting to supplement synthetic LHRH agonist contraceptive treatment with enough testosterone to preserve libido without stimulating sperm production.

Unfortunately, blocking natural LHRH secretion with exogenous synthetic LHRH can have adverse sexual effects not involving testosterone. In Chapter 29, we will describe the positive sexual effects shown by LHRH itself. When sexual activity is anticipated, natural LHRH secretion is increased to facilitate sexual approach. Disrupting natural LHRH secretion with synthetic analogues could interfere with spontaneous sexual anticipatory behavior.

The periodicity of human LHRH secretion is approximately 90 minutes. If this frequency is changed, or if there is too little or too much LHRH available for optimum pulsatile frequency and amplitude, Leydig-cell testosterone production decreases, causing, in turn, a decrease of sperm production. For LHRH replacement therapy, special pumps that reproduce the 90-minute periodic rhythm of natural LHRH secretion must be worn.

ANDROGENS IN AGING MEN

Although testosterone levels for subgroups of healthy men over age 60 have been shown to remain stable, typically both total testosterone and free testosterone levels decline in men over this age (Kaiser & Morley, 1994; Vermeulen, 1991, 1994). One recent longitudinal study of a large community population of men aged 40 to 80 reported a decrease of total serum testosterone by 0.4% per year and a decrease of free serum testosterone at 1.2% per year (Gray, Feldman, McKinlay, & Longcope, 1991). The decreases were steeper over age 60 than under age 60. Testosterone decreases in older men can be attributed to a decrease in gonadal production from Leydig cells, a decrease in adrenal production, and apparent dysregulation of hypothalamic-pituitary gonadotropin secretion (GnRH) (Kaiser & Morley, 1994; Vermeulen, 1994).

Decreased gonadal production may be due to a decreased number of Leydig cells, impaired testicular blood circulation, impaired steroid biosynthesis, and decreased response to human chorionic gonadotropin (GnRH) stimulation (Vermeulen, 1994). Insufficient GnRH secretion in response to lowered gonadal testosterone production is unexplained, but has been partly attributed to impaired timing of pulsatile gonadotropin release or decreased pulsatile amplitude; a decrease in the cellular mass of the hypothalamic GnRH pulse generator; inhibition by glucocorticoids in response to normal stress and slow, degenerative disease; diminished pituitary luteinizing hormone (LH) response to GnRH; and increased prolactin (Kaiser & Morley, 1994; Vermeulen, 1994).

An increase in estrogen levels in men during aging may decrease the amplitude of LH pulses from the pituitary or cause increased sex hormone-binding globulin (SHBG), which binds overall testosterone and disproportionally decreases free testosterone (Vermeulen, 1994). Note that estrogen acts chiefly at the pituitary level on LH pulse amplitude, while testosterone acts chiefly at the hypothalamic level on pulse frequency of GnRH (Vermeulen, 1994). Vermeulen (1991) reviews past studies on testosterone levels in male aging, noting varied conclusions; but the present consensus is that testosterone does decline at least past age 60, though individual variations are great.

The evidence for a male "climacteric" due to decreased testosterone between ages 40 to 55 (Solstad & Garde, 1992) is still questionable and certainly insufficient for instigation of widespread testosterone supplementation for treatment of symptoms such as neurasthenia, lack of energy, decreased muscle and bone mass, decreased libido, and weakened erection (Vermeulen, 1994, concisely describes these symptoms often attributed to supposed androgen deficiency). The negative side effects on health of such testosterone supplementation, including a decrease in good HDL cholesterol, prostate growth, and insulin resistance, could be tragic.

The best study of changes in various steroids and steroid metabolites was reported by Belanger et al. (1994), who measured a cross-section of 2,423 healthy men aged 40 to 80. The decline in DHEA/DHEAS was continuous and steep, but there was no decline in progesterone or estradiol and even a slight, significant increase in cortisol (see Chapter 9 for a discussion of the possible negative effects of such changes). Decreases in levels of androstenedione and testosterone were about half those of DHEA/DHEAS and appeared to be significant only after age 60. Quite remarkably, dihydrotestosterone (DHT) remained unaltered or even increased after age 60, despite lowered levels of total testosterone, suggesting that 5-alpha-reductase enzyme activity, which metabolizes testosterone to peripheral DHT, may increase progressively with aging. If such an increase in reductase exists, it would account for prostatic growth with aging, particularly over age 60. It would also justify more widespread prophylactic use of 5-alpha-reductase inhibitors (finasteride—Proscar—is currently available) to prevent such an imbalance in the androgen system, which could foster prostatic hypertrophy and other, as yet undiscovered, pathologies resulting from an increase in DHT compared to the levels of other androgens.

TESTOSTERONE AND AGGRESSION

Testosterone is a prototypical sex hormone, the "fuel" of libido. As noted, during fetal and neonatal development, testosterone secretion differentiates the organism away from the female prototype, thus separating the sexes. Testosterone's action is best understood from the perspective of its active role in creating and maintaining this separation. Basically, sex hormones are divided into male sex hormones (androgens) and female sex hormones (estrogens). Progesterone is a reproductive hormone that appears to be symbiotic with estrogens but antagonistic to androgens. Perhaps 21st-century physiology will establish categories beyond the gross dichotomization of male/female. In humans, this dichotomy creates and maintains life. Testosterone and its derivatives maintain and express this dichotomy, in contrast to other hormones that usually transcend this dichotomy.*

This differentiating aspect of testosterone is absolutely crucial to understanding its sexual

*Elsewhere we have proposed oxytocin as a peptide hormone/neurotransmitter that mediates sexual behavior for both males and females—even to the point of transcending the testosterone-estrogen/male-female polarity. Other peptides and transmitters appear to align themselves at either the active/testosterone pole or the passive/estrogen pole.

properties. While female sex requires accommodation for fertilization and mothering to occur, male sex requires active aggression, which is inextricably tied to sexuality. Aggressive behavior is inherently social. An animal biting off its own foot is not be considered aggressive or dominating. In fact, self-directed aggression is correlated with a decrease in testosterone; increased testosterone precipitates aggression toward others. To be aggressive, the animal must act outside of itself to mark his separateness as a male. Indeed, when a male is blocked from autonomous social expression due to defeat in fighting other males, his testosterone levels drop. At that point, he may turn upon himself, often in a pathological manner.

High levels of testosterone are established and maintained by winning and dominance (Kemper, 1990). Indeed, testosterone levels can serve as a barometer of winning, success, assertion, and dominance (McCaul, Gladue, & Joppa, 1992). Albert, Dyson, Walsh, and Wong (1988) have proposed three types of aggression: defensive aggression (response to attack or provocation), predatory aggression (directed toward obtaining food), testosterone-dependent aggression (most evident in attacks on unfamiliar or subordinate males and in sexual mating). Competitive situations typically generate testosterone-dependent aggression. Many other studies have reported that testosterone levels increase in winners and decrease in losers.

Mazur and Lamb (1988) found increased testosterone in young adult men who won tennis matches and decreased testosterone in those who lost. They also found that lack of a clear-cut victory or that winning *by chance* (as in a lottery) resulted in no change in testosterone. Kreuz, Rose, and Jennings (1972) found that testosterone levels declined during the difficult and oppressive early stages of military officer candidate training, but increased with graduation. Along similar lines, successful execution of parachute jumps by military trainees caused increased testosterone (Ellertsen, Johnsen, & Ursin, 1978), but initial frightening and awkward jumps caused decreased testosterone (Davidson, Stefanick, Sachs, & Smith, 1978).

In male monkey groups, males who become dominant show elevated testosterone, while those who are attacked into submission show lowered testosterone (Mendoza, Lowe, Davidson, & Levine, 1979; Rose, Bernstein, & Gordon, 1975). However, once dominance, status, and rank become stable, differences in testosterone decrease (Mendoza, 1984). Infusions of testosterone—or even castration—may not cause any immediate change in this stable hierarchy. Apparently, testosterone differences only appear when competition or challenges are actually occurring.

Since a male animal's testosterone level may increase the attractiveness of his odor cues to females (Ferkin, Sorokin, Renfroe, & Johnston, 1994), there may be a sexual advantage to maintaining high testosterone levels through competitive or aggressive encounters (as long as the male wins). Castration decreases or eliminates the attractiveness of a male animal's odor to females; testosterone replacement restores the attractiveness to females (Ferkin et al., 1994) Ferkin castrated male meadow voles (small rodents) used as odor "donors" and implanted capsules in them containing four different levels of replacement testosterone. Testosterone replacement increased the attractiveness of male odors to female voles in a dose-dependent manner. However, male-female dominance hierarchies are not the same in humans as in animals and male odor cues indicating aggressive competitiveness may be repulsive to many women.

The interconnection between aggression and sexual behavior is more obvious in lower animals than in humans. For instance, a male stickleback's sexual behavior is preceded by aggressive encounters. First, the male establishes a territory in which he is dominant.* When other animals enter the male's territory, the male chases them away. If the intruder does not retreat, the male launches an aggressive attack. A male intruder resists the attack either by retreating or fighting back (fight or flight). How-

***Territory* implies an awareness of space and boundaries. The establishment, protection, and defense of boundaries is characteristic of the male's tendency to distinguish himself as separate by excluding other animals, except those that do not threaten autonomy (i.e., females).

ever, a female intruder typically remains passive. This passivity under attack signals the male that the intruder is female and triggers a switch into sexual behavior.

Tentative circling allows better evaluation of the female intruder. If cues are appropriate, there is progression to a sequence of more direct sexual actions until copulation and ejaculation occur. Stickleback mating involves this complementary action and reaction, activity versus passive receptivity in dynamic interaction.

Burris, Gracely, Carter, Sherins, and Davidson (1991) have shown that testosterone in human males may reduce the sense of touch as measured by reduced tactile sensitivity in response to mild vibration applied to either the finger or the penis. The authors note that prior research has shown that the finger is generally more sensitive than the penis to vibrotactile stimuli. Untreated hypogonadal males showed greater sensitivity at both the finger and penis sites than men with normal testosterone levels. Subsequent chronic treatment over 12 months of five out of six of these hypogonadal men with replacement testosterone enanthate progressively decreased perceived intensity of vibratory touch stimuli applied to the penis but not to the finger (counter to the authors' initial expectations). Apparently, the touch differential is greatest for men deprived of testosterone for several years or more (untreated hypogonadal men). Steiness (1957) has shown that women are slightly more sensitive to vibratory touch stimuli than men. (It should be noted that while increased touch sensitivity would encourage and enhance cuddling, at the same time it would be detrimental to aggressive defense and fighting behavior.) Given this sensitivity differential, women who are given supplemental testosterone for decreased libido should be monitored for any decrease in touch sensitivity that negatively affects sexual responsiveness and tactile pleasure.

TESTOSTERONE REPLACEMENT THERAPY (TRT) IN MEN

Testosterone was first recognized as a sex hormone at the turn of the century (Bayliss & Starling, 1904), but strictly controlled experimental studies of testosterone supplementation date back little more than a decade. Prior to 1979, a multitude of studies reported correlations of thought and behavior patterns with testosterone levels. Later work found that increasing testosterone in men with normal values but without exceeding normal levels (300–1,200 ng/dl) did not significantly alter sexual behavior (Davidson & Rosen, 1992). One interpretation of this finding that, if a man has normal levels of testosterone, increasing those levels does not enhance sex. By contrast, if there is a testosterone deficiency, replacement to achieve normal levels can make a dramatic difference. Another interpretation of these data derives from the fact that testosterone exists in two forms—free and bound—with the free form functioning as the active molecule. No matter how much total testosterone is increased, if the increase occurs in the bound fraction, enhancement of sexual function is unlikely. Nevertheless, there are no studies showing that raising free testosterone within the normal range has any more impact than testosterone supplementation. Also, exogenous testosterone administration may lack impact on sexual function because it is not administered in a proper pulsatile fashion to be coded effectively into body chemistry. Rather, it may simply form a residual inactive pool.

The use of simplistic measurements to evaluate functional potency has been ubiquitous in the study of male sexual behavior (i.e., more testosterone, more sexual function; less testosterone, less sexual function), but it is inadequate for evaluating the complexities involved. Beyond the evident finding that supplemental testosterone can reverse the loss of sexuality due to subnormal levels, little has been learned about the relationship of testosterone to male sexual behavior, except that even substantial variations in normal testosterone levels seem to have surprisingly little effect on sexual thought and behavior.

Studies of healthy normal men, in which endogenous testosterone was experimentally suppressed and testosterone levels were manipulated with exogenous testosterone treatment, have shown that normal sex drive, function, and activity is maintained equally in men returned to low borderline testosterone levels (e.g., above 250 ng/dl) or to much higher testosterone levels (e.g., above 750 ng/dl) (Bagatell, Heiman, Rivier, & Bremmer, 1994; Buena et al., 1993). Similarly, treatment of 13 impotent men who had low borderline testosterone levels with biweekly 200 mg injections of testosterone enanthate (an appropriate, conventional replacement dose) produced improvement in only one of the men (and only on a sexual questionnaire, not on RigiScan nocturnal tumescence monitoring) (Gilbert, Graham, & Regan, 1992). Carani et al. (1990) have shown that oral testosterone undecanoate (TU) treatment of 14 impotent men with borderline low testosterone levels improved sexual function in men with subnormal low free testosterone levels, but not in men with normal free testosterone levels (oral TU treatment increased both total and free testosterone, and the increase in free testosterone was much greater in the group with initial subnormal free testosterone).

Sexual desire and initiative are deficient or insufficient in men who have subnormal testosterone levels. Sexual function is enhanced when testosterone supplements are given to men (usually by injection) with abnormally low testosterone (below 300 ng/dl) (O'Carroll, Shapiro, & Bancroft, 1985). Although the capacity for erection is not dependent on testosterone (erection is a mechanical hydraulic vasodilation response mediated chiefly by adrenergic neurotransmitters as well as acetylcholine and various peptides), low sex drive can cause avoidance of opportunities to become erect.

Due to the evidence that erectile function can be retained in castrates, Kinsey discounted the importance of testosterone in sexual function (Kinsey, Pomeroy, Martin, & Gebhard, 1953), claiming that castration has "little or no effect on the sexual responsiveness of half or more of the males." However, careful observation over many years has revealed that most castrated men show a clear decline in sexual desire and response. Kinsey's denial of the impact of castration on sexual function is a reflection of the general failure to recognize as sexual dysfunction anything but the complete loss of erection and ejaculation.

Proof of the essential role of testosterone in male sexuality has accrued over the last 15 years. The dose-response relationship between testosterone and sexual function has been studied either directly with exogenous testosterone administration or indirectly by correlating endogenous levels of testosterone with behavior or thoughts. For example, treatment of young men (at least 15 years old) with hypogonadotropic hypogonadism (low testosterone due to insufficient hypothalamic-pituitary gonadotropin secretion) with either six months of testosterone enanthate or six months of human menopausal gonadotropin (hMG-Pergonal equivalent to 75 IU of LH and 75 IU or FSH) produced equivalent increases in self-reported frequency of ejaculation, ratings of libido, and nocturnal penile tumescence (NPT) event duration (Clopper, Voorhess, MacGillivray, Lee, & Mills, 1993). Burris, Banks, Carter, Davidson, and Sherins (1992) treated six profoundly hypogonadal men aged 25 to 40 on an inpatient basis with either biweekly 200 mg testosterone enanthate (n = 3) or human gonadotropins (Pergonal or Pregnyl) (n = 3). Significant increase in NPT to normal levels required between six and 12 months of treatment, even though serum testosterone levels rose to an asymptote even higher than shown by normal men within the first three months.

Prior to initiation of hormone replacement in the Clopper et al. 1993 study, the hypogonadal men showed elevated ratings of depression, anger, fatigue, and confusion, all of which decreased during treatment. However, the treated hypogonadal men continued to show higher depression scores at the end of 12 months compared to normal controls. Both serum total and salivary testosterone (salivary assumed representative of free testosterone levels) have been found to be lower in severely depressed men compared to controls (Davies et al., 1992). Similarly, Levitt and Joffe (1988) found 20% lower free testosterone in 12 depressed men. Driscoll and Thompson (1993) point out that the decline in testosterone with aging may be exaggerated in depressed men.

Steiger, Von Bardeleben, Wiedemann, and Holsboer (1991) measured nocturnal secretion of cortisol and testosterone in 12 depressed male patients during the initial stage of severe depression prior to drug treatment and after recovery and the end of drug treatment. Testosterone was depressed to the low end of the normal range (400 ng/dl, with 300 ng/dl considered the threshold normal level) and cortisol was elevated. During recovery, testosterone increased and cortisol decreased, despite no change in sleep patterns. Sexual response was not measured, but the authors wonder whether a decrease, even within the normal range, in depressed men would account specifically for lowered libido and inhibited or absent sexual response.

Testosterone replacement therapy studies conducted by Julian Davidson in the United States and John Bancroft in Scotland have demonstrated that hypogonadal men often achieve normal erections in response to erotic films and to their partners' sexual advances, despite a lack of nocturnal and spontaneous daytime erections. Davidson, Camargo, and Smith (1979) published the first double-blind controlled trial of testosterone replacement therapy. Comprehensive evaluation of six hypogonadal men included detailed daily logs of all forms of sexual activity as well as spontaneous sexual events. Clear and precipitous increases in sexual function occurred in five of the six men within a few weeks of receiving a single injection of testosterone (as measured by erections, coitus, and nocturnal erections). While 400 mg of testosterone enanthate consistently resulted in increased erection, 100 mg often showed no effect. The current recommended dose of testosterone enanthate is 200–300 mg every three weeks. Clear sexual improvement after an injection usually requires more than a week to manifest. Men who experience immediate benefit are thought to be experiencing a placebo effect.

Subsequent controlled testosterone replacement therapy studies in hypogonadal men confirmed that testosterone restored or facilitated sexual activity, including erection, orgasm, ejaculation, and nocturnal erections (Salmimies, Kockott, Pirke, Vogt, & Schill, 1982; Skakkebaek, Bancroft, Davidson, & Warren, 1981). Patient self-assessments during testosterone replacement therapy showed improved sexual desire and interest and an increase in sexual thoughts and fantasies. A general improvement in mood typically accompanied the increased sexual desire.

Testosterone replacement for hypogonadal men does not invariably reverse impotence. Segraves, Schoenberg, and Ivanoff (1983) found that nine of 52 (15%) patients with complaints of erectile impotence had abnormally low testosterone (defined as below the rather high normal minimum of 376 ng/dl used at their clinic). Five of the men chose to receive testosterone replacement therapy treatment (200 mg depo-testosterone every two weeks). However, none recovered erectile function, despite a return to normal or high testosterone levels.

Bancroft and Wu (1983) found that the erection response to pornographic films did not differ among eight hypogonadal men and eight normal controls. Apparently, the pornographic films supplied sufficient sexual stimulation to the hypogonadal men. Furthermore, testosterone replacement therapy in hypogonadal men did not increase erections in response to pornographic films. In contrast, fantasy-induced erections were smaller and slower to develop in hypogonadal men and improved with testosterone replacement therapy.

Kwan, Greenleaf, Mann, Crapo, and Davidson (1983) found normal erectile responses to erotic films and fantasy in six hypogonadal men. While nocturnal erections and spontaneous daytime erections increased with testosterone replacement therapy (200 or 400 mg testosterone enanthate), no change occurred in erectile responses to film or fantasy. However, increases in sexual feelings and sexual acts were reported by three of the men.

A man sitting in a laboratory strapped, wired, and monitored is unlikely to show increments in testosterone in the rather passive experience of voyeuristic masturbation. The reliance of academic sex research on such nonsocial and psychologically inappropriate contexts for sexual measurements is good reason to wonder whether their conclusions apply to sex with a partner. Unfortunately, this limitation is often overlooked by the researchers themselves, who erroneously generalize their findings. Studies in monkeys and men have often shown that masturbation without interpersonal sexual interaction does not increase testosterone levels (Fox, Ismail, Love, Kirkham, & Loraine, 1972; Keverne, 1979), while intercourse with a partner usually does.

The consideration of the couple as the sexual subject preserved some of the basic dynamics of sex in Masters and Johnson's studies. Testosterone dynamics are best observed within the context of interpersonal attraction and contest of wills.

The essential cause of decreased sexual response and activity in hypogonadal men seems to be due primarily to a lack of desire (libido) and sensory excitement than to a lack of capacity:

> Anecdotally, untreated hypogonadal men complain of erectile problems though the effects of the powerful stimulus of erotic films shows that the erection mechanism is intact. They can have erections to satisfy their partners, but it may be little more than a chore; the decreased libido apparently leads to a secondary decrease in erectile performance during sexual situations, due probably to lack of interest or pleasure. (Davidson, 1986a)

Eyal, Ish-Shalom, Hoch, and Hochberg (1988) studied a group of hypogonadotrophic hypogonadal men treated with testosterone replacement therapy for two to eight years. Hormonal and sexual measurements were taken at two-week intervals following testosterone injections. Testosterone levels were highest at week 2, then declined from week 4 to 8. Erection strength peaked at week 4 and declined thereafter. Sexual desire remained heightened through week 6. Regardless of these changes, sexual relations remained infrequent throughout the study. Thus, despite obvious benefits from testosterone replacement in many hypogonadal men, improvement in sexual function frequently does not occur, suggesting a need for further examination of other factors. The lack of sexual desire and response may be caused by insufficient activity of other neurotransmitters and peptides, which are more difficult to measure than testosterone.

Lack of response to testosterone replacement might indicate a need for concurrent sex therapy. In fact, the sexual problem in a hypotestosterone man is a combination of lack of desire and inadequate stimulation, then sex therapy even without testosterone replacement can restore sexual activity through cognitive and behavioral means. However, full sexual response and enjoyment would be achieved only when the testosterone deficit was corrected. Conversely, a man with little to stimulate him sexually may notice no more than a return of nocturnal erections during testosterone replacement therapy. Sexual sensitivity and response capacity may be improved with no overt manifestations, due to a simple lack of sexual stimulation.

Testosterone supplements can also be used to enhance bromocriptine effects for more effective treatment of impotence due to hyperprolactinemia. Testosterone potentiates dopamine sexual effects (Dallo, Lekka, & Knoll, 1986) and inhibits prolactin release (Sinha, Gilligan, & Barkley, 1984). It also has a synergistic effect with dopamine in brain sex centers such as the medial preoptic nucleus.

TESTOSTERONE SUPPLEMENTS

Testosterone supplements are usually in the form of long-acting testosterone esters (enanthate, cypionate), which allow gradual release and are slowly metabolized by the liver. Oral forms of testosterone include mesterolone (Proviron), fluoxymesterone (Halotestin), and methyltestosterone (Virilon, Testred) and testosterone undecanoate.

Methyltestosterone, Fluoxymesterone

Methyltestosterone can have all the problematic side effects of testosterone, including liver damage, increased cholesterol, weight gain, gynecomastia (due to metabolism to estrogens), edema, acne, and prostate hypertrophy. Doses of 10–50 mg/day are used for treatment of testosterone deficiency. Fluoxymesterone has similar side effects and is given in doses of 5–20 mg/day. Due to their hepatoxic and other dangerous side effects, oral methyltestosterone and fluoxymesterone are not recommended for long-term testosterone replacement therapy in men (Nieschlag & Freischem, 1982). However, both drugs are available in the United States for this use; whereas testosterone undecanoate and mesterolone, which are not toxic to the liver, have not been approved for use in this country.

Though treatment of hypogonadal men with oral methyltestosterone is considered ineffective and dangerous in the United States (NIH Consensus Conference on Impotence, 1993), many generic preparations of oral methyltestosterone are commercially available and no doubt used by many men for testosterone replacement or supplementation. Morales, Johnston, Heaton, and Clark (1994) treated 22 hypogonadal impotent men for 30 days with one of two commercial preparations of oral testosterone. Supraphysiological levels of total testosterone were shown for all patients, but there was a significant *decrease* in free testosterone with the majority of men showing decreases. Only two of the 22 men reported complete recovery of sexual function, and visual analogue scales showed no significant changes in energy, mood, or well-being. Morales et al. (1994) note that oral androgens account for 75% of the legal androgen market in North America.

Testosterone Undecanoate

The chief oral form of testosterone for men is testosterone undecanoate, which is a fatty acid ester absorbed from the intestines into lymphatic system lacteals, bypassing the liver (Nieschlag & Freischem, 1982). Marketed in Europe by Organon as Restandol, Andriol, and under various other names, testosterone undecanoate is available to U.S. physicians who request it for use with patients who specifically need an oral form of treatment. Because gastrointestinal absorption is unpredictable, doses can be difficult to control. Injectable testosterone is usually preferred for its potency and avoidance of liver metabolism. Also, testosterone injections are far less expensive. However, a valuable role for oral testosterone remains; for example, men with a borderline testosterone deficiency may refuse replacement therapy due to the inconvenience and discomfort of injections.

Many of the early placebo-controlled studies of testosterone replacement therapy were done with testosterone undecanoate. Benkert, Witt, Adam, and Leitz (1979) treated 13 men who had inadequate erections but normal testosterone levels with 120 mg/day testosterone undecanoate for eight weeks compared to 16 given placebo. Five testosterone undecanoate patients (38%) reported improvement, but eight placebo patients (50%) also reported improvement. With such high placebo response rates, the possibility of finding significant differences is low. (Studies of men with low sexual desire and hypogonadism show far lower placebo response rates.)

Skakkebaek et al. (1981) reported an unusually comprehensive study of using testosterone undecanoate (160 mg/day) for two months versus placebo. Plasma testosterone increases with testosterone undecanoate were sometimes rather small, not reaching normal levels in many patients. Nonetheless, there were significant improvements on all measures of sexual interest and behavior. Sexual desire increased during the first week (surprisingly early) and ejaculations became more frequent by the second week. General increases in well-being also occurred during testosterone undecanoate treatment, including decreased tension, hostility, and fatigue. After testosterone withdrawal, sexual desire decreased followed by subsequent ejaculation failures. These results indicated that assessing the efficacy of testosterone replacement therapy by measuring serum levels of total testosterone achieved is not adequate. (Perhaps isolating free testosterone would have provided meaningful results.)

Increases in sexual thoughts and arousal have been reported to occur dose-dependently with testosterone undecanoate (40–160 mg) in hypogonadal men (O'Carroll et al., 1985). Luisi and Franchi (1980) found significant increases compared to placebo in desire, erections, and ejaculations during treatment of 12 primary hypogonadal men with four weeks of 120 mg/day testosterone undecanoate. Daily doses of 120–160 mg/day testosterone undecanoate (60–80 mg taken twice a day) proved effective treatment.

Cantrill, Dewis, Large, Newman, and Anderson (1984) have shown that a dose of 160 mg/day of testosterone undecanoate produces the equivalent of 100 mg of testosterone which has to be metabolized by the liver (the normal production rate of endogenous testosterone is 7 mg/day). As noted, gastric absorption of testosterone undecanoate from the stomach is quite variable and may differ from patient to patient. Average levels of testosterone produced by 160 mg/day testosterone undecanoate were less than half that produced by 250 mg testosterone injections every three weeks. A particular concern is that abnormally high levels of dihydrotestosterone (peripheral sex organ effects) and DHT to T ratios may occur in some testosterone undecanoate-treated patients, suggesting a possibility that prostate growth may be encouraged (Cantrill et al., 1984).

Mesterolone

The special properties of oral mesterolone (Proviron) are that it is not metabolized to estrogens (aromatized), does not suppress gonadotropin secretion (LHRH-LH, FSH), and causes minimal liver toxicity (Barwin, 1982). Since mesterlone does not suppress gonadotropin secretion, its spermatogenic effect is more reliable than other androgen supplements (Barwin, 1982); indeed, it is used for the treatment of insufficient spermatogenesis. However, a recent placebo-controlled study showed that 150 mg/day mesterolone over a full year did not increase pregnancies produced by infertile men, despite a significant increase in the motility and proportion of normal spermatozoa (Gerris, Peeters, Comhaire, Schoonjanes, & Hellemans, 1991).

The androgenic potency of mesterolone is less than other testosterone supplements, but it is free of many androgenic side effects. Since it is not aromatized to estrogens, it does not cause gynecomastia or other potential estrogenic effects, including tumor/cancer promotion.

Mesterolone has been shown by Vogel, Klaiber, and Broverman (1985) to function as an antidepressant in men, with far fewer side effects than amitriptyline. However, the antidepressant effect shown in this study was rather small and very high doses (150–550 mg/day) were required. (As a testosterone supplement, mesterolone is often used in doses ranging from 50 to 150 mg.) Since testosterone acts as a MAO-A inhibitor, similar to estrogen, it should have some antidepressant effects (however, its MAO-inhibiting effect is quite weak compared to MAO-inhibitor antidepressants). It also functions symbiotically with activating neurotransmitters and peptides such as dopamine and vasopressin. In a placebo-controlled study, Kaiser et al. (1978) found that mesterolone (75 mg/day) could be used to treat what they considered to be the male climacteric or menopause in men between the ages of 45 and 60. They described this syndrome as characterized by unusual fatigability, listlessness, diminished productivity and disinclination to work, increased irritability, physical hypersensitivity, and poor concentration and memory. Serious depression and reduced sexual function are not considered characteristic, but there is some indication of decreased libido and reduced desire for sexual activity. When mesterolone was compared to placebo, it significantly improved activity and performance, extroversion, and masculine self-image including assertiveness, but did not alter neuroticism, anxiety, irritability, depressed mood, or psychovegetative symptoms such as disturbed sleep, restlessness, headaches, dizziness, bothersome cardiac and skin sensations. Side effects of mesterolone were minor.

Combination Treatment

Vogel's and Kaiser's studies suggested that mesterolone may be used in conjunction with other antidepressants, stimulants, herbal, and vitamin supplements to alleviate neurasthenic symptoms and clinical depression. Androgens may also be useful in the treatment of decreased libido when they are used with other sexual stimulants such as yohimbine or dopaminergic agents. The Federal Drug Administration has discouraged use of combination treatments with drugs which do not have clearly reproducible efficacy when used alone. However, the integrated functioning of hormones, peptides, neurotransmitters, vitamins, and diet are intrinsic to natural human physiology, suggesting that treatments involving combinations of interacting drugs should be investigated.

TESTOSTERONE DELIVERY SYSTEMS

Injections

Injectable testosterone (depo-testosterone) comes in two forms: testosterone enanthate and testosterone cypionate. The injection method bypasses the liver, thus avoiding toxicity. It is usually used in men because it is difficult for them to achieve sufficiently high levels orally. Oral testosterone or, more recently, implantable pellets, are the current preferred methods for women. However, injection appears to be the most effective and safe method for both men and women.

Mechanical injection pens with the syringe needle propelled by touching a button and needle-less jet injection guns are available to facilitate this procedure. Jet injection avoids needlestick injuries and may be acceptable to patients who are clumsy or fear needles. The testosterone fluid is propelled out of the syringe gun by a $C0_2$ cartridge with a force sufficient to penetrate the skin. Jet injection has even been used in France for intracavernosal penile injections to induce erection (Lemaire, Bailleul, Sister, Demaine, & Buvat, 1990). The Biojector 2000 Needle-Free Jet Injection System has also been used successfully in a small pilot trial for intracavernosal injection and is widely used for injections to diabetic and multiple sclerosis patients (personal communication, Robert Bennett, 1994).

Jet injection of testosterone for both women and men should increase the acceptability of testosterone supplementation or replacement during the 1990s (its use for in vitro fertilization programs, which may require a long series of daily injections, is particularly promising). At this time, the jet injection guns cost over $700, so it is likely to be used only by doctors; however, individuals may be able to rent these guns from doctors for short-term use, and business companies may buy an injection gun for administration to their employees by a company doctor or nurse.

Transdermal Patches

Within the past few years, the use of transdermal patch delivery systems for drugs such as nitroglycerin, clonidine, scopolamine, estradiol, and nicotine has become routine. The transdermal therapeutic testosterone patch Testoderm became commercially available in 1994 (Alza Pharmaceuticals, 1994). Intended for men with low testosterone levels, it is a self-adhering patch applied daily to the testicular scrotal skin. A new patch must be applied each morning, the scrotum must be shaved, and the patch should be removed before bathing or swimming. Different sizes deliver different sequential amounts of testosterone within each day of use. Further information is available from the manufacturer (Alza Pharmaceuticals, 800-634-8977). The rise and fall of testosterone absorbed from the daily patches better resembles the normal circadian variation of natural testosterone secretion. Patch administration to the scrotal skin is necessary for adequate testosterone absorption; however, newer patches are being developed for application to other body areas, such as the abdomen and thigh (Meikle et al., 1993).

A major advantage of the transdermal patches is that testosterone levels can be titrated to acceptable normal ranges without the exaggerated and unpredictable increases and decreases in concentration and consequent emotional highs and lows that occur with injections. Furthermore, since a bolus of testosterone is not injected, sequestered, metabolized, and released from tissues, there is relatively little metabolism of testosterone to estradiol and other androgenic-estrogenic metabolites which can cause undesirable side effects. With the Testoderm patch, steady-state testosterone levels are not reached until three weeks following initiation of treatment (Alza, 1994). A 12-week treatment study with hypogonadal men showed significant increases in mood, energy level, and sexual thought frequency by week three and further improvement to an asymptote at week nine (Alza, 1994). While spontaneous erections increased dramatically, there was no increase in sexual intercourse and only a small increase in orgasms by weeks nine through 12.

Removability of the patches at any time allows testosterone to be quickly withdrawn if toxic psychological (e.g., aggression, psychoses, euphoria) or somatic (e.g., allergic reaction, headache) occur. A potential drawback is that excessive local dihydrotestosterone might be produced because the scrotal skin contains such a high level of 5-alpha reductase activity, potentially aggravating prostatic hypertrophy and prostatic cancer. The patch has been tested in some subjects for months and years with no prostatic hyperplasia noted (Cunningham, Cordero, & Thornby, 1989; McClure, Oses, & Ernest, 1991), but other effects of high concentrations of dihydrotestosterone in the genitals are unknown. While cholesterol levels are decreased with patches, both HDL and LDL are reduced, so that the HDL/LDL ratio does not change.

Sublingual Linguets

Sublingual testosterone is available in the United States under the name of Testoral. When testosterone linguets are placed underneath the tongue, they are absorbed directly into the bloodstream, bypassing the intestine. Dosing is more consistent, but linguets do not achieve blood levels as high as injectable testosterone and are consequently less popular. However, for those with borderline testosterone values, they are more convenient and better tolerated.

Carrier Drugs

Brain-targeted carrier drugs have been developed and have entered early clinical testing (Greer, 1988). A water-soluble active drug substance is attached to a special lipid-soluble molecule that easily passes through the blood-brain barrier. Once inside the brain, this special molecule is oxidized by enzymes, splitting off the water-soluble active drug substance. The inactive nontoxic lipid-soluble carrier passes back through the blood-brain barrier into the body and is excreted in the urine. A small portion of the drug-carrier system does not enter the brain and is apparently not converted within the body; it, too, is excreted in the urine. Various body chemicals, including hormones, neurotransmitters such as dopamine and GABA, peptides, and antiviral agents, could be attached to such carrier vehicles.

Bodor and Farag (1984) have described and tested a brain-specific drug-carrier system containing testosterone. Apparently, most beneficial psychotropic actions of testosterone occur within the brain in both men and women (e.g., stimulation of sex drive, stimulation of feelings of confidence and assertiveness, and facilitation of other activating brain substances).

Peripheral androgenic effects caused by currently available testosterone preparations (such as cholesterol/lipid changes, liver damage, prostatic hyperplasia, and virilizing excesses) have prevented widespread use of testosterone outside of the small endocrinological specialty of testosterone replacement for hypogonadism in men and rare gynecological problems in women. The brain-specific testosterone-carrier systems being developed by Bodor and others could avoid these adverse peripheral effects and present the possibility of using testosterone or other androgens as psychotropic drugs. Delivery targeted directly into the brain would also allow further study of hormonal/peptide actions within the brain.

On the basis of the assumption that testosterone increases human male sex drive through conversion (aromatization) to estradiol (as it often does in lower animals such as rats [Anderson, Simpkins, Brewster, & Bodor, 1987]), this form of estrogen is being investigated as a treatment for low sex drive in men. At present, the most active clinical testing appears to be utilizing an estradiol brain-specific carrier-drug system called CDS-E2 (Anderson, Simpkins, Brewster, & Bodor, 1988; Estes, Brewster, Simpkins, &

Bodor, 1987). One proposed use of this brain-estradiol drug is for stimulation of male sex drive and initiative (but not sexual response itself). The development of both brain-delivered estradiol and brain-delivered testosterone for human clinical use would finally allow sophisticated investigation of the psychotropic and sexual actions of these hormones in both men and women. At that point, sexual pharmacology would enter another research "galaxy" altogether—one with enormous clinical potential for expanding our knowledge of male/female differences.

CONCLUSIONS

Experimental understanding of the pharmacological profile of testosterone is changing. It is becoming increasingly clear that testosterone, originally believed to be a male hormone, plays a meaningful role in female sexuality, although that role has not yet been completely delineated. It is also apparent that testosterone is not the only "chemical switch" that governs sexuality. Sexual desire and response are increased or decreased in various ways by a complex interaction of body chemicals, including peptides, neurotransmitters, and hormones. The prevalent notion that sex hormones exclusively control sexual behavior is out-of-date today.

Lowering testosterone levels with synthetic LHRH analogues has shown that testosterone is required more for sexual desire than for potency. Since we now have the means to lower testosterone safely and reversibly by LHRH agonist treatment without direct antiandrogen receptor blockade, the extent and nature of testosterone's role in maintaining sexual desire should soon be clarified by well-controlled longitudinal studies.

Testosterone has been liberally prescribed for men with sexual dysfunctions, whether or not they have endogenous decreased levels. So far, it appears that testosterone is clinically effective for sex drive only in hypotestosterone males. The use of testosterone in men, however, is not without complications. These complications include prostatic hypertrophy, stimulation of prostatic cancer, precipitation or aggravation of hypertension, and liver damage. In spite of these serious side effects, testosterone has been over-prescribed for men by many of the same physicians who under-prescribe estrogen in women. A medical double standard appears to be operating, since these two hormones with relatively comparable side effects are used in such opposite patterns.

With the development of "cleaner" androgens that have fewer peripheral side effects, and the use of new methods of delivery directly into the brain that have the potential to avoid virilizing side effects, testosterone treatments for both men and women sexes will be re-evaluated.

9

Dehydroepiandrosterone (DHEA/DHEAS)

OBJECTIVES

- To describe the physiology and metabolism of this mysterious hormone, including male/female differences
- To examine drugs that either inhibit or stimulate DHEA production
- To consider the role of DHEA in sexual function
- To explore its potential role in facilitating longevity

Dehydroepiandrosterone—DHEA—is the most abundant circulating steroid in the human body, yet its functions remain largely unexplored by researchers to date. DHEA also is the dominant hormone produced by the fetus, in amounts from 200 to over 400 times greater than concentrations of progesterone and testosterone, 100 times greater than the level of androstenedione, and over 800 times greater than the levels of estradiol and estrone (Stone, Fair, & Fishman, 1986).

This mysterious sex hormone, which displays comparable activity in both sexes, has been disregarded due to the finding that its androgenic potency is only 3% of that possessed by testosterone. Furthermore, it has not been demonstrated to generate masculine behaviors typical of testosterone; and, unlike estrogen and progesterone, it is not associated with the menstrual cycle.

DHEA and its conjugated sulfate DHEAS are secreted by the inner regions of the adrenal gland. In the adrenal gland, cholesterol is metabolized by certain enzymatic processes to pregnenolone. Pregnenolone is metabolized either to DHEA and DHEAS or to progesterone and cortisol. The uterine level of DHEAS is 40 times the level of unconjugated DHEA. Pregnenolone-sulfate, which has some actions similar to DHEAS, is the next highest uterine steroid. It occurs in the human uterus and placenta at high concentrations, and is thought to assist the birth process in some way. Though DHEA and DHEAS levels and metabolism differ, their physiological effects appear similar.*

DHEAS serves as a precursor to other estrogenic and androgenic steroids. It is metabolized peripherally to estrogen, various androgens, androsterone, and possibly significant sexual pheromonal substances in the skin. The sexual effects of DHEA are fascinating and still somewhat mysterious, due to the limited research thus far devoted to studying this complex hormone. Particularly intriguing is its action as a neurosteroid and its stimulation by bupropion, which was first identified in a research study performed by the authors in 1984. This study is described in detail in Chapter 27.

After describing the physiology and metab-

*This chapter will concentrate on DHEA; however, DHEA and DHEAS are two forms of the same hormone. For brevity, the hormone will be referred to as DHEA; but DHEA/DHEAS or each separately will often be used for the sake of accuracy.

olism of DHEA, we will review the effects of various drugs and medications on DHEA levels. Table 9.1 summarizes the functions and interactive characteristics of DHEA/DHEAS.

DHEA is secreted episodically throughout the day in a manner similar to cortisol. Both DHEA and cortisol adrenal secretion are stimulated by ACTH. However, since DHEA and cortisol levels may change independently, there appears to be a separate factor responsible for regulating DHEA secretion. For instance, in certain disease states, DHEA levels may decrease, while cortisol remains unchanged or increases. Cortisol levels usually remain constant as one grows older; DHEA levels peak between ages 25 and 30 and thereafter decline steadily, so that levels are quite low by age 60.

Unconjugated (nonsulfated) DHEA can change rapidly. When stimulated by corticotropin (ACTH) administration, DHEA in the human adrenal may increase 20 to 100 times without any immediate change occurring in DHEAS (Feher, Szalay, & Szilagyi, 1985; Vaitukaitis, Dale, & Melby, 1969). These dramatic and rapidly shifting levels make the clinical effects of DHEA elusive and difficult to identify.

By contrast, the level of DHEA-sulfate (DHEAS) is stable throughout the day. In fact, DHEAS is one of the few steroid hormones free of the circadian and other cyclic changes which complicate measurement of other hormones. With dexamethasone suppression, DHEA levels decrease more than DHEAS levels. The metabolism of free adrenal DHEA to DHEAS is apparently rather slow.

Since DHEA levels often change independently of cortisol, Parker and Odell (1979) have postulated a separate adrenal androgen-stimulating hormone distinct from pituitary ACTH. Though both are adrenal steroids, the changes of DHEA and cortisol in opposite directions indicate that they may have separate brain-releasing factors and/or that cortisol reciprocally inhibits DHEA during the physical stress of trauma and disease. During chronic disease or aging, DHEA levels decrease but cortisol levels remain the same or increase. DHEA also changes independently of testosterone. For instance, digoxin increases DHEA and estradiol but lowers testosterone (Neri, Aygen, Zukerman, & Bahary, 1980). It is interesting that DHEA itself has digitalis-like properties similar to digoxin. Also, while prolactin may cause increased production of DHEA, DHEA does not cause a rise in prolactin.

Sexual hormone responses in animals are usually analyzed at the hypothalamic level only, using fairly simple and externally measurable

Table 9.1 *The Functions and Interactive Characteristics of DHEA/DHEAS*

Increased DHEA	*Decreased DHEA*	*Substances that Increase DHEA*	*Substances that Decrease DHEA*
Protects immune function	Associated with degenerative diseases	Prolactin	Glucocorticoids
Inhibits carcinogenic tumors	↑ cardiovascular disease	Bupropion	Carbamazepine
Promotes bone growth	50% in ovarian cancer	Digoxin	Phenytoin
Opposes glucocorticoid toxicity	In breast cancer 9 years prior to diagnosis	Trilostane	Phenobarbital
Promotes weight loss	Stress ↓ DHEA ↑ cortisol	Amlodipine	Norethindrone
↑ energy utilization	↑ osteoporosis	Nitrendipine	Medroxyprogesterone
↓ conversion of energy to stored fat	↓ in obese humans	Diltiazem	Ketoconazole
↓ cholesterol		Metformin	Cimetidine
↓ LDL and body fat		Tobacco	Aminoglutethimide
Vigorous exercise ↑ DHEA			Flutamide
			Lovastatin
			Alcohol
			Insulin

copulatory and masturbatory behavior. With DHEA, the investigation may have to be far more sophisticated to discover functionally significant actions related to sexual desire and behavior. In many ways, DHEA activity appears more characteristic of limbic neurotransmitters, including acetylcholine, GABA, and excitatory amino acids, than to other sex hormones. The emergence of high levels of DHEA production from the adrenal glands has accompanied the evolutionary development of the limbic system to the dominant position found in primates and especially in humans. Consequently, the sexual actions of DHEA must be considered within the context of limbic interactions with the hypothalamus as well as in the lower brain.

THE NEUROSTEROID CONNECTION

Animal research has revealed that DHEA/DHEAS persist in the brains of male and female rats and monkeys after surgical or pharmacological elimination of adrenal and gonadal steroid secretion (Robel et al., 1984). Therefore, they must be independently produced within the brain itself as neurosteroids. Discovery of substantial DHEA/DHEAS levels in the rat brain contrasts with minimal production in rat adrenals. Pregnenolone and pregnenolone sulfate, steroid precursors to DHEA/DHEAS, also exist independently in the brain as neurosteroids. Thus, the brain can supply itself with these hormones and may be considered an endocrine organ.

Neurosteroids can be produced from the glia surrounding nerve cells, white matter, and/or from as yet unidentified glandular nuclei. The brain contains the enzymes and sulfatase necessary for DHEA/DHEAS metabolism. As steroid precursors, DHEA/DHEAS and pregnenolone and pregnenolone sulfate may be incorporated directly into cell membranes in a manner similar to cholesterol.

It is unclear to what extent these brain neurosteroids are supplemented from the peripheral circulation and endocrine glands. (In contrast, brain testosterone and corticosteroids appear to come mostly from peripheral circulation and glands, crossing the blood-brain barrier to bind to specific brain areas.) Although the actions and functions of DHEA/DHEAS, pregnenolone, and pregnenolone sulfate in the brain are unknown, preliminary studies (Robel et al., 1991) have shown them to be present in levels much higher than other sex steroid hormones (testosterone, estrogens) in all areas of the brain. Lanthier and Patwardhan (1986) also found that the brain levels of free DHEA and pregnenolone were higher than DHEAS and pregnenolone sulfate, in contrast to the peripheral circulation, where DHEAS and pregnenolone sulfate levels are much higher. Though only three male and two female brains were studied, free DHEA was strikingly higher in females than in males, particularly in the hypothalamus and limbic structures. It should be noted that studies of human brains have questionable relevance because they must be done from autopsy of brains, usually from elderly patients, in which peripheral DHEA/DHEAS has dropped to minimal levels.

Production of large amounts of DHEA/DHEAS from the adrenal gland only occurs consistently in humans, and the limbic area where neural DHEA/DHEAS appears to be concentrated has greatly expanded in humans. For these reasons, one may anticipate a greater and more complex role for neural DHEA/DHEAS in humans than in rats.

The excitatory nature of DHEA/DHEAS, pregnenolone, and pregnenolone sulfate has been shown by a research group in France, including Etienne-Emile Baulieu (RU-486 developer) and Paul Robel, who found that these neurosteroids may act as excitatory neuroregulators in the central nervous system, existing in balance or opposition to inhibitory CNS neuroregulators such as GABA (and perhaps endogenous "benzodiazepines") and progesterone derivatives (Baulieu et al., 1984; Baulieu et al., 1987; Robel et al., 1984; Robel et al., 1991). For example, these neurosteroids were found to facilitate seizure activity similar to GABA/benzodiazepine antagonists and to activate limbic structures.

With regard to sexual desire and behavior in rats, DHEA/DHEAS, pregnenolone, and pregnenolone sulfate neurosteroids have excitatory effects on septum and medial preoptic neurons (Carette & Poulain, 1984), which promote active and pleasurable sexual behavior and reactions. When male rats in their home cage are exposed to the scent of receptive female rats for seven days, DHEA/DHEAS, pregnenolone, and pregnenolone sulfate neurosteroids increase in the amygdala and hypothalamus (Robel et al., 1984). No changes occur in blood concentrations, however. Robel and Baulieu (1985) hypothesized that DHEA or pregnenolone may have "a role in perception and/or integration of the scent of the opposite sex in the central nervous system."

Similar levels of neural DHEA/DHEAS, pregnenolone, and pregnenolone sulfate have been found in male and female rats when the females are near or in estrus, decreasing to lower levels during diestrous when females are not sexually active or receptive.

The fact that DHEA/DHEAS, pregnenolone, and pregnenolone sulfate promote excitation and facilitate seizure-like activity in the septum suggests that they can also facilitate orgasm, which is at least partly generated in the septum. Currently, there is no information about how these neurosteroids interact with or are influenced by more well-known sex steroids such as testosterone or estrogen, or how their actions may differ between females and males.

Augmentation of neural DHEA/DHEAS, pregnenolone, and pregnenolone sulfate during sexual excitation may occur with no change in blood levels outside the brain. Since vasopressin has excitatory actions on the limbic structures where these neurosteroids are most active, can raise peripheral DHEA/DHEAS levels, and increases during the sexual response, it is conceivable that vasopressin and neural DHEA/DHEAS are mutually activated during sexual behavior. Melatonin, which suppresses sexual behavior and gonadal activity, has been suggested by Robel et al. (1991) to inhibit neurosteroidal activity in a rhythmic manner related to lighting conditions (melatonin increases during darkness).

Neural DHEA/DHEAS, pregnenolone, and pregnenolone sulfate (1) act as picrotoxin-like GABA antagonists in the brain; (2) inhibit benzodiazepine binding; (3) counteract the GABA-activated chloride conductance which causes tranquilization and sleep; (4) facilitate seizure; and (5) can reduce sleep time (Robel et al., 1991).

In addition, DHEA/DHEAS inhibit the action of GABA agonists, while alcohol potentiates GABA agonists. Neural progesterone derivatives generally have actions opposite to those of DHEA/DHEAS, pregnenolone, and pregnenolone sulfate (i.e., they are inhibitory).

It appears that neuroendocrine steroidal regulation probably is chiefly mediated by glutamate transmission and excitatory/inhibitory amino acids, rather than by amine neurotransmitters and peptides (Van den Pol, Wuarin, & Dudek, 1990). Although glutamate neurotransmission has received very little attention, exciting research on the interaction of neurosteroidal and glutamate/amino acid transmission has been reported by Maria Majewska (Majewska, 1987; Majewska, 1990; Majewska, Demirgoren, & London, 1990; Majewska, Mienville, & Vicini, 1988). The prominent excitatory and/or inhibitory effects of steroids shown in this research has suggested that stress, immunity, brain-cell homeostasis, and cell degeneration are important foci for DHEA/DHEAS, pregnenolone, and pregnenolone sulfate actions. Activity and states studied by Majewska include anesthesia, seizure activity and its association with long-term potentiation of learning and memory, trauma, premenstrual tension, and postpartum depression. Majewska's research has also suggested elaborate interactions of neurosteroids with GABA in the control of sexual behavior and male/female differences relating to this behavior. The sexual effects which occur with GABAergic medications may be far more subtle and complex than current notions of sexual dysfunction allow. DHEA/DHEAS sexual effects may be expected to be similarly subtle and complex.

The psychobiological intricacies of limbic function mandate that attention be directed to the continual interplay of mind-body responses. As a sex steroid hormone, DHEA/DHEAS activity encompasses the more subtle and interactional sexual factors common to both females and males (in contrast to the polarized and sexually overt behavior and reactions characteristic of testosterone and estrogens).

PERIPHERAL ACTIVITY

DHEAS and its derivatives are substantially higher in fat from the breasts and pubic region than in fat from the abdomen. Estradiol and many androgen derivatives have the same concentrations in the fat of both areas (Deslypere, Verdonck, & Vermeulen, 1985).

One function of DHEAS is to provide a source for peripheral androgenic and estrogenic hormones within the skin itself. DHEAS penetration into skin tissue is limited due to its sulfate form, which is not well-absorbed from the blood into peripheral tissue. Instead, DHEAS has much of its peripheral effects through metabolizing into androgen and estrogen derivatives that are well-absorbed by the skin. While DHEAS itself therefore would not have a pheromonal or smell potency, its derivatives potentially could. Androstenediols, for example, have become known as sex pheromones/attractants/repellents.

The conversion of DHEA/DHEAS to testosterone or androgen represents the action of a "prehormone pair": the secretion of a precursor substance, which is then converted by peripheral tissue to a potent hormone (Horton & Lobo, 1986). This prehormone/precursor pairing allows high levels of potent hormones to effect target tissues (e.g., genital skin), while the hormonal effects in the general circulation are limited to the effects of precursor prehormones like DHEAS.

Human skin actively participates in both the synthesis and breakdown of DHEAS (Parker, 1989). Indeed, many of the sex steroids produced in the skin are dependent upon a vast array of enzymes that mediate their metabolism and the different kinds of cell structures within the skin (sebaceous glands, apocrine glands, other sweat glands, hair follicles, epidermis, and dermis which contains collagen and capillary networks). In most skin areas, estradiol (E2) is converted to estrone (E1). In the vaginal mucosa, more estradiol than estrone is produced due to the presence of special protein receptors. Since DHEAS is especially abundant in the genital area, it is probably converted to estradiol to a greater extent in the genitals than in the blood and other skin areas.

The large amount of DHEA secreted by humans is unique, even though the adrenals of some other primates, particularly apes (chimpanzees), secrete considerable levels. Blood DHEAS levels in adult men are 100 to 500 times higher than testosterone levels (Labrie et al., 1990). Labrie has suggested that the huge contribution of non-gonadal DHEA expands the concept of endocrinology beyond the limited notion of hormones being released into the circulation to act on distant target organs/tissues. He has described three additional levels of hormone activity: *paracrine* (hormone acting on neighboring cells), *autocrine* (hormone active on its own cell surfaces), *intracrine* (hormone active inside its own cell). These additional levels of hormone activity are particularly appropriate for the "endocrinology of skin." Pheromones provide chemical contact communication that links us to one another. By definition, a pheromone is a chemical substance secreted externally by one organism (or person) that causes a specific reaction in receiving organisms of the same species. There is good reason to believe that DHEA/DHEAS play a part in skin sensation, touch, and pheromonal contact, although this role has not yet been confirmed. The skin is virtually awash in an abundant variety of steroid hormones derived from DHEAS. With continued investigation of human skin steroidal activity, our understanding of sexuality will expand beyond the circumscribed regions of sexual hormones and genitals. Recognition of the sexual possibilities of touch and smell in humans could lead to the discovery of pheromonal activity that may be missing in couples and individuals who lack physical intimacy.

The sex hormone concentrations in skin and other peripheral tissue are usually different from those in the blood. Even with equivalent blood levels of sex hormones, there are large individual differences in peripheral responses. For example, different skin sensitivity to testosterone metabolites may explain why there is decreased body hair in Japanese people, despite normal testosterone levels. Consideration of DHEAS and other prehormones in relation to their transformation into more active metabolites is necessary for an understanding of peripheral hormone effects.

MALE/FEMALE DIFFERENCES IN DHEA

In contrast to the notable gender-related differences in testosterone and estrogen levels, DHEA levels in females are quite close to male levels. DHEA is produced chiefly in a non-sexual organ (the adrenals) rather than in the sexually differentiated gonads. It is secreted in major amounts only in non-human primates and humans. One could speculate an evolutionary role in the liberation of female sexual drive from the ebb and flow of estrus (ovulatory period of heightened sex drive controlled by the female hormone estrogen) to a sex hormone state more equivalent to the continuously active male sex drive. Non-human primate and human females are not bound to the cycle of estrogen/progesterone for sexual receptivity, even though receptivity may still increase at the time of ovulation or at estrogen peaks. However, there is probably a major hormonal difference between non-human primates and women, because only in women can the ovaries be removed without routinely predictable reduction of sexual desire. One might conclude that human female sexual desire has shifted somewhat from estrogen to androgen influence (from the ovaries to the adrenals).

Unfortunately, there is no conclusive evidence that DHEA has an effect on sexual drive in women or men. Though it rises precipitously prior to and during puberty and declines with aging, its fluctuations have seldom been studied in regard to sexual drive and behavior. A recent six-month study by Morales, Nolan, Nelson, and Yen (1994) found overall increases in subjective well-being with daily 50 mg DHEA supplementation in men and women between 40 and 70 years old, but no specific change in libido. However, well-being was assessed by an open-ended questionnaire, while libido was measured with a visual analogue scale that may have been insensitive to moderate changes.

During the early 1960s, DHEA was identified as a sex hormone in women. Masters and Johnson attributed the lack of decline in female sexual desire after menopause in part to continued secretion of androgens such as DHEA from the adrenals. The early studies in this area were conducted by Waxenberg and his colleagues at the Sloan-Kettering Cancer Research Institute (Waxenberg, 1962; Waxenberg, Drellich, & Sutherland, 1959; Waxenberg, Finkbeinter, Drellich, & Sutherland, 1960). During the 1950s, the sexual effects of cancer disease and surgery (including radical mastectomy, colostomy, and hysterectomy) were investigated at Sloan-Kettering. In the initial study, Waxenberg et al. (1959) interviewed 29 women (mean age = 51) who had undergone removal of both their ovaries and adrenals to stop the spread of metastatic breast cancer. Twelve women had reported a total lack of sexual desire and activity even before removal of the ovaries and adrenals. In the remaining women still experiencing some sexual desire, removal of the ovaries and adrenals resulted in a decrease in sexual desire in 14 of the 17 (10 experienced a total decrease to zero). All 17 women experienced a decrease in sexual activity; seven experienced a total decrease to zero; 10 experienced some decrease. Of 12 women with preoperative sexual responsiveness, all but one experienced a decrease (nine experienced a total decrease to zero).

A subgroup of seven women had had their ovaries removed one to five years prior to undergoing adrenalectomy. Two of these women experienced no sexual change after oophorectomy, three experienced some decrease, and two were already at a zero level prior to oophorectomy. After adrenalectomy, four of the five women experienced a total loss of sexual desire and responsiveness. Since the more serious decline in sexual desire occurred only with removal of the adrenals, Waxenberg concluded that "the androgenic hormones of adrenal origin play a critical part in maintaining the patterns of sexual behavior in the human female."

Results of the Waxenberg study are limited by the small number of subjects, by the compounding effect of disease progression on adrenal functioning, by the compounding effect of fatigue occurring with adrenal removal, and by the absence of subjects who had undergone only adrenalectomy (the surgery resulted in loss of both the ovaries and adrenals). Furthermore, there are other adrenal androgens (chiefly androstenedione and testosterone) that have sexual effects separate from changes that occur with DHEA (about 50% of androstenedione and 25% of testosterone production comes from the adrenals).

Ordinarily, after adrenalectomy, cortisol is the only hormone replaced with supplements. By default, adrenal androgens remain at low levels. An interesting observation by Waxenberg (1962) was that the few women who experienced sexual interest after adrenalectomy-oophorectomy showed a change in preference from direct genital gratification to more diffuse gratification derived from affection and overall physical closeness.

In girls at puberty, Udry (1988) found that levels of free testosterone and adrenal androgens (including DHEA, DHEAS, and androstenedione) were significant hormonal predictors of sexual desire and non-coital sexual behavior (e.g., fantasy and masturbation). It may be that social and conditioned gender restraints are responsible for this lack of significant correlation to actual intercourse. However, some of these restraints would also apply (perhaps even more intensely) in regard to masturbation.

NIMH/NIH studies have found no significant correlations in females between pubertal hormones and affective states such as depression. However, negative correlations of DHEA/DHEAS with aggressive behavior and positive correlations of androstenedione and estradiol with verbal aggression have been reported in adolescent girls (Paikoff & Brooks-Gunn, 1991). It is interesting that in adolescent girls, progesterone has been positively correlated with impatience and aggression (Udry & Talbert, 1988). Progesterone and GABA play an opposite role to DHEA in many bodily processes, and paradoxical aggression due to progesterone or GABA potentiation (e.g., with benzodiazepines) occurs more often in females than in males.

DHEAS levels are very high in the fetus during pregnancy, serving as an estrogen precursor and other unknown functions. First pregnancies are followed by a permanent decrease in DHEA and DHEAS (Key, Pike, Wang, & Moore, 1990). Consequently, DHEA and DHEAS levels are generally lower in parous than in nulliparous women. A relation between this drop in DHEA to postpartum depression or to a decrease in libido and sexual attraction to mates has not been investigated.

Despite the general assumption that there is no change in adrenal androgens with menopause, since they do not come from the ovaries, it is clear that DHEA decreases during perimenopause and continues to decrease during postmenopause in conjunction with aging (Rozenberg, Ham, Bosson, Peretz, & Robyn, 1990).

Increased or abnormal sexuality in women may be seen in the adrenal virilizing syndrome (e.g., adrenogenital syndrome), which is caused by excess ACTH secretion and abnormally high levels of adrenal androgens (Young, 1983). Heightened libido and sexual fantasizing may also be due to pubertal changes. Disturbed sexual behavior and extremes of sexual activity may occur.

DHEA IN ANIMALS

DHEA production from the adrenals is not significant in rodents; consequently, most of the research investigating the sexual effects of DHEA in animals has been conducted on non-human primates, which is expensive and therefore less abundant. DHEA mechanisms have evolved from monkeys through apes to humans, so that the application of research on monkeys to humans, while valuable, is not direct.

Furthermore, monkeys are typically tested for sexual behavior in natural colonies rather than in unnatural, isolated, caged-pair tests (e.g., Wallen et al., 1986; Wallen & Winston, 1984). In natural environments, most putative "aphrodisiacs" (including testosterone, LHRH, deprenyl, L-dopa, and yohimbine) fail to alter sexual behavior significantly (Chambers & Phoenix, 1989). Consequently, lack of evidence for a DHEA adrenal androgen sexual effect in monkeys and apes does not indicate that DHEA would not be sexually active in other circumstances, for example, with either humans or rats. More serious criticisms of these studies are that adrenal suppression or removal is not equivalent to an isolated change in DHEA.

Recent research in animals has not supported Waxenberg's observation of a positive sexual effect of adrenal androgens in human females (Dixson, 1987; Everitt & Herbert, 1971; Everitt, Herbert, & Hamer, 1972; Lovejoy & Wallen, 1990; Nadler, Wallis, Roth-Meyer, Cooper, & Baulieu, 1987; Wallen et al., 1986; Wallen & Winston, 1984). Waxenberg and the animal researchers claim that their findings are relevant to illuminating the nature of DHEA sexual actions, but the full scope of this hormone is not known.

DHEA SUPPLEMENTATION

Prostate Cancer

Although some hormone treatments of prostate cancer show greater efficacy when adrenal androgens as well as gonadal androgens are pharmacologically suppressed (Labrie et al., 1988), adrenal androgens alone are unlikely to promote prostate hypertrophy or cancer (Oesterling, Epstein, & Walsh, 1986). In fact, DHEA has been shown to inhibit cancerous tumor growth in rodents (Schwartz, Pashko, & Whitcome, 1986). If DHEA has a testosterone-like effect, it is probably not due to DHEA itself but to its metabolism into testosterone. Van Weerden et al. (1990) found that the adrenal androgen androstenedione, but not DHEA, induced growth in human prostatic tumor tissue transplanted into mice. Bartsch, Greeve, and Voight (1987) further implicated androstenedione in prostatic hypertrophy by showing that it is the chief adrenal precursor for active androgens in the human prostate. DHEA conversion to testosterone in prostate tissue was not detected. DHEA stimulation of prostate activity has been demonstrated in rats (Labrie et al., 1989, 1990). However, even in rat prostates, androstenedione is more than twice as potent as DHEA (Bruchovsky, 1971).

Given the lack of direct evidence for DHEA stimulation of abnormal prostate growth, DHEA supplementation in men should not be precluded without definitive research that addresses this issue. However, men on DHEA therapy should be monitored regularly for prostate growth, and men with prostatic hypertrophy should not be treated with DHEA until more information is available.

Obesity

DHEA/DHEAS supplementation has been shown to consistently decrease obesity in mice and rats with no apparent toxic effects. Yen, Allan, Pearson, Acton, and Greenberg (1977) showed that DHEAS decreased lipogenesis in mice *despite no change in food intake*; benefits were lost when DHEAS was withdrawn. Cleary, Shepherd, and Jenks (1984) have shown reduction of obesity, decreases in weight gain, decreases in fat cells and fat tissue weights, and decreases in cholesterol with DHEA/DHEAS supplementation, with no reduction in food intake. They have hypothesized that DHEA induces a "futile cycle of fatty acid metabolism" (recylation), leading to enhanced energy utilization and decreased conversion to stored fat.

Whatever the mechanism, DHEA seems to cause a shift in metabolic utilization of dietary energy, rather than a reduction of energy (i.e., food) intake. Of special importance to obesity-related diabetes or hyperinsulinemic disorders, DHEA supplements in rats lower insulin levels by as much as 40% without any increase in glucose levels, indicating that the insulin becomes more efficient and/or needed in lower doses (Cleary & Zisk, 1986; Mohan & Cleary, 1989). Abnormal glucose metabolism in diabetic mice has also been corrected by DHEA (Muller

& Cleary, 1985). Interestingly, testosterone has the opposite effect: It increases insulin requirements, not to mention abdominal fat deposits.

There is evidence that DHEA supplementation has greater effects in female animals than in males. For example, much of Cleary's work cited above utilized female mice and rats. Tagliaferro, Davis, Trachon, and van Hamont (1986) found that changes in body composition in rats were greater in females than in males. DHEA supplementation increased thermogenesis (burning of calories and fat), resting heat production, and otherwise decreased fat synthesis and storage to an equal extent in male and female rats. A study of rhesus monkeys has shown double the amount of DHEAS in lean females compared to spontaneously obese females, but no difference in DHEAS levels between obese and lean males (Kemnitz, Goy, Flitsch, Lohmiller, & Robinson, 1989). In this study, obese female monkeys with excess abdominal fat showed hyperinsulininemia, which was not found in lean females. The relationship of hyperinsulininemia in the obese females to lower DHEAS was not examined.

There has been little investigation of specific differences in DHEAS levels in obese humans or of the effects of DHEA/DHEAS supplements. Sonka (1976) found DHEAS production to be lower in obese humans; vigorous exercise such as running in women (Baker et al., 1982) and swimming in men (Brisson, Quirion, Ledoux, Raiotte, & Pellerin-Massicotte, 1984) has been demonstrated to elevate DHEAS levels for several hours. It would be interesting to study whether such DHEAS increases occur in obese humans after exercise. Nestler, Barlascini, and Clore (1988) found that DHEA supplementation in men decreased low density lipoproteins (LDL) and body fat over a period of 30 days. Other researchers with whom we have spoken indicated that they found no reduction of weight in humans treated with DHEA supplements for various illnesses including multiple sclerosis. DHEA supplementation has been used in women to treat breast cancer, and there has been no mention of weight changes in these studies.

The incidence of androgenic side effects in women treated with DHEA/DHEAS is unclear. Hidvegi, Feher, Feher, Koo, and Fust (1984) used DHEAS to treat hereditary angioneurotic edema, with none of the typical signs of adverse masculinization that occur with other androgens. Another finding that may restrict DHEA treatment in humans is elevated levels of cholesterol in the liver during DHEA supplementation.

Osteoporosis

Decreased levels of DHEA/DHEAS have consistently been correlated with lowering of bone mineral content due to aging and menopause (Nordin et al., 1985; Rozenberg, Ham, Bosson, et al., 1990; Taelman, Kaufman, Janssens, & Vermeulen, 1989; Wild, Buchanan, Myers, & Demers, 1987; Wild, Buchanan, Myers, Lloyd, & Demers, 1987). In Europe DHEA/DHEAS use as hormonal supplements for menopause has been encouraged by the possibility of inhibiting the progression of osteoporosis. Since both estrogen and androgens can foster bone growth and maintenance, DHEAS may function in this regard both as an androgen and as a precursor for estrogen. Early research reported that conjugated estrogen supplements (but not the synthetic ethinyl form) significantly increased DHEAS levels (Abraham & Maroulis, 1975), but more recent studies have found these increases to be less than previously reported (Cumming, Rebar, Hopper, & Yen, 1982).

While the correlation of lower DHEAS levels to bone loss (particularly in the spine), is definite, there is as yet no evidence that a decreased DHEAS *causes* the bone loss. Some investigators have suggested a stimulatory effect of DHEAS on bone formation regardless of the cause of bone loss (Taelman et al., 1989). DHEAS may indirectly prevent bone loss (and muscle atrophy) by opposing the erosive effects of cortisol, which are indicated by the severe osteoporosis experienced with long-term use of glucocorticoid steroids or with the excessive endogenous glucocorticoid levels of Cushing's disease (Falduto, Czerwinski, & Hickson, 1990; Lukert & Raisz, 1990; Prummel, Wiersinga, Lips, Sanders, & Sauerwein, 1991). Glucocorticoid treatment reduces both DHEAS and testosterone (Jennings, Andersson, & Johansson, 1991).

Since DHEA decreases with age and reaches very low levels over age 50 in both men and women, one might expect associated osteoporosis to occur in men as well. Although conventional medical opinion does not consider this to be a significant problem in men, most research and treatment regarding osteoporosis has been conducted in women. More subtle but nonetheless serious changes may occur in men. While women can take estrogen supplements to alleviate bone decline, there is no hormonal treatment available at this time for men over 50 experiencing accelerated bone loss. Since men are adversely effected by estrogen and testosterone is often contraindicated, DHEA supplementation could be a possible alternative treatment for preventing the development of osteoporosis.

DRUGS INHIBITING DHEA

Oral Contraceptives

Oral contraceptives generally lower DHEA/DHEAS levels (Gaspard et al., 1984; Klove et al., 1984; Vermeulen & Thiery, 1982), apparently due to progestogen (Lobo, 1988). Oral contraceptives with the progestogen norethindrone (Ortho-Novum, Ovcon, Tri-Norinyl) decrease DHEA/DHEAS more than the more androgenic progestogens, norgestrel or levonorgestrel, contained in many triphasic formulations (Tri-Levlen, Triphasil, Nordette) (Gaspard et al., 1984; Klove et al., 1984).

Both norgestrel and levonorgestrel can cause unpleasant androgenic side effects such as acne and hirsutism in some users. Though levonorgestrel reduces DHEA/DHEAS less than norethindrone, its much greater progesterone-like actions and its suppressive action on estrogen can cause as much or more sexual problems than norethindrone. Beneficial actions of estrogen on vaginal epidermal keratinization, urinary tract conditions, and skin composition and lubrication may be blocked by levonorgestrel, though there is no current research documenting this interference. Levonorgestrel oral contraceptions are in wider use in Europe than in the United States. The novel five-year subdermal progestogen implant, Norplant, contains this synthetic form of progesterone.

Estrogen and Progestogens

Early reports indicated that estrogen supplementation increased DHEAS, but more recent studies have found no change or even decreases. The 10-to-12-day addition of progestogens to estrogen supplements, currently used to decrease the incidence of endometrial cancer, usually consists of medroxyprogesterone (Provera), which has a potent suppressive effect on DHEA/DHEAS. Sexual desire also may be severely depressed by Provera, although this side effect of Provera use is rarely addressed. Norgestrel progestogens, which are more often added to estrogen supplements in Europe, may be less sexually suppressive than Provera, although direct comparisons show little difference (Fraser, Padwick, et al., 1989).

P-450 Enzyme Inhibitors

The antifungal drug ketoconazole (Nizoral) potently reduces DHEA/DHEAS, mainly through inhibition of the P-450 enzymes necessary to metabolize DHEA/DHEAS (Lobo, 1988). Other P-450 enzyme inhibitors also reduce DHEA/DHEAS. Cimetidine (Tagamet), which is chemically similar to ketoconazole, apparently lowers DHEA/DHEAS by blocking these enzymes, but is far less potent in this respect than ketoconazole (see Chapter 24). Aminoglutethimide (Cytadren), which is used in the treatment of prostate cancer to suppress adrenal androgens by inhibiting the P-450 enzymatic conversion of cholesterol to pregnenolone, potently suppresses DHEA/DHEAS. Other antiandrogens, such as flutamide and cyproterone acetate (Belanger, Labrie, Dupont, Brochu, & Cusan, 1988; Lambert, Mitchell, & Robertson, 1987), and the cholesterol-lowering drug lovastatin (Mevacor) (Engelhardt, Gore-Langton, & Armstrong, 1988) appear to decrease DHEA/DHEAS specifically through inhibition of 17–20 desmolase adrenal enzyme activity.

Glucocorticoid and Progesteronal Steroids

Synthetic glucocorticoids such as dexamethasone and prednisone (Lobo, 1988) and progestogens such as medroxyprogesterone (Provera) and megestrol (Megace) severely lower DHEA/DHEAS levels. In terms of natural metabolism in the adrenal gland, cholesterol-pregnenolone is metabolized either to cortisol and progesterone or to DHEA/DHEAS. When cortisol and progesterone production is blocked by inhibition of the enzyme 3-beta hydroxysteroid dehydrogenase, excessive levels of DHEA/DHEAS may be produced. Conversely, as cortisol levels rise during stress and chronic illness, DHEA/DHEAS levels are decreased.

Anticonvulsant Drugs

The high incidence of nonseizure-related fractures occurring in male and female epileptic patients may be due to the DHEAS-lowering effect of anticonvulsant drugs (Kraus et al., 1983). Carbamazepine (Tegretol), phenytoin, and phenobarbital all reduce DHEA/DHEAS (Connell, Rapeport, Beastall, & Brodie, 1984; Isojarvi, Pakarinen, Ylipalosaari, & Myllyla, 1990; Levesque, Herzog, & Seibel, 1986). Only sodium valproate (Depakene) appears to leave DHEA/DHEAS levels unaffected (at therapeutic doses) (Isojarvi et al., 1990; MacPhee, Larkin, Butler, Beastall, & Brodie, 1988). Generally anticonvulsant drugs lower DHEAS during chronic treatment, but cause no change in testosterone, free testosterone, and estradiol (Isojarvi et al., 1990). DHEAS levels in untreated male and female temporal-lobe epileptics are no different from those in normal subjects (Levesque et al., 1986). Decreased sex drive during anticonvulsant therapy has been attributed to reduction of DHEAS, since other androgens such as testosterone are not reduced (Connell et al., 1984; Isojarvi et al., 1990; MacPhee et al., 1988). Aminoglutethimide, which is now used to control prostate cancer through suppression of adrenal androgens, was originally used as an anticonvulsant to treat epilepsy, but was found to be too toxic.

Alcohol

Alcohol injection can potently and rapidly reduce brain levels of DHEA/DHEAS within 30 minutes, and recovery to normal levels takes about four hours (e.g., Becker et al., 1988); chronic alcohol-induced cirrhosis is characterized by lowered DHEAS. Women alcoholics free of cirrhosis have reduced DHEAS as well as women with non-alcoholic cirrhosis (Becker et al., 1991). Jasonni et al. (1983) found lower DHEAS levels in women alcoholics with cirrhotic liver disease, despite an increase in the other main adrenal androgen, androstenedione. Similarly, male alcoholics with cirrhosis may have higher androstenedione but lower DHEAS (Becker et al., 1991). Since DHEAS is the only sex hormone that decreases substantially and progressively before the age of 60, the low levels of DHEAS found in female and male alcoholics (Becker et al., 1988; Becker et al., 1991) indicate a premature aging effect.

Nicotine

DHEAS is measured chiefly for diagnosis and treatment of virilization in women (i.e., hirsutism and acne). However, Barrett-Connor and Khaw (1987) found higher mean levels of DHEAS for current male smokers aged 30 to 80 in a large cohort study. DHEAS levels remained significantly higher when adjusted for age and body mass index (BMI). Androstenedione and estrogen levels were also significantly higher in male smokers versus nonsmokers. The significantly higher mean DHEAS levels in the male cohort reported in 1987 remained when the number of men was later expanded from 590 to 986 (Barrett-Connor, 1988).

Any hormonal health or sexual advantage

of higher DHEAS levels in smokers would be cancelled by a concurrent increase in cortisol (besides the direct adverse sexual effects of smoking). Smoking increases ACTH, adrenal androgens, progesterone, and cortisol (Yeh & Barbieri, 1989). Smoking also increases vasopressin (Chiodera & Coiro, 1990), which has been shown to increase DHEAS and to be inhibited by cortisol. There is some possibility that smoking-induced increases in DHEAS may contribute to the approximate 5% lower weight in smokers, currently attributed to metabolic factors.

DRUGS STIMULATING DHEAS

Bupropion (Wellbutrin), trilostane (Modrastane), and epostane are among the few drugs shown to selectively increase DHEAS. Recently metaformin and calcium-channel blockers have also been shown to increase DHEAS in some circumstances.

Bupropion

Bupropion has seizurogenic activating properties, but contrary to current clinical perceptions, they are only slightly greater than those of most other approved antidepressants. Due to its affinity for sigma receptors, bupropion may have an excitatory effect on glutamate amino acid transmission, which in turn may facilitate sexual and orgasmic sensations in people who have experienced deficits in this area. The confluence of effects of DHEA/DHEAS, bupropion, and limbic activation characterized by theta rhythms thus appears to be involved in a potentiation of sexual desire and response. In addition, the sexual stimulant drug l-deprenyl, which activates copulation and ejaculation in rats, also selectively induces EEG theta in rats (Nickel, Schulze, & Szelenyi, 1990). At the present time, practically nothing is known about the biochemical triggers and nature of orgasm. Further research on DHEA, sexual stimulant drugs, and theta rhythms is needed to analyze orgasm in the context of sexual psychopharmacology.

There are surprisingly few drugs known to increase DHEAS levels. For this reason, we were surprised to find that bupropion (Wellbutrin) increased DHEAS in women during our sexual dysfunction treatment trial (see Chapter 27). As far as we know, bupropion is the only antidepressant that increases DHEAS. Any chemical change discovered due to bupropion is of particular interest, because its mechanism of action is imperfectly understood. It has been shown to effect known neurotransmitter/hormone/peptide receptors minimally except for the dopamine uptake transporter. However, DHEAS is rarely measured. We were interested in measuring it in our study to explore its possible contribution to sexual function.

Unfortunately, the makers of bupropion, Burroughs Wellcome, did not pursue further monitoring of DHEAS levels in other clinical protocols, even those involving treatment of sexual dysfunction—further reflecting the extent to which sex hormone consequences of psychotropic drugs are overlooked by both drug companies and the Federal Drug Administration. Without additional monitoring of DHEAS levels during bupropion treatment, we cannot confirm our findings through others' research. We consider the rise in DHEAS meaningful in our study because (1) it clearly occurred in women treated with drug rather than with placebo; (2) it was positively correlated with recovery from sexual dysfunction; (3) it reversed when bupropion-treated women were switched to placebo; and (4) no changes occurred in the many other sex hormones and steroids measured.

Increased levels of DHEAS may cause some women to experience irresistible but transient physical sensations as DHEAS reaches a peak level in the vagina before the body's hormonal feedback system has the opportunity to adjust to this increased tissue level. Since DHEAS is metabolized to estrogens, and estrogens sensitize receptors to sexually active peptides like oxytocin, DHEAS could also increase sexual touch potency indirectly.

No significant change in DHEAS levels occurred in male subjects taking bupropion, either in the sexual dysfunction-low sex drive protocol or in our subsequent trial of bupropion as a treatment for impotence (see Chapter 27). However, our male sexual dysfunction subjects were, on the average, older than our female subjects (mid-40s in men versus mid-30s in women). It would be interesting to study the DHEAS response to bupropion in young men between the ages of 20 and 30, before DHEAS has begun its decline during aging.

The increase of DHEAS in subjects taking bupropion was apparently not related to the dopaminergic properties of bupropion. *Anti*dopaminergic neuroleptic drugs have been found to increase DHEAS, but this increase could have been an indirect effect of increased prolactin (Oseko et al., 1986).

We have hypothesized that DHEAS is in some way related to EEG theta activity, which is increased not only by antidopaminergic neuroleptics but also by dopamine D_1 receptor stimulation. Differences in dopamine receptor subtypes D_1 and D_2 have been reviewed by Ongini and Longo (1989). Possibly, the dopamine-2 (D_2) receptor lowers DHEAS (DHEAS is lowered when hyperprolactemia is treated with the D_2 agonist bromocriptine), just as it decreases theta activity, inhibits inositol phosphate (IP_3) activity, inhibits adenylate cyclase, and decreases sensitivity to seizure.

In contrast, the rarely studied dopamine-1 (D_1) receptor increases theta activity, increases IP_3 activity, increases adenylate cyclase, and increases seizure sensitivity. The D_1 receptor may also increase DHEAS, possibly in conjunction with excitatory amino acid activation in the limbic system. As a dopamine uptake-inhibitor, bupropion may increase the activity of both D_1 and D_2 receptors. A possible excitatory amino acid effect through bupropion's action on the sigma receptor could reinforce the action of the D_1 receptor leading not only to an increased sensitivity to seizure, but also to an increase in DHEAS activity.

As a sexual stimulant the interrelationship of bupropion with DHEAS and theta rhythms (which are triggered by orgasm) should be explored. Interestingly, the sexual stimulant l-deprenyl also generates theta, while d-amphetamine suppresses theta (Nickel et al., 1990). The effect of l-deprenyl on DHEA has not been studied.

The fascinating association of bupropion with DHEAS and sexual function has encouraged our investigation of the site where substances act in the brain, leading to our interest in the limbic system. Our extended consideration of DHEAS as a sex hormone in this book reflects its possible stimulatory actions on sex and health, even though the literature on DHEAS is sparse.

Trilostane and Epostane

Trilostane (Modrastane) increases DHEA/DHEAS by blocking 5-beta-hydroxysteroid dehydrogenase (3B-HSD) enzymatic metabolism of the precursor steroids pregnenolone and DHEA to progesterone and cortisol (Komanicky, Spark, & Melby, 1978). Essentially, synthesis of cortisol and progesterone is blocked and, consequently, there is more precursor available for DHEA/DHEAS synthesis. Trilostane decreases the excess cortisol production of Cushing's disease. The hypothalamic-pituitary-adrenal axis apparently adjusts itself so that cortisol and progesterone do not fall below normal levels, but DHEA/DHEAS continue to be elevated. The 17–20 desmolase pathway to DHEA becomes a safety valve absorbing excessive cortisol and progesterone production precursor.

Whereas P-450 enzyme inhibitors can reduce DHEA/DHEAS by blocking the 17–20 desmolase enzyme path, trilostane increases DHEA/DHEAS by blocking the alternate 3B-HSD enzyme path.

Though the ovaries and testes also possess important 3B-HSD enzymes, specific changes or adverse effects of trilostane have not been found in the gonads. Semple, Weir, Thomson, and Beastall (1982) found no changes in sexual desire or response in ten male volunteers given trilostane for four weeks.

Many drugs that affect hormone activity do so by affecting enzymes rather than blocking or stimulating receptors. The counterparts to such enzymatic mechanisms in amine neurotransmitter drugs are the MAO-A and MAO-B enzyme inhibitors such as phenelzine (Nardil) for both MAO-A and MAO-B, deprenyl (Selegiline) for MAO-B, and clorgyline for MAO-A. Manipulation of body chemistry by enzymatic alterations instead of direct actions on receptors affords increased flexibility and perhaps is more natural. However, the resultant metabolic effects may be less specific than with the use of receptor agonists and antagonists.

Enzymatic activity also shows essential sex differences that could be responsible for unpredictable reactions. The sex differential is reduced with age: Enzymatic activity in men slowly shifts during aging to that characteristic of women (a return to the female mode from which males deviate during fetal growth). Due to major sex differentials, it is essential that enzyme-changing drugs be carefully tested in both women and men.

Trilostane has been investigated (in England) for the treatment of breast cancer in postmenopausal women (Beardwell et al., 1983; Beardwell, Hindley, Wilkinson, John, & Bu'-Lock, 1985; Williams et al., 1987). However, its apparently small effect on breast cancer seems to be due to inhibition of the conversion (aromatization) of adrenal androgens (primarily androstenedione) to estrone, rather than to its inhibition of 3B-HSD, which results in DHEAS elevation (Beardwell et al., 1985). The fatigue, lethargy and nausea experienced by many breast-cancer patients treated with trilostane are reminiscent of, but less severe than, the side effects of aminoglutethimide and ketaconazole, which are used in the treatment of prostate cancer. Aminoglutethimide and ketaconazole block adrenal cortisol and progesterone; they also lower DHEA/DHEAS levels by inhibiting P-450/17-20D enzymes.

Assessment of the clinical effects of trilostane-induced DHEAS elevation is confounded by its effects on progesterone and cortisol. The hypothalamic-pituitary-adrenal axis appears to compensate for trilostane's 3B-HSD block, so that normal cortisol and progesterone levels are maintained. The increase in DHEA/DHEAS may reduce or inhibit progesterone/cortisol effects. We might speculate that many negative effects of adrenal androgens, such as hirsutism and prostate growth, might be due to androstenedione rather than to DHEA/DHEAS. Alterations in trilostane's chemical structure may eventually yield a drug which specifically and precisely stimulates an increase in DHEA/DHEAS. Inhibition of 3B-HSD enzymatic action, properly modulated, may be an excellent way to increase DHEA/DHEAS. However, if enzymatic metabolism to DHEA/DHEAS itself is reduced by aging, merely decreasing competitive metabolic pathways may be insufficient to cause a notable increase. Direct DHEA/DHEAS supplementation or direct stimulation of the inner regions of the adrenal gland producing DHEA/DHEAS may be necessary when there has been a decrease in physiological reactivity.

The tumor promoter 12-0-tetradecanoyl-13-acetate (TPA) has an opposite enzymatic effect to trilostane: enhancing 3B-HSD and possibly inhibiting 17-alpha and 17–20 desmolase enzymes. These enzymatic changes cause increases in progesterone and corticosterone synthesis and reduction in DHEA/DHEAS synthesis in cultured human adrenocortical cells (McAllister & Hornsby, 1987). Pathological changes in adrenal steroid production due to endogenous TPA-like substances possibly causing cancer growth might be limited or reversed by use of trilostane.

Epostane, a different version of trilostane with similar chemical actions, can safely induce termination of the fetus by decreasing progesterone (Crooij et al., 1988). Epostane acts through progesterone inhibition in a manner similar to the notorious abortion pill RU-486 (mifepristone), which blocks progesterone and cortisol by a more direct receptor antagonist mechanism. Epostane is not available in the United States; but trilostane, which is, may have a similar abortive action, though it has not been tested for this controversial application.

INSULIN-DHEA DYNAMICS

There is an inverse relationship between insulin and DHEAS: Elevated insulin levels or insulin administration decrease DHEAS in men and women; elevated DHEAS in men is associated with decreased insulin, though not glucose tolerance, indicating a decrease in unhealthy insulin resistance (Beer, Jakubowicz, Beer, & Nestler, 1994; Diamond, Grainger, Laudano, Starick-Zych, & Defronzo, 1991). DHEAS levels are typically lower in disease states associated with insulin resistance or hyperinsulinemia such as hypertension (Nestler, Beer, Jakubowicz, & Beer, 1994). Insulin has been shown in humans to inhibit the adrenal 17,20-lyase enzyme necessary for DHEA production (Nestler, McClanahan, Clore, & Blackard, 1992).

Treatment of obese hypertensive men with the dihydropyridine calcium channel blockers amlodipine (Norvasc) or nitrendipine (Baypress, not available in the United States) decreased both hyperinsulinemia and insulin resistance while increasing DHEAS levels, indicating that the elevated DHEAS could have been responsible for the decrease in insulin pathology (Beer, Jakubowicz, Beer, Arocha, & Nestler, 1993; Beer, Jakubowicz, Beer, & Nestler, 1993). However, treatment of obese, hypertensive postmenopausal women (n = 13) with the nondihydropyridine calcium channel blocker diltiazem (Cardizem) lowered insulin levels by almost 50% without any increase in DHEAS, suggesting that this beneficial effect on insulin in women was not due to a change in DHEAS levels (Beer et al., 1994). However, none of the female postmenopausal patients was on estrogen replacement therapy, which conceivably could reduce sensitivity to, or potency of, DHEA.

Twenty-one-day treatment of both normal and obese hypertensive nondiabetic men with the proven antidiabetic drug metformin (available in the United States in 1995 and currently available throughout the world, usually under the brand name of Glucophage) has been shown by Nestler et al. (1994) to increase DHEAS by 48% in obese hypertensive men and by 80% in nonobese normotensive men. Furthermore, DHEAS increases showed a positive correlation with decreases in insulin levels. Nestler et al. (1994) point out that there is a progressive, age-related decrease in DHEAS in humans and an age-related increased prevalence of insulin resistance and hyperinsulinemia, indicating that DHEAS supplementation may prevent or ameliorate insulin-related pathology in diabetic and/or hypertensive older men and women. It should be noted that, in contrast to the beneficial effect of DHEAS, testosterone typically increases insulin resistance (Buffington, 1991; Polderman, Gooren, Asscheman, Bakker, & Heine, 1994).

Similar to DHEA, growth hormone and insulin-like growth factor-1 (IGF-1) also decrease over age 35, with possible negative effects on health (Corpas, Harman, & Blackman, 1993). Chronic three-month placebo-controlled treatment of both men (n = 13) and women (n = 17) aged 40 to 70 with 50 mg/day physiologic replacement doses of DHEA has been shown to produce increased IGF-1 and decreased IGF-1 binding protein (IGFBP-1) in the treated group but not in the placebo group) (Morales, Nolan, Nelson, & Yen, 1994). The decrease in IGFBP-1 increased free IGF-1 available for metabolic homeostasis (Morales, Nolan, et al., 1994). Furthermore, improvements in well-being, including increased energy, more relaxed feeling, improved mood, and stress tolerance, were noted in both men and women treated with DHEA.

TRANSCENDENTAL MEDITATION

The association of DHEA/DHEAS with limbic system activity has been reinforced by findings that Transcendental Meditation (TM) may increase blood levels of DHEAS (and even prevent decreases with aging) compared to non-practicing control groups (Glaser, Brind, Eisner, & Wallace, 1986). DHEAS levels were measured in 252 men and 74 women who were experienced practitioners and compared to levels in 799 men and 173 women who were not practitioners. Results were analyzed by sex and age. Mean DHEAS levels were higher in women in each of five age groups, but levels were higher only in men over 40 years old. No significant differences were found between younger (under 40 years old) and controls. Mean DHEAS levels were 47% higher in TM women over 45 and 23% higher in TM men over 40. Adjustments for diet, obesity, and exercise could not account for the significant DHEAS differences. DHEAS levels in the older practitioners were comparable to levels found in controls five to ten years younger.

Schneider et al. (1989) found that type-A behavior scores were inversely related to DHEAS levels (i.e., DHEAS levels became lower as type-A scores rose). However, in 15 age-matched men who had practiced Transcendental Meditation for about 12 years, type-A behavior scores were positively related to DHEAS levels. The immune system enhancement sometimes shown in experienced meditators (Smith, G.R., et al., 1989) may be due in part to increased DHEAS activity.

These two studies, both conducted at Maharishi University, indicated that long-term Transcendental Meditation practice may increase DHEAS levels, perhaps by decreasing stress that lowers DHEAS.

In another study with male subjects conducted at Maharishi University (Hill, Wallace, Walton, & Myerson, 1989), serotonin and prolactin were found to be decreased during actual meditation. Years of TM practice were inversely related to prolactin levels, and type-A behavior scores were positively related to prolactin levels. Opposite effects of Transcendental Meditation on DHEAS in comparison with prolactin would be in accord with opposite effects on sex. DHEAS increases sexual responsiveness; prolactin decreases sexual responsiveness. However, such opposite sexual effects could be confounded by the fact that prolactin itself tends to increase DHEAS levels.

The studies at Maharishi University, which reported increased DHEAS among TM practitioners, used experienced meditators of Tantric Yoga, which is intended to focus on sexual energy (Kundalini). Proficient meditators demonstrated increased EEG theta power during meditation, which peaked during Samadhi states (Corby, Roth, Zarcone, & Kopell, 1978). Such a finding would suggest that meditation increases both EEG theta and DHEAS, indicating limbic activation.

Tantra meditators often report energy bursts or "rushes" during meditation which are suggestive of orgasmic sensations. Corby et al. (1978) has also shown that the most proficient Tantra meditation subjects ("experts") had increased theta power in their EEGs during normal consciousness outside of meditation states. Studies of Zen masters with 22 to 55 years of training have shown that there is a switch into rhythmical EEG theta activity in the final and highest stage of meditation (Echenhofer & Coombs, 1987). Kissin (1986) has suggested that altered states of consciousness involve activation of theta activity in the limbic septum and hippocampus and he associated limbic activation with sexual euphoria and orgasm. Heath (1963) has shown that stimulation of the septum in humans elicits sexually pleasurable sensations resembling orgasm.

The limbic areas activated by meditation may also be activated by DHEA/DHEAS (Carette & Poulain, 1984). Experienced TM meditators show higher levels of DHEA/DHEAS than nonmeditator controls. Thus, DHEA/DHEAS can be associated with sensations felt during meditation, and these sensations can in turn be associated with human orgasm. The abundant evidence of excitatory limbic actions of DHEA/DHEAS, pregnenolone, and pregnenolone sulfate has suggested that increases in limbic theta power during meditation are in some way associated with DHEAS, which appears to be increased by regular practice of meditation. It is possible that study of the relationship between DHEA/DHEAS and limbic theta power could reveal information on the nature of orgasm in particular and sexual activation in general.

LONGEVITY, DISEASE, AND DHEA

DHEA/DHEAS appears to be a "healthy" steroid that enhances the quality of life and promotes longevity. The association of lowered DHEAS levels with degenerative disease and mortality has proved to be remarkably consistent, especially considering that DHEA/DHEAS is a mysterious sex hormone with unknown functions currently measured chiefly by dermatologists to diagnose pathological hyperandrogenic states. Research has shown that DHEA/DHEAS clearly decreases during aging, times of chronic stress, and in the presence of disease. Indeed, its decline could be a catalyst for illness and aging. Although we do not have enough data to ascertain cause-and-effect relationships, we do know that DHEA decreases as these conditions worsen (see Table 9.2).

Semple, Gray, and Beastall (1987) measured

adrenal steroid levels in acutely ill (less than two weeks) and chronically ill (more than two weeks) patients versus healthy controls. DHEAS levels dropped extremely low in the chronically ill patients (although another adrenal androgen, androstenedione, did not change), but not in the acutely ill patients. Parker, Levin, and Lifrak (1985) compared adrenal hormone levels in the severely ill. Cortisol levels were consistently elevated and DHEA/DHEAS levels were lower. Parker hypothesized that during serious illness, there is a shift in the metabolism of adrenal pregnenolone toward glucocorticoids and away from DHEA/DHEAS.

Abnormally high levels of glucocorticoids compromise immune function and bone growth. They also cause degenerative loss of neurons, particularly in the hippocampus, which is essential to cognitive function and memory (Sapolsky, Krey, & McEwen, 1986). In contrast, DHEA can protect immune function, inhibit carcinogenic tumors, decrease toxic actions of glucose and lipids, promote bone growth, and oppose glucocorticoid neurotoxicity (Regelson, Loria, & Kalimi, 1988; Schwartz et al., 1983; Schwartz, Fairman, Polansky, Lewbart, & Pashko, 1989). DHEA also inhibits the tumor-promoter TPA and excess glucose-6-phosphate dehydrogenase (G-6-PDH), which is an enzymatic factor in cell proliferation and carcinogenic activation (Cleary et al., 1984; Marks & Banks, 1960; Schwartz, Hard, Pashko, Abou-Gharbia, & Swern, 1981).

Female breast cancer is associated with lowered DHEA/DHEAS and low urine concentrations of the DHEA metabolites androsterone and etiocholanolone (Schwartz et al., 1983). In a prospective study of women aged 30 to 59, Bulbrook, Hayward, and Spicer (1971) found lowered DHEA metabolites up to nine years prior to cancer diagnosis; a greater risk for developing breast cancer was associated with below normal DHEA metabolites.

Barrett-Conner, Khaw, and Yen (1986) found that older men (aged 50 to 80) with higher DHEAS levels lived longer and showed a lowered incidence of heart disease. A 100 mcg/dl increase in DHEAS level was associated with a 36% reduction in death from any cause and a 48% reduction in death from heart disease. Subsequent studies by Barrett-Conner and Khaw (1987) replicated the inverse relation of DHEAS to death and heart disease for older men.

However, these studies inexplicably found the reverse relationship in older women (aged 60 to 80). Death and heart disease in women was *greater* with higher DHEAS levels. The difference in ages between male and female cohorts (men 50 to 80; women 60 to 80) might account for some of this apparent sex difference, with differences in normal DHEAS levels between 50 and 60 more indicative of accelerated aging or degenerative disease states than the minimal levels reached beyond age 60. Rozenberg, Ham, Caufriez, et al. (1990) found lower DHEAS in gynecology clinic female inpatients, compared to outpatients between the ages of 40 and 60, but undifferentiated low levels in female patients older than 60.

In other studies, lower DHEAS levels in women were associated with higher risk factors for cardiovascular disease. In a random survey of a normal community sample of men and women between 20 and 70 years old (Nafziger, Herrington, & Bush, 1991; Nafziger, Jenkins, Bowlin, & Pearson, 1990), DHEAS levels were significantly and positively correlated to the cardiovascular protective factors of high-density lipoproteins (HDL) and apolipoprotein A in men but not in women. However, DHEAS levels in women were significantly and inversely related to the cardiovascular risk factors of cholesterol, low-density lipoproteins (LDL), apolipoprotein B, and triglycerides.

In a large study of hormonal differences between healthy and diseased men aged 40 to 70, Gray et al. (1991) found significantly lower DHEAS level in diseased men (9% lower), and a 22% lower DHEAS level in men with heart disease alone. Diseased men were defined by the presence of one or more of the following factors: obesity, alcoholism, prescription medication, prostate problems, and chronic diseases such as cancer, heart disease, diabetes, or ulcer.

DHEAS levels are lower in diabetic men, despite normal levels of androstenedione and cortisol (Ando, Rubens, & Rottiers, 1984). Ando, Rubens, and Rottiers (1985) suggested that

Table 9.2 *Disease and Degenerative States Associated with Lowered DHEA/DHEAS Levels*

Disease	*Research*
Alzheimer's disease	Sunderland et al., 1989
Anorexia nervosa	Winterer et al., 1985
Lupus autoimmune dysfunction (systemic lupus erythematosus)	Jungers et al., 1982; Lahita, Bradlow, Ginzler, Pang, & New, 1987
Rheumatoid arthritis	Cutolo et al., 1984; Cutolo, Balleari, Giusti, Intra, & Accardo, 1991; Feher & Feher, 1984
Graves' disease	Ahmad, Penhale, & Tatal, 1985
Cholecystectomy surgery	Semple et al., 1987
Burn injuries	Lephart, Baxter, & Parker, 1987; Semple et al., 1987
Intensive care	Wade et al., 1988
Ovarian cancer	Heinonen, Koivula, & Pystynen, 1987
Pre-surgery patients	Parker, Levin, & Lifrak, 1985
Hypothyroidism	Bassi et al., 1980
Chronic obstructive pulmonary disease	Semple, Beastall, Gray, & Thompson, 1983

the progressive decrease of DHEAS levels in diabetic males indicates an accelerated process of aging due to diabetes. Interestingly, DHEAS levels have not been found to be decreased in diabetic women (Nyholm et al., 1989).

One of the chief effects of aging is difficulty in adapting to or recovering from physical stress. Adaption and recovery require the participation of all body parts and functions, from molecular enzymatic reactions to large muscle activity. With less physiological resilience, more damage is incurred during times of stress. Rhythmic processes lose their exactness and coordination; the body cannot go as fast or act as precisely as it did when young. The optimal range and margins for error are reduced, so that the body reacts progressively less successfully. If an athlete is injured at the age of 20, he may recover within a few days or even play through the injury; but if injured at 40, recovery may take weeks and is often incomplete. A 20-year-old punk rocker can survive a night of blasting music with only a mild, lingering buzz; a 40-year-old rocker might take days to get over the aural fatigue and suffer a severe headache as well as actual neural damage. It is not yet clear that reduced DHEA is cause for decreased recovery or if decreased recovery shifts body metabolism away from production of DHEA, perhaps to better "allocate resources."

Due to recent intense research in biotechnology, the beneficial effects of DHEA on the immune system has become particularly impressive. DHEA supplementation corrects negative cytokine interleukin-6 (IL-6) function in aged mice (Daynes et al., 1993) and enhances positive human T-cell interleukin-2 (IL-2) activity (Suzuki, Suzuki, Daynes, & Engleman, 1991). Immune dysregulation leading to insufficient immune function during old age is characterized by increased IL-6 production and decreased IL-2 production (Weksler, 1993). Treatment of old mice with DHEAS has resulted in increased antibody response to foreign antigens and reversal of dysregulated cytokine production by T-cells (Weksler, 1993). Tissue metabolites of DHEA have also been suggested to be involved in the immune response of various tissues in mice (Morfin & Courchay, 1994).

Many positive findings involving DHEA and immunity may not as yet have been published due to proprietary considerations crucial to biotech company research and testing. A recent placebo-controlled study in 11 healthy postmenopausal women ($n = 11$) treated with physiologic 50 mg/day micronized DHEA for three weeks showed decreased IL-6 and enhanced natural killer-cell number and cytotoxity (Casson et al., 1993). DHEA treatment trials in HIV patients are currently being conducted (Dyner et al., 1993).

Multitudinous studies of various disease and degenerative states have reported correlations with lowered DHEA/DHEAS levels.

CONCLUSIONS

Despite the fact that there is far more DHEA/DHEAS in the body than testosterone, estrogen, or progesterone, these more abundant substances generally have been ignored in research on emotional and sexual behavior. By emphasizing the importance of DHEA/DHEAS (as well as acetylcholine, GABA, excitatory amino acids, and vasopressin) on a level equivalent to testosterone, estrogen, and progesterone, we hope to shift attention to the neural mechanisms that influence sexual desire and activity. The benefit of this attentional shift could be the integration of cognitive psychology and therapy with research focusing on the concrete physiological areas of pain, pleasure, aggression, and other components of sexual behavior.

Investigation of DHEA and its multidimensional role in sexuality and longevity could lead to the discovery of other critical substances involved in the complex interaction of mind and body, of cognition and stress, and sexual fantasy, desire, and behavior (not to mention love and intimacy). Simplistic preoccupation with identifying "aphrodisiacal" hormones could then yield to more mature and useful applications of sexual pharmacology research and treatment.

Part III

SUBSTANCE USE AND ABUSE

10

Alcohol

OBJECTIVES

- To summarize the physiological impact of alcohol abuse
- To identify gender-related differences in effects of alcohol on sexual function
- To explore the impact of alcohol abuse on longevity
- To overview treatment alternatives

The distinction between alcohol use and abuse is not well-defined medically. In lay terms, the social drinker, the problem drinker, and the chronic alcoholic are regarded as distinct categories that tend to remain stable throughout life. However, one phase often develops into the other, progressively, over time. There are many classification systems for determining alcohol abuse. Some diagnostic systems utilize demonstrable physiological changes to determine degree of alcohol-induced damage: tissue damage, hormonal aberrations, and mental disturbances identified in the patient. Others evaluate the effects on behavior and ability to function at work and in relationships. For instance, Dr. Joseph Pursch, the Medical Director of the Addiction Institute in Costa Mesa, California, uses a behavioral, not physiological, definition of alcoholism: A person is an alcoholic if his/her consumption of alcohol disrupts the lifestyle on any level—financially, on the job, in relationships, or by creating a criminal record ("Driving Under the Influence"). In other words, if a man consumes only two drinks but experiences enough disinhibition to beat his wife, even though he is technically a light drinker, he would be considered an alcoholic under Pursch's definition.

There are also numerous theories regarding the root cause of alcoholism, ranging from developmental experiences to genetic determinants. Medicine cannot satisfactorily explain why some "social drinkers" progress to alcoholism and others do not. Individual, sexual, and ethnic differences in metabolism and endocrine reactions to alcohol intake are complex and insufficiently investigated.

Brain damage is clearly a consequence of chronic alcoholism, but the scope and degree of deterioration are not fully defined, nor is the point at which these consequences become irreversible. The memory defects of Korsakoff's syndrome (alcoholic dementia) involve actual tissue death in these limbic areas. A better understanding of alcohol-induced changes in limbic mechanisms, acutely and chronically, could tell us a great deal about the sexual effects of this drug. The expectancy variables associated with alcohol (what people think will happen when they drink) involve these limbic areas where cognitive and social cues interact (the amygdala, frontal cortex, septum, hippocampus, entorhinal cortex, and nucleus accumbens). The stimulation of aggression and the muting of anxiety during social interactions involve the amygdala. Alcohol reduces anxiety and causes sedation through GABA receptor activation similar to benzodiazepines. At least part of alcohol's relaxing and inhibitory action is due to GABA activation. Consequently, when benzodiazepines (e.g., Valium) are unavailable, alcohol may be used to reduce panic attacks and phobic tendencies.

The purpose of this chapter is to focus on those aspects of alcoholism that specifically pertain to sexual function and dysfunction. There are marked, gender-related differences associated with alcohol abuse. Sexual dysfunction increases precipitously with age in male alcoholics. A study by Jensen (1984) found that sexual problems are present chiefly in alcoholic men over 40. In contrast there was no sexual effect of age in female alcoholics or in male and female controls. Although alcoholic women did not notice any adverse sexual effects from the medications used adjunctively during withdrawal and recovery, the large number (50%) of men who related sexual dysfunction to medication begun during withdrawal has suggested a major sex-linked factor usually ignored in sexual evaluations of recovering alcoholics.

Our clinical experience with recovering male alcoholics has revealed that chlordiazepoxide (Librium) often causes sexual dysfunction (lack of desire and ejaculation). It could be assumed that the frequent use of chlordiazepoxide and other benzodiazepines by recovering alcoholic women will cause subtle if indefinite sexual problems. While male and female alcoholics share many characteristics, their behavioral and physiological profiles are actually quite different. The scope of these differences has not been generally appreciated in medicine and will therefore be highlighted throughout this chapter. For example, the sexual consequences of alcohol consumption are different in men and women. While blood alcohol levels are increasing, both men and women may experience positive sexual dividends – psychological, via disinhibition; physiological, due to various neurotransmitter effects or hormonal factors (a transient increase in dopamine and an LH surge). As blood alcohol levels reach intoxicating doses, however, sexual responsiveness is blunted in both men and women. At this point, the sexual consequences become quite dissimilar: Men are less able to participate sexually, whereas women may become more receptive and compliant. Women can be sexually exploited in this condition, while men ordinarily cannot, without an erection. With increased intoxication, sexual function in both sexes usually becomes irrelevant. Men can neither get erect nor ejaculate; women are unable to experience orgasms. The sedating effect of alcohol may lead to "blackouts," stupor, or unconsciousness.

Doses of alcohol are expressed in various units for research study reports. Nonintoxicating doses are about 0.06 blood alcohol level (BAL) or below. The legal limit for alcohol intoxication in various states ranges from 0.08 to 0.10 blood alcohol level. Social drinkers become moderately intoxicated at doses from 0.10 to 0.15 and grossly intoxicated at about 0.20 or above. Chronic alcoholics may not become noticeably intoxicated until reaching over 0.15 to 0.20 blood alcohol level. Corresponding doses and body concentration levels reported in the literature in various units are approximately as follows:

$$0.025\%\ \text{BAL} = 25\ \text{mg}/100\ \text{ml blood} = 25\ \text{mg}\%$$

An approximate blood alcohol level of 0.15 would occur when a 150-pound person consumed three mixed drinks in the space of one to two hours.

THE EFFECTS OF ALCOHOL ON SEXUAL FUNCTION IN FEMALES

Female sexual response is not as readily observable as a male response (erection and ejaculation), so that meaningful physiological deficits are hard to identify. Whether alcoholism causes direct physical damage to women's sexual "circuits and organs" is not known yet. However, we do know that gynecological disease is far greater in alcoholic women than in nonalcoholic women and that such diseases may compromise the function of genital nerves and tissues.

Acute alcohol intake has not been shown to cause significant hormonal changes in young, healthy, nonalcoholic women tested under laboratory circumstances. Careful studies have shown no significant reductions in serum testosterone, luteinizing hormone, follicle stimulating hormone, or estradiol (McNamee, Grant, Ratcliffe, & Oliver, 1979; Mendelson, Mello, & Ellingboe, 1981).

Slight elevations of prolactin found during the descending limb of the blood alcohol curve might be an artifact resulting from the nausea often experienced by women administered a large dose of alcohol over a relatively short period of time (Mendelson et al., 1981). Interestingly, women do not experience the clear reduction of testosterone that men experience after administration of high doses of alcohol; alcohol may not be as damaging to ovaries as it is to testicles, or more ovarian damage may be necessary before testosterone production is affected. The difference might also be due to more adequate adrenal compensation in women than in men.

While alcohol may facilitate a woman's sexual receptivity, it also obscures her memory of what actually occurs during sex. Prospective studies have not been conducted in women alcoholics while they are still drinking; rather, most studies of sexual functioning depend on women's reports during detoxification and rehabilitation, during which time they have a very limited recall of their responsiveness while alcoholic. Studies performed specifically to examine the impact of alcoholism on sexual function in women are confounded by factors such as different drinking patterns (bingeing versus heavy daily drinking), differential influences of the menstrual cycle (women with PMS often drink more heavily premenstrually), defective memory, increased diseases of the reproductive tract, liver, and gonads, as well as the immediately disabling and sedative effects of alcohol itself.

In an excellent clinical examination of female alcoholic sexual dysfunction, Forrest (1983) estimated that 70–80% of alcoholic women entering psychotherapy are found to have secondary orgasmic dysfunction and approximately 15% have never experienced orgasm (primary dysfunction).* Masters, Johnson, and Kolodny (1988) have estimated 30–40% difficulty in sexual arousal and 15% difficulty in achieving orgasm in alcoholic women. (In alcoholic men they estimated 40% erection problems and 5–10% retarded ejaculation.) This percentage is considerably higher than the figures usually cited for alcoholic women (about 5–10%, with no difference from female control groups).

Murphy, Coleman, Hoon, and Scott (1980) evaluated sexual dysfunction by self-report questionnaire in 74 female alcoholic inpatients at a rehabilitation center and a halfway house. They also provided a 12-session sexual enhancement program. Of the 74 women, 31% had had no sexual intercourse during the prior six months; 74% had never masturbated or had stopped masturbating; 29.7% reported little or no sexual desire; and 28.4% reported orgasm from intercourse less than 50% of the time. However, when evaluation was limited to those women who had been sexually active during the prior six months, substantial numbers reported both positive (49%) and negative effects (41%) of alcohol on sexual arousal and alcohol on sexual performance and response. Overall, the frequency of sexual problems reported by the alcoholic women was not significantly different from that found in a nonclinical sample. However, since many of the women revealed sexual problems during the 12-session enhancement program, the authors believed that the women had minimized their initial reports of sexual dysfunction.

In a retrospective study relying upon women's memory and judgment, Apter-Marsh (1984) studied 61 middle-class, well-educated former female alcoholics with a mean age of 40 and a mean length of sobriety of 4.2 years. The women reported that frequency of intercourse had been

*Alcoholic women who enter therapy may be considerably more sexually dysfunctional than alcoholic women not requiring therapy. Lower-class women often cannot afford therapy or their husbands may forbid it. Abusive alcoholic husbands may be particularly opposed to therapy for their alcoholic wives. Tragically, these women usually have very high levels of sexual dysfunction compounded by severe sexual physical and emotional trauma.

highest during active drinking (2.2 times a week), much lower during early abstinence (1.1 times a week), and improved somewhat later during sobriety (1.3 times a week). However, although intercourse was more frequent during active drinking, their ability to reach orgasm was reduced compared with later sobriety.

Jones and Jones (1976) noted that transient genital feelings were sometimes experienced unexpectedly by volunteer women subjects (who were neither alcoholic nor sexually dysfunctional) given small amounts of alcohol in laboratory studies. Subjects spontaneously reported genital sensations as blood alcohol levels reached the 0.04% level on the ascending curve. The sensations were described as "clitoral tingling or itching," with warm feelings in the groin area. Sensations dissipated within 10 to 15 minutes. Although the sensations were often intense, they did not occur in every drinking session. This initially aphrodisiacal effect of alcohol may be attributed to the potentiation of luteinizing hormone releasing hormone and a rise in estradiol, as well as to disinhibition and impairment of judgment.

Impact of Expectations

Many women expect alcohol to facilitate sexual arousal. They may report increased sexual arousal even when they receive tonic water that they think (incorrectly) contains alcohol (Wilson & Lawson, 1976a, 1978). Physiologically, alcohol progressively decreases a woman's vaginal response (vasocongestion, lubrication) as ingestion exceeds one alcoholic drink. In fact, decreased vaginal responses have been reported even at modest doses (Wilson & Lawson, 1978). Nevertheless, women will expect and report greater sexual arousal as drinking increases, despite evidence that their vaginal response is decreasing. Wilson and Lawson (1976a) measured vaginal response by use of a photoplethysmograph inserted into the vagina, which assesses blood volume and pressure changes by measuring differences in light reflections. Vaginal responses decreased as alcohol levels increased toward intoxication levels. Nevertheless, these women predicted that they would become more aroused as alcohol blood levels increased and self-reports after testing affirmed this prediction.

A similar contradiction between subjective and objective sexual arousal measurements was noticed by Malatesta, Pollack, Crotty, and Peacock (1982). Eighteen female college students masturbated to orgasm while attached to measuring devices. Subjective sexual arousal and orgasmic pleasure increased at higher alcohol levels, despite a decrease in physiologic response. The researchers reported decreased vaginal blood measures, longer time to orgasm, and decreased intensity of orgasm at blood levels that were all under the legal limit (0.08% to 0.10% BAL). Increasing levels of intoxication caused a corresponding delay in orgasm during masturbation as well as decreased subjective intensity of orgasm. Measured vaginal blood volume also decreased. However, despite the physiological impairment defined by objective measurements and the subjective experience of decreased orgasmic intensity, the female subjects reported greater sexual arousal and more pleasure during orgasm as alcohol intake increased.

In an extensive study, Barbara Leigh (1990) showed that women's expectations in regard to the effects of alcohol on sexual responsiveness influenced whether they drank as a prelude to sex. Women who expected decreased nervousness with alcohol were twice as likely to initiate sex as women who had less anticipated effect. Heavier drinkers expected alcohol to enhance sex and decrease nervousness significantly more than lighter drinkers.

In a sample of sexually well-adjusted women, drinking heavily clearly induced less sexual desire and enjoyment than drinking lightly (Wilson & Lawson, 1976a). However, sexual desire and enjoyment were believed to increase with increasing alcohol intake. While women usually believed that drinking did not influence frequency of sexual activity (64.2%), more women reported that they engaged in sex more frequently when drinking (22.4%) than when not drinking (13.4%) (Harvey & Beckman, 1986).

There are two particularly informative studies pertaining to women and alcohol which are worth reviewing in more detail. The most comprehensive and properly conducted survey of women's experience of alcohol was a 1981 national investigation of drinking habits conducted by Sharon Wilsnack, Richard Wilsnack, and Albert Klassen (Klassen & Wilsnack, 1986; Wilsnack, Klassen, & Wilsnack, 1984; Wilsnack, Wilsnack, & Klassen, 1987).

Nine hundred and six women over 21 years old were chosen according to statistically proper sampling procedures as nationally representative. They were given a self-administered questionnaire, which they filled out privately, and a personal but structured interview, which included questions similar in nature and wording to those used by Kinsey in his sex surveys (Kinsey et al., 1953). Of the 120 interviewers from the National Opinion Research Center, 116 were women. None reported any history of alcohol-related problems or expressed moral objections to alcohol use. A considerable part of the interview questionnaire was devoted to ascertaining family history, physical health, psychological problems, social experiences, obstetric and gynecological problems, and drug use other than alcohol. (We will only review the sex and alcohol questions here.) For purposes of comparison, a large and representative group of men was also included in the survey.

Subjects were assigned to different groups, depending upon how much they drank. They were considered moderate to heavy drinkers if they reported four or more drinks per week of beer (12 ounces), wine (4 ounces), or liquor (1 ounce). Each drink was estimated to contain slightly less than one-half ounce of alcohol.

Abstainers were those who had consumed no alcohol for the past year (n = 72) or had never drunk alcohol (n = 145). Light drinkers drank less than four drinks per week and had consumed at least one drink in the past week. Moderate drinkers drank more than three drinks per week, but less than two drinks daily. Heavy drinkers drank an average of two drinks or more per day. A group of women with a history of previous drinking, who had abstained over the prior 30 days, was also included. A group of women with a history of periodic binge drinking of at least six drinks per day was also examined but not included as a designated group.

The number of women in each group is shown below:

Abstainers past 12 months	= 217 (24%)
Abstainers prior 30 days	= 73 (8%)
Light drinkers (less than 0.22 oz./day)	= 247 (27%)
Moderate drinkers (between 0.22 and 0.99 oz./day)	= 261 (29%)
Heavy drinkers (1 or more oz./day)	= 108 (12%)

Responses of each group are summarized in Table 10.1 (from data given by Klassen and Wilsnack, 1986). The majority of women reported that they were less sexually inhibited on alcohol and felt closer and more open with others. Nearly half found sexual activity more pleasurable when they drank. These positive effects tended to be more frequent in the heavy drinker group. (Note that no questions asked if sexual activity was ever less pleasurable or less intense.)

The subgroup of heavy drinkers was more likely to feel less sexually inhibited while drinking (80%). Relatively few women had become "sexually forward" (20–28%) or less particular in their choice of sexual partners (4–12%) while drinking, though these behaviors were more frequent among heavy drinkers. The majority of women reported that aggressive sexual advances had been made toward them by "another drinker," indicating that women are more often bothered by male drinkers rather than themselves instigating sexually provocative behavior.

Among abstainers and light drinkers, fewer had ever masturbated (37-39%) than among moderate drinkers, heavy drinkers, or temporary abstainers. The widest difference between abstainers and drinkers was recorded for the item dealing with premarital sex: only 18% of the abstainers approved of premarital sex, compared to 74% of heavy drinkers.

Moderate drinkers generally showed the lowest frequency of sexual problems or dysfunction. Heavy drinkers who averaged four drinks daily reported more lack of sexual interest than

Table 10.1 *1981 National Survey of Alcohol Drinking in Women*
Percent (%) Positive Response to Sex Questions
Modified from Klassen and Wilsnack, 1986

	Abstainers	*Temporary Abstainers (past 30 days)*	*Light Drinkers (<0.22 oz/day)*	*Moderate Drinkers (0.22–.99 oz/day)*	*Heavy Drinkers (1 oz or more/day)*
When Drinking					
Less inhibited about sex			56	63	68
Sex more pleasurable			40	47	56
Feel closer to partner/other			61	60	67
Easier to be open with others			64	73	81
Ever became sexually forward			20	21	28
Less particular in partner choice			4	11	12
Aggression from another drinker			61	58	58
Sex History					
Never interested/enjoy sex	8	6	3	1	5
Never orgasm with intercourse	5	5	6	5	7
Intercourse orgasm < 1/2 time or never	26	27	25	20	28
Intercourse pain (vaginismus)	16	22	19	13	14
Partner wants more sex	55	70	56	39	44
Ever masturbate	31	52	37	49	56
Premarital sex not wrong	18	35	42	52	74
Had intercourse before marriage	27	45	49	60	53

the total subgroup of heavy drinkers (10% versus 5% overall); those who drank six or more drinks per day at least three times a week reported a lack of sexual interest at 15% (versus 5% overall) as well as a higher incidence of orgasm failure during intercourse (12% versus 5% overall).

One impression gained from this survey was that moderate levels of drinking (more than three drinks per week but less than two drinks daily) were associated with normal sexual adjustment. Interestingly, moderate levels of drinking have been also associated with greater longevity than with histories of abstinence or heavy drinkers (De Labry et al., 1992).

The size and representativeness of the sample make these results particularly impressive. Unfortunately, the lack of specific questions eliciting information about current sexual adjustment and levels of sexual activity lessened the usefulness of the survey. Additional questions on sexuality appeared to have been asked but not reported. It is not clear whether many of the differences between groups are significant.

Other findings not summarized in Table 10.1 included more frequent experiences of depression in the group of heavy drinkers: at least one two-week period of depression was reported by 61% of this subgroup, compared to 38% of long-term abstainers. Suicide attempts were also associated with heavy drinking (0.2% in long-term abstainers, 5% in women who consumed two to four drinks daily, 10% in women who consumed four drinks or more per day, and 24% in women consuming six or more drinks at least three days a week). It is not clear from this study whether depression and suicidal tendencies lead to heavy drinking or the reverse.

Another useful research project (Beckman, 1979) studied 103 women who had no history of alcoholism or psychiatric disorders. Twenty-nine percent desired intercourse more when drinking and 32% enjoyed intercourse more when drinking. Beckman also studied another group of 120 alcoholic women. Of these, 57% desired intercourse more when drinking, 55% enjoyed intercourse more when drinking, and 55% engaged in intercourse more when drinking. However, these alcoholic women reported significantly less sexual satisfaction than normal or psychiatric control groups.

In 1986, Harvey and Beckman conducted a detailed study using daily logs of alcohol intake and sexual activity kept by 69 nonalcoholic woman social drinkers (aged 18–34) recruited from a college population. The study was limited to women reporting alcohol consumption at least twice a week, but not consuming over three drinks per day. The subjects had never been treated for alcohol abuse. One criterion was a stable heterosexual relationship, with sexual activity occurring at least once a week. Since the study was also investigating lapses in contraceptive use due to alcohol, women using permanent contraception (such as birth control pills, intrauterine devices, or tubal ligations) were excluded, as were those with menstrual cycle irregularities, histories of mental illness, or histories of using recreational drugs other than alcohol.

Thus, these women were a normal healthy group free of influences which would otherwise interfere with normal sexual activity. They were mainly white (87%), young (mean age of 24), highly educated (81% had had two or more years of college, 60% were undergraduates, and 36% were graduate students). For contraception, 83% used a diaphragm, 13% used condoms, and 4% used a cervical cap. Sexual activity and alcohol consumption were measured over two or three menstrual cycles (mean of 2.8 cycles) by daily logs.

Alcohol use with sexual activity was defined as alcohol consumed four hours or less before sex. Drinking condition was split into three categories: no alcohol, moderate alcohol (three or fewer drinks), and heavy alcohol (more than three drinks).

Results (in Tables 10.2 and 10.3) failed to show any significant effects of alcohol on sexual arousal, pleasure, or orgasm. The only significant difference between groups was reported in the category of female-initiated sexual activity, which occurred twice as often without alcohol than with it. Since the data were collected prospectively by daily logs rather than retrospectively, the lack of significant effect on sexual arousal or pleasure was particularly intriguing, considering that in the heavy alcohol condition of more than three drinks some degree of intoxication would be present. This failure to find effects of alcohol on sexual function indicated that retrospective accounts of alcohol effects may not be accurate. Furthermore, as described in the laboratory expectancy studies of women (Wilson & Lawson, 1976a, 1978), the physiological sexual response may decrease even as women subjectively experience greater sexual arousal.

While a decrease of female-initiated sexual activity when drinking was noted in this study, data on total occurrence of sexual activity oddly were not reported, even though the authors speculated that the decrease in female-initiated activity while drinking may have been due to an increase in male-initiated sexual activity. With-

Table 10.2 *Subject Evaluation of Sexual Effects of Drinking by Daily Logs*

	No Alcohol	*Moderate Alcohol*	*Heavy Alcohol*
Self-rating sexual arousal (ns)	3.67	3.72	3.93
Self-rating sexual pleasure (ns)	3.82	3.81	3.89
% Orgasm during sexual activity (ns)	66	66	61
Daily female-initiated sexual activity ($p < 0.001$)	0.78	0.32	0.41
Contraceptive nonuse (% occasions)	23.1	19.2	23.1

Data from Harvey and Beckman, 1986.

Table 10.3 *Percent Comparison of Sexual Effect of Drinking**

	When Drinking a Little	*When Drinking a Lot*	*When Not Drinking*	*Does Not Matter*
Desire sexual activity most	44.8	16.4	4.5	34.3
Enjoy sexual activity most	32.8	1.5	19.4	46.3
Engage in sexual activity most	13.4	9.0	13.4	64.2

*By post-study questionnaire.
Data from Harvey and Beckman, 1986.

out this additional information, the decrease in female-initiated sexual activity with alcohol is difficult to interpret, even though it is likely to be cited as evidence of a negative effect of alcohol on sexual function. At most, this finding indicated that the stereotype of drinking women being sexually provocative was not necessarily true for well-adjusted women in active and stable sexual relationships.

Impact on Relationship

A woman portrayed as drinking is perceived by both women and men to be less attractive, more sexually available, and more likely to have sex compared to a nondrinking woman (George, Gournic, & McAfee, 1988). Alcohol-induced sexual activity in women may cause loss of self-esteem, anxiety, distress from lack of self-control, and exposure to sexual and physical abuse as well as to sexually transmitted diseases—factors which invariably impact intimate relationships (Schuster, 1988). The contributing factors to relationship problems compounded by alcoholism are attachment dependencies, poor communication between partners, the increased probability of aggression and abuse, and undermining of the emotional and sexual bond between partners. Alcoholic women are more likely to be single or divorced (Schuster, 1988); perhaps the inability to respond sexually in a satisfying manner is one component of the failed relationships. Given the possibility of aggressive effects of alcohol in women as well as in men, the alcoholic woman may attribute all of her problems, including her sexual inadequacies, to her male partner and be especially cruel and deprecating. In effect, all the problems that plague ordinary relationships are exaggerated when alcoholism is involved.

Another major obstacle is the difficulty of distinguishing primarily sexual effects from changes in relationship dynamics which determine sexual desires and response. An intoxicated woman may feel more sexual desire and be more sexually assertive but be less attractive and desirable to the partner. With both chronic and acute alcohol abuse, general attractiveness may decrease and there may be a loss of respect from her "respectable" sexual partners and sexual exploitation by abusive partners.

Obstetric, Gynecological, and Menstrual Complications of Alcohol

The prevalence of heavy drinking in women outpatients of obstetric and gynecology clinics is about three times higher than in the general community (Russell & Bigler, 1979). Wilsnack et al. (1984) reported that 77% of alcoholic women (compared to 35% of controls) experienced hysterectomy, infertility, miscarriages, or other pregnancy complications. Pelvic inflammatory conditions primarily due to sexually transmitted diseases were reported in 50% of the alcoholic sample, compared with 10% in controls (Jensen, 1984).

There is a higher prevalence of hysterectomy and complications such as infections and bleeding in women alcoholics. Felding, Jensen, and Tonnesen (1992) identified these complications in 80% of women who drank more than five drinks daily compared to 13% of women who drank fewer than two drinks daily. Heavy drinking apparently compromises both natural immune defenses and hemostatic control. More serious complications such as gynecological surgery other than hysterectomy, pregnancy problems including miscarriage, stillbirth, and prematurity, and birth defects were significantly greater among women who consumed six or more drinks at least three to five days a week.

Menstrual disorders are also prevalent in alcoholic women. Amenorrhea or irregular menstrual cycles has been found in as high as 85% of chronic female alcoholics (Hugues et al., 1980). In a well controlled residential ward setting, Mendelson and Mello (1988) reported that women who drank more than three drinks a day generally experienced menstrual cycle disruption. To explore the cause for such disruption, Mendelson et al. (1992) administered luteinizing hormone releasing hormone (LHRH) intravenously, simultaneously with alcohol or placebo; they found consistent increases of estradiol with alcohol and LHRH, but not with placebo and LHRH. Chronic alcohol-induced increases in estradiol could reduce LHRH secretion and cause amenorrhea or irregular cycles, because ovulation is dependent upon appropriate signaling by the LHRH mid-cycle rise and fall. These alterations could reflect pathological changes in estradiol due directly to alcohol intake or indirectly to changes in liver function and to dysregulation of the ovarian-hypothalamic/pituitary feedback circuit.

Menstrual cycle disruption by alcohol may also occur due to chronic excess activation of the hypothalamic-pituitary-adrenal axis. In animals (monkeys and rats), administration of corticotropin-releasing-factor (CRF) has been shown to inhibit the pulsatile secretion of LH and FSH (Teoh, Mello, & Mendelson, 1994). Excess CRF can also be expected to inhibit sexual desire and activity in animals and humans.

The percentage of women who experienced dysmenorrhea, heavy menstrual flow, and premenstrual discomfort increased with increased alcohol intake among drinking women (Mendelson et al., 1992). Conversely, drinking has been reported to increase in 67% of menstruating alcoholics during the premenstruum (Belfer, Shader, Carroll, & Harmetz, 1971; Podolsky, 1963).

Moderate alcohol use of up to one drink per day may be beneficial for postmenopausal women receiving no estrogen replacement therapy, since estradiol levels are significantly increased (Gavaler & Rosenblum, 1994). At this moderate level of alcohol intake, there is no increased risk of liver disease or breast cancer in postmenopausal women.

Eating Disorders and Alcohol Use

Excessive alcohol use is frequently associated with eating disorders, indicating that both involve deficient impulse control. In various studies, excessive alcohol use has been reported in 6–50% of bulimic women and 6–23% of anorectic women (Krahn, Gosnell, & Kurth, 1994). In a study by Beary, Lacey, and Merry (1986) comparing 20 alcoholic women to 20 bulimic women, 35% of the alcoholics reported a prior major eating disorder and 50% of the bulimics reported excessive alcohol use. Eating disorders frequently precede alcohol abuse. Excessive alcohol use has been found to increase from 14–20% prior to onset of bulimia and to 41–49% after bulimia onset (Krahn et al., 1994). By age 35, 50% of bulimic patients may use alcohol excessively (Hatsukami, Mitchell, Eckert, & Pyle, 1986), indicating that alcohol abuse is a frequent concomitant or alternative to dieting and food bingeing. Food deprivation has been shown to be a potent stimulus to alcohol dependence in monkeys and rats (Carroll & Meisch, 1984). Krahn et al. (1994) found a strong association between dieting and prevalence of alcohol use in a questionnaire survey of 1,796 female freshman college students.

THE EFFECTS OF ALCOHOL ON SEXUAL FUNCTION IN MALES

Alcohol is both a drug and a carbohydrate food that is extensively metabolized within the testes, probably causing testicular tissue damage and malnutrition. With just a few drinks, most men experience transient boosts in sex drive and sociability. With continued drinking, however, erection and ejaculation abilities systematically decrease in a dose-related fashion, to a point of total dysfunction. (There is always the exception to the general rule: Some men are impotent when sober and can *only* participate in sexual activity when drinking.)

Lemere and Smith (1973) reviewed their extensive clinical experience with an estimated 17,000 alcoholic male patients over a time period of 36 years. They noted that 8% remained impotent after detoxification; after several years of sobriety, 50% of these alcoholics recovered normal erectile function, but the remaining 50% remained partially or fully impotent, despite generally strong sexual desire. While such impotence is often attributed to hypogonadism consequent to alcoholism, the preservation of sexual desire indicated that testosterone levels were sufficient—at least within the central nervous system.

The persistence of impotence may be caused by a combination of factors: testosterone receptor degeneration; estrogenic dominance; enzymatic and metabolic pathology in the lower intestine, liver, and gonads; or gonadal tissue damage.

Testosterone

Reduced normal levels of testosterone have been found in alcoholics (e.g., Huttunen, Harkonen, Niskanen, Leino, & Ylikahri, 1976; Liegel, Fabre, Howard, & Farmer, 1972). While testosterone levels often increase after extended abstinence, damage to testosterone receptors, the gonads, and the liver may remain, particularly in men over 40. Intoxicating doses of alcohol (BAL of 0.10 or above) were shown to lower testosterone levels in healthy nonalcoholic male volunteers (Cicero, 1980; Gordon, Altman, Southren, Rubin, & Lieber, 1976; Mendelson, Mello, & Ellingboe, 1977).

In a study of male alcoholics (Mendelson & Mello, 1988) in a residential ward setting, overall mean testosterone levels decreased from 555 ng without alcohol to 383 ng during a ten-day alcohol-available period. Levels returned to normal when subjects voluntarily ceased drinking. The researchers concluded that both chronic alcohol abuse and acutely intoxicating doses can decrease testosterone; however, an acute moderate dose of alcohol causes no change. They also noted that, when alcohol intake is high enough to decrease testosterone levels, cortical output of luteinizing hormone releasing hormone (LHRH) and luteinizing hormone (LH) usually increases, providing a sexual surge.

Moderate doses of alcohol can increase epinephrine and norepinephrine activity, particularly in the hypothalamus (Linnoila, Mefford, Nutt, & Adinoff, 1987), thereby priming LHRH release. Since sexual desire may be instigated by LHRH secretion alone, alcoholics may feel an increase in sexual desire even as testosterone levels decline. Testosterone levels do not rise in response to LHRH/LH until consumption of alcohol ceases. Because alcohol did not block the LHRH/LH rise, and because testosterone levels did not respond to the LHRH stimulation, Mendelson and Mello (1988) concluded that alcohol-induced reductions in testosterone occur peripherally in the gonads and the liver. Furthermore, the LHRH/LH response may result in transiently higher testosterone levels during withdrawal. "Roller-coasting" of this kind probably dysregulates the LHRH/LH testosterone feedback circuit unpredictably. A further imbalance occurs in the adrenal steroid production characterized by increased cortisol and decreased DHEAS (Ylikhari, Huttunen, & Harkonen, 1980).

In a previous study Mendelson et al. (1977) measured the effect of acute alcohol intake in 16 healthy nonalcoholic male volunteers (aged 21–26). Testosterone levels fell significantly during the ascending limb of the blood alcohol curve. Depression of testosterone was greatest at peak blood alcohol levels, even while LH levels increased. During the descending limb of the blood alcohol curve, LH levels decreased and testosterone level remained decreased. Additional studies by Mendelson and Mello (1988) have shown that euphoria and sexual feelings were felt most powerfully during ascending and peak blood alcohol levels, despite descending testosterone levels.

Since successful sexual experience can increase testosterone production, while unsuccessful intercourse can potentially depress it, achieving only a weak erection or no erection at all while under the influence of alcohol could render subsequent sexual experiences even more difficult. On the other hand, if sexual function is "successful," it also can promote LHRH secretion, so that a combination of alcohol intake, LHRH secretion, and sexual activity under optimal circumstances conceivably could condition an aphrodisiac response to alcohol. Like alcohol itself, this alcohol-sex combination is subject to abuse, tolerance, and eventual dysphoria.

Since endocrine responses to alcohol are variable and subject to individual and circumstantial differences, failure to find reduced testosterone with acute or chronic alcohol administration is relatively common (Bannister, Handley, Chapman, & Losowsky, 1986; Huttunen et al., 1976; Linnoila, Prinz, Wonsowicz, & Leppaluoto, 1980; Sparrow, Bosse, & Rowe, 1980; Ylikahri et al., 1978). Jensen and Gluud (1985) found that cirrhotic patients who were otherwise healthy showed comparable sexual function to an age-matched sample of healthy alcoholics, despite abnormally low levels of free serum testosterone. Testosterone levels were no different between sexually functional and dysfunctional cirrhotic alcoholics. Lindholm et al. (1978a, 1978b) found no hormonal differences between alcoholics with or without cirrhotic liver disease. Liegel et al. (1972) measured normal testosterone levels in abstinent alcoholics, decreased testosterone while drinking at intoxication levels, and increased levels during early alcohol withdrawal.

In a study by Couwenbergs (1988), a decrease in dihydrotestosterone (DHT), the peripheral form of testosterone considered to be responsible for secondary sex characteristics, was particularly noticeable and most severe shortly after alcohol intake. In other studies, dihydrotestosterone often increased shortly after alcohol intake due to the accelerated metabolism of testosterone. Long-term studies of alcoholic abuse usually have shown a decline in DHT, which could be responsible for the hypogonadism and peripheral demasculinization often noted in alcoholics. Though 5-alpha-reductase enzyme activity, a prerequisite for DHT production, increases shortly after alcohol intake, prolonged alcohol consumption is associated with a decrease in 5-alpha-reductase activity (Gordon, Southren, & Lieber, 1979). Sex-hormone-binding-globulin (SHBG), which binds testosterone and decreases its availability, is typically elevated by chronic alcohol intake in association with increased estrogen levels (Lindholm et al., 1978b).

Despite the number of studies indicating a testosterone-suppressing effect of alcohol, testosterone reduction does not account for the sexual dysfunction associated with male alcoholics. It appears that localized gonadal tissue damage in conjunction with brain damage are largely responsible for these effects. Sexual dysfunction associated with alcohol can also be due to the diseases caused or aggravated by alcohol abuse (i.e., diabetes, heart disease, peripheral neuropathy).

Erectile Dysfunctions

Wilson and Lawson (1976b) found that a low dose of alcohol (0.25 g/kg) facilitated erection to erotic stimuli in men. This effect appears to be attributable to a psychological factor of disinhibition rather than to a physiological mechanism per se (although, as noted previously, a transient increase in LHRH/LH may be responsible). The facilitation of sexual response is temporary and quickly replaced by progressive dysfunction, involving the loss of erection and inhibition of ejaculation that is directly related to the dose of alcohol.

The direct impact of alcohol on erection has been measured in awake subjects with visual erotic stimuli (VES) tests and with nocturnal penile tumescence (NPT) sleep studies (Briddel & Wilson, 1976; Farkas & Rosen, 1976; Langevin et al., 1985; Wilson & Lawson, 1976b). Actual erectile performance during intercourse has been assessed only indirectly from patient reports. Direct measurements (the use of strain gauges around the penis—penile plethysmography) are intrusive and have usually recorded penile tumescence, not rigidity. Integrated tumescence-rigidity monitors have become available only recently.

Visual erotic stimuli tests are conducted in laboratories on subjects fitted with measurement devices that evaluate sexual reactions to erotic stimuli compared to neutral stimuli. The interpretation of these studies, however, is not straightforward. Since normal erections to visual erotic stimuli have been noted in patients with deficient or castrate testosterone levels, who fail to show normal erection during sleep, intercourse, or masturbation, it appears that the strong pornographic content of these stimuli can be sufficient to compensate for the decreased sexual excitement typically experienced by men with abnormally low levels of testosterone.

Also, the "erection-on-demand" results of visual erotic stimuli testing may be more attributable to the novelty of being strapped to an apparatus, receiving alcohol, watching explicit material chosen and presented by otherwise respectable university authorities, and being monitored by a white-coated scientist. Indeed, volunteers for such studies have been shown to have special characteristics not representative of the general population (Nirenberg et al., 1991).

Facilitation of erection has been demonstrated with 0.025 to 0.05 BAL (Farkas & Rosen, 1976; Langevin et al., 1985). Penile stimulation studies conducted with alcohol and visual erotic stimuli generally have shown that there is either no difference or a slight, nonsignificant decrease of erection at 0.06 BAL (Briddel et al., 1978; Farkas & Rosen, 1976; Lansky & Wilson, 1981; Rubin & Henson, 1976; Wilson & Lawson, 1976b). At levels of 0.06 and above, erectile decreases usually appear and become more noticeable as subjects become intoxicated (Briddel & Wilson, 1976; Farkas & Rosen, 1976; Rubin & Henson, 1976). Rubin and Henson (1976) found reliable decrements in erection in most subjects with BAL between 0.106 and 0.156, the moderate intoxication range for social drinkers. The researchers found no significant relationship between how subjects believed alcohol would affect erection and the measured effects. Since these studies measured only passive erection to erotic pictures, the resilience and robustness of erection were inadequately determined.

Alcohol seems to impair erection more when the subject is distracted or circumstances make it difficult to limit attention to sexual gratification. Wilson, Niaura, and Adler (1985) tested erection using a dichotic listening paradigm: an erotic tape played in one ear; an involved cognitive task requiring responses was played in the other ear. In this situation, a nonintoxicating dose of alcohol significantly decreased erection during a more complex version of the cognitive task, but did not interfere when the task was relatively simple. Since audiosexual stimuli may be less stimulating than visual stimuli, ineffective sexual stimulation (rather than alcohol) may have accounted for decreased erection during the complex cognitive task condition.

Ejaculatory Dysfunctions

Clinical observations of alcoholic patients have shown a 23–25% rate of retarded ejaculation (Jensen, 1984). This difficulty in achieving orgasm/ejaculation reflects the anesthetic and sedative action of alcohol as well as significant inhibition of limbic centers that process sensation and generate psychological tension. A lessening of tension and inhibitions through limbic inhibition may also lessen positive attentive sexual cognitions as well as receipt and excitation from physical sensations.

One study by Malatesta, Pollack, Wilbanks, and Adams (1979), which has never been replicated independently, involved volunteer subjects who masturbated to orgasm/ejaculation while exposed to erotic pictures. Time to ejaculation was five to six minutes at BAL, about 10 minutes at 0.06 BAL, and 13 minutes at 0.09 BAL. The time limit for completion was 16 minutes. Ten of 24 subjects failed to ejaculate within this time limit at 0.06 to 0.09 blood alcohol levels. Though there was no measurement of erection, subjective reports at 0.06 to 0.09 BAL noted decreased sexual arousal, decreased pleasure and intensity of orgasm, and increased difficulty in achieving orgasm. Retarded ejaculation was also noted in three of four alcoholics tested at between 0.09 and 0.10 levels, despite their prior belief that such moderate intake would not affect their sexual arousal.

It should be noted that the sexual stimuli in these laboratory studies may be far less exciting than real-life interpersonal sexual encounters. In Malatesta et al.'s study, subjects were wired and strapped with multiple electrodes to allow measurement of genital EMG activity and heart rate—a most atypical sexual situation. Since these situations are so unusual and the sexual response so sensitive, replication is essential.

Nocturnal Penile Tumescence Studies

Sleep studies conducted with alcoholic subjects have identified nocturnal penile tumescence erection deficits. However, these deficits do not occur with nonintoxicating doses of alcohol. Snyder and Karacan (1981) conducted sleep study on 26 sober, detoxified chronic male alcoholics (mean age = 40, mean years alcoholic = 7.2) compared to age-matched healthy controls. None of the alcoholic patients reported sexual dysfunction (decreased desire, erection, or orgasm/ejaculation) and all liver, renal, and endocrine tests were normal. Total nocturnal tumescence time did not differ between groups, but former alcoholics showed diminished tumescence (80–100% of full erection) and more semitumescence (20–80% of full erection) than control subjects.

In a prior study by Karacan (Karacan, Snyder, Salis, Williams, & Derman, 1980), alcoholic patients (mean age = 50.8) complaining of impotence similarly showed no difference in total nocturnal penile tumescence time, but had fewer full tumescence episodes (0.8 versus 2.7 in matched controls) and more partial tumescence episodes (2.8 versus 1.0 in controls). Only three of the six impotent alcoholics showed complete absence of full sleep erections.

Paradoxical Effects

Differences in autonomic response may explain why some men function sexually *only* when drunk. Finn and Pihl (1987, 1988) identified differences in autonomic response in nonalcoholic men at high risk for alcoholism by family history. Evidently, the autonomic hyperactivity of these men was dampened by alcohol (which is opposite to the effect on normal men). Given that excessive adrenergic reactivity (the epinephrine response) is a frequent cause for failure to achieve or maintain an erection, the high-risk man may find that he can get and maintain an erection better with alcohol than without.

Normal men will experience increased adrenergic reactivity (shown by increased heart rate) under the influence of alcohol, which usually hinders erection. For individuals with panic/phobia disorder, which causes autonomic overreactivity, alcohol may similarly reduce excess adrenergic reactions, allowing satisfactory sexual performance.

ALCOHOL, SEX, VIOLENCE, AND EXPECTANCY

Alcoholism has been identified in 35–50% of child abusers (Orford & Vellman, 1990). The rate of alcohol dependence in incestuous fathers has ranged from 20–70% and most alcoholic fathers are intoxicated when incest occurs (Forrest, 1983). As adults, victims of abuse may suffer from alcoholism. Various studies of incest or sexual abuse/molestation have indicated that 33–50% of women treated at alcohol and substance abuse clinics were sexually abused as children (Schuster, 1988).

Alcohol is also consumed by 30–70% of rapists prior to rape assaults and is frequently associated with abusive marital incidents (Abbey, Ross, & McDuffie, 1994; Evans, 1986). Among college students, 30–74% of males and 29–53% of females involved in sexual assaults have been found to be drinking alcohol prior to the incident (Abbey, Ross, & McDuffie, 1994).

Sexual benefits resulting from the belief that one has consumed alcohol may be accompanied by increased aggression. Lang (1981) reported that male heavy drinkers were more aggressive when they believed they had consumed alcohol, even when they actually received placebo. Subjects were more verbally abusive in social interactions and gave longer duration, high-intensity shocks to investigators when given the opportunity. Lang, Goeckner, Adesso, and Marlatt (1975) previously had shown that subjects would deliver greater duration and intensity of shocks to mock opponents if they believed they had consumed alcohol.

Briddel et al. (1978) reported that erection could be increased in male social drinkers exposed to videotapes showing rape and sadistic aggression, due solely to the belief that they had consumed alcohol whether they had or not. Similarly, George and Marlatt (1986) found that the alcohol expectancy effect was manifested in increased viewing time for sexually violent slides and sexual slides, but not for sexually neutral slides. The expectancy effect was greatest for the sexually violent slides and, in particular, for the most deviant scenes depicted. Preference for the sexually violent slides increased along with the increased viewing times when alcohol was expected. With intoxicating doses of alcohol, direct pharmacological effects were more pronounced than expectancy effects. However, both expectancy and direct consumption of alcohol increased aggression.

In the study by Briddel et al. (1978), male subjects who thought they received alcohol (but actually received tonic water) showed greater erection than those thinking they had received only tonic water. In a study by Briddel and Wilson (1976), three different tapes were used as tests: tapes portraying mutually enjoyable heterosexual intercourse, forcible rape, and nonsexual sadistic aggression. Results with actual alcohol intake (mean BAL = 0.03%) did not differ from those with tonic water alone. Subjects who believed they had consumed alcohol showed equal penile tumescence in response to the forcible rape and mutual heterosexual tapes; whereas subjects who believed they had consumed only tonic water showed less tumescence to the rape tape than to the heterosexual tape. The alcohol expectancy-induced increase in sexual response was greater with the rape and aggression tapes than with the normal intercourse tape. Aspects of sexual arousal other than erection (such as heart rate, skin temperature, and subjective perceptions) also increased in subjects who believed they had consumed alcohol.

Case Report

A male patient in his mid-sixties was referred to me by the criminal court system for evaluation and treatment of the alleged sexual abuse of his grandson. "Phil" denied these events, vehemently declaring that he treasured this child and *under no circumstances* would harm him.

Phil had a serious problem with alcohol, complete with a lengthy history of drunk driving offenses that included accidents involving physical injury to himself and others. As a result, he had been required by the court to take Antabuse on a daily basis. However, according to his wife he had been skipping his pills and was bingeing on alcohol periodically.

In an effort to understand the family relationships, I arranged an interview with his son and daughter-in-law, the parents of the child involved. The son readily volunteered that when he was a boy, his father had sodomized him on a regular basis when drunk. Phil never abused him when he was sober, however. The sexual abuse continued for about five years and was extended to his younger brother, whom he had tried to protect from his father's sexual rages. The son acknowledged his confusion about the fact that when sober his father was emphatically homophobic, exclaiming in disgust whenever the subject came up in conversation or in the media. Although the son viewed his father as a hopeless hypocrite, he still had great affection for him in his sober state. The younger son confirmed these experiences. I also interviewed the grandson, who was less articulate due to his youth, but was able to describe the sexual approaches of his grandfather quite specifically.

Having interviewed numerous sex offenders, I had little doubt that the sexual abuse had occurred, but I was disturbed by the sincere denial of the elder man. To resolve this matter to my satisfaction, I arranged for a family meeting that included the two grown sons and their father. The sons confronted him with the details of the sexual abuse. Instead of denying it or confessing with remorse, he angrily demanded from his sons, "Why didn't you tell me I had done these terrible things? How could you keep it from me?"

His sons were stunned. "But *you* did it! We naturally assumed you knew!" I watched their father crumble before my eyes. He was in extreme distress, crying angry tears, indicating that he had absolutely no recollection of any of these events and was horrified at the thought that he could behave in this abhorrent way. Nonetheless, he believed his sons were telling the truth, which was torturous for him. According to them, the only time he was abusive was when he drank, and it appears that his sexual assaults occurred during alcoholic blackouts—that he had no conscious access to these memories after the event.

In his sober personality, Phil and his wife were Buddhists, pacifists, and gentle people. Alcohol dramatically affected Phil's physiology, resulting in abusive behavior for which he had no conscious recall.

It is difficult to describe adequately the subjective experience of observing this family interaction. I can only say that once confronted by his sons, the father did not hesitate to believe them. He was not defensive; he was shocked and deeply saddened. The interaction felt extraordinarily genuine to me and gave me a frightening insight into the relationship between alcohol and sexual trauma, and the potential for sexual abuse without recall.

ADDITIONAL PHYSICAL AND PSYCHOLOGICAL SYMPTOMS

In addition to the sexual and emotional problems associated with alcohol that have already been addressed, there are a number of physical and psychological symptoms common to both men and women that affect sexual function secondarily.

Korsakoff's Syndrome

Permanent physiological and neurological damage can occur from chronic alcoholism (Ryan & Butters, 1980). While hypothalamic-pituitary activity seems to be relatively well-preserved in mild alcoholism, degeneration in the limbic system can occur, causing "short circuits" in the brain sex centers for command, thought, and sensation (e.g., amygdala, septum, hippocampus, entorhinal cortex, nucleus accumbens, and extensions to the frontal cortex). In severe cases, the memory loss characteristic of Korsakoff's syndrome appears.

Certainly, the degeneration experienced in the limbic area, which in some alcoholics progresses to Korsakoff's syndrome, would only worsen schizophrenic or schizo-affective tendencies that also involve limbic dysfunction.

Cirrhosis

Chronic excess alcohol intake typically leads to cirrhosis and other liver diseases, which can result in the loss of male sexual desire through a decrease in testosterone and increase in estrogen. Liver damage and enzymatic alterations lead to changes in androgen metabolism, increased clearance of testosterone from the blood, and decreased clearance of estrogen (Van Thiel, Gavaler, & Schade, 1985). There is increased hepatic release of the weak androgen, androstenedione, which is converted to the sexually inactive estrone form of estrogen (Van Thiel, 1977). Aromatase activity which converts testosterone to estrogens, is increased by alcohol (Gordon et al., 1979).

Alcohol decreases DHEAS (e.g., Becker et al., 1988, 1991b) and chronic alcohol-induced cirrhosis is characterized by lowered DHEAS. Women alcoholics free of cirrhosis have reduced DHEAS, as do women with non-alcoholic cirrhosis (Becker et al., 1991a). Jasonni et al. (1983) found lower DHEAS levels in women alcoholics with cirrhotic liver disease, despite an increase in the other main adrenal androgen, androstenedione. Similarly, male alcoholics with cirrhosis may have higher androstenedione but lower DHEAS (Becker et al., 1991).

Gynecomastia

High estrogen levels, accompanied by increases in sex-hormone-binding globulin and decreases in free testosterone (resulting in a lower estrogen to testosterone ratio), often lead to gynecomastia (Chopra, Tulchinsky, & Greenway, 1973; Farnsworth, Cavanaugh, Brown, Alvarez, & Lewandowski, 1978). Gynecomastia as well as hypogonadism occur more frequently in patients with alcohol-induced liver disease than in patients with non-alcoholic liver disease (Mendelson & Mello, 1988). Estrogenic substances in beer and wine cause different hormonal metabolites than those shown after ingestion of "hard" liquor (Couwenbergs, 1988), but differences in the rate of gynecomastia have not yet been shown between consumers of beer, wine, or hard liquor.

Infertility

A major cause of male infertility is gonadal deficiencies caused by alcohol abuse. Some degree of testicular atrophy, involving a loss of normal germ cells and a generation of grossly abnormal germ cells (Van Thiel, Gavaler, Lester, Loriaux, & Braunstein, 1975), is found in about 70% of male alcoholics. Atrophy has been associated partly with vitamin A and zinc deficiencies (McClain, Van Thiel, Parker, Badzin, & Gilbert, 1979). Severe reduction of spermatogenesis has been shown in 30% of alcoholics (Brzek, 1987; Lindholm et al., 1978a) and abnormally low motility in 23% (Brzek, 1987). Degenerate morphological changes in spermatozoa are common, including sperm-head breaks, curling of the tail, and midsection distension (Van Thiel, Gavaler, Eagon, & Lester, 1980).

The direct toxic effect of alcohol often occurs in the absence of liver disease (Cicero, Bell, Meyer, & Badger, 1980; Gordon et al., 1979; Mendelson & Mello, 1979). Oxidative metabolism of alcohol involves reduction of nicotinamide adenine dinucleotide enzyme reactions to nicotinamide adenine dinucleotide. Consequently, the amount of the enzyme available for testicular steroidogenesis is reduced. Both alcohol and its metabolite acetaldehyde inhibit various microsomal enzymes involved in steroidogenesis and gonadal tissue maintenance (Chiao, Johnston, Gavaler, & Van Thiel, 1981; Cicero et al., 1980; Johnston, Chiao, Gavaler, & Van Thiel, 1981).

THE IMPACT OF ALCOHOLISM ON LONGEVITY

Alcohol basically liquifies cell membranes. When such disordering of cell membranes becomes chronic, a situation resembling the body's breakdown during old age is created. Since alcohol is a food as well as a drug, its metabolism critically affects the lipid and enzymatic environment of cell membranes, which may lead to disordering and degeneration of target organs with high cholesterol metabolism, such as the liver and testicles.

Wood and Strong (1986) have extensively reviewed the similarity of membrane changes with chronic alcohol use to those found during old age. Since membrane structure and function during aging is already deteriorating and vulnerable, excessive alcohol use will contribute to advanced cell pathology.

Spontaneous abortion, intrauterine growth retardation, and birth defects clearly increase with even moderate alcohol use (greater than two drinks per week) during pregnancy (Teoh et al., 1994). Fetal alcohol syndrome (FAS) resulting from heavy alcohol use during pregnancy is associated with decreased sex-hormone-binding globulin (SHBG), decreased total testosterone and DHEAS, but increased free testosterone and androstenedione (Ylikorkala, Stenman, & Halmesmäki, 1988).

While shifting operations in limbic areas probably modulate sexual effects in healthy social drinkers, the chronic alcoholic is more likely to show signs of brain and body aging, fatigue, and exhaustion. Studies of sexual dysfunction in "healthy" alcoholics have shown a clear age effect, with dysfunction becoming frequent as men pass the age of 40 (Jensen, 1984; O'Farrell, Choquette, & Birchler, 1991). Since DHEAS is the only sex hormone that decreases substantially and progressively with age before 60, the low levels of DHEAS found in female and male alcoholics (Becker et al., 1988; Becker, Gluud, Farholt, et al., 1991) indicate such a premature aging effect. Particularly strong effects of alcohol in limbic areas and in the gonads may also cause premature aging and dysregulation in these "sexual" areas of the body.

Cognitive therapy may repair some of the damage done to the limbic areas, but sexual changes in older alcoholics are increasingly irreversible. Older dysfunctional alcoholics may also have symptoms that resemble Alzheimer's disease within the genital sexual circuit. Drugs with the potential to alleviate sexual dysfunction (such as bupropion or yohimbine) may have their primary effect in the brain; the peripheral effects of these drugs appear limited, so that their efficacy will be limited by the extent of physiological and gonadal damage which has occurred.

Ryan (1980) reported that the performance of alcoholics on several learning and memory tasks was comparable to normal controls who were ten years older. Alcoholics showed less deficiency on tasks utilizing over-learned rote responses than on tasks requiring visual-perceptual skills, abstract reasoning, and learning and memory abilities in general (Ryan & Butters, 1980). Holden, McLaughlin, Reilly, and Overall (1988) found that alcoholics performed at a mental age seven years advanced over age-matched controls, replicating prior studies that had shown premature cognitive aging in alcoholics. Such learning and cognitive deterioration indicates damage to those limbic mechanisms that mediate learning, memory, and discrimination.

Lishman, Jacobson, and Acker (1987) found that older alcoholics with relatively short abuse and dependence histories suffered the same degree of brain deterioration shown by younger alcoholics with longer abuse and dependency histories. Alcohol-induced physical deterioration can be partly prevented by a healthy diet, which may protect against toxic lipid peroxidation in cell membranes.

Brain shrinkage is probably more important to sexual response than testicular shrinkage in aging. Brain weight has been shown to decrease 30 to 100g with chronic alcoholism. Further, brain water content increases with chronic alcohol use, as it does with aging (Smith, J.A., et al., 1985). Alcohol-induced sexual deterioration is not simply a matter of genital toxicity and hormonal aberrations. Both brain and body tissue and function are damaged. However, it would not be inaccurate to tell male alcoholics that alcohol goes directly to their testicles, causing damage, so that their genitals age before they do. (Men often are more motivated by explicit threats to their sexual potency than to warnings of damage to their general health.)

HEALTH BENEFITS OF MODERATE ALCOHOL CONSUMPTION

As bothersome as the finding may be to those who have observed the damage due to irresponsible alcohol use, moderate alcohol consumption of one to two drinks per day, in sample populations without evident current poor health, appears to have certain definite health benefits compared to abstaining, including decreased heart disease and even decreased mortality (De Labry et al., 1992; Friedman & Klatsky, 1993; Gaziano et al., 1993; Renaud & De Lorgeril, 1992; Sheehy, 1992). Studies showing these benefits have now eliminated explanation by other confounding variables, and many have followed health status in cohort samples for 10–20 years. Apparently, the original finding that alcohol use was cardioprotective was by Wilens (1947), who noted from autopsies that chronic alcoholics who died before age 50 had less atherosclerosis than nonalcoholics. The cardioprotective effect of alcohol has been shown for both men and women, for beer, wine, and liquor. There have been similar findings in the elderly and in smokers and non-smokers (Renaud & De Lorgeril, 1992). Furthermore, from the evidence of healthy community cohorts, rates of overall mortality may be reduced as much or more than heart disease rates (De Labry et al., 1992). Note that these health benefits are often shown in samples chosen to exclude obvious alcohol-induced illness, though antiatherosclerotic prevention is found even among chronic alcoholics with severe cirrhosis of the liver. The relation between alcohol and heart disease is U-shaped: Higher rates of heart disease are correlated with either complete abstinence or excessive drinking (three or more drinks per day are correlated with the highest rates of heart disease and mortality) (De Labry et al., 1992; Gaziano et al., 1993). Moderate alcohol intake also decreases the rate of gallstone disease (Friedman & Klatsky, 1993).

The mechanisms of alcohol's cardioprotective action include an increase in beneficial high-density lipoprotein (HDL) and an antithrombotic effect from a decrease in platelet aggregation (Gaziano et al., 1993; Renaud & De Lorgeril, 1992). Postmenopausal women may benefit from low-to-moderate alcohol use (up to one drink per day) due to an increase in estrogen levels (Gavaler & Rosenblum, 1994). However, the cardioprotective effect of moderate alcohol intake appears to be significantly less than that of estrogen replacement therapy (in the region of 10–40% decreased risk of heart disease with moderate alcohol compared to a 40–50% decreased risk with estrogen replacement).

TREATMENT ALTERNATIVES

For acute alcohol detoxification, substitute medications (a selection of benzodiazepines and various other tranquilizers and sedatives) are important and sometimes necessary to preserve life. Many drugs have been investigated in terms of their ability to reduce the craving for alcohol. (Antabuse has been available for a considerable time, but is used less widely than it was a decade ago; it does not affect the craving for alcohol, but induces nausea, vomiting, and other acutely distressing symptoms when consumed in conjunction with alcohol.) It used to be common practice to continue patients on a variety of psychotropic medications after detoxification to help them cope with underlying neuroses and psychopathologies. Currently, however, most alcohol rehabilitation centers strongly recommend using no drugs whatsoever subsequent to detoxification.

Selective Serotonin Reuptake Inhibitors (SSRIs)

In a series of studies during the 1980s, a group of researchers at the University of Toronto, including Claudio Naranjo and Edward Sellers, showed that SSRIs decreased alcohol consumption in both alcoholics and nonalcoholics. The work of this group and others was extensively reviewed by Galanter (1987) in a comprehensive edited volume (chapters by Naranjo and Sellers; Zabik; Gill and Amit; Gorelick). Unfortunately, the doses of SSRIs needed to reduce alcohol consumption are usually much higher than those required to treat depression (60 mg fluoxetine compared to 20 mg fluoxetine). Such high doses increase both side effects and cost. More importantly, although drinking is reduced, it is rarely eliminated. Consumption may decrease 15–25%, from a daily mean of six to eight drinks to five to seven drinks (Naranjo, Bremner, Poulos, & Lanctot, 1992). Although this difference compared to placebo is often significant, it indicates that most alcoholics will not receive clinically meaningful benefit from SSRIs. Furthermore, while the number of abstinent days typically increases from one to two days to three to four days, the relatively small decrease in overall mean daily consumption indicates that alcoholics drink somewhat more on non-abstinent days, apparently increasing the risk of bingeing episodes. Despite this marginal facilitation of abstinence, however, the use of SSRIs in alcoholics may have other benefits, such as reductions in depression, panic, phobia, obsessive and compulsive thoughts and actions, and aggressive, acting-out behavior.

Treatment with SSRIs may be more effective

in women, who often drink as a result of psychological disorders treatable by SSRIs. Sexual side effects and sedation from SSRIs seem particularly obvious in men, while nausea is frequent and often intolerable in both women and men. Failure to recognize and treat SSRI-induced sexual dysfunction may lead to covert noncompliance by patients. Often lowering the SSRI dose below a particular threshold for sexual response is all that is required.

The most common sexual side effect of SSRIs in men is retarded orgasm/ejaculation and inability to achieve orgasm despite prolonged erection and penetration. Both partners may become fatigued or even exhausted before completion of intercourse, due to the male's inability to climax. Compulsive sexual activity, a frequent concomitant to alcoholism, may be reduced or eliminated. Although the sexual effects in men usually occur at the beginning of SSRI treatment, they may not manifest until six months to a year after starting treatment. Though sexual drive, arousal, sensation, and climax may be decreased in women by SSRIs, they are somewhat compensated by increased feelings of relaxation and emotional closeness during sexual activity.

Alcohol, opiates, benzodiazepines, and serotonergic drugs all can cause neurological changes involving loss of sensation, decreased pain, and sedation. A decrease in physical sexual sensitivity and response is characteristic of all these substances. Therapeutically, these substances can often substitute for one another. For instance, panic disorder patients who cannot get benzodiazepines (e.g., Valium, Xanax) from their doctors often resort to alcohol in desperation. These patients often can be safely treated with SSRIs such as fluoxetine (Prozac), fluvoxamine (Luvox), or paroxetine (Paxil). Indeed, a fortunate indirect effect of the widespread use of Prozac is that many doctors who refuse to prescribe scheduled benzodiazepines realize that Prozac or Paxil is often efficacious as a treatment for panic and phobia, so that their patients need not resort to alcohol. Since Prozac may itself cause intolerable anxiety, particularly in women, Luvox or Paxil appears from our clinical practice to be more appropriate for treatment of panic and phobia.

Antabuse

When Antabuse (disulfiram) was first introduced as a means of treatment for alcoholism, it was administered at considerably higher doses than it is today. Troublesome side effects included a prominent garlic taste in the mouth, retinopathy, and reports of impotence. The reports of impotence associated with Antabuse were problematic because they were all from alcoholic patients and it was not possible to determine whether the sexual dysfunction was due to long-term physiological effects of alcoholism or to Antabuse treatment. In recent years, the accepted dose of Antabuse has decreased five-fold and associated sexual problems appear to be minimal. However, the early reputation Antabuse developed for causing sexual dysfunction lingers, often making noncompliance an issue.

Of interest is the fact that reports about the adverse sexual side effects of Antabuse apply to men but not to women. However, research methodologies have clouded the validity of the finding. For example, one difficult study to interpret by Jensen (1984) reported on the sexual side effects of disulfiram, which was sometimes used in conjunction with either chlordiazepoxide or chlorprothixene, both of which are known to cause sexual dysfunction independently. Sixty-three percent of the male alcoholics experienced sexual dysfunction compared to 10% of the controls. Fifty percent of the male patients were taking chlordiazepoxide (Librium) or chlorprothixene. However, it was not clear how many of the patients experiencing sexual dysfunction were on both tranquilizer and Antabuse. Without controlled groups of abstinent alcoholic men not on Antabuse, and men on Antabuse but not tranquilizer, no definitive conclusions could be drawn.

The lack of adverse sexual effects in alcoholic women who were taking both disulfiram and chlordiazepoxide or chlorprothixene is perplexing, but may reflect the difficulty of documenting sexual dysfunction in women.

CONCLUSIONS

Alcoholism is a debilitating medical disease involving a process that appears to be indistinguishable from premature aging. In addition to the high prevalence of liver disease in both male and female alcoholics, gynecomastia, atrophied testicles, infertility, and feminization may occur in males; menstrual disorders, pelvic inflammatory disease, hysterectomies and other complications associated with indiscriminant sexuality, and a diathesis toward bleeding disorders are found in women. There is some debate in the literature regarding the effect of alcohol on testosterone. We feel that the weight of evidence demonstrates a depressant effect on this hormone.

No one knows with certainty at what point reversible changes due to chronic alcoholism become fixed and permanent. Certainly, changes begin affecting certain limbic structures in the brain from the first few drinks. At what point irreversible damage occurs remains unknown. In end-stage alcoholism, some patients develop Korsakoff's syndrome, which involves a devastating degeneration of brain tissue with associated confabulation and behavioral disorders.

Alcohol seems to share inhibitory properties with GABA, benzodiazepines, opiates, and serotonin. However, despite the similarities of certain actions of alcohol, the sexual effects differ dramatically despite their common overall depression of sexual function. Alcohol stimulates sexual desire at low doses, but decreases erection and orgasm at intoxicating doses. Serotonergic drugs chiefly inhibit desire and orgasm, but not erection (except secondary to loss of desire and orgasm). The sexual effects of benzodiazepines are much more subtle, involving decreased sensitivity and reactivity and increased receptivity. Opiate sexual effects essentially involve a transient dopaminergic LH surge, followed by a shutdown of the entire sexual circuit. Some opiates themselves become a substitute for sexual pleasure.

The balance and function of endogenous opioid transmission is disturbed and often irreversibly impaired by chronic abuse of alcohol or opiates. Whether inhibitory or excitatory to sexual arousal, endogenous substances exhibit a natural balance, which can be compromised by exogenous drugs. Recovery from alcoholism probably involves a long process of healing the endogenous opioid system.

The link between alcohol and sexual function, while behaviorally clear, remains a complex one with unknown variables. In spite of physiological decreases in intensity of sexual response, men and women generally describe their sexual encounters as improved with increasing levels of alcohol. Because irritability, aggression, and belligerence increase with the disinhibiting effects of alcohol, child sexual abuse, incest, battery, spousal abuse, and rape are strongly associated with alcohol abuse. Apparently, whatever basic need is satisfied by alcohol may also be satisfied by sex, which itself can become compulsive and addictive. Some aspects of the primal forces involved in the use and abuse of alcohol are no doubt common to sexual arousal and its abuse. In order to effectively prevent and treat these addictions, we must better understand why people want or need these highly abused drugs. In the interim, facilitating the relationships and sex lives of alcohol/substance abusers is an important aspect of rehabilitation that is sometimes overlooked.

11

Nicotine and Caffeine

OBJECTIVES

- To identify the sexually toxic effects of nicotine
- To identify the negative effects of nicotine on reproduction
- To evaluate the impact of caffeine on sexual function

Smoking has clearly identifiable effects on sexual function, particularly on the erection. Nicotine is a vasoconstrictor that diminishes blood flow to both the brain and the penis, and simultaneously increases the outflow from the penis, effectively promoting impotence (Padma-Nathan & Payton, 1986) and erectile insecurity. In addition, smoking promotes atherosclerosis in both sexes, thus compromising blood flow to the pelvis even further (Rosen et al., 1991). Although the vasoconstrictive aspects of smoking can be expected to affect women to some degree, they are not as vulnerable to negative vascular sexual effects as are men.

Smoking may improve sex drive through several mechanisms. While smoking does not appear to increase testosterone, it does increase DHEA and dopamine, while decreasing serotonin—and any of these mechanisms can favorably impact sex drive. Yet smoking also alters hormones and chemicals in a manner that is sexually unfavorable to sexual functioning. For example, it increases cortisol and progesterone, which generally diminish sexual responsiveness. Smoking also has been found to impede reproduction in both men and women.

Given the extent to which smoking compromises sexual function, especially in men, it is remarkable how little attention is paid to this habit by sex therapists and physicians dealing with sexually dysfunction in patients. Also given the impact smoking has on fertility in both sexes, infertility treatment approaches might benefit from including aggressive stop-smoking programs.

Coffee is one of the most popularly enjoyed beverages throughout the world. People drink it to wake up, to stay awake, to sober up. Most drinkers would scoff at the suggestion that their morning cups of coffee had addictive potential. In the future, however, it is possible that products containing caffeine will be categorized as being as addictive and unhealthful as we currently view nicotine. Some day, both of them may even become controlled substances. Not too long ago, smoking was considered a habit, not an addiction. Will coffee be the next on the list? Not long ago, cocaine was used as an ingredient in Coca-Cola and in over-the-counter medicines and tonics. Should the fact that caffeine has replaced cocaine give us any food for thought? Are they, perhaps, "chemical cousins" of an addictive sort?

THE EFFECTS OF NICOTINE ON SEXUAL FUNCTION

- diminishes blood flow to brain
- diminishes blood flow to penis
- increases venous outflow from penis
- causes impotence

- increases arteriosclerosis
- passive smoking may be harmful to sex

The extent of sexual dysfunction caused by smoking is most clearly seen by observing its effect upon erection. Smoking has been shown to contribute to many organic factors involved in impotence: degeneration of arteries and nerves leading into the penis and to the interior penile muscle and other tissue, and inadequate operation of venous blockade and drainage.

Even "passive smoking" can harm sexual function—at least in dogs. In a study by Juenemann et al. (1987), six healthy dogs were exposed to cigarette smoke released slowly near their noses and mouths. With cavernosal nerve electrostimulation sufficient for erection without smoke exposure, five of six dogs failed to show full erection after inhaling smoke from two or three cigarettes. Decrease in blood flow through the internal pudendal artery and almost complete lack of venous restriction were observed. The same effect was noted with intravenous injection of nicotine.

Thus, smoking acutely reduces blood inflow while increasing blood outflow (venous leak). With chronic exposure, smoking can actually destroy the penile tissues which mediate erection. Indeed, the prevalence of erectile dysfunction is disproportionally high among smokers (Virag, Bouilly, & Frydman, 1985). Up to 90% of patients with obstructive peripheral vascular disease are smokers (Condra, Surridge, Morales, Fenmore, & Owen, 1986). Brain vascular function is also compromised by smoking. Compared to nonsmokers, subarachnoid hemorrhage is 11 times more likely to occur in those who smoke more than one pack a day and four times more likely in those who smoke up to a pack a day (*Psychiatric Times*, 1991). Stroke risk has been shown to be greatest within three hours of smoking a cigarette and decreases thereafter.

Impotence

A recent epidemiological study of the relation of smoking to impotence (Manning, Klevens, & Flanders, 1994) received widespread media attention by affirming that cigarette smoking was an independent risk factor for impotence. Data from a cross-sectional survey of 4,462 U.S. Army Vietnam-era veterans aged 31 to 49 showed a prevalence of 2.2% impotence among *never smokers,* 2% among *former smokers,* and 3.7% among *current smokers*. Impotence was determined by a positive response to the question: "Have you experienced persistent difficulty in getting a satisfactory erection for sexual purposes within the last year?" The difference in impotence rate between current smokers and nonsmokers remained statistically significant after adjustment for other confounding factors, such as vascular disease, psychiatric disease, substance abuse, and marital status. However, examination of the data on other factors associated with current smokers (more not married, more substance abuse, and more psychiatric disorders) suggested that these factors could have greatly contributed to the higher impotence rate among current smokers. Oddly, neither number of cigarettes smoked daily nor years of smoking were significant predictors of impotence in current smokers. Prior to this study, there were already ample diagnostic urological studies in the literature showing a direct pathological effect of smoking on erectile functioning.

Alvaro Morales' research group at Queens University in Kingston, Canada has thoroughly investigated smoking-induced impotence (Condra et al., 1986). In a sample of 178 impotent clinic patients, 58.4% were current smokers (versus a 38% population estimate), and 81% were either current or ex-smokers (versus a 58% population estimate). The percentage of heavy smokers (more than 25 cigarettes per day) in this sample was more than twice that of normal non-impotent population estimates (about 10–15% versus about 3–7% for the general population). Smokers had significantly lower penile blood pressure than nonsmokers and smokers were more likely to have abnormally low penile blood pressure (an indication of organic impotence) (one in four smoking patients versus one in eight nonsmoking patients).

Padma-Nathan and Payton (1986) at Boston University found a 78% prevalence of smoking among 1,011 impotent patients compared to

31% in the general male population of Massachusetts. The variable of smoking was more strongly associated with lower penile blood pressure measures than the variables of hypertension, diabetes, or age. Furthermore, a higher papaverine infusion rate was necessary to maintain erection in chronic heavy smokers, indicating either reduced blood inflow from arteries or increased venous drainage.

More specific pathways of smoking toxicity were identified by Irwin Goldstein's Boston University research group (Rosen et al., 1991). Using a sample of 195 clinic impotence patients, they found that cigarette smoking was associated with atherosclerosis in the internal pudendal artery that supplies the erection. Risk for atherosclerosis increased with increased smoking: 15% increase for those who had smoked 5 pack-years (a product of the number of packs smoked per day times the years they were smoked: e.g., 1 pack/day × 5 years = 5 pack-years), 31% increase for 10 pack-years, and 72% increase for 20 pack-years. Common artery disease also increased steadily: 8% increase for 5 pack-years, 17% for 10 pack-years, and 37% for 20 pack-years. For each additional pack-year of smoking, pudendal artery disease increased by 3% and common artery disease increased by 2%.

Smoking also appears to render penile nerves and tissues more vulnerable to irritation and trauma, regardless of the cause. Mersdorf et al. (1991) examined the penile tissue of 59 impotent men who were implanted with penile prostheses. The number of cavernosum smooth muscle cells was reduced in smokers, alcoholics, and hypertensive men, with the greatest reduction found in smokers. Loss of sinusoidal endothelial linings was found in all groups, but was most pronounced in alcoholics who smoked. A considerable amount of vasodilating substances (e.g., EDRF or nitric oxide) comes from the endothelial lining during erection; additionally, axion nerve tissue was often decreased and replaced by collagen fibrosis.

Reduced erection with smoking has also been demonstrated by Glina, Reichelt, Leao, and Dos Reis (1988). Twelve chronic smokers between the ages of 22 and 65 were given papaverine injection erections (1) without smoking or (2) after smoking two cigarettes. Direct measurement of erectile intracavernous pressure using a 100 mg injection showed significantly less pressure in subjects who had smoked two cigarettes. All 12 men obtained full erections without smoking, but only four of the 12 obtained full erections after smoking.

The negative effect of smoking on erection has also been demonstrated in men viewing erotic films (Gilbert, Hagen, & D'Agostino, 1986). Forty-two cigarette smokers aged 18 to 44 were assigned to one of three groups: (1) high-nicotine cigarettes, (2) low-nicotine cigarettes, (3) a hard candy control group. Smoking two high-nicotine cigarettes significantly decreased the rate of penile diameter change compared to that for the other groups. High-nicotine cigarettes also caused significantly more vasoconstriction than low-nicotine cigarettes or the control group. Maximum tumescence was not affected by smoking.

Nocturnal Penile Tumescence (NPT)

The effects of chronic smoking on sleep erections have been identified by Karacan and Williams' sleep research group (Hirshkowitz, Arcasoy, Karacan, Williams, & Howell, 1992). These investigators reviewed the records of 800 patients who had been evaluated for impotence at their clinic. Of the 800 patients assessed with NPT monitoring, 314 were cigarette smokers. Smokers were broken down into three groups: (1) 1–19 cigarettes a day, (2) 20–39 a day, and (3) more than 40 a day. The total minutes of sleep erections and penile rigidity were significantly decreased in group 3 and nonsignificantly decreased in the group 2 compared to group 1. Patients in group 3 also lost tumescence more quickly.

Other measures of autonomic function included responses to deep breathing and supine-to-standing blood pressure regulation. The decrements caused by smoking still existed after statistical adjustment for age, diabetes, and otherwise poor health. The premature detumescence found in group 3 indicated that venous outflow resistance was decreased. Penile blood pressure showed only small mean decreases as number of cigarettes per day increased. The bulbocavernosus reflex latency, as well as the number of sleep erections, did not differ between groups.

In another study, diagnosis of erectile dysfunction with papaverine injection tests indicated that 9 of 28 (32%) men with venous leakage were smokers, but only 1 of 14 (7%) men without venous leaks was a smoker (Lowe, Schwartz, & Berger, 1989). Finally, a study by Elist, Jarman, and Edson (1984) of 20 smokers with erectile dysfunction and no NPT erections showed that abstinence from smoking for six weeks resulted in recovery of NPT erectile activity in seven of the 20 patients.

Forsberg, Gustavii, Hojerback, and Olsson (1979) likened the effect of smoking to the peripheral vasoconstriction that occurs with propranolol beta-blocker treatment. They reported that four males with erectile dysfunction—two smokers and two treated with propranolol—returned to normal function after smoking and propranolol were discontinued. Additionally, the penile blood pressure index, which initially indicated peripheral vascular insufficiency, returned to the normal range.

HORMONAL AND OTHER CHEMICAL CHANGES

Although early reports indicated that testosterone levels were lower in smokers than nonsmokers (Briggs, 1973; Shaarawy & Mahmoud, 1982), later studies showed conflicting findings. Condra et al. (1986) found that levels of testosterone, luteinizing hormone (LH), and prolactin were no different in smokers than in nonsmokers. Similarly, Tsitouras, Martin, and Harman (1982) found no difference in testosterone levels between 183 smoking and nonsmoking elderly men, and Handelsman, Conway, Boylan, and Turtle (1984) found no differences related to smoking in 119 healthy sperm donors. Other large studies have found even higher levels of both total and free testosterone in smokers than in nonsmokers (Deslypere & Vermeulen, 1984). Smoking men between the ages of 30 and 79, followed longitudinally in the California Rancho Bernardo cohort study, showed significantly higher levels of DHEAS and androstenedione than nonsmokers, even after adjustment for age and obesity (Barrett-Connor, 1989). Testosterone levels were nonsignificantly higher in smokers, but the testosterone-estrogen ratio was reduced due to increased levels of estradiol and estrone in smokers. Contrary to Barrett-Connor's findings, most studies report an antagonistic effect of smoking on estrogen actions, despite no significant change in overall estrogen levels (Berta, Frairia, Fortunati, Fazzari, & Gaidano, 1992). For instance, Kiel, Baron, Anderson, Hannan, and Felson (1992) found that smoking eliminates the protective effect of postmenopausal oral estrogen replacement therapy against osteoporosis.

Cardiovascular studies of men aged 35 to 60 also have found significantly higher levels of testosterone and androstenedione in smokers than in nonsmokers (Lichtenstein et al., 1987). Androgen levels were higher for both light and heavy smokers. Although any possible sexual benefits of increased androgen levels in male smokers probably would be cancelled out by a negative impact of increased cortisol and corticotropin-releasing-factor (CRF) (Fuxe, Andersson, Eneroth, Harfstrand, & Agnati, 1989), the risk of prostatic hypertrophy is reduced in smokers from 10–50% (Morrison, 1990), perhaps due to decreased prolactin, which typically is found in long-term smokers (Baron, Bulbrook, Wang, & Kwa, 1986).

There is abundant evidence that smoking has a thermogenic sympathomimetic action (Moffat & Owens, 1991), so that significant weight gain occurs when smoking is stopped, even with no increase in caloric intake. On average, weight gain after smoking cessation is greater in women than in men (Williamson et al., 1991); and the nervous tension engendered by complicated weight reduction plans targeted for women, along with willful reduction of food intake, may actually cause greater relapse to smoking (Hall, Tunstall,

Vila, & Duffy, 1992). The adverse effects of smoking on sexual function have already been documented.

Chronic elevation of cortisol due to habitual heavy smoking can be expected to eventually cause degenerative changes in the body, the brain, and the immune system (Sapolsky, Krey, & McEwen, 1986). Although DHEAS and vasopressin are beneficially raised by smoking, similar benefits might be achieved without smoking by supplementation with nasal vasopressin (Diapid) and DHEA. Consequently, long-term benefits may occur for smokers who have managed to quit smoking if these supplements are used.

Barrett-Connor, Khaw, and their colleagues found that smokers had higher DHEAS levels than nonsmokers in their well-publicized longitudinal Rancho Bernardo cohort study of men and women between the ages of 50 and 80 (Barrett-Connor, 1988; Khaw, Tazuke, & Barrett-Connor, 1988). In a sample of 233 women aged 60 to 80, current smokers had significantly higher adrenal androgens, DHEAS (43% more), and androstenedione when adjusted for age and weight. However, this sample of women also showed increased mortality correlated with higher DHEAS levels, in contrast to the decrease of mortality previously reported for cohort men with higher DHEA levels. It was not clear whether current smoking was causally related to increased DHEAS levels and higher death rates.

Friedman et al. (1987) found almost twice as much DHEAS (88% more) in postmenopausal women smokers versus nonsmokers. Key et al. (1991) found 33% more DHEAS in postmenopausal women smokers than nonsmokers, but DHEAS levels were 5% lower in smokers when adjustment was made for age and body mass index. If bupropion is confirmed to raise DHEAS levels in women, then women smokers could enjoy slightly higher DHEAS, slightly lower weight, and less depression if they were treated with bupropion during withdrawal from smoking.

Fuxe et al. (1989) have reviewed the effects of smoking on corticosteroids and various peptides. Cigarette smoking was first recognized to increase cortisol levels in 1961 (Fuxe et al., 1989). Subsequent studies have shown both acute and chronic smoking to increase cortisol and the hypothalamic-pituitary releasing factors CRF and ACTH (Fuxe et al., 1989). The increase in peptide releasing factors appears to occur through stimulation of nicotinic cholinergic receptors. Other peptides similar to or derived from ACTH are also increased by smoking, particularly vasopressin and beta-endorphins. Smoking may increase prolactin acutely, but generally prolactin levels are lower in chronic smokers than in nonsmokers (Fuxe et al., 1989). Both increases and decreases in LHRH/LH and growth hormone have been found in smokers. Acute smoking may increase LHRH in the medial preoptic sex center, suggesting one way in which smoking might stimulate sex drive mentally, despite its toxic action on genital sexual responses (Fuxe et al., 1989).

The apparent overexcitation from "binges" of cigarette smoking (being "wired") appears due to an excessive adrenal response, particularly oversecretion of cortisol, CRF, epinephrine, and norepinephrine. Rapid smoking of two high-nicotine cigarettes, which has been shown to reduce erection in laboratory studies, reliably elevates cortisol (Meliska & Gilbert, 1991). However, in many subjects, nausea, malaise, and shakiness may accompany this adrenal response, perhaps contributing to the acute rise in prolactin that sometimes occurs with rapid smoking of a number of cigarettes (prolactin secretion is a response to nausea and vomiting).

Self-reported decreases in self-reported drowsiness have been associated with the first few cigarettes of the day by both male and female smokers (Meliska & Gilbert, 1991). This initial, excitatory effect of smoking is accompanied by elevations in cortisol and beta-endorphins. Though not measured by the researchers, increases in vasopressin, dopamine, norepinephrine, and epinephrine, with decreases in serotonin, may also contribute to this temporary state of arousal.

Norton, Brown, and Howard (1992) examined EEG changes in 11 male smokers over the course of smoking a cigarette. Initially there was a reduction in alpha waves (indicating arousal), but there was an increase in alpha (decrease in arousal) towards the end of the cigarette. Additionally, in moderate nicotine smokers there was an initial shift toward left-hemispheric activation, which decreased as right-hemispheric activation occurred toward the end of the cigarette. Higher nicotine doses from smoking were associated (measured by residual butt analysis) with greater shifts towards right-hemispheric activation and greater decreases in subjective arousal. Furthermore, lower nicotine doses were associated with increases in theta-wave power, while higher doses were associated with decreases in theta-wave power. As discussed in Chapter 9 on DHEA, we consider the theta EEG rhythm to be an intrinsic aspect of sexual arousal and orgasm. The authors of this study believe that initial lower-dose nicotine smoking stimulates activation of a left hemisphere "go" system and the sedative effect of more smoking and higher nicotine doses increases activation of a right hemisphere "no go" system.

Meliska and Gilbert (1991) hypothesized that female smokers may be more depressed and experience more negative effects than do nonsmokers, so that smoking would offer transient relief from their abnormally low level of arousal. As with prolactin (e.g., Baron et al., 1986), short-term, acute elevations in stimulating body chemicals may be negated by long-term reductions typical of exhaustion subsequent to overstimulation (down-regulation).

Recent studies have shown that depression frequently plays a role in cigarette smoking (Anda et al., 1990; Breslau et al., 1993a; Glassman et al., 1990). In a large national survey, Anda et al. (1990) found that the prevalence of current smokers increased as depression scores increased, and the incidence of smokers quitting decreased as depression scores increased. The incidence of quitting cigarette smoking after nine years of follow-up was 9.9% for depressed smokers and 17.7% for nondepressed smokers. Breslau et al. (1993a) found that a history of depression increased the risk of progression to nicotine dependence and that people with a history of nicotine dependence had a higher rate of first incidence of depression followed longitudinally during the study. Glassman et al. (1990) point out that antidepressants may be a key facilitator of smoking cessation, given the high rate of depression in smokers and the dysphoric effects of quitting. Additionally, female patients with panic disorder compared to community controls studied by Pohl, Yeragani, Balen, Lycaki, and McBride (1992) have shown a higher prevalence of smoking prior to panic onset (54% versus 35%) and higher prevalence of current smoking (40% versus 25%). Breslau, Kilbey, and Andreski (1993b) have found that nicotine-dependent smokers are more vulnerable to depressive and anxious psychopathology than nondependent smokers.

Chronic nicotine intake in rats increases dopamine release in the nucleus accumbens (NACC), an effect that does not show tolerance, indicating that this dopamine effect is a reinforcing factor for continued smoking. Chronic nicotine treatment of rats also potentiates behavioral responses to dopaminergic drugs (Suemaru, Gomita, Furuno, & Araki, 1993). Dopaminergic stimulation in the NACC can increase sexual desire as well as compete with sexual activity which, in turn, increases NACC dopamine activation. Bupropion may be an excellent substitute for smoking, since it appears to preserve dopamine activation while minimizing the weight gain and depression often experienced during withdrawal. The stimulating actions on dopamine and beta-endorphins could account for the addictive quality of smoking. Hopefully, recognition of NACC dopamine activation by smoking will lead to a better understanding of the attraction to this particular addiction. Since sexual activity as well as bupropion can stimulate NACC dopamine, satisfactory sexual activity during smoking withdrawal may lessen the craving for smoking.

The complex mix of chemical actions triggered by smoking suggests both positive and negative sexual effects. Stimulation of ACTH, DHEAS, androstenedione, LHRH, GH, vasopressin, acetylcholine, epinephrine, and dopamine, as well as lowered prolactin and serotonin, could have a positive impact on sexual function. However, heightened levels of cortisol, CRF, and beta-endorphins, as well as excessive levels of norepinephrine and epinephrine, could also dampen the response. Furthermore, higher levels of estrogen would adversely affect male sexual responsiveness. Despite these hormonal and chemical changes, the negative effects of smoking on male sexual function seem predominantly due to damage to vascular and genital tissue.

EFFECTS OF NICOTINE ON REPRODUCTION

The effects of smoking on reproduction are summarized in Table 11.1.

Vicizian (1968) found that the percentage of motile sperm decreased from 69% in nonsmokers to 57% in smokers who consumed one to 10 cigarettes a day, and to 49% in those who smoked more than 30 cigarettes a day. Lower sperm counts and a higher percentage of abnormal sperm were found in smokers by Evans, Fletcher, Torrance, and Hargreave (1981), but not by Godfrey (1981). In 11 of 12 studies reviewed by Stillman, Rosenberg, and Sachs (1986), sperm density was reduced in smokers by an average of 22% and the proportion of motile sperm was reduced by about 17%. A more recent meta-analysis review by Vine, Margolin, Morrison, and Hulka (1994) indicates that sperm density in smokers is, on the average, 13–17% lower than in nonsmokers. However, in the majority of studies reviewed, changes in sperm density were not statistically significant but reflective of large variation among individuals. Furthermore, reductions in sperm density were not significantly correlated with number of cigarettes smoked per day.

Unfortunately, proper epidemiological studies of effects of smoking on sperm parameters have yet to be conducted. Findings have often been reported for small selected samples, usually from infertility clinics. Degenerative and disease factors usually associated with smoking, such as malnutrition and alcohol and drug abuse, are often not factored out. When Holzki, Gall, and Hermann (1991) selected a sample of 50 nonsmokers and 40 smokers, excluding men having any health or injury problems that could be related to lowered sperm, there were no significant differences between smokers and nonsmokers in sperm count, density, morphology, or motility.

The fact remains that smoking is often accompanied by various diseases and degenerative conditions. The constriction of blood flow in the penis, which has been shown in smokers, and the decrease in tissue oxygenation by smoking, suggest a toxic effect on all gonadal tissue. Peripheral anterial disease is also strongly related to lifetime smoking (Shabsigh, Fishman, Schum,

Table 11.1 *Adverse Effects of Nicotine on Reproduction*

In Females

Infertility (Tokuhata, 1968)
Amenorrhea (Petersson, Fries, & Nillius, 1973)
Vaginal bleeding (Hammond, 1991)
Irregular menses (Hammond, 1991)
Urinary infections (Boyce, Schwartz, & David, 1976)
Cervical cancer (Clarke, Hatcher, McKeown-Eyssen, & Lickrish, 1985)
Early menopause (Kaufman, Slone, Rosenberg, Miettinen, & Shapiro, 1980; Surgeon General, 1990)
Spontaneous abortion (Stillman et al., 1986)
Tubal (ectopic) pregnancy (Surgeon General, 1990)
Premature birth (Simpson, 1957)
Pregnancy complications (Surgeon General Report, 1990)
Fetal growth reduction and low birth weight (Surgeon General, 1990)

In Males

Lower sperm density (Evans et al., 1981; Stillman et al., 1986)
Lower proportion of motile sperm (Stillman et al., 1986; Vicizian, 1968)
Abnormal sperm (Evans et al., 1981; Surgeon General, 1990)
Impotence factors (Surgeon General, 1990) including:
- atherosclerotic peripheral vascular disease
- vasoconstriction
- disturbed prostaglandin production
- increased platelet aggregation
- increased estrogen levels
- lower penile blood pressure index

& Dunn, 1991; Surgeon General, 1990). Smoking should certainly be avoided by couples with infertility problems.

Infertility has been observed in female smokers (Stillman et al., 1986; Surgeon General, 1990). Tokuhata (1968) found infertility in 21% of smoking women compared to 14% of nonsmokers and a 46% increased risk of infertility in a cohort sample of 2,016 women. An increase in urinary tract infections (chiefly urethritis), from 13% in nonsmokers to 25–30% in women smoking over 30 cigarettes per day in a sample of 3,074 women attending an infertility clinic (Boyce et al., 1976), indicates that infections or trauma may compromise gonadal function in smokers.

However, smoking may help to maintain a normal endometrium. Franks, Kendrick, and Tyler (1987) found that smoking was associated with a 70% reduced risk of endometrial cancer among estrogen users and a 50% reduced risk among nonusers of estrogen in menopausal women aged 40 to 55. The risk for women who smoked and took estrogen replacement was no greater than the risk for women who did not smoke and did not take estrogen supplements. Perhaps a smoking-induced elevation of DHEAS and androstenedione adrenal androgen levels contributes to this observed decreased risk of endometrial cancer (Barrett-Connor, 1988; Key et al., 1991; Yeh & Barbieri, 1989).

Urinary incontinence is a key, bothersome factor often involved in female sexual dysfunction. Bump and McClish (1992) found that cigarette smoking increases the risk of genuine urinary stress incontinence in women by 2.5-fold, independent from other known risk factors. The risk increased to five-fold for women who smoked more than a pack a day. To determine what was responsible for this greatly increased risk of stress incontinence, Bump and McClish (1994) gave complete urogynecologic exams to 71 female smokers (mean age = 44) and 118 nonsmokers (mean age = 51) with pure genuine stress incontinence. Surprisingly, smokers had stronger urethral sphincters with greater functional length and maximum closure pressure than nonsmokers. However, smokers also produced greater increases in abdominal and bladder pressure with coughing, which apparently resulted in greater pure stress incontinence than nonsmokers, despite their significantly stronger urethral sphincters.

Women smokers appear to experience an earlier onset of menopause. Kaufman et al. (1980) showed a dose-related onset of menopause that varied from 49.4 years in nonsmokers to 48 years in light (1–14 cigarettes per day) smokers and 47.6 years in heavy (15 or more cigarettes per day) smokers. Such an advance in a natural marker of aging such as menopause indicates that smoking, like alcohol, causes premature aging of body tissues due to the abnormalities created by use of such substances.

The United States Surgeon General's report in 1990 detailed various adverse effects of smoking on maternity, including spontaneous abortion, tubal (ectopic) pregnancy, other pregnancy complications, premature birth, and reduced fetal growth. Some of these effects were attributed to the decreased blood flow and reduced availability of oxygen to the fetus caused by the vasoconstrictive properties of smoking.

THE EFFECTS OF CAFFEINE ON SEXUAL FUNCTION

Caffeine is the most widely used drug in the world. Over 85% of all Americans drink caffeine daily, with an average intake of 200 mg per day (Gilbert, 1984). Though widely believed to be a phosphodiesterase inhibitor that extends excitatory adrenergic synaptic action, caffeine only inhibits phosphodiesterase at doses far higher than normal daily consumption (Stoner, Skirboll, Werkman, & Hommer, 1988). Though a sympathetic nervous system activator, it is not an adrenergic stimulant. Caffeine is a purine derivative, a methylated xanthine; its activating effect is chiefly due to antagonism of adenosine receptors (Biaggioni, Paul, Puckett, & Arzubiaga, 1991; Spealman, 1988). Adenosine is a ubiquitous purine involved in nervous system transmissions. It decreases numerous excitatory processes in the body, including blood pressure, catecholamine release, CNS activity, urine output, renin release, lipolysis, respiration, and in-

Table 11.2 *Caffeine Content of Common Drinks*

Caffeine appears, in varying amounts, in a range of products. Most experts recommend not exceeding "moderate" consumption of caffeine—about 200 to 300 milligrams (mg) a day. Coffee and tea doses, 5-ounce cup, unless noted.

Drip coffee	110–150 mg	Percolated coffee	64–124 mg
Instant coffee	40–108 mg	Decaffeinated coffee	2–5 mg
1-minute brew tea	9–33 mg	3-minute brew tea	20–46 mg
Instant tea	12–28 mg	Iced tea (12-ounce)	22–36 mg

From *Editor's Choice*
Accompanies October 1990 *Mayo Clinic Nutrition Newsletter*

testinal peristalsis. Thus caffeine increases these bodily functions by inhibiting adenosine activity.

Stimulant effects of caffeine include cortical arousal, reticular formation (attentional) activation, vagal and vasomotor stimulation, elevated muscle tension, and increased metabolic rate (Smith, Davidson, & Green, 1993). Caffeine also increases production of norepinephrine, epinephrine, dopamine, serotonin, and cortisol. Smith et al. (1993) showed that caffeine usage increased both tonic and phasic arousal, which facilitated recall task performance. Females showed greater overall facilitation than males and greater facilitation on novel tasks, while males showed increased facilitation on repetitive tasks.

Generally, the arousal effect of caffeine follows an inverted-U principle of optimum performance at intermediate levels and decreased performance when under-aroused (bored or fatigued) or over-aroused (anxious or hyperactive). This means that a moderate amount of caffeine/coffee may have a beneficial effect, but performance degenerates as intake increases. Although caffeine can cause a mild stimulant effect in normal volunteer subjects, it generally does not change mood, produce feelings of euphoria or well-being, or serve as a positive reinforcer (Stern, Chait, & Johanson, 1989). At very high doses, most subjects found that it produced unpleasant anxiety, while a few reported feeling pleasantly stimulated rather than anxious. A contradictory opinion has been offered by Griffiths and Woodson (1988), who argued that under appropriate conditions caffeine could serve as a reinforcer, and that with chronic use it could create dependence in animals and humans. Hughes et al. (1992) also found that caffeine served as a reinforcer in moderate coffee drinkers at moderate but not at very high, doses; also, headaches and drowsiness increased self-administration of caffeine.

Most people do not realize that caffeine is used as a powerful pesticide and also heightens the effectiveness of other pesticides. According to Dr. James Nathanson, Department of Neurology, Massachusetts General Hospital, Boston, low doses of caffeine make insects "hyperactive and uncoordinated." Large amounts kill them. In fact, caffeine is such an effective, biodegradable pesticide that it is being considered for broad use. Spray-on caffeine solutions may soon be used commercially to protect crops.

As little as 250 mg per day of caffeine (about two or three cups of coffee) can cause restlessness, nervousness, excitement, insomnia, flushed face, diathesis, gastrointestinal disturbance, muscle twitching, rambling flow of thought, tachycardia or cardiac arrhythmia, periods of inexhaustibility, and psychomotor agitation (Dews, 1982). In addition, drinking five or more cups of coffee a day more than doubles the risk of heart problems, according to researchers at Johns Hopkins Medical School (LaCroix, Mead, Liang, Thomas, & Pearson, 1986). The Johns Hopkins group used a large number of subjects and a lengthy study period, collecting data at five-year intervals for 25 years. Caffeine is also known to aggravate certain existing disorders. More than 75% of all physicians recommend caffeine-free diets for patients experiencing anxiety, insomnia, panic disorder, arrhythmias, fibrocystic disease, palpitations, tachycardia, or esophagitis (Hughes, Amorie, & Hatsukami, 1988), as well as for pregnant women (caffeine inhibits fetal growth) (Fenster, Eskenazi, Swan, & Windham, 1991).

Caffeine appears to elevate the LDL fraction of cholesterol, which is associated with an increase of risk of heart disease. To the extent that caffeine contributes to arteriosclerotic heart disease, caffeine is certainly not facilitative of sexual performance in the male (Superko, Bortz, & Williams, 1991). A recent study has shown a possible link between coffee and bone fractures in middle-aged women (Hemenway, Colditz, Willett, Stampfer, & Speizer, 1988). Among 85,000 nurses at Brigham and Women's Hospital and Harvard Medical School, there were 65 hip fractures over a six-year period. Women who drank four or more cups of coffee a day experienced three times as many hip fractures as women who drank less coffee. It was found that caffeine can cause calcium to be lost in urine, and impedes coordination.

Caffeine reduces cerebral blood flow by constricting blood vessels in the brain (Cameron, Modell, & Hariharan, 1990). When caffeine is withdrawn after chronic use, blood vessels dilate as a rebound effect, producing headaches. The vasoconstricting action may be due to the blocking of adenosine, which dilates blood vessels. It is not known whether habitual caffeine intake reduces penile blood flow through vasoconstriction; but it has been shown that adenosine induces erection by powerfully relaxing smooth muscle tissue when injected directly into the cavernosum (Takahashi et al., 1990), while caffeine induces smooth muscle contraction in vascular tissue (Karaki, Ahn, & Urakawa, 1987). It is possible that caffeine reduces adenosine-induced vasodilation, resulting in decreased resting penile tone and decreased erectile tumescence rigidity.

In a study of psychotic inpatients, symptoms lessened during a period of decaffeinated coffee use and worsened when patients were again drinking caffeinated coffee (DeFreitas & Schwartz, 1979). Consequently, caffeine may worsen sexual perversions, which may be involved in psychotic or schizophrenic behavior.

Due to its strong diuretic effect, caffeine can cause or exacerbate urinary incontinence, thus decreasing sexual function through urinary-genital sensitivity as well as mental anxiety. However, because it mimics dopaminergic stimulants, caffeine may also positively affect sexual function by making individuals more alert and awake. In 1991, a small report was published through the media suggesting that coffee enhanced the sex lives of older men. If wakefulness is an advantage in sex, coffee may well add the "kick" needed to interest one in sexual participation. Otherwise, it is a doubtful "aphrodisiac."

12

Opioids

OBJECTIVES

- To identify the sexual effects of opioids in addicts and non-addicts
- To explore the impact of treatment alternatives on sexual function

Opiates is the term applied to exogenous pharmaceuticals that stimulate opioid receptors; *opioids* is a more general term that includes both exogenous and endogenous opiate-like substances. Endogenous opioids include enkephalins, spread diffusely throughout the body, and endorphins. The best-known endorphin is beta-endorphin, which is found at relatively high levels in sex-related brain areas such as the hypothalamus and pituitary. There is no question that opioids decrease sexual responsivity; however, the extent to which different opioids cause sexual dysfunction and the range of individual susceptibility to these negative sexual effects vary. Since endorphins exist naturally in the body, they may have some positive sexual effects not seen with exogenous opiate substances. Some patients do report sexual benefits from opiate use. At low doses, a transient positive impact similar to a low dose of alcohol may be experienced. Individuals abusing high doses of opiates may also develop a tolerance to some of the adverse side effects.

Prior to the Harrision Narcotic Act in 1914 controlling opiate use, more women than men used opiates (1.4 to 2 times more), often prescribed by physicians to treat "female troubles" (Abel, 1984). Subsequently, less toxic prescription medications such as benzodiazepines, non-steroidal pain-relievers, and serotonergic drugs (e.g., tryptophan and Prozac) have served in place of opiates and barbiturates. Despite the adverse sexual effects of many of these newer "therapeutic depressants," most are less inhibitory sexually than are opiates.

Current popular mythology promotes the notion that endogenous (naturally occurring) opioids have positive sexual effects (Hawkes, 1992). However, satisfactory evidence supporting the validity of endorphin-enhanced sex is virtually nonexistent. Indeed, although naturally occurring endorphins may provide a sense of well-being and relaxation, perhaps even facilitating greater receptivity, they most probably have an analgesic effect on sexual sensations. Nonetheless, the popularity of the notion of sexual bliss from endogenous endorphins is itself an indication of the potential for sexual abuse and dependency—a danger that has been well described by Patrick Carnes (1989).

Pain relief from opiates may make sex possible if illness and debility are not too great. However, due to the potential for dependence, extended medical use is recommended only in cases of intractable pain (i.e., cancer). Sexual desire and response are usually inhibited in patients with severe pain, as are most aspects of behavioral performance. Such limitation has been labeled the "pain brake" by Zenz, Strumpf, and Tryba (1992). Although sexual activity may lessen pain temporarily or at least distract attention from it (perhaps with the help of endorphins), more often pain blocks sexual responsivity as well as therapeutic attempts to resolve sexual dysfunction. In patients with less severe chronic pain, the effects of opiates on sexual function are less clear. Opiates given "as needed" are often abused, particularly in elderly patients. They may be taken with other inhibitory drugs such as benzodiazepines and excessive alcohol, which in combination effectively inhibit sexual feelings.

The chief sexual benefit of opioids is the delay of orgasm/ejaculation in men. Indeed, one motivation for heroin use among young men is to prolong sexual activity in order to please or impress their sexual partners (J. Mendelson, personal communication, 1981). Eventually, however, opioid use leads to sexual dysfunction. The extent to which endogenous opioids contribute to ejaculatory control is unknown. Since copulation involves a degree of pleasurable stress, some endorphin secretion may be needed to balance the secretion of excitatory substances such as epinephrine, dopamine, oxytocin, and amino acids.

For women, adequate endorphin secretion in combination with serotonin and estrogen may prevent nervousness and promote receptivity to the more aggressive aspects of copulation. Although endorphins are credited with facilitating attachment and touch, in actuality they inhibit oxytocin release, which mediates touch behavior (Leng & Russell, 1988; Racke et al., 1991; Van Wimersma Greidanus & Ten Haaf, 1985).

Pfaus and Gorzalka (1987) have written a remarkably comprehensive review of the negative effects of opioids and opiates on sexual desire and response and the positive effects of opioid antagonists in humans and animals. Absent in this review, however, were studies of commonly prescribed pain-relievers such as codeine, oxycodone, hydromorphone, and propoxyphene. Changes in sexual desire and function with these prescribed opiates used by non-addict patients to treat pain remain undocumented.

INHIBITION OF TESTOSTERONE

Perhaps the clearest indication of the negative effects of opioids on sexual function is their inhibitory action on testosterone. Opioids lower testosterone and testosterone administration can lower endorphin levels. The opiate antagonist naloxone increases testosterone in rats, nonhuman primates, and man (Cicero, 1980; De Feo et al., 1986; Gilbeau, Almirez, Holaday, & Smith, 1984).

One way opioids inhibit testosterone production is by suppressing luteinizing hormone release (LHRH/LH). Endogenous opioid peptides inhibit LHRH/LH and testosterone stimulation (Gilbeau et al., 1984); naloxone injection can release LHRH/LH and testosterone from this inhibitory influence. Injection of beta-endorphin into men can suppress LH secretion (Reid, Quigley, & Yen, 1983); injection of beta-endorphin antiserum increases circulating LH (Petraglia et al., 1985). In the rat, castration increases beta-endorphins and subsequent testosterone replacement reduces beta-endorphins (Almeida, Nikolarakis, & Herz, 1987). Castration also increases the sensitivity of genital tissues to the inhibitory action of morphine (Miranda et al., 1985). In women and female rats, estrogens and/or progesterone increase central beta-endorphin activity, while androgens decrease brain beta-endorphin concentrations (Genazzani, et al., 1992).

Positive sexual effects associated with increases in endorphins may occur as a result of opioid stimulation of dopamine in brain reinforcement centers, which also may account in part for opiate abuse and dependency. Negative and positive interactions of opioids with dopamine reinforcement activity must be investigated further to determine specific sexual benefits of endorphins.

Fabbri, Ulisse, et al. (1989) have demonstrated that the beta-endorphin localized in male Leydig cells and seminal vesicles is stimulated by corticosteroid releasing factor (CRF), which is also present in the testes and has a local inhibitory action on testicular production of testosterone. Stress-induced CRF may simultaneously increase beta-endorphins and lower testosterone. The consequent elevation of beta-endorphins also may inhibit Sertoli cell function as well as Leydig cell androgen production necessary for spermatogenesis. Six months of treatment with naltrexone, an opioid antagonist, increased sperm count and motility as well as actual fertility (pregnancy induction) in a 32-year-old infertile male with oligozoospermia of unknown origin (Fabbri et al., 1989).

Testosterone is associated with increased nocturnal penile tumescence (NPT); opioids are associated with decreased NPT. Young men (24 years old, average) versus middle-aged men (49 year old, average) have greater NPT tumescence time, higher total and free testosterone, and lower beta-endorphin levels (Murray, Fettes, Wyss, Cameron, & Sciandini, 1988). Constant infusion of the opioid antagonist naloxone in young men over a 24-hour-period increased luteinizing hormone secretion and testosterone levels (Delitala et al., 1983). It is not known whether older men would have the same response. Beta-endorphins are lower in prepubertal and elderly humans than in pubertal, young, and middle-aged humans (Genazzani et al., 1984). When testosterone levels are chronically low, opioids are also low and naloxone does not stimulate an increase in luteinizing hormone or testosterone.

It is important to keep in mind that the reciprocal actions of opioids and testosterone exist within a modulated integrated feedback circuit that involves other hormonal, peptide, and neurotransmitter factors. For instance, epinephrine injection can cause a fall in circulating testosterone akin to a stress reaction, whereas opioids reduce sympathetic tone, thus decreasing the stress reaction (Maric et al., 1987). In this way endogenous opioids can sometimes prevent a prolonged decrease in testosterone by blocking increased, stress-induced epinephrine release. In the long run, normal testosterone levels may modulate normal opioid levels in a natural balance. However, there is much more involved than a simple reciprocal relationship between testosterone and opioids. Administration of exogenous opiates may cause this reciprocal balance to break down, so that the androgen-producing circuitry is abnormally suppressed.

ANIMAL RESEARCH

Since endorphins may be addictive and, as peptides, are not well absorbed, research on their sexual consequences in humans is limited. Therefore, we must depend heavily on animal research data, which may or may not generalize to humans.

Findings in monkeys have indicated either negative or nonsignificant effects of endorphin stimulation on sexual function (e.g., Crowley, Hydinger, Stynes, & Feiger, 1975). Endorphin stimulation of and synergy with endogenous substances to sexual response such as prolactin, and endorphin suppression of positive sexual substances such as testosterone, luteinizing hormone releasing hormone (LHRH), and oxytocin occur in both humans, monkeys, and rats.

There is overwhelming evidence of negative sexual effects following endorphin stimulation in rats. Research findings on sexual changes due to endorphin administration in rats are shown for females and males in Table 12.1. Beta-endorphin, with fibers originating from the hypothalamic arcuate nucleus, is particularly active in the rat MPO sex center and in the amygdala, where it appears to influence sexual approach or avoidance. McGregor and Herbert (1992a, 1992b) found that infusion of beta-endorphin into the male rat amygdala suppresses or retards approach to an estrous female, but does not interfere with copulation once it begins. Some of this sexual approach deficit appears due to a deficit in processing olfactory cues specific to sexually receptive females (McGregor & Herbert, 1992b).

OPIATES AND ALCOHOL

Some researchers have reported that alcohol alters the metabolism of endogenous opioid peptides in a complex manner (Ollat, Parvez, & Parvez, 1988). A single dose of alcohol given to rats stimulated the release, synthesis, and utilization of beta-endorphins (Gianoulakis & Barcomb, 1987). Other researchers, however, have been unable to verify a stimulatory effect of alcohol on endogenous opiates, particularly when lower doses were used (Jorgensen & Hole, 1986). The opiate antagonist naloxone can reduce alcohol craving (Froehlich, Harts, Lumeng, & Li, 1986) and the depressive effect of

Table 12.1 *Sexual Function in Rats Inhibited by Endorphin Stimulation*

Female Rats

Lordosis and active proceptive sexual behavior suppressed; suppresion is reversed by naloxone or naltrexone (Meyerson, Berg, & Johansson, 1988; Sirinathsinghji, 1984, 1985, 1986; Sodersten, 1990; Sodersten, Forsberg, Bednar, Eneroth, & Wiesenfeld-Hallin, 1989; Weisner & Moss, 1984, 1986a, 1986b)
Maternal behavior disrupted (Bridges & Mann, 1990)
Oxytocin release inhibited (Haldar, Hoffman, & Zimmerman, 1982)
Prolactin levels elevated (Barden, Merand, Rouloux, Garon, & Dupont, 1981; Herbert, 1989; Leadem & Yagenova, 1987)
Exploratory social contacts reduced (Weisner & Moss, 1986b)

Male Rats

Copulation (mounting, intromission, ejaculation) suppressed (reversed by naloxone or naltrexone) (Hughes, Everitt, Herbert, 1987; Mandenoff, Bertíere, Betoulle, & Apfelbaum, 1986; McIntosh, Vallano, & Barfield, 1980; Melis, Stancampiano, Gessa, & Argiolas, 1992; Meyerson & Terenius, 1977)
Mounting and intromission impeded (Meyerson, 1981)
Sexual satiation, fatigue, and refractory state characterized by high levels of endorphins (Murphy, Bowie, & Pert, 1979)
Prolactin reduced (Ragavan & Frantz, 1981)
Beta-endorphin levels increased by exogenous factors (shortened daylight or injections of anti-gonadal melatonin) associated with sexually refractory states (Herbert, 1989)
Beta-endorphin levels increased by castration; reduced by testosterone replacement (Herbert, 1989)

alcohol (Jeffcoate, Herbert, Cullen, Hastings, & Walder, 1979; Jefferys, Flanagan, & Volans, 1980).

Comparing breeds of alcohol-preferring rats to non-preferring rats has revealed that alcohol-preferring rats have a dysfunction in the endogenous opiate system, causing excess or unreliable opiate reactivity. Enkephalin levels are considerably greater in the hypothalamus of alcohol-preferring rats (Froelich et al., 1986). Morphine can increase alcohol craving (Reid & Hunter, 1984), while naloxone can reduce it (Froehlich et al., 1986; Reid & Hunter, 1984).

In chronic human alcoholics as well as children born from alcoholic mothers, the plasma levels of met-enkephalin are reduced by almost 50%, indicating possible degeneration in the opiate system or substitution of alcohol metabolites at opiate receptors (Govoni et al., 1983). During alcohol withdrawal, the plasma levels of met-enkephalins increase; levels of beta-endorphins decrease in plasma but increase in brain fluid CSF (Anokhina, Panchenko, Kogan, & Brosen, 1985). Alcohol stimulation of endogenous opioid activity is sometimes attributed to the liver metabolite tetrahydroisoquinoline, which binds to opioid receptor sites. Persons genetically prone to alcoholism produce more tetrahydroisoquinoline in their livers when they drink. It has been suggested that "born" alcoholics have an opioid deficiency that results in a craving for alcohol and the opiate activity it stimulates (Aguirre, Del Arbol, Raya, Ruiz-Requena, & Irles, 1990).

Both the reinforcing property of alcohol and the physical withdrawal symptoms are similar to those experienced with opiate dependence. Tetrahydroisoquinoline effects no doubt involve excitatory amino acid transmission (similar to PCP, "angel dust," actions). Until we know more about excitatory amino acid function and its interaction with opioid peptides, the effects of tetrahydroisoquinoline as well as those of other alcohol metabolites will not be fully appreciated.

EFFECTS OF OPIATES ON THE SEXUAL FUNCTION OF ADDICTS

Since opiates cause physiological dependence and withdrawal, the term *addict* is appropriate to describe those who are dependent upon opiates. Equating opiate dependence with other substance dependence such as nicotine, as is the current fashion, may cause an underestimation of the severe dangers involved. Opiate dependence is a deadly, numbing disease that destroys overall health and threatens personality integrity. Sexual deficiencies in addicts are secondary to this system-wide degeneration. Nonetheless they bear discussing, particularly as they pertain to rehabilitation.

Opiates have direct adverse effects on sexual functioning. The most noticeable initial effect of opiates is the inhibition of orgasm/ejaculation; in addition, subsequent severe decreases in desire and response also occur.

Even in the addict community, heroin is regarded as a drug that decreases or replaces sexual pleasure (Gay, Newmeyer, Perry, Johnson, & Kurland, 1982). From histories of 500 male and female heroin addicts, David Smith and his colleagues at the Haight-Ashbury clinic (Smith, D.E., et al., 1982) determined that, while improvement in sexual function may occur initially, a decrease in orgasm/ejaculation and sexual desire inevitably follows with prolonged use. During its use, heroin may cause a rush even more pleasurable than orgasm. With withdrawal, spontaneous erection and ejaculation often occur as a result of extended inhibition during prior heroin use. These sexual "overshoots" of withdrawal are usually experienced dysphorically, since they are not under the patient's control.

Some addicts attempt to titrate heroin use for sexual benefits. For instance, males with premature ejaculation may note delayed ejaculation with low doses, but loss of erection at higher doses. Females may be assumed to benefit from relaxation, disinhibition, and relief from dyspareunia at low doses, but experience anorgasmia and lack of sexual desire at higher doses. Although tolerance to testosterone inhibition may occur with continued heroin use, sexual difficulties or disinterest seem to increase with chronic use beyond six to 12 months.

Smith et al. (1982) and others (e.g., Mendelson, Mendelson, & Patch, 1975) have noted that sexual difficulties also occur on methadone maintenance and, in fact, that sexual dysfunction is a frequent cause for discontinuing the treatment. Male patients on higher methadone doses (80–150 mg/day) frequently reported sexual deficits and showed reduced testosterone levels; however, these negative effects may not be present at lower doses (10–60 mg/day). Addicts interviewed by Smith and his colleagues reported sexual deficits at high doses of all opiates including methadone, codeine, oxycodone (Percodan), hydromorphone (Dilaudid), and propoxyphene (Darvon). Sexual dysfunction in female addicts may lessen during methadone substitution, but improvement may be due predominantly to low doses and medical, social, and nutritional supervision (not to mention the absence of impure heroin injections).

Among 11 of 15 women experiencing decreased sexual desire and activity during heroin use, half showed sexual improvement when switched to methadone (Abel, 1984). Smith et al. (1982) noted frequent sexual dysfunction prior to heroin addiction (28% in men and 47% in women), which increased to 37% in men and 58% in women during heroin use. Abnormal menstrual cycles or amenorrhea have been found to increase from 5–7% to 65–90% during heroin addiction, with severe problems occurring within one to two years of use and resolution occurring within one to 12 months of withdrawal (Abel, 1984). Reversal of amenorrhea usually occurs during methadone maintenance and the improved health and nutritional circumstances that accompany it. However, sexual dysfunction often continues during methadone maintenance despite lifestyle improvements (e.g., Martin et al., 1973), requiring sexual therapy that is often unavailable. Additional psychiatric problems that continue with withdrawal or methadone maintenance include depression, lack of self-esteem, anxiety, phobia, and panic.

Within the last few years, buprenorphine (Buprenex) has been used increasingly instead of methodone, due to less severe side effects and less withdrawal symptoms (Nigam, Srivastava, Saxena, Chavan, & Sundarem, 1994). While buprenorphine seems preferable to methodone (or heroin), it is expensive and not yet widely available. Furthermore, while withdrawal may be far less frequent with buprenorphine, and relatively mild when it does occur (Nigam et al., 1994), there is a high probability of abuse. For combination heroin-cocaine addicts, buprenorphine often relieves dysphoric withdrawal symptoms, but doctors treating such addicts have told us that buprenorphine does not replace the cocaine high, which maintains craving and relapse in these "highball" cocaine-heroin users.

EFFECTS OF ALTERNATIVE TREATMENTS ON SEXUAL FUNCTION

The blood pressure medication clonidine, which has a normalizing, regularizing, and hyperpolarizing action, is an adequate treatment for the physical symptoms of opiate withdrawal. Serotonergic drugs such as trazodone (Desyrel), fluoxetine (Prozac), and some tricyclic antidepressants can be used to the reduce opiate dose used daily or as a substitute for opiate treatment. As noted, although most of these drugs (with the exception of trazodone) depress physical sexual sensations, they have fewer negative effects on sexual desire and response than opiates. Trazodone was originally used in Italy to treat pain; in Europe, pain relief is still perhaps its chief indication. In the United States, it is only approved for treatment of depression. Adjunctive use of trazodone can be used to lessen the dose of mild opiates (such as codeine) used for chronic pain; it also can be used as a sleeping pill due to its strong sedative action and to treat depression resulting from opiate treatment of chronic pain. Use of SSRIs such as fluoxetine (Prozac), fluvoxamine (Luvox), and sertraline (Zoloft) also help reduce pain and the obsessive-compulsive tendencies that accompany some pain symptoms. Opiates generally do not affect the psychiatric aspects of pain and, in fact, add to compound psychiatric disturbance by generating dependency, abuse, and sexual dysfunction.

Naloxone and naltrexone are the most common opiate antagonists available. Naloxone (Narcan, Talwin) has a short course of action of a few hours and must be injected; naltrexone is longer-acting (20 to 40 hours), orally active, and widely available. The search for clinical applications of naltrexone, other than its limited use in opiate withdrawal programs, has been disappointing. Since opiate actions can decrease sexual function, it may be assumed that these drugs, which block opiate action, can reverse sexual deficits due to endogenous opiate activity. One promising application is as a treatment for impotence and retarded orgasm.

Positive sexual effects of naloxone, which facilitates dopamine and oxytocin-induced penile erection and yawning (Melis et al., 1990), have been observed in groups of sexually normal and sexually sluggish rats (Serra, Collu, & Gessa, 1988). However, naloxone and naltrexone have failed to produce any increase in sexual activity when tested in sexually active and sexually deficient rhesus monkeys (Abbott, Holman, Berman, Neff, & Goy, 1984). In fact, sexual activity of the active male monkeys was reduced by both opiate antagonists.

Although endorphin/opioid antagonists such as naloxone and naltrexone rarely induce sexual activity in humans, transient sexual stimulation from these antagonists during opiate withdrawal has been noted in certain individuals (e.g., Mendelson, Ellingboe, Keuhnle, & Mello, 1979). Though spontaneous erection and ejaculation are often noted in men during naloxone-precipitated withdrawal (Mendelson et al., 1979), there has been little investigation of normal or sexually dysfunctional patients. While naloxone has not been reported to cause sexual changes in normal subjects, the longer-acting oral naltrexone produced spontaneous erection in three of eight normal male subjects (50 mg/day) (Mendelson et al., 1979) and restored erectile function in six impotent patients (25–50 mg/day) (Goldstein, 1986).

When naloxone infusion (1 mg/kg) was combined with oral yohimbine administration, Charney and Heninger (1986) noted erections in six normal male subjects tested in a study for panic disorder. Erections started five to ten minutes after naloxone infusion, became full and lasted for 60 minutes or more. However, there was no associated increase in sexual drive or pleasure; in fact, the patients generally became anxious, nervous, nauseated, shaky, and dysphoric. Naloxone alone produced only partial erections lasting about 30 minutes in three subjects. None of four female subjects reported any change in sexual function or feelings with naloxone alone; but one of the four women, given naloxone combined with yohimbine, noted increased sexual drive lasting about 60 minutes without any change in lubrication, orgasm, or other sexual effects. Women subjects experienced the same dysphoric symptoms as men.

Fabbri, Jannini, et al. (1989) reported therapeutic effects of naltrexone treatment (50 mg/day) for two weeks on psychogenically impotent patients between the ages of 25 and 50. No effect was shown for placebo. However, the study was single-blind (the investigators knew which subjects received naltrexone or placebo). Consequently, results could have been due to investigator bias. Full erection was reported by 11 of the 15 impotent men, and there was an increase in full erections for coitus from 0.25 per week to 1.25 a week (0.5 per week on placebo). All naltrexone patients noted increased sleep erections and spontaneous erections. No changes in sex drive were reported. The authors wrote that "most of the patients reported that naltrexone treatment . . . improved their sexual function after the first day of treatment"—a finding difficult to interpret, since only an average of one to two useable erections occurred over an entire week. The lack of any noticeable placebo effect in this study is contrary to the findings of most double-blind impotence treatment trials (e.g., Benkert, 1973). Follow-up of patients after a subsequent two months without drug treatment showed that five of the 11 positive responders were still functioning normally. It should be noted that the two-week treatment period was too short to allow evaluation of full therapeutic benefits. Since several aspects of this study limit its usefulness, replication in a larger, well-controlled study would be helpful.

It appears that naltrexone stimulates erection in both normal and impotent men, but there is no firm evidence that such stimulation is sufficiently enduring for therapeutic efficacy. Improvement in sexual desire or orgasm/ejaculation has yet to be reported, and positive sexual effects in women have only rarely been noted. Lastly, the dysphoric psychological and physical symptoms experienced in both opiate-dependent men and women by naltrexone use make its usefulness as a treatment for opiate-induced sexual dysfunction doubtful. Some researchers have suggested that luteal phase dysphoria may be due to abnormally low endorphin levels in women with PMS (Facchinetti et al., 1987); but Chuong and Hsi (1994) could not demonstrate any central beta-endorphin changes in PMS patients.

CONCLUSIONS

In future studies, prescription opiates should be investigated for sexual effects and should be compared with alternative pain and anxiety suppressants. Unfortunately, the probability of the Federal Drug Administration encouraging such investigation, or drug companies financing such clinical research, is not likely, due to the hesitancy to perform controlled research in humans using addictive drugs, whether prescribed or illegal.

13

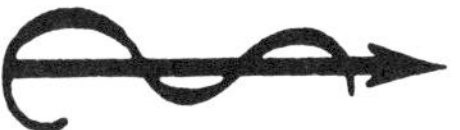

Marijuana and Other Illegal Drugs

OBJECTIVES

- To identify the effects of marijuana on sexual function and on sex hormones
- To identify the effects of marijuana on reproduction
- To review the sexual side effects of hallucinogens, amphetamines, and cocaine

Marijuana, called *cannabis sativa*, is a hemp plant native to central Asia. The active ingredient is considered to be tetrahydrocannabis (THC). Other cannabinoids include *cannabidiol* and *cannabinol*. While these other cannabinoids may influence physiological effects, psychoactive properties have not been described. Other names for marijuana used in various countries include *ganja* in Jamaica, *hashish* in the Middle East, *bhang* in India, *kabak* in Turkey, *ma* in China, and *kif* in North Africa. Common names used in the United States include *grass, joints, reefers, hash*, and *Mary Jane*. Sometimes called the "foreplay drug," the aphrodisiac reputation of marijuana is centuries old; for example, it is mentioned in the *Arabian Nights* and the *Materia Medica of Dioscorides;* it is recognized in Ayurveda (Hindu) medicine as a means of stimulating sex drive; and it is traditionally used by practitioners of sexual-based Tantra yoga. Concern about sexual promiscuity induced by marijuana use emerged in the United States during the 1930s and still exists to some extent today. A superb, comprehensive review of the impact of marijuana on sexual function has been written by Ernest Abel (1981).

From the testimony of users, marijuana is the gentlest and kindest of the so-called "aphrodisiacs." A five-year review of 800 men and 500 women between the ages of 18 and 30 reported that 83% of males and 81% of females believed that marijuana enhanced sexual enjoyment but did not improve sexual "performance" (erection, lubrication, orgasm, or ejaculation) (Kolodny, Masters, & Johnson, 1979). Rather, it increased relaxation, sociability and openness to others, and enhanced touch and comfort between partners during sexual activity. Kaplan (1974) has suggested the following sexual benefits of marijuana smoking:

- heightened receptivity to and interest in erotic activity
- stimulation of erotic thoughts
- increased sensual and erotic feelings
- altered time and touch perceptions (which enhance sexual feelings)
- disinhibition and relaxation of behavioral restraints and aversiveness
- decrease of aggressive attitudes

The prolonged sense of time, intensification of touch, perception, and attentiveness to sexual partners seem to highlight the sexual enhancement facilitated by marijuana use. However, with marijuana, apparently less is more. High doses resulting in marijuana intoxication and consequent sedation will interfere with sexual activity. In a questionnaire survey conducted by Koff (1974) involving 251 college students (123 males and 128 females between the ages of 17 and 24), 58% of females and 39% of males believed that marijuana increased sexual desire, while 60% of males and 43% of females believed it enhanced sexual enjoyment. Similarly, 60% of males and 47% of females felt that it increased partner satisfaction from sexual activity. Sexual desire and enjoyment was increased more with one joint (61% and 59%) than with two or more joints (42% and 39%). With two or more joints, decreases in sexual desire and enjoyment were reported by a greater number of males (over 10%) than females, possibly indicating that females feel more comfortable with the relaxing, intoxicating, and disinhibiting effects of marijuana, while males may be bothered by loss of erection. Ten percent or less believed that it decreased sexual desire or enjoyment.

In another study, Halikas, Weller, and Morse (1982) presented extensive information on the sexual practice of marijuana users in Wisconsin. During 1969–70, they interviewed 100 regular marijuana users and 50 nonusers. Follow-up interviews were conducted in 1975–1977 on 97 users and 35 nonusers. Regular use was defined as two to three times per week over more than two years. Users were less likely to be married than nonusers and more likely to be living with lovers or alone. Users had their first intercourse at a younger age and were more likely to have had postpubertal homosexual experiences, though very few were homosexual or bisexual. Thirty-three percent of the users reported using alcohol or drugs before their first sexual intercourse, compared to none of the nonusers. However, 33% of nonusers had experienced undesired intercourse while intoxicated, usually with alcohol. Among the users, marijuana was used before intercourse more frequently than alcohol, though intoxication prior to intercourse was more often associated with alcohol than marijuana.

A summary of Halikas et al.'s results follows:

- In 12–27% of males and 3–16% of females, marijuana increased sexual responses, including duration of intercourse, number of orgasms, or ability to repeat intercourse. Most of the subjects (60–90%) reported no effect of marijuana on these aspects of sexual activity. Only 2–3% of males and none of the females reported decreases due to marijuana use.
- Marijuana enhanced the quality of orgasm in 58% of males and 37% of females; none felt that it decreased orgasm quality.
- Sexual desire for familiar partners was increased by marijuana use in 50% of males and 60% of females.
- Sexual desire for unfamiliar partners was increased in 43% of males and 14% of females.
- Over 50% of both females and males reported that marijuana enhanced touching and physical closeness.
- Sensory stimulation (smell and sight) was enhanced in 7–11% of females and 11–23% of males.
- Marijuana was considered a mild aphrodisiac by 35% of users and a strong aphrodisiac by 8% of male users and 11% of female users.
- Sexual pleasure and satisfaction increased in 76% of female users and 70% of male users.
- Feelings of emotional closeness and intimacy were increased in 63% of females and 46% of males.

Although marijuana increased sexual desire, quality of orgasm, touching, and physical closeness in the majority of these marijuana users, the quantity of sexual activity was increased only infrequently. Opinions on the sexual benefits of marijuana may be connected to its frequency of use. Fisher and Steckler (1974) found that sexual pleasure from marijuana was claimed by 70% of daily users, 58% of regular users, 34% of occasional users, and 25% of past users. Interest in the sexual effects of marijuana seems to decline steeply with age (past 25 to 30) and transition from peer-group culture to stable domestic relationships. Tolerance to negative effects of marijuana use occurs with frequent regular use and the extent of dependence or addiction is unknown.

Patients at the Haight-Ashbury Free Medical Clinic during the 1970s generally felt marijuana enhanced sexuality far more than alcohol, barbiturates, amphetamines, cocaine, amyl nitrate, psychedelics, or heroin (e.g., Gay & Sheppard,

1972). Sexually abusive aspects of marijuana use are often associated with concurrent use of these other drugs. Intoxication ("getting stoned") is perhaps the most negative sexual aspect of marijuana use, since sexual attention and performance may be decreased. Marijuana intoxication has a dampening sexual effect; "getting stoned," however, is the major motive for its use. The sedation and antianxiety properties of marijuana appeal to individuals, particularly women, who would tend to find benefits in benzodiazepine use. Some general sexual effects of marijuana are similar to those of benzodiazepines, though more complex, pronounced, and noticeable.

Marijuana use by women is more associated with social/interpersonal relationships than is use by men (Lex, 1994). There is a strong "husband and friend effect," wherein marijuana use is associated with cooperation and comfort with a husband and/or friends who use marijuana. Therefore, marijuana use may facilitate intimacy and sexual reciprocity within these relationships and decrease sharply when these relationships are broken or change (a baby is a whole new relationship). Women who are particularly heavy marijuana users also typically use alcohol and other illicit drugs, and exhibit tension, anger, fatigue, and confusion (Lex, 1994).

EFFECTS OF MARIJUANA ON SEX HORMONES

Widely publicized studies by Kolodny and his colleagues (Kolodny, Lessin, Toro, Masters, & Cohen, 1976; Kolodny, Masters, Kolodner, & Toro, 1974), which reported that acute and chronic marijuana smoking reduced testosterone in men, have not been replicated in other studies. Furthermore, the reported decreases in testosterone still left testosterone levels within the normal range. Kolodny's group (Dornbush, Kolodny, Bauman, & Webster, 1978) later found that chronic marijuana use increased testosterone and decreased prolactin in women. However, these findings were not replicated by Mendelson, Ellingboe, Kuehnle, and Mello (1978).

A tightly controlled study by Mendelson, Kuehnle, Ellingboe, and Babor (1974), which included constant residential ward control of diet as well as observation of casual and heavy users, showed no change in testosterone levels due to marijuana. Schaefer, Gunn, and Dubowski (1975) found no change in testosterone levels with acute and chronic administration of tetrahydrocannabis. Further studies (Cushman, 1975; Hembree, Zeidenberg, & Nahas, 1976) also failed to show any effect of marijuana on testosterone levels. Block, Farinpour, and Schlechte (1991) reviewed numerous studies in this area and concluded that, despite occasional changes noted in various sex hormones, generally no changes were found in testosterone, luteinizing hormone, and follicle stimulating hormone, with unpredictable changes noted in prolactin (perhaps associated with nausea). Block et al. (1991) also compared levels of sex hormones in healthy male (n = 93) and female (n = 53) users (average age of 24) to nonuser controls; no hormonal differences were shown in infrequent, moderate, or frequent users.

EFFECTS OF MARIJUANA ON REPRODUCTION

- negative effects on fertility of both sexes
- adverse fetal effects
- menstrual cycle disturbances

Extensive evidence indicates that chronic marijuana use has indirect negative effects on fertility in both men and women. Decreased sperm counts and motility as well as abnormal sperm have been reported in male users (Hembree et al., 1976; Hembree, Nahas, & Huang, 1979; Issidorides, 1980; Kolodny et al., 1974). Adverse effects on spermatogenesis are probably due to a direct toxic action on gonadal cell function, enzymatic processes, and the germinal epithelium of testicular tissue (Hembree et al., 1976; Husain & Lame, 1984). Direct adverse effects on fertility have not been shown, which means that pregnancy can still occur despite damaged sperm. However, birth defects may be expected to occur.

Marijuana use during pregnancy can adversely affect the fetus. Neurobehavioral and physical abnormalities in the newborn resembling fetal alcohol syndrome have been verified (Hingson et al., 1982; Zuckerman et al., 1989), as has increased frequency of premature births (Gibson, Baghurst, & Colley, 1983; Tennes, 1984). Since marijuana is often used with other drugs, especially alcohol, reproductive effects are compounded (Abel, 1981).

OTHER ABUSED DRUGS

Information on the sexual effects of non-alcohol, non-prescription drugs, both legal and illegal (hallucinogens, amphetamines, cocaine, and barbiturates*) is sparse and unreliable. The fact that these abused drugs are often used in combination further confounds research attempts to isolate the sexual effect of any one particular drug. The way in which these drugs are ingested, the circumstances in which they are used, the dose, time periods, and duration of their use, all are uncontrolled variables that may contribute to their impact on sexual function. Often the circumstances of their use and the associated intoxication effects preclude any accurate report from users on sexual side effects. Finally, since research subjects are usually drug addicts and multiple drug users, funding is not readily available from the government or private sources.

Hallucinogens

LSD, "ecstacy," "mushrooms," "angel dust," and amphetamines are all hallucinogens. While they operate via slightly different mechanisms, they have a common impact on subjective reality: altering and distorting perceptions to the point of full-blown hallucinations. Although these hallucinations are induced for their excitement and mind-expanding value, nightmarish "bad trips" have also been associated with these drugs. LSD-induced hallucinations have caused individuals to plummet to their deaths, believing they can fly; head-banging and cerebrovascular accidents have resulted in deaths from MDMA (ecstacy); PCP (angel dust) and ketamine have been associated with intensely violent episodes involving the police (abusers have been shot when authorities were unable to subdue them). Mescaline, peyote, and other mushrooms seem to be a quieter experience.

Hallucinogens are supposedly the ultimate in "sexual" drugs. The intoxicated states (however mystical) that occur with hallucinogens involve severe alterations in dopamine, serotonin, and excitatory amino acid activity. Phencyclidine (PCP, angel dust), for example, incites potent activity at glutamate receptors, apparently inducing psychoses by altering excitatory amino acids. Given the strong impact of these neurotransmitters on sexual function, both extremely positive and negative sexual effects may be expected to occur.

The circumstances surrounding hallucinogen use often include personal or social situations that encourage sexual freedom and experimentation. To the extent that sensory-perceptual and imaginative capacities are heightened or expanded, sexual activity may also be enhanced and intensified. Thus the pleasure that occurs during hallucinogenic episodes may incorporate sexual activity—however, it may also derive from utterly mundane pastimes such as watching paint dry!

The positive and negative effects of hallucinogens on sexual functioning resemble those that occur with stimulants (Chapters 23 and 26) and marijuana use (described previously), except that these effects may be telescoped into a very brief period of time. The acute and transient intensification of sexual sensations during hallucinogenic use may be described, rightly enough, as "ecstasy" or "agony." However, to the extent that the body is disabled during hallucinogenic episodes, sexual performance may be impossible or absurdly awkward. Body coordination necessary for sexual activity can be undermined by frequent hallucinogen use. Mann (1968) labels the sexual responses accompanying hallucinogenic use as "sensory and illusory platonic affections." He concluded that hallucinogenic drugs were "incapacitating," causing "bizarre visual distortions" that tend to impede sexual arousal and function.

---

*Barbiturates are discussed extensively in Chapter 19.

As with most drugs, excessively high doses of hallucinogens have dangerous and disabling physical and mental effects. Unfortunately, the desire and temptation "to excess" is characteristic of hallucinogen use.

Amphetamines*

Although amphetamines may be considered aphrodisiacs by some drug abusers, any actual sexual improvement seems to be the indirect product of overall stimulation/activation. Reviewing sexual findings from six commonly cited studies of stimulant abusers, Angrist (1987) found that 29 of 116 abusers reported greater intensity in sexual drive and sensations, while 10 reported decreased sexual feelings; and 75 reported no effect on sexual functioning. Even in those individuals who experience intense sexual stimulation on amphetamines, tolerance and subsequent exhaustion are likely to occur with long-term abuse. Hostility and aggression due to amphetamine abuse, may increase individual assertiveness and decrease sexual inhibitions. The amphetamine assertiveness effect is characterized by intoxication and indiscriminate behavior rather than increased confidence and heightened self-esteem. For women, atypical assertiveness may serve as a short-term advantage, but it may also incite hostility in males.

At best, sexually pleasurable effects similar to those experienced with dopaminergic stimulants (see Chapter 26) are typical of initial acute and transient use of amphetamines. However, the chemical changes involving "overdrive" of neurotransmitter release eventually lead to temporary or permanent neural exhaustion. In short, it may be assumed that these pleasure neurons "burn out," leaving behind a diminished capacity for pleasure, sexual arousal, and sexual function. The extreme sympathetic arousal that occurs during use of stimulants often causes vasoconstriction of genital tissue, reducing or preventing sexual sensations. Furthermore, because the intensity of the drug experience itself often exceeds the intensity of sexual intercourse, extended use of the drug frequently replaces the desire for sexual stimulation.

Cocaine

Cocaine, much like alcohol and benzodiazepines, can impair judgment and lead to indiscriminate sexual behavior. Through its dopaminergic effect, cocaine has a pronounced effect on sex drive in both men and women; ironically, it also simultaneously inhibits orgasm in both sexes. Men often appreciate this effect as a sexual advantage (lasting longer), whereas women may find themselves at a disadvantage: intense arousal but increasing difficulty achieving orgasm. There is a fine line between the amount of cocaine that sustains erection by inhibiting orgasm and the amount that causes absolute impotence. It is not long before the man who abuses cocaine may become completely impotent, even though his sexual interest may remain.

CONCLUSIONS

In the hierarchy of drugs subject to abuse, cocaine has a well-deserved reputation as a transient sexual stimulant. At light to moderate doses, it can increase sex drive through dopamine activity and inhibit orgasm; with increased use, impotence and anorgasmia are predictable. By contrast methamphetamine ("crystal") and other amphetamines have a street reputation for sexual benefits that appears to be less well-deserved and certainly more transient. At low doses marijuana appears to intensify sexual experience, but intoxication severely dampens interest, participation, and performance. Hallucinogens have little direct impact on sexual function. However, hallucinogenic episodes are so mentally and physically debilitating that the focus and coordination ordinarily required for sexual participation are generally lacking.

---

*Amphetamines are discussed further in Chapter 23.

Part IV

ANTIHYPERTENSIVES

14

Sexual Side-Effect Research

OBJECTIVES

- To summarize the history and development of sexual side-effect research
- To compare results from studies with different methods and samples
- To identify problems with sexual side-effect research
- To propose a standard approach for future studies

Because antihypertensive medications were the first drugs recognized to cause sexual dysfunction as part of their side-effect profile, most of the sexual side-effect research has been focused on their investigation. Sixty million patients in the United States have been diagnosed with hypertension and are under various forms of treatment. Many of these patients are asymptomatic and otherwise healthy. However, since a common cause of hypertension is atherosclerosis (narrowing of the arteries throughout the body), which can cause impotence without the addition of any medication, there is a higher incidence of sexual problems among untreated hypertensives than among the general population. The fact that hypertension predominantly affects men at earlier ages than women also results in the most obvious and visible manifestation of sexual problems—mainly impotence, which is easily recognized by patients. Once hypertension is diagnosed, antihypertensive treatment typically continues for life. This long-term treatment results in the emergence of sexual deficits over time.

Research studies dating from the 1970s to the present have gradually defined the sexual consequences of this class of medication. The few large controlled longitudinal studies of antihypertensives paved the way for the evaluation of other drugs. Information on sexual side effects comes from many research sources, ranging from single patient anecdotal reports to comprehensive long-term placebo-controlled trials, which include symptom checklists and in-depth quality-of-life interviews. Given that antihypertensives are typically used for extended time periods, sexual effects eventually become so evident that they are not easily ignored.

A list of the top 20 prescription drugs in the United States is published each year. From the 1990 rankings (*American Medical News*, 1991), it is apparent that antihypertensive use exceeds all other prescription treatments except antibiotics. According to data from *Pharmacological Data Services* and *American Druggist*, seven antihypertensives ranked in the top 20 (see Table 14.1).

Patterns of prescribing drugs change from year to year, based on the development of new drugs as well as new information about old drugs (particularly in regard to side-effect profiles).

In a study of physician drug preferences from 1987 to 1989 (Bostick, Luepker, Kofron, & Pirie, 1991), antihypertensive prescribing patterns emerged. The popularity of diuretics as first drug of choice decreased considerably, while the popularity of angiotensin-converting enzyme (ACE) inhibitors increased; beta-blockers were being

Table 14.1 *Top 20 Prescription Drugs (United States Pharmacies, 1991)**

1. Amoxil (amoxicillin)	11. *Vasotec (enalapril)*
2. Lanoxin (digoxin)	12. *Tenormin (atenolol)*
3. Zantac (ranitidine)	13. *Procardia (nifedipine)*
4. Premarin (conjugated estrogen)	14. Ortho-Novum 7/7/7
5. Xanax (alprazolam)	15. *Capoten (captopril)*
6. *Dyazide (hydrochlorothiazide)*	16. Naprosyn (naproxen)
7. *Cardizem (diltiazem)*	17. Tagamet (cimetidine)
8. Synthroid (levothyroxine)	18. *Calan (verapamil)*
9. Ceclor (cefaclor)	19. Prozac (fluoxetine)
10. Seldane (terfenadine)	20. Ortho-Novum 1/35

*Antihypertensive drugs are italicized.
From *American Medical News*, March 4, 1991. Data sources: *Pharmaceutical Data Services* and *American Druggist*.

replaced by medications with fewer undesirable side effects. Among antiulcer drugs Tagamet began to fall in popularity, replaced by Zantac in large part due to their differing effects on sexual function.

It is important to note that prescribing patterns in the United States do not reflect patterns in other countries. Prescribing patterns around the world and in different regions and settings within the United States are influenced by economic factors, not just medical considerations. Weiland et al. (1991) have reported that in Germany, beta-blockers are still overwhelmingly preferred as the first-step antihypertensive drug, and calcium channel blockers are far more popular than ACE inhibitors. Even in the United States, older drugs such as beta-blockers, diuretic combinations, and methyldopa are still preferred in most hospitals and clinics.

OVERVIEW OF RESEARCH ON SEXUAL SIDE EFFECTS

As studies of treatment protocols have improved, sexual side effects have been discovered and demonstrated to be a major problem. Unfortunately, these side effects are still not adequately acknowledged or considered by physicians or by large health providers (such as the Veterans Administration hospital system). Until recently, sexual side effects were addressed primarily through anecdotal communication among physicians; very little published information existed on this topic. Even less was communicated to patients. Mechanical disturbances in male function were usually the only side effects reported under the general term "impotence." More subtle manifestations of dysfunction in men, such as decreases in sexual desire, were rarely acknowledged. In women, where sexual compromise is less noticeable, little was even noted. Even as the quality and frequency of monitoring sexual effects has increased, scientific attention still focuses predominantly on male sexual disorders—in particular, erection and ejaculation dysfunctions. Even for men, many sexual problems are simply not referenced: sex drive disorders, orgasm without ejaculation, retarded ejaculation, painful ejaculation, retrograde ejaculation, or ejaculation without orgasm.

A few landmark studies illustrate how the field of pharmacology has evolved. Although most of these studies involved antihypertensives, the principles apply equally well to any drug. Concentrating exclusively on male sexual dysfunction as measured by erectile function and lack of ejaculation, the 1973 Bulpitt and Dollery questionnaire survey (Bulpitt & Dollery, 1973) was the first study to include sexual side effects in the side effect analysis. However, it failed to correlate the sexual symptoms with drug or dosage.

The British Medical Research Council (MRC) study reported in 1981 investigated the sexual effects associated with diuretics, propranolol, and placebo (MRC, 1981). Although it was a large-scale single-blind study including both men and women, only men were questioned about sexual issues. The study demonstrated that impotence was a common consequence of antihypertensive medications and contradicted earlier studies by providing evidence that diuretics were twice as harmful to erectile function as propranolol.

The Hypertension Detection and Follow-up Program (HDFP) (Curb et al., 1985; Davis, Ford, Remington, Stamler, & Hawkins, 1986), conducted in the United States, further contributed to the body of knowledge concerning sex and prescription drugs. This study found that adverse sexual side effects were the most common complaint of patients taking thiazides and reserpine and/or methyldopa and sometimes hydralazine. While this study included both men and women, female sexual dysfunction was not reported.

The captopril "quality-of-life" study (CQL), published in the *New England Journal of Medicine* in 1986 (Croog et al., 1986), was the key trend-setting study to investigate sexual side effects: It was the first to expand the concept of side effects beyond specific sexual dysfunctions to include sexual dissatisfaction and discontentment. It also included sexual questions for both sexes.

Quality-of-life was a term used by epidemiologists in the 1970s to evaluate the effects of health care and disease treatment on patients with chronic illness. Christopher Bulpitt in England applied the quality-of-life concept advantageously to drug side effect monitoring. Quality-of-life determinations are conducted chiefly by epidemiologists and public health specialists who work in conjunction with physicians, usually in large, multi-site studies. The quality-of-life approach transforms side-effect information gathered by questionnaires into summary indexes concerning various aspects of life (e.g., work, sex, leisure, medical complaints). These indexes are conducive to broad statistical generalizations, which can give the studies an authoritative appeal. However, it is very difficult to know just what the index scores actually represent. Separate sexual aspects, such as orgasm, desire, erection, amount of sexual activity, and sexual satisfaction, often are combined into an overall index score (a summary number noted to increase or decrease, significantly or insignificantly), which tells the reader little about how the drug actually affects the patient's sexuality. Thus quality-of-life studies are difficult to interpret and the information provided may not be as useful for practical management of drug therapy as it appears at first glance.

Furthermore, while there is promise that drug therapy can be measured against reliable standards of well-being, the quality of these measurements are suspect when the most sexually toxic antihypertensive drugs (e.g., methyldopa, propranolol, reserpine) often show no significant sexual side effects. Skeptics use the term "data-dredging" pejoratively, to describe the possible manipulation of the enormous amount of data to support almost any point of view with some statistical authority (Feinstein, 1988; Koplan, 1991).

Unfortunately, the quality-of-life questionnaires do not pass the "propranolol test." Sexual side effects with propranolol are well documented. When comparative tests do not identify sexual dysfunction with propranolol, it can be concluded that something is wrong with the methodology of the study. Although the 1986 CQL questionnaire (Croog et al., 1986) did identify differences between captopril and methyldopa or propranolol, even as a demonstration it was barely sufficient. Sexual dysfunction differences between drug groups were significant only when diuretic was added. Using diuretics adjunctively, only "problems in gaining erection" showed a significant difference between captopril and propranolol. No significant differences between drugs were found for interest in sex, maintaining an erection, or ejaculation. The predictable difference between captopril and methyldopa was not identified.

A particularly valuable study, the Trial of Antihypertensive Interventions and Management (TAIM), compared drug therapy with or without diet therapy, demonstrating that some of the adverse sexual consequences of various drugs could be minimized by adjunctive therapies such as weight loss programs and low-sodium diets (Wassertheil-Smoller et al., 1991).

The key research in drug side effects has had such a profound influence on our current understanding of sexual side effects and the assessment of other drug categories that it warrants a closer look. As we proceed through the literature reviews of various drugs, it is wise to bear in mind that most large drug trials are sponsored by drug companies hoping to demonstrate that their drug is the preferred alternative. Positive data from trials can be selectively published, while negative effects go unreported.

BULPITT AND DOLLERY QUESTIONNAIRE SURVEY, 1973

The first researchers to demonstrate the sexual consequences of antihypertensive medications were two British doctors, Christopher Bulpitt and C. T. Dollery. Bulpitt's specialty was the monitoring of chronic disease as a public health problem, while Dollery specialized in clinical pharmacology. Bulpitt and Dollery devised the first comprehensive side effect questionnaire, which was self-administered in a cross-sectional survey of 477 male and female patients being treated at a local hypertension clinic by various doctors with various medications and combinations of medications. (As such, it was an epidemiological inquiry characterized by drug treatments rather than a direct side effect inquiry.) Medication groups reflected the prevailing prescribing practices of the time: 51 were on diuretic alone, 220 on methyldopa and diuretic, and the remaining were on propranolol and reserpine, and various adrenergic ganglionic blockers.

Questions on sexuality included impotence, failure of ejaculation, and frequency of sexual activity. The questions did not address whether the symptoms started before or after taking the medication. The patients were asked, "Since the last visit, have you been troubled by ______?" A typical sexual question was, "During sexual intercourse are you troubled by failure to sustain erection or pass semen?" The results of the questionnaire survey were published in 1973 in the *British Medical Journal*. In 1974 the Bulpitt and Dollery questionnaire was published in the *Journal of Chronic Disease* (Bulpitt, Dollery, & Carne, 1974), together with an unprecedented epidemiological review of the results by age, sex, race, marital status, and medical status. The main weakness of this survey was the exclusion of women from the sexual questionnaire and the absence of established relationship between the sexual dysfunction and the onset of drug treatment. The relationship to drug therapy was addressed in a later study (Bulpitt, Dollery, & Carne, 1976); the exclusion of women from sexual questions, however, continued.

Bulpitt and Fletcher published an excellent review of quality-of-life studies in 1990, entitled: "The Measurement of Quality of Life in Hypertensive Patients: A Practical Approach." Questions concerning sexual desire are included for both women and men in their current quality-of-life questionnaires, although the scope of these questions remains unfortunately limited.

BRITISH MEDICAL RESEARCH COUNCIL TRIAL, 1981

In 1981, physicians of the British Medical Research Council (MRC) published the results of a large prospective study investigating adverse reactions to diuretics, propranolol, or placebo (drug groups, n = 495; placebo, n = 539). Bulpitt and Dollery's side-effect questionnaire was adapted for this study, the objective of which was to determine if measurable benefits occurred when mild hypertension (diastolic blood pressure of 90 to 109) was treated with drugs compared to no treatment. Patients (aged 35 to 64) with the same degree of illness were randomly assigned to one of three groups: those receiving thiazide diuretic (bendroflumethiazide, 10 mg); those receiving propranolol (160–320 mg); or placebo. Both male and female patients were included, but again, the women were not asked sexual questions. The studies were single-blind (doctors knew which drugs patients were taking, but patients did not). Patients were carefully monitored for over two years. Results were determined by calculating side effects over equivalent time periods represented by patient-years (number of patients multiplied by years on drug).

The use of proper experimental and statistical procedures distinguished the MRC trials from most prior antihypertensive studies. Doctor bias was reduced by use of self-administered questionnaires, allowing the patients to participate directly in the medical evaluation. The incidence of side effects was determined by responses to questions during the study and by drop-out rates. Results indicated that:

- 8.3% of the withdrawals from the study were due to impotence*;
- 36% of impotence withdrawals occurred within the first three months;
- 87% of impotence withdrawals occurred within the first year.

Patients who were monitored beyond the initial two-year evaluation point continued to show withdrawal rates due to impotence (Dollery, 1987). Reports of impotence from the placebo group also increased (from 8.9% to 10.1%), which could represent the progression of atherosclerosis in penile arteries or reflect the rate of impotence in the general population. The impotence withdrawal rates showed that diuretics caused almost twice as much impotence as propranolol, a finding which contradicted the prevalent clinical impression. For example, Laganière, Biron, and Robert (1986) reported 5.2% sexual dysfunction on propranolol as compared to 3% on thiazides and 2.4% on chlorthalidone. Even a physician particularly knowledgeable about the sexual side effects of antihypertensive "guesstimated" 13–23% side effects on propranolol versus 3–9% on thiazide diuretics (Wartman, 1983). Until Dollery's study demonstrated otherwise, diuretics were not believed to cause sexual problems.

The discrepancy between the results of the MRC trial and "common practice" opinion may be accounted for by the fact that patients were randomly assigned to drug conditions in the MRC, whereas in common practice patients with less severe illness are more likely to receive diuretics than propranolol. By eliminating this bias in drug assignment, the MRC allowed a more objective analysis. Currently, bendroflumethiazide and other diuretics are generally used in lower doses than were used in the MRC study, due in some part to the MRC side effect findings.

The treatment of hypertension in the elderly (65 and over) was studied at a later date. In a separate MRC trial, elderly patients were randomly assigned to one of the three groups: diuretic (Moduretic/Moduret), the beta-blocker atenolol (Tenormin), or placebo (MRC, 1987). Early evaluation of patients on drugs for three to 24 months showed that withdrawal rates in the diuretic and beta-blocker groups were approximately equal, compared to no withdrawals in the placebo group. Women were still not questioned about sexual effects.

HYPERTENSION DETECTION AND FOLLOW-UP PROGRAM, 1986

The Hypertension Detection and Follow-up Program (HDFP) was the first comprehensive evaluation of antihypertensive side effects in a large prospective trial. Curb and his colleagues published surveillance figures of adverse sexual effects from the large extended study which was begun in 1973 by a national council of cardiologists at 14 sites in the United States (Curb et al., 1985; Curb, Maxwell, Schneider, Taylor, & Shulman, 1986). The goal of the study was to determine whether over five years antihypertensive therapy would reduce all-cause mortality in the general patient community. Like the MRC research, there was random assignment to drug group; however, there was no placebo condition. Side effect questionnaires were completed by physicians, study coordinators at the 14 sites, and the patients themselves. Treatment occurred from 1973 to 1979 and subsequent follow-up evaluations were completed in 1982.

Over 90% of patients had mild to moderate hypertension (90–114 diastolic), with 72% in the mild range (diastolic blood pressure, 90/104). Reflecting common clinical practice, a three-step protocol was used: All patients were started on

*Impotence was usually reversible within a few weeks after drug withdrawal.

the long-acting thiazide diuretic chlorthalidone; if blood pressure was not controlled in 12 weeks, either reserpine or methyldopa was added; if blood pressure still was not controlled, the vasodilator hydralazine was added.

Yearly interviews of patients conducted in their homes by nontherapist interviewers, standard office questionnaires for patients, and information from doctors and therapists were analyzed in the final determination of side effects.* Notably, adverse sexual reactions to the drugs were reported in about 6% of patients—*more than any other class of side effects*, except for upper gastrointestinal symptoms (which also occurred in 6% of patients). Lethargy, depression, and dizziness occurred in about 4% of patients. Sexual side effects were also the most common cause for drug discontinuation among male patients (8.3% compared to 6.2% for lethargy and 6.5% for gastrointestinal complaints). The diuretic chlorthalidone caused as much impotence as reserpine or methyldopa (4.4%). Decreased sex libido was somewhat greater with reserpine and methyldopa (2.0% and 1.6%) than on diuretic (1%). Calculated as rate per 1,000 patient-years to correspond to MRC figures, the impotence rate with the diuretic chlorthalidone was 14.0 compared to 19.6 for the diuretic bendroflumethiazide in the MRC study. Both studies demonstrated that diuretics alone can cause impotence comparable to drugs like reserpine and methyldopa. Only six female patients out of 2,529 discontinued drug usage due to sexual side effects. Although decreased libido was evaluated, its incidence was not reported for women.

CAPTOPRIL QUALITY-OF-LIFE STUDY, 1986

The large pharmaceutical company, Squibb, sponsored many small studies of its new antihypertensive drug, captopril (Capoten). Since these studies showed few side effects and even some health benefits, Squibb decided to take a quality-of-life approach, which could be expected to show the side-effect profile of captopril to the best advantage. Since sexual dysfunction, which was one of the major antihypertensive side effects, did not appear to occur with captopril, the company had the wisdom to realize that, with the quality-of-life documentation, this sexual advantage could be effectively marketed. The captopril quality-of-life study (CQL) included hypertensive male patients treated with captopril, methyldopa, or propranolol over a sufficiently long time (six months) for most effects to appear (Croog et al., 1986). Comparison with the two sexually toxic antihypertensives, methyldopa and propranolol, practically ensured a favorable outcome for captopril.

The sexual component of the CQL inventory was called the Sexual Symptoms Distress Index and notably excluded female sexuality. Four questions regarding reduction of sexual desire, problems obtaining erection, problems maintaining erection, and problems with ejaculation were asked. Patients were questioned at the end of 24 weeks by nurses and "technical health personnel" who were not otherwise involved in patient care. Although these independent interviewers were considered best able to conduct a structured and unbiased interview, there is no indication that they had the experience or training to ask sexual questions appropriately or to interpret sexual responses correctly.

The results of the CQL study, which were published in the *New England Journal of Medicine*, attracted enormous attention, much of it due to a mammoth advertising campaign by Squibb. Lack of negative sexual effects were touted as a core feature of captopril's quality-of-life advantage. Even though there were few statistically significant differences in sexual side effects between the three antihypertensive drugs (captopril, methyldopa, or propranolol), the consistent indication that captopril caused *none* of the sexual problems that occurred with methyldopa and propranolol was very impressive.

The chief contribution of the CQL study was to focus attention on sexual side effects as an

*This eclectic approach was possible due to the cooperation of public health specialists and physicians treating the hypertensive patients.

important health issue that should be a major consideration in prescribing practices. The chief flaw of this study was its omission of female sexuality. The perspective that sexual well-being is essential to quality of life was further emphasized in a major follow-up report by Sydney Croog (Croog, Levine, Sudilovsky, Baume, & Clive, 1988), who carefully analyzed the study's findings on sexual side effects and related them to overall well-being.

TRIAL OF ANTIHYPERTENSIVE INTERVENTIONS AND MANAGEMENT, 1991

The Trial of Antihypertensive Interventions and Management (TAIM) study made a major contribution to the understanding of medication side effects by measuring the impact of drugs on sexual function in the context of other treatment approaches. Drug research and treatment often disregard additional clinical, nonpharmacological therapies that could be equally or perhaps more effective. Rather than promoting a complementary integration of therapies, drug studies are often instrumental in creating this either/or polarization. Examination of drug and nondrug therapies in combination, as was accomplished by TAIM, is necessary to evaluate this integrative approach fairly.

In TAIM, a placebo-controlled, double-blind, random assignment trial, sexual side effects were measured for three drugs under three different diet conditions: usual diet (no change); a weight-loss program including weekly group therapy with nutritionists; and a low-salt diet (Wassertheil-Smoller et al., 1991). The drugs tested were the long-acting diuretic chlorthalidone (Hygroton), the beta-blocker atenolol (Tenormin), and placebo. Male and female patients all had mild hypertension only (diastolic blood pressure, 90/100) and were 110–160% over their ideal weights. They could be treated over a limited time with placebo without health risk, and they were suitable for diet therapy.

This study introduced major improvements in the evaluation of sexual dysfunction. Important advances in study design included: Sexual side effects and sexual satisfaction were evaluated from questionnaires answered by both female and male patients; sexual effect questions included inability to have orgasm and loss of sexual interest in addition to erection ratings. Questionnaires were given at baseline and after six months of treatment; improvement and decline were measured by comparing the six-month ratings to the baseline ratings.

Findings on women's experience of sexual problems were published in general terms. Sexual problems worsened for 24% of women treated with the diuretic chlorthalidone in the usual diet group, whereas only 5% of the chlorthalidone-treated weight-loss group developed any difficulties. In fact, significant worsening of sexual problems did not occur in either the weight-loss or low-salt diet therapy conditions regardless of drug treatment. Not surprisingly, addition of the diet therapy minimized the negative sexual effects found to occur with diuretic treatment alone. However, when all diet therapy conditions were averaged for women patients, there were no significant differences in sexual deterioration among placebo, diuretic, or beta-blocker.

Sexual deterioration (predominantly, decreases in erection) in male patients occurred with the diuretic only when the usual diet condition prevailed. For male patients with the usual diet, sexual function worsened 28.9% on chlorthalidone, 12.8% on atenolol, and only 2.9% on placebo. Diuretic-treated male patients in the weight loss program actually showed some sexual improvement. Overall, for all the diet group males patients combined, sexual function worsened for 17% on chlorthalidone, 11% on atenolol, and 7% on placebo.

Patients treated with diuretic under their usual diet conditions showed substantially increased glucose intolerance. In the weight-loss diet group, glucose intolerance was reduced with all drugs and sexual deterioration did not occur with any drug. This successful combination of diuretic treatment with weight-loss therapy demonstrated that nondrug therapies can be used to minimize or eliminate sexual side effects ordinarily associated with pharmacological interventions.

IS DISEASE OR DRUG THE CAUSE OF SEXUAL SYMPTOMS?

A consistent complaint of reviewers is that sexual dysfunction due to drug is difficult to distinguish from sexual dysfunction caused by the underlying disease. For example, hypertensives experience more sexual dysfunction than normals, even without the drug (see Table 14.2).

A "best estimate" of impotence in nontreated hypertensives was derived from baseline data on the men entering the American Hypertension Detection and Follow-up Program discussed previously. The baseline data at trial entry (before trial drug), broken down by age, race, and previous treatment with antihypertensives, were reported by Kraus et al. (1983). Impotence (defined in this study as decrease in sexual ability) existed in 19% of untreated hypertensives and in 32% of those treated with medication. Since this figure of 32% is virtually identical to the Bulpitt-Dollery 1973 survey study of men on diuretic and other antihypertensives, it can be assumed that drug treatment caused 13% (32 minus 19) of men to develop impotence. The Bulpitt-Dollery 1973 figure of 32% has repeatedly been given in reviews as the high end figure for impotence due to diuretics. However, since about 19% of hypertensives would be impotent without drug treatment, only 13% impotence should be attributed to diuretics. The 13% impotence figure is in accord with the MRC figure of 13% for propranolol. Bansal (1988) recalculated the MRC patient-years figure into a percent of total patients. With this recalculation, the impotence rate was 16.2% for diuretic, 13.8% for propranolol, and 8.9% for placebo.

Bauer et al. (1978) showed nearly equivalent impotence rates for diuretic and propranolol treatment (14% on diuretic and 11% on propranolol). When an additional antihypertensive was added to either diuretic or propranolol in Bauer's study, impotence incidence rose to 20–23%. The 23% figure with propranolol combination therapy was equivalent to that found in Hogan's 1980 study. The impotence figure for normotensive men under 40 is estimated to be approximately 10% (Bansal, 1988). With a 19% impotence rate for nontreated hypertensive men, it appears that the impotence rate in untreated hypertensive men is roughly twice that of normotensive men (19% versus 10%). Inde-

Table 14.2 *Sexual Dysfunction in Hypertensives (Treated and Untreated)*

Symptom	*Normotensives*	*Hypertensives Untreated*	*Hypertensives Treated*	*Reference*
Impotence	6.9%	17.1%	24.6%	Bulpitt et al., 1976
		22.1%	40.6%	Croog et al., 1988
		19%	32.1%	Kraus et al., 1983
	10%	20%	20%	Bauer, Baker, Hunyor, & Marshall, 1978
Erection dysfunction		23.3%	38.4%	Croog et al., 1988
Ejaculatory dysfunction	0%	7.3%	25.6%	Bulpitt et al., 1976
		17.2%	29.8%	Croog et al., 1988
Decreased desire		33.7%	43.4%	Croog et al., 1988
Sexual dysfunction	3%	13%		Dimenas, Wiklund, Dahlof, Lindvall, & Olofsson, 1989
	4%		13%	Hogan, Wallin, & Baer, 1980

pendent figures by Bulpitt and Bauer chart this base impotence rate for hypertensives between 17% and 20%. These figures gathered in different countries are consistent with the 19% figure. The 10% figure for normotensive men accurately reflects various incidence reports on population impotence base rate. Additional impotence due to diuretic and/or older antihypertensive drugs runs about 13%.

Hopefully, these impotence figures (10% in normals, 19% in hypertensives, 32% in drug-treated hypertensives) will remove confusion from historical reviews of the literature. All three figures—32% reported by Bulpitt and Dollery (1973), 23% reported by Hogan et al. (1980), and 13–16% noted by MRC (1981)—can now be seen to support the 13% figure correlating impotence to antihypertensive treatment.

CRITIQUE OF CURRENT RESEARCH

A literature that provides a range of 0–80% for the incidence of sexual side effects (Papadopoulos, 1980) leaves much to be desired. An average between these low and high figures becomes the best compromise under the circumstances. Unfortunately, findings are often taken out of context via statistical manipulation. For example, a 34% methyldopa-erection incidence was included in a respected review (Bulpitt & Dollery, 1973) and then was repeatedly cited as authoritative, with or without qualification. Eventually, these figures appear to take on a life of their own; they are cited without attention to how they were derived or what they represent.

Further reducing the accurate reporting of sexual side effects is the practice of calculating incidence over the entire number of patients studied. Two cases of impotence in a sample of 20 patients would be described as a 10% occurrence—misleadingly low—because ten of the patients were women and five of the men were not sexually active. The correct figure for impotence actually would be 40% (two of five). The incidence noted in the literature would be incorrect by a factor of four.

Study design and execution often leave a lot to be desired. If patients are asked how well they are functioning sexually at the time of the study, instead of what changes have occurred since initiating drug treatment, it is difficult to determine whether the reported effect is due to a pre-existing condition or to the drug. The association of a sexual side effect with a drug is determined simplistically by how many patients experience the symptom. For example, the percentage of patients on drug *X* who report impotence is then compared to "normal" rates (historical control). A statistical significance test is made between the incidence with patients on drug *X* to the incidence of those on drug *Y* or on a number of other drugs. Alternately, drug *X* incidence is compared to placebo incidence, to incidence among normals, or to incidence at baseline prior to initiation of drug *X* treatment (it is surprising how often baseline rates and tests are not taken). A more scientific but underutilized research option is to use patients as their own controls, thus avoiding arcane comparisons of incidence rates from various populations. Developing a separate control group is fraught with problems, beginning with defining what is sexually normal.

When patients are questioned directly about the effects of a drug, then the nature and duration of the symptom can be ascertained. However, survey epidemiology, which contains set questions within limited parameters, continues to be the most popular research method. Consequently, side-effect reviews present a hodgepodge of incidence rates and then usually note how confusing the differences are among the various findings. At the root of the problem, however, is the use of superficial methods and over-reliance on statistical analysis. An additional problem of survey research is that other conditions that commonly impair sex (such as various diseases, alcohol and drug abuse, and other medications) are not identified in these studies. Furthermore, the significance of the lack of an available sex partner is rarely appreciated.

The precise nature of the terms used is highly important for comparison and clarity. A 1975 methyldopa study (Alexander & Evans, 1975) showed a 7% spontaneous report of erection *failure*, but asking patients about erection *diffi-*

culty resulted in a figure of 53%. The 53% erection *difficulty* could later be cited incorrectly as a 53% erection *failure*. The erection failure figure is typically the only one used, since it is absolute, easy to record, not subjective, and obviously mechanically significant. Determining just how much erectile "difficulty" has to occur for it to be cited as a side effect is not generally addressed and the continuum of difficulty is ignored. The insidious progression of sexual side effects through the years from minor to notable and consistent difficulty is not usually recognized, recorded, or reported.

Without a clear definition of sexual side effects, it is difficult to compare the various research results, except in the most general sense. Even the meaning of the sex term *drive* varies from study to study. In addition, authors of review articles change the original terminology to support their positions. Hypothetically, 27% "sexual difficulties" in an original article may later be cited as "27% impotence" or as "27% ejaculation failure." Incidence "not recorded" tends to become incidence "not occurring." The "lack of ejaculation" commonly observed with phenoxybenzamine has been referred to as "retrograde or retarded." In addition to being glaringly incorrect, the distinction between male orgasm and ejaculation is not even recognized. The sexual event itself is usually not retarded: orgasm typically occurs when it should. The problem is that there is no *ejaculation* (Money & Yankowitz, 1967). Since no semen was passed given the lack of ejaculation, phenoxybenzame was once considered a possible form of birth control.

In spite of emerging data to the contrary, for a considerable time diuretics were regarded as sexually benign drugs. With further study, however, it has become clear that their adverse sexual effects are equal to or greater than some of the most sexually toxic drugs in the antihypertensive class. Finally, given that women's sexuality is largely ignored and that sexual effects are noted in men only when extreme and debilitating, the reported rate of negative sexual effects in any study could be expected to be falsely low or absent.

CONCLUSIONS

Clinical research on the sexual side effects of drugs is still in its infancy.

Some progress has been made; we are somewhat more sophisticated today in identifying the impact of antihypertensive drugs on sexual function then we were 20 years ago. Key lessons and problems learned from this area of research include:

- Sexual dysfunction side effects may manifest only in trials of six months or more.
- Sexual side-effect studies rarely investigate or identify female problems, suggesting that women experience fewer adverse sexual effects when, in fact, they are not being evaluated at all.
- Quality-of-life questionnaires generate considerable data but few significant differences and may be less sensitive than the 1973 Bulpitt-Dollery side-effect questionnaire.
- Sexual side effects are more likely to appear if they are considered separately, rather than within an overall index score, so that incidence figures can be determined.
- Clear and consistent standards must be established specifying the type of sexual dysfunctions to be considered and the definitions used.
- The rate of sexual dysfunction contributed by underlying disease conditions should be established and controlled for in the study design.
- Whenever possible, sexual partners should be included in the study questionnaire or interview.
- Masturbatory patterns should be assessed. Interviews and questionnaires almost never include questions about masturbation, yet changes in this area are one of the most reliable indicators of sexual function. Furthermore, masturbation patterns are one of the few ways to assess sexual function in patients without partners.
- While placebo-controlled trials are not

necessary to identify that a particular drug causes a problem, with the newer, cleaner drugs available, the sexual side effects are more subtle and consequently more difficult to ascertain without placebo for comparison.

- Drug side-effect studies must include an assessment of alcohol use/abuse and illegal drug use and abuse.

Masters and Johnson's (1966) detailed description of the sexual response cycles in men and women serves as an excellent model for investigating the physiological effects of drugs. Unfortunately, drug side-effect researchers have not used this standard to advantage. Instead of integrating the medical and psychological sciences, which was the focus of Masters and Johnson's work, drug side-effect studies have evolved more in the direction of a social science with epidemiological overtones. It would be far more useful to monitor the course of 30 couples on a drug than to administer superficial questionnaires to 3,000 patients, with no individual interviews.

Even though most of the existing studies do not incorporate all of these recommendations, they nonetheless have considerable value. In spite of the inconsistencies in definition and number of sexual dysfunctions, the cumulative effect shown by the studies is fairly consistent. While the studies may disagree about the precise rate of dysfunction, they generally agree that the medication in question causes some degree of dysfunction.

The extensive clinical studies that have been performed on antihypertensive drugs have not been performed on other classes of medication. However, progression to the sexual evaluation of all drugs is inevitable, as physicians become more aware of noncompliance issues and as patients continue to demand medical care without sexual compromise.

15

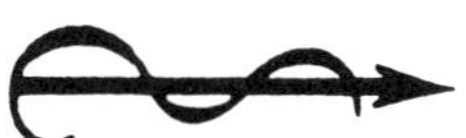

Diuretics, Reserpine, Methyldopa, Guanethidine

OBJECTIVES

- To illustrate the adverse sexual consequences of most diuretics, even when used alone
- To identify the most sexually benign diuretic
- To compare and contrast diuretics with reserpine, methyldopa, and guanethidine in relation to sexual function
- To suggest alternative treatments less toxic to sexual functioning

Diuretics are used extensively to treat hypertension, sometimes as monotherapy, but more often together with other antihypertensive drugs. They are also widely prescribed for fluid retention, as with congestive heart failure, or for more benign conditions such as bloatedness from premenstrual tension or ankle edema from a variety of causes ranging from heart conditions to plane rides. Most physicians prescribe diuretics fairly liberally under the misguided notion that they have few, if any significant, adverse sexual side effects. Although recent research has documented the opposite, this information is not yet widely known clinically.

Because diuretics are often prescribed with other heart medications which have adverse sexual consequences, the problem is magnified. Cardiac conditions can be so life-threatening that sexual problems become irrelevant. However, noncompliance with medication is also a serious problem when sexual side effects are present. Patients are not always sensible and cooperative about taking medications that detract from what they consider to be an important aspect of their lives. In these cases concurrent counseling is important to ensure compliance with the prescription regimen. Physicians too readily assume that, due to age or disease, patients are no longer concerned with sex.

Fortunately, in the majority of cases alternative medications that are not sexually debilitating are available. Too often, patients do not receive the dual benefits of these drugs—effective health care without sexual compromise—because so little information is available to help physicians distinguish between the sexual properties of the various drugs available.

Reserpine, methyldopa and guanethidine were among the earliest antihypertensive drugs developed and widely prescribed. Since they have been in use for quite some time, a great deal of research and clinical information is available. Examining this body of research, however, reveals inconsistent and contradictory conclusions. Therefore, no single study should be evaluated in isolation. The conclusions offered about the various antihypertensive drugs are based on an analysis of the pertinent literature available, taking into consideration the size of the studies, the quality of the research design, the nature of the questions asked and the manner in which they were posed, and the background of the investigators. Table 15.1 summarizes the characteristics and side effects of diuretics.

Table 15.1 *Profile of Commonly Used Diuretics*

Class of Drug	Daily Dose
Thiazide-type	
Bendroflumethiade (Naturetin)	2.5–5 mg
Chlorthalidone (Hygroton)	12.5–50 mg
Chlorothiazide (Diuril)	12.5–500 mg
Hydrochlorothiazide (Hydrodiuril, Esidrex, etc.)	12.5–50 mg
Indapamide (Lozol)	2.5 mg
Methyclothiazide (Enduron)	2.5–5 mg
Trichlormethiazide (Naqua)	1–4 mg
Loop diuretics	
Bumetanide (Bumex)	0.5–10 mg
Furosemide (Lasix)	40–320 mg
Potassium-sparing	
Amiloride (Midamor)	5–10 mg
Spironolactone (Aldactone)	25–100 mg
Triamterene (Dyrenium)	50–200 mg
Combinations	
Aldactazide (hydrochlorothiazide + spironolactone)	1–2 tablets
Dyazide (hydrochlorothiazide + triamterene)	1–2 tablets
Maxzide (hyrdochlorothiazide + triamterene)	1 tablet
Moduretic (hydrochlorothiazide + amiloride)	0.5–1 tablet

COMMON INDICATIONS

Hypertension   Congestive heart failure   Edema

MECHANISMS OF ACTION (GENERAL)

Increases urinary excretion of water and salt
Blocks reabsorption of electrolytes in renal tubule
Promotes excretion of electrolytes

MECHANISMS OF ACTION (SEXUAL)

Positive
Increased estrogens (female)

Negative
Increased estrogens (male)
Increased prolactin
Decreased zinc

DIRECT SEXUAL SIDE EFFECTS

Desire disorders (in both sexes)
Erection difficulties

Breast disorders
- Gynecomastia

INDIRECT SEXUAL SIDE EFFECTS

Discomfort caused by constipation, indigestion, nausea, pain, rash/itching, urinary problems (incontinence, nocturia)
Neurological disturbances resulting in dizziness, fatigue, pain, paresthesia, sedation, weakness
Vascular disturbances resulting in orthostatic hypotension, peripheral vasodilation
Endocrine disturbances precipitating or aggravating diabetes

SEXUAL CONTRAINDICATIONS/BENEFITS

Avoid with prior condition of
Desire disorders (both sexes)
Impotence

May be useful for
Lubrication

ALTERNATIVES

Preferred thiazides
Indapamide (Lozol)
Hydrochlorothiazide (Hydrodiuril)

Preferred loop diuretic
Furosemide (Lasix)

Preferred alternative drug class
Calcium channel blockers

DIURETICS

Thiazide diuretics have been used to treat hypertension since 1957 and were used routinely as adjuncts to the early antihypertensives (reserpine, guanethidine, hydralazine, and methyldopa). When diuretics began to be used as monotherapy for mild hypertension (often to avoid negative side effects of other antihypertensives), their adverse metabolic effects became more apparent (Jaffe, Haitas, & Seftel, 1987). These effects include:

- decreased potassium (blood and tissue)
- decreased magnesium (blood and tissue)
- decreased calcium metabolism
- hyperuricemia (risk factor for gout)
- increased glucose level or glucose intolerance
- altered insulin release
- increased total and LDL-cholesterol
- increased triglycerides

Even though potassium supplements can correct deficits due to diuretics, tissue concentrations of potassium and magnesium may remain depressed. The patient may require up to three different medications: diuretic, potassium supplement, and a supplementary antihypertensive. (The potassium deficit can sometimes be minimized by adding a potassium-sparing diuretic.) Because of the severe sexual side effects associated with most diuretics, which are becoming more widely recognized among physicians, prescribing patterns are slowly shifting toward other antihypertensives as the first drug of choice.

Despite the availability of newer antihypertensives, diuretics continue to be a treatment of choice for hypertension, particularly in the elderly and in African-Americans: Diuretic efficacy may increase in the elderly, unlike other antihypertensives; and high salt sensitivity and tissue concentration in the presence of greater blood volume in African-Americans may justify diuretic treatment (Moser, 1989). Although monotherapy with other antihypertensives is often sufficient in African-Americans, there is no doubt that diuretics increase efficacy and are often essential for adequate blood pressure control.

The British Medical Research Council studies (MRC, 1981) described in the previous chapter reported that more sexual dysfunction occurred on diuretic than on beta-blockers – an unexpected finding that startled many doctors and is still considered by many to be peculiar to the MRC trial, in spite of confirmatory evidence. For example, the TAIM quality-of-life trial (also discussed in the previous chapter) reported that diuretic could have more severe sexual side effects than beta-blockers (Wassertheil-Smoller et al., 1991). This study further indicated that diuretics that were prescribed to patients who continued on their usual diet caused sexual problems and increased serum glucose, whereas negative sexual effects did not occur in patients on diuretic in conjunction with a weight-reduction diet that also reduced hyperglycemia. In some cases, diuretics can induce diabetes, as defined by hyperglycemia. Since the incidence of impotence and neuropathy is common with diabetes, any chronic hyperglycemic state should be investigated when sexual dysfunction is present.

Sexual Side Effects

Substantial sexual effects on sexual functioning have been noted for diuretics in all major large trials (Curb et al., 1985). The sexual side effects found for diuretics were equal to or greater than those found for methyldopa, propranolol, and reserpine. Furthermore, in the Multiple Risk Factor Intervention Trial (MRFIT), Geissler, Turnlund, and Cohen (1986) found sexual dysfunction in 41% of men treated with the diuretic chlorthalidone, compared to 16% in an untreated control group.

Poloniecki and Hamilton (1985) surveyed men and women on diuretics combined with propranolol or other conventional antihypertensives such as methyldopa or prazosin hydrochloride. Forty-eight percent of the men and 23% of the women complained of sexual impairment due to the diuretic/antihypertensive medications. Although sexually inactive patients were eliminated from the sample, no figures were provided on what percentage of the total they comprised. If all patients were counted, then a low sexual side-effect incidence might reflect that a majority of the patients simply had no sexual behavior to report.

Lowering the dosage does not necessarily remove these effects. For example, the TAIM diet trial showed a 28% erection deficit with the lowest dose (25 mg) of chlorthalidone (Wassertheil-Smoller, et al., 1991).

Male/Female Differences

Although there is inadequate information on gender-related benefit and risk differences of diuretics, it is known that diuretics can have an estrogenic effect that is positive for women but negative for men (Rose, Underwood, Newmark, Kisch, & Williams, 1977). For example, thiazides have been shown to decrease osteoporosis and hip fracture in women (La Croix et al., 1990). However, high doses of thiazide (50 mg), with consequent metabolic effects, may be necessary for this benefit, which is rapidly lost when the drug is discontinued. Chronic diuretic use by women for various discomforts such as excessive weight, water retention, and premenstrual syndrome can be of value, but long-term, daily use should be avoided. In men, excess estrogen causes gynecomastia and feminine distribution of body fat, decreases sexual desire, and can cause impotence.

Chlorthalidone

Among the diuretics, chlorthalidone (Hygroton) seems to be the worst offender. A major difference between chlorthalidone and other thiazides is its long duration of action (25 to 48 hours). In the HDFP trial (Curb et al., 1985, 1986), incidence of withdrawal from the study due to impotence with chlorthalidone was 14 per 1,000 patient-years, compared to withdrawal due to impotence with chlorthalidone of 4.4% in the MRC studies (MRC, 1981). The incidence of impotence was greater with chlorthalidone than with the antiandrogen, spironolactone.

No case reports of impotence due to chlorthalidone were reported until 1980. It is possible, however, that the 80% sexual dysfunction figure reported for methyldopa in 1976 by Pillay (1976) was due to the concurrent use of chlorthalidone. (This figure is far higher than what has been reported in other methyldopa research.) Stessman and Ben-Ishay (1980) reported five cases of impotence in patients on 100 mg chlorthalidone. Two of the patients had previously been treated with thiazides without negative sexual effects. Geissler et al. (1986) found sexual dysfunction with low-to-moderate doses of chlorthalidone (11–50 mg) in a large, placebo-controlled trial of middle-aged men, 42 to 65 years old. After six months of treatment, 42% (8/19) of those treated with chlorthalidone showed decreased sex drive or erectile function, compared to 16% (5/31) of controls. The conclusions of this study were more reliable than most previous research in this area because the methodology included an adequate period of time (six months) for measurement and patients were asked direct questions about sexual changes.

Taken together, the results of the TAIM study (Wassertheil-Smoller et al., 1991) and Geissler et al. (1986) provided strong evidence that chlorthalidone causes impotence at normal therapeutic doses. Although no noticeable sexual dysfunction was noted overall by women using chlorthalidone in the TAIM study, when the "usual diet" condition was considered separately (i.e., when there was no additional diet therapy), both men and women on chlorthalidone reported a 25% increase in sexual problems. Until direct comparisons of the sexual side effects of chlorthalidone to other diuretics are documented, chlorthalidone use should be minimized.

There is further evidence that low chlorthalidone doses often cause psychological problems that would usually not be attributed to diuretic use. Since diuretics tend to be used widely among the elderly, these psychological and sexual problems will often be attributed to aging. Consequently, they will be left untreated or treated with sexually toxic antidepressants such as amitriptyline (Elavil) and fluoxetine (Prozac).

Hydrochlorothiazide

A recent study by Chang et al. (1991) indicated that hydrochlorothiazide (HCTZ) (Hydrodiuril, Esidex) treatment may cause as much sexual dysfunction as chlorthalidone. Chang and his colleagues conducted a large, placebo-controlled, quality-of-life trial investigating diuretic effects in 176 men. Six different medication conditions were compared for a two-month period: (1) 50 mg HCTZ; (2) 50 mg HCTZ plus potassium-sparing diuretic; (3) 50 mg HCTZ plus potassium supplement; (4) 50 mg HCTZ plus potassium/magnesium supplement; (5) 50 mg chlorthalidone; and (6) placebo. Mild to moderate deficits in sexual desire and erectile function were reported by a substantial number of men in all the diuretic groups. Only one of 23 placebo patients reported sexual dysfunction.

Far more sexual dysfunction was reported in confidential self-report questionnaires than in response to queries by doctors. Of those patients reporting sexual dysfunction to their doctors, 50% said that the problems were new and 72% attributed them to the medication. No differences between diuretic and placebo were found for other quality-of-life factors such as psychological well-being, mood, ability to work, alertness, and social/recreational functioning. The sexual dysfunction appeared to be a direct drug effect, not secondary to psychological or physical symptoms caused by the diuretics. The dose of 50 mg used in all groups is larger than the 25 mg dose used for mild hypertension.

Indapamide

Indapamide (Lozol) is an excellent alternative to thiazide diuretics. Used since the 1970s in Europe, it has recently been approved for use in the United States. Though derived from thiazide-type diuretics, it has an indole ring structure that attenuates contractile responses to angiotensin II, norepinephrine, electrical stimulation, and calcium influx. It may have therapeutic actions similar to calcium channel blockers and ACE inhibitors and therefore can serve as monotherapy for hypertension. Nevertheless, its strongest action is as a diuretic.

In a 12-week quality-of-life trial (Pirrelli & Nazzaro, 1989), indapamide (2.5 mg/day) decreased symptoms of anxiety, depression, and obsessive/compulsive/phobic responses, whereas chlorthalidone (25 mg/day) increased these indices. A review by Clarke (1991) summarized the clinical advantages of indapamide compared to other antihypertensive drugs: Indapamide does not cause weight gain, does not increase cholesterol or triglycerides, and does not disturb glucose balance. In common with the loop diuretic furosemide (Lasix) and the ACE inhibitors, it increases vasodilating prostaglandins, including PGE_2 and prostacyclin, which serve to protect body tissue. The mild calcium-blocking action of indapamide, generally free of calcium channel-blocker side effects (like flushing and headache), suggests that it may be preferable to calcium channel blockers as monotherapy. In addition, indapamide has a smooth muscle relaxing effect and antispasmogenic properties greater than thiazides but less than loop diuretics (furosemide, bumetanide). Finally, its lack of hyperglycemic effects and its prostaglandin action make indapamide suitable for diabetics. All in all, the availability of a safe diuretic alternative like indapamide is a valuable resource for hypertension treatment.

In a 30-subject 12-week quality-of-life study by Lacourciere (1988) that compared the effects of indapamide (2.5 mg/day) and captopril (12.5–50 mg/2 x day), indapamide received ratings similar to captopril in the areas of well-being and lack of negative sexual effects. Indeed, according to this study, sexual side effects with indapamide appeared to be no higher than with captopril. While it is too early to ascertain indapamide's side-effect profile (fatigue is often reported), it is clear that this drug has a wide range of applications and may be safer than other antihypertensives.

Other open trials have shown an increase in

well-being in patients on indapamide who were previously treated with other antihypertensive medications. Werning, Weitz, and Ludwig (1988), for example, studied 149 elderly male and female patients (mean age = 67) who had experienced lack of sex drive and reduced sexual activity when treated with various antihypertensives. When they were switched to 12 weeks of indapamide treatment (2.5 mg/day), sexual activity and drive improved in 85% of the patients. Similarly, Guez, Crocq, Safavian, and Labardens (1988) studied 30 patients (mean age = 52.5), most of whom were on prior antihypertensive medications until placed on placebo for a three-week observation period. When treated with 2.5 mg/day indapamide for 12 weeks, symptoms such as discomfort, fatigue, anxiety, headaches, and concentration difficulties significantly decreased. Sexual drive and activity were not affected, however.

Spironolactone

Spironolactone (Aldactone) is a potassium-sparing anti-aldosterone diuretic that causes sexual problems in both men and women (Stevenson & Umstead, 1984). These sexual problems are more noticeable in men because they manifest as impotence and gynecomastia (Greenblatt & Koch-Weser, 1973). Spironolactone is sometimes used to treat hirsutism in women, but sex drive is often sacrificed in the process. Since spironolactone is an antiandrogen, sexual side effects can be expected, especially with larger doses. There is no dependable information on the sexual effects of other potassium-sparing diuretics such as amiloride (Midamor) or triamterene (Dyrenium). However, they appear to cause sexual problems comparable to thiazides.

Furosemide

Furosemide (Lasix) is a loop diuretic that may be efficacious when thiazide diuretics are inadequate. It can increase the release of vasodilator prostaglandins (Gerber, 1983), and potassium depletion does not occur. There are few sexual side effects reported with this drug, despite its widespread use.

Alternatives

In summary, diuretics appear to cause as much impotence as the most sexually toxic beta-blocker, propranolol. Chlorthalidone (Hygroton), in particular, should be avoided whenever possible. Its primary advantage is its extended duration of action, which may itself be a key factor in its toxicity. Due to its antiandrogen properties, spironolactone should also be avoided. Hydrochlorothiazide (Hydrodiuril, etc.) appears to be as safe as any other popular diuretic. When necessary, it is best used at the lowest dose possible (sometimes less than 25 mg). For conditions in which a stronger diuretic action is needed, use of indapamide (Lozol) or furosemide (Lasix) is recommended for minimal adverse effects on sexual function. Lastly, calcium channel blockers have some diuretic action that has made them a popular alternative for treatment of African-Americans.

Since diuretics alone have such a negative sexual impact, their use most probably impairs erectile function when added to sexually benign antihypertensive drugs such as captopril, atenolol, prazosin, and the calcium channel blockers. Therefore, avoiding older drugs and beta-blockers will not prevent a substantial risk of antihypertensive-induced impotence, unless diuretics are also avoided. In general, the use of diuretics increases the impotence rate by about one-third when added to single-drug therapy. Given the various negative metabolic effects of diuretics, their ubiquitous use should be reduced. Diuretics cannot be justified as prophylactic treatment for patients with mild hypertension.

RESERPINE

Reserpine (Serpasil) was one of the first drugs derived from a plant to be used in Western medicine. Subsequently, many naturally derived substances have been replaced by synthetic drugs, which now dominate psychopharmacology. Enlightened medical practitioners view reserpine as an example of the toxic drug effects that characterized the "Dark Ages" of pharmacology. Its derivation from plants—and, in particular, from rauwolfia alkaloids, which may have psychedelic properties—reinforced its image as a dinosaur drug superseded by synthetically derived pharmaceuticals through the evolution of modern science. Since reserpine effectively controls blood pressure, it was used widely until the discovery and acceptance of these newer synthetic antihypertensives. It is still widely used in developing countries and among poorer populations where cost is a primary consideration. Most side effects, with the exception of its sexual and depressive actions, can usually be limited by dosage adjustment.

Reserpine exerts its therapeutic effect by depleting neuronal stores of catecholamine neurotransmitters: norepinephrine, dopamine, and the indolamine serotonin. Given that reserpine depletes catecholamines and can cause severe depression, psychiatrists in the 1960s hypothesized that depression was due to depletion of catecholamines (Schildkraut, 1965). The notion of insufficient catecholamines as an explanation of one form of depression seemed sensible and easy to understand. This catecholamine depletion theory dominated antidepressant research and development for many years. Reserpine's reduction of sympathetic cardiovascular function could be viewed as providing less "fuel" (depleted catecholamines) to drive the blood pressure "pump" (heart), resulting in lower pressure in the "pipes." Sedation, psychological depression, and other side effects due to this "fuel" reduction were tolerated in exchange for its antihypertensive effect.

Some physicians view negative sexual side effects as a minor price to pay, especially since reserpine is used predominantly among the elderly, for whom, it is assumed, sexual function is no longer important. Unfortunately, reserpine can have negative sexual side effects far more severe than those ordinarily associated with aging. Many elders treasure their sexual function and consider its absence no small sacrifice. Table 15.2 summarizes the characteristics and side effects of reserpine.

Sexual Side Effects

The undesirable sexual side effects of reserpine are probably more numerous than acknowledged in the literature. Although a basic handbook on antihypertensives reported only a 1% incidence of sexual dysfunction with reserpine (McMahon, 1978), most of the literature has shown its sexual side effects to be comparable to sexually toxic antihypertensives like propranolol (Inderal), methyldopa (Aldomet), clonidine (Catapres), or moderate-dose thiazides. The unfavorable comparison with these other drugs confirms the sexual toxicity of reserpine, as will become clear in this section.

Adverse sexual effects are most apparent with reserpine after many weeks or several months of treatment (beyond the common four to six weeks of conventional drug research trials), explaining the low incidence rates reported by some studies. These effects, however, are believed to be readily reversible upon drug discontinuation. When there is a specific sexual complaint, the doctor can try reducing the dosage. In fact, over the years, reserpine's recommended dosage has decreased from 1 mg or more to 0.1 to 0.25 mg daily.

Because there are no obvious side effects such as the block of ejaculation impairment that occurs with sympathetic ganglion-blocking drugs, subtle effects such as lack of sexual interest and responsiveness may be overlooked. As noted, one of the most debilitating side effects of reserpine is depression (Schildkraut, 1965), a symptom often not recognized until it is so severe that the patient requires antidepressant medication. The sexual repercussions of depression and, perhaps, additional antidepressant medication are cumulative.

Three important comparative surveillance studies on sexual side effects of reserpine were conducted by the Veterans Administration (VA, 1972, 1977, 1984). Unfortunately, in these studies reserpine was used in combination with diuretics, making it impossible to isolate those effects attributable solely to reserpine. In the 1977 study of propranolol, a 14.3% rate of impotence was reported with propranolol and thiazide, versus a 10.7% rate for reserpine and thiazide. In

Table 15.2 *Profile of Reserpine (Serpasil)*

	Daily Dose 0.05–0.25 mg
COMMON INDICATIONS	
Hypertension	
Agitated psychotic states	
MECHANISMS OF ACTION (GENERAL)	
Depletes amine stores in neurons	
Reduces vasoconstricting catecholamines and indolamines	
MECHANISMS OF ACTION (SEXUAL)	
Positive	*Negative*
Decreased serotonin (5-HT)	Decreased adrenergic ($alpha_1$) activity
	Decreased dopamine
	Decreased LHRH
	Increased prolactin
DIRECT SEXUAL SIDE EFFECTS	
Desire disorders (in both sexes)	Breast disorders
Erection difficulties	• Gynecomastia
Ejaculation retarded	• Galactorrhea
Orgasm delayed or blocked	• Pain/tenderness
Menstrual disorders	
Amenorrhea	
INDIRECT SEXUAL SIDE EFFECTS	
Discomfort caused by dryness of skin, mouth, mucous membranes, nasal stuffiness, edema, hypothermia, shortness of breath, indigestion, nausea, rash/itching, weight gain	
Mood/disorders resulting in anhedonia, anxiety, depression, nervousness	
Neurological disturbances resulting in dizziness, fatigue, sedation, sleep disturbances, muscular weakness	
Vascular disturbances resulting in arrhythmias, headache, orthostatic hypotension, peripheral vasodilation	
SEXUAL CONTRAINDICATIONS/BENEFITS	
Avoid with prior conditions of	*May be useful for*
Impotence	Premature ejaculation
Ejaculatory problems	
Anorgasmia	
Menstrual disorders	
Depression	
ALTERNATIVES	
ACE inhibitors	Atenolol (Tenormin)
Calcium channel blockers	Bisoprolol (Zebeta)

Bulpitt and Dollery's 1973 questionnaire study of antihypertensive side effects, there were no recorded differences in impotence side effects between diuretic with reserpine, diuretic with methyldopa, or diuretic alone. Similarly, there were no differences noted in "ejaculation failure." Despite the claim that there were no differences in sexual side effects between these antihypertensives, however, they reported 32–36% rate of impotence and 14–18% ejaculation failure, which was clearly higher than most other studies investigating these drugs. Apparently, higher figures were due to the fact that the questionnaire was answered by the patients instead of the doctors. As noted, patients generally volunteer more sexual information when they answer questionnaires directly.

Another major comparative side-effect surveillance study on reserpine, the Hypertension Detection and Follow-Up Program (HDFP) (Curb et al., 1985, 1986), was described in the previous chapter. When treatment with diuretic alone was not adequate, reserpine was the next drug of choice. Drug dosage was not reported until a later paper which noted a range of 0.1 to 0.25 mg a day, the conventional low therapeutic dose (Curb et al., 1986). In the HDFP trial, 183 men discontinued the drug because of sexual problems, compared to six women. The sexual problem recorded for men was usually impotence. The nature of the women's sexual side effects apparently was not investigated. Adverse sexual effects due to reserpine and diuretic were no different from those due to methyldopa or diuretic alone. Table 15.3 summarizes the research on the sexual side effects of reserpine.

Male/Female Differences

Interest in including women in the HDFP study developed primarily because reports of breast cancer related to reserpine coincided with the start of the study (Kewitz, Jesdinsky, Schroter, & Lindtner, 1977).

Although no increased risk of breast cancer with reserpine was identified, other side effects were sufficient to cause patients to discontinue treatment. Of more than 2,500 women studied in this detailed five-year study, 22.9% of the African-American women and 33.7% of the caucasian women discontinued drug treatment due to various side effects not noted as sexual.

Alternatives

The combination of sexual problems and depression is sufficient to discourage the use of reserpine. Unless a patient's condition responds to no other alternatives or economic factors play a limiting role, reserpine should be avoided. Fortunately, many alternatives to reserpine currently exist. Among beta-blockers, atenolol (Tenormin) and bisoprolol (Zebeta) are preferable to reserpine, but are more expensive and still may have noticeable sexual side effects. Calcium channel blockers have shown minimal sexual side effects, but some cause fatigue and discomfort (e.g., nifedipine, verapamil); diltiazem (Cardizem) and newer calcium blockers such as amlodipine (Norvasc) are preferred. The ACE inhibitors and alpha-blockers (e.g., prazosin) are the best alternatives.

METHYLDOPA

Methyldopa (Aldomet) is a synthetic antihypertensive drug that was introduced in the late 1950s as an alternative to direct adrenergic blocking drugs such as guanethidine and reserpine. Some $alpha_2$ agonist action has been identified, but the mechanisms underlying other properties, such as alteration of dopaminergic activity, remain undefined. Although the precise mechanism of its action is unclear, methyldopa appears to blunt adrenergic activity through regulatory control centers in the brain. Table 15.4 summarizes the characteristics and side effects of methyldopa.

Sexual Side Effects

Some publications suggest that methyldopa presents few sexual difficulties. However, the weight of the evidence documents extensive sexual side effects with this drug.

Compared to the side effects of guanethidine and reserpine, methyldopa initially appeared to be sexually benign. Since the peripheral adrenergic ganglion is not directly blocked by methyldopa, it was thought that ejaculation would not be inhibited. Without catecholamine depletion (as occurs with reserpine), there would be less reduction of sex drive secondary to severe depression. And, indeed, methyldopa's negative effect on ejaculation appeared minor compared to guanethidine, and its depressive effects seemed less severe than reserpine.

Early drug studies investigating methyldopa reported few sexual side effects even with higher

Table 15.3 *Reserpine Sexual Side Effects*

Method	*Reserpine Alone*	*Reserpine + Other Drugs*	*Other Drugs*	*Source*
Doctor report (SE)	Impotence: 1%			McMahon, 1978
Questionnaire	SSE: 5%			Curb et al., 1985, 1986
Doctor report + checklist (SE)		+ **Misc drugs** Impotence (early): 29% Impotence (chronic): 21%	**Placebo** Impotence (early): 28% Impotence (chronic): 23%	VA, 1972
Questionnaire		+ **Diuretic** Impotence 10.7%	**Propanolol** Impotence: 14.3%	VA, 1977
Survey questionnaire	Impotence: 33% Ejaculatory dysfunction: 14.3%		**Methyldopa** Impotence: 36% Ejaculatory dysfunction: 18.5% **Diuretic** Impotence: 32% Ejaculatory dysfunction: 18.5%	Bulpitt & Dollery, 1973

SE = side effect; SSE = sexual side effect (unspecified)

doses. Dollery and Harington (1962) found 3%; Johnson, Kitchin, Lowther, and Turner (1966) found 2–5% impotence, and, in a review of 19 literature reports, McMahon (1978) found only 1% incidence of impotence and ejaculation failure. In some studies in which methyldopa was compared to other antihypertensives, no sexual effects were noted (e.g., McMahon, 1978). However, symptoms including gynecomastia, hyperprolactinemia, and lactation were reported early in clinical use (Husserl & Messerli, 1981). Fatigue, lethargy, adverse cognitive alterations and mood changes (depression) were also identified (Papadopoulas, 1980). Reports of galactorrhea, gynecomastia, and amenorrhea have identified methyldopa's antagonism of dopamine and its ability to elevate prolactin level. For instance, Lamberts (1983) showed prolactin elevations in five of eight men treated with a relatively low dose (750 mg/day) of methyldopa. Three of the five men complained of loss of sex drive or impotence, which was resolved when bromocriptine was added to normalize the prolactin levels.

Although the literature indicated that methyldopa was generally equivalent to other antihypertensives (including diuretic alone) in its impact on sexual function, many doctors began to note marked adverse sexual effects in their clinical practices. Newman and Salerno (1974) reported sexual deficiencies in sex drive, erection, or ejaculation in 26% of patients treated with methyldopa; however, these difficulties disappeared soon after switching the patients to propranolol.

Table 15.4 *Profile of Methyldopa (Aldomet)*

Daily Dose
500–2,000 mg

COMMON INDICATIONS
- Hypertension
- Schizophrenia

MECHANISMS OF ACTION (GENERAL)
- Infterferes with enzymatic conversion to dopamine and serotonin
- Generates transmitter substances that block norepinephrine

MECHANISMS OF ACTION (SEXUAL)

Negative
- Decreased adrenergic ($alpha_1$) activity
- Increased adrenergic ($alpha_2$) activity
- Decreased dopamine (DA)
- Decreased LHRH
- Increased opioids
- Increased prolactin

DIRECT SEXUAL SIDE EFFECTS
- Desire disorders (in both sexes)
- Erection difficulties
- Ejaculation retarded
- Orgasm delayed or blocked
- Breast disorders
  - Gynecomastia
  - Galactorrhea
  - Pain/tenderness

INDIRECT SEXUAL SIDE EFFECTS

Discomfort caused by constipation, dryness of skin, mouth, mucous membranes, edema, indigestion, nausea, rash/itching, urinary problems (nocturia), shortness of breath, weight gain

Mood disorders resulting in anhedonia, depression

Neurological disturbances resulting in cognitive deficit, dizziness, fatigue, sedation, tremor, muscular weakness

Vascular disturbances resulting in hemolytic anemia, arrhythmias, angina, orthostatic hypotension

SEXUAL CONTRAINDICATIONS/BENEFITS

Avoid with prior condition of
- Desire disorders
- Ejaculatory disorders
- Anorgasmia
- Depression

May be helpful for
- Hypersexuality?

ALTERNATIVES
- ACE inhibitors
- Calcium channel blockers
- Prazosin (Minipress)
- Atenolol (Tenormin)

In the literature the range of methyldopa's adverse effect on sexual functioning varies from zero to 80% (see Table 15.5). Almost 700 general practitioners who responded to a survey request to name the most frequent side effects they associated with each of eight antihypertensive drugs reported 35.3% sexual problems with methyldopa (Laganière et al., 1986). The next highest drug associated with sexual problems was clonidine, followed by propranolol and prazosin (see Table 15.6).

Numerous other studies have reported nega-

Table 15.5 *Methyldopa Sexual Side Effects*

Method	*Methyldopa Alone*	*Methyldopa + Other Drugs*	*Other Drugs*	*Source*
Doctor report (SE)	Impotence: 30% Ejaculatory dysfunction: 8%			Bauer, Hull, Stokes, & Raftos, 1973
Survey of general practitioners	SSE: 35.3%		**Clonidine** SSE 7.2% **Propranolol** SSE: 5.2% **Prazosin** SSE: 0.5%	Laganière et al., 1986
Physicians' reports	SSE: 14–33%		**Propranolol** SSE: 13–23% **Prazosin** SSE 1–5%	Wartman, 1983
Questionnaire		+ **Diuretic** SSE: 13%	**Diuretic** SSE: 9%	Hogan et al., 1980

Questionnaire		+ **Diuretic** Impotence: 35.7% Ejaculatory dysfunction: 18.5%	**Diuretic** Impotence: 31% Ejaculatory dysfunction: 13.6% **Reserpine + Diuretic** Impotence: 33% Ejaculatory dysfunction: 14.3% **Guanethidine + Diuretic** Impotence: 66.7% Ejaculatory dysfunction: 41.2% **Bethanidine + Diuretic** Impotence: 54.5% Ejaculatory dysfunction: 60%	Bulpitt & Dollery, 1973
Questionnaire	Impotence: 20%	+ **Diuretic** Ejaculatory dysfunction: 7%	**Diuretic** Impotence: 20% Ejaculatory dysfunction: 9% **Propranolol alone & with diuretic** Impotence: 11–14% Ejaculatory dysfunction: 7–9%	Bauer et al., 1978
Doctor interview		+ **Chlorthalidone** Impotence: 80% Ejaculatory dysfunction: 0%		Pillay, 1976
Doctors' clinical observations		+ **Diuretic** (assumed): 26%		Newman & Salerno, 1974
Patients' spontaneous reports		+ **Diuretic** Erectile failure: 7%		Alexander & Evans, 1975
Patients' elicited reports		+ **Diuretic** Erectile problem: 53%		Alexander & Evans, 1975

SE = side effect; SSE = sexual side effect (unspecified)

Table 15.6 *Sexual Side Effects Commonly Associated with Antihypertensives*

Drug	*Sexual Side Effects*	*Fatigue & Weakness*
Methyldopa	35.3%	24.2%
Clonidine	7.2%	
Propranolol	5.2%	29.2%
Prazosin	0.5%	
Metoprolol	25.1%	
Diuretics		23.0%

Data from Laganière et al., 1986.

tive sexual side effects associated with methyldopa. For example, Bulpitt and Dollery's study (1973) found impotence and ejaculation failure rates for methyldopa comparable to diuretic alone and to reserpine plus diuretic. However, guanethidine plus diuretic and bethanidine plus diuretic showed almost twice the incidence of both impotence and ejaculation. Other fatigue symptoms such as depression, hypertension, sleepiness, and asthenia were equally prevalent with methyldopa, reserpine, or diuretic alone, but somewhat less with guanethidine. Rosen, Kostis, Jekelis, and Taska (1994) found a decrease in firmness of erection after four weeks of methyldopa treatment in a placebo-controlled investigation of antihypertensive sexual effects, despite no changes noted for atenolol, propranolol, dyazide, or placebo. Hogan et al. (1980) reported increased sexual problems with methyldopa. Using a self-administered questionnaire, the researchers surveyed 381 men on methyldopa and diuretic, 287 men on diuretic alone, and 177 clinical controls. This questionnaire contained a more detailed exploration of sexual function than most of this era, and some of the questions were later used to advantage in the Captopril Quality-of-Life study discussed in the previous chapter (Croog et al., 1986). (For example, questions investigated loss of interest in sex, inability to achieve erection, inability to maintain erection, and inability to ejaculate.) The negative sexual effects of methydopa may not be as severe as generally assumed. In the Croog et al. (1986) study of 626 men, methyldopa and propranolol caused more dropouts due to side effects than captopril. The predominant symptoms were fatigue and lethargy, which may indirectly but significantly affect sexual function. Trial withdrawals due to sexual problems appeared virtually identical for the three drugs tested in this study: five for captopril and six each for methyldopa and propranolol. No significant differences between groups were found using the study's Sexual Symptom Distress Index to evaluate sex drive, gaining and maintaining an erection, and ejaculation.

With the addition of a diuretic, the only significant differences between groups (captopril, methyldopa, or propranolol) was in gaining erection and the total index score. Sex drive, maintaining erection, and ejaculation showed no significant differences. (Differences that did occur were mainly due to propranolol rather than methyldopa.) Thus, the conclusion could easily be made that methyldopa is relatively free of adverse sexual effects, even when comprehensively evaluated over an extended period.

However, quality-of-life differences between captopril and methyldopa or propranolol were demonstrated in the CQL study in men over 50 years old as specific changes from baseline. The sexual data were gathered in interviews conducted not by the physicians but by "interviewer staff consisting of registered nurses or medical administrative and technical health personnel." These interviewers were not involved in patient care, not trained in sexual therapy, but were trained for standardized survey-type interviewing.

Unfortunately, the CQL study allows for sufficient "data-dredging" to prove almost any point. The manufacturers of methyldopa and propranolol could interpret the results to show that there were no significant differences in sexual side effects among the three drugs and that their drugs were as sexually benign as captopril. In fact, the lack of significant differences between methyldopa and captopril was in contrast to most other findings in this area of research (see Tables 15.5 and 15.6).

In conclusion, methyldopa is now known to have a dysfunctional effect on sexual desire and response. However, given the failure to consider any but the most severe sexual effects, differences in the drug's sexual impact on men and women cannot be evaluated. The percentage of sexual problems thought to be associated with methyldopa may be approximately five times greater than with any of the other drugs. Indirect sexual side effects (mainly fatigue and weakness) attributed to methyldopa are also high. Diuretics, which are frequently used in association with methyldopa, intensify this fatigue and weakness. Yet, because this information is not widely known among physicians, methyldopa has remained, undeservedly, a mainstay of hypertension treatment.

The disparities among the studies examined in this section raise questions about the quality of the research designs and methodologies. For example, various literature reviews on the sexual side effects of methyldopa assumed that the appropriate questions were asked in a proper fashion—which is not a valid assumption. In the Bulpitt and Dollery 1973 survey, patients on reserpine had intercourse only six times a year as compared to 27 times a year on methyldopa and 42 times on diuretic alone. Yet, the incidences of impotence and failed ejaculation were reported as the same in all three conditions and have been noted as being no different in several reviews. Obviously, either reserpine was used to treat only sexually inactive patients or reserpine radically decreased the frequency of sexual activity. Clearly, analysis of methyldopa's sexual side effects well illustrates the complexities involved in interpreting available data.

Alternatives

The preponderance of clinical evidence strongly indicates that methyldopa causes sexual problems comparable to propranolol, guanethidine, and reserpine. Taking into consideration the other adverse side effects of methyldopa, it should not be the first drug of choice and, ideally, should be used only when it is the best or only drug effective for a particular patient. Better alternatives include ACE inhibitors, calcium channel blockers, prazosin, and some of the newer beta-blockers like betaxolol or bisoprolol.

GUANETHIDINE

Guanethidine (Ismelin) was a popular antihypertensive until newer drugs became available. It is a peripheral adrenergic ganglion depletor that can inhibit or altogether block ejaculation, making it a potent sex-offender drug.

Sexual Side Effects

Bauer et al. (1973) compared methyldopa to guanethidine: Twenty-eight men on long-term guanethidine and diuretic treatment were compared with 27 men on methyldopa and diuretic. Thirteen men were withdrawn from guanethidine treatment due to side effects or ineffectiveness; eight were withdrawn from methyldopa, six due to side effects. Guanethidine patients reported hypotension, diarrhea, drowsiness, and fatigue. These same side effects occurred less frequently with methyldopa, but eight men on methyldopa experienced severe depression. Over 30% of both groups of patients showed decreased sex drive or mild to marked impotence. Eleven guanethidine patients reported lack of ejaculation; nine reported impaired ejaculation. Two of 24 methyldopa patients showed impaired ejaculation. Upon termination of medication, all men recovered normal or "near normal" erectile and ejaculatory function.

The results of Bauer et al.'s study tended to confirm the physiological interpretation of the sexual effects of these drugs: that peripheral adrenergic depletors such as guanethidine probably block ejaculation to some degree in the majority of men (and most probably inhibit orgasm in women), while methyldopa only occasionally impairs orgasm/ejaculation (probably through a central mechanism) and moderately decreases sex drive and/or erection. However, the sexual effects of guanethidine and methyldopa both involve decreased adrenergic activity and, therefore, both may result in decreased sex drive, erec-

Table 15.7 *Profile of Guanethidine (Ismelin)*

Daily Dose
10–50 mg

COMMON INDICATIONS
Hypertension

MECHANISMS OF ACTION (GENERAL)
Decreases peripheral resistance and vasoconstriction
Inhibits release and/or reuptake of norepinephrine
Depletes norepinephrine from intraneuronal vesicles

MECHANISMS OF ACTION (SEXUAL)

Positive	*Negative*
Increased cholinergic activity	Decreased adrenergic ($alpha_1$) activity
	Decreased adrenergic ($beta_2$) activity

DIRECT SEXUAL SIDE EFFECTS

Desire disorders (in both sexes)	Orgasm difficulties
Erection difficulties	• Premature ejaculation
• Priapism	• Retarded ejaculation
• Impotence	• Anorgasmia

INDIRECT SEXUAL SIDE EFFECTS
Discomfort caused by edema, nausea, urinary problems (incontinence), weight gain, shortness of breath

Mood disorders resulting in depression

Neurological disturbances resulting in dizziness, fatigue, neuropathy, paresthesia, sedation, muscular weakness

Vascular disturbances resulting in peripheral vasodilation, angina, orthostatic hypotension

SEXUAL CONTRAINDICATIONS/BENEFITS

Avoid with prior condition of	*May be useful for*
Desire disorders	Premature ejaculation
Ejaculatory problems	
Anorgasmia	
Priapism	
Depression	

ALTERNATIVES

$Alpha_1$ blockers	Calcium channel blockers	ACE inhibitors

tion, orgasm, and ejaculation. Table 15.7 summarizes the characteristics and side effects of guanethidine.

Sexual Benefits

Money and Yankowitz (1967) reported lack of ejaculation in 12 patients treated with guanethidine and determined that five of the 12 experienced orgasm despite the lack of ejaculation. Kedia and Markland (1975) also found that orgasm could occur without ejaculation. As a result, some doctors have suggested using guanethidine as a male contraceptive, indicating an unjustified confidence in its sexual innocuousness. Furthermore, the effects of guanethidine on ejaculation and orgasm are not clearly dose-related and are unpredictable; therefore, it is not useful as a contraceptive.

Alternatives

Preferable alternatives to guanethidine include prazosin or other $alpha_1$ blockers, calcium channel blockers, and ACE inhibitors.

16

Beta-Blockers, $Alpha_1$ Blockers, $Alpha_2$ Agonists

OBJECTIVES

- To identify sexual problems associated with these drugs
- To suggest better alternatives

This group of antihypertensives—beta-blockers, $alpha_1$ blockers, and $alpha_2$ agonists—has prominent adverse sexual complications. All of the drugs decrease adrenergic (sympathetic) activity to some degree. Some beta-blockers have the double impact of decreasing sympathetic activity while indirectly increasing serotonin, thereby reducing sex drive and impairing erection and, possibly, ejaculation. Even eyedrops containing beta-blockers (in both liquid and oral forms, used for the treatment of glaucoma) can be devastating to sexual drive and functioning. All beta-blockers, however, are not the same; some are kinder to sexual function than others. Beta-blockers also can cause clinical depression so severe that antidepressant medication is required.

$Alpha_1$ blockers and $alpha_2$ agonists are curiously alike. Both decrease adrenergic ($alpha_1$) activity: $alpha_1$ blockers directly; $alpha_2$ agonists by negative feedback on $alpha_1$ activity. $Alpha_2$ agonists, while increasing adrenergic ($alpha_2$) activity, have a variety of other undesirable sexual mechanisms, such as decreasing vasoactive intestinal peptide (VIP). In addition, while $alpha_2$ agonists can be relatively benign at low doses, they have pronounced sexual side effects at high doses, comparable to those of methyldopa and guanethidine.

Of the two alternatives, $alpha_1$ blockers have the lowest sexual side-effect profile, but can still cause both direct and indirect sexual dysfunction via impotence, priapism, inhibited ejaculation, fatigue, and weakness. $Alpha_1$ blockers have been tried unsuccessfully as a treatment for premature ejaculation. Interestingly, labetolol (with both $alpha_1$ and some beta-adrenergic blocking activity) lowers blood pressure from the usual peak occurring at orgasm. This has interesting treatment implications for those rare patients who experience headaches during orgasm.

The drugs discussed in this chapter were developed by pharmaceutical companies in an effort to replace the less tolerated antihypertensives. The intention was to minimize side effects of all sorts, while achieving equal or better therapeutic potency. When these drugs were first released, the picture was promising. However, after decades of use it is clear that profound side effects do occur. Some of the most troublesome are sexual dysfunction and depression. However, when sex-sparing alternatives are not suitable, sophisticated use of these medications can still serve patients well.

BETA-BLOCKERS

Propranolol was the first beta-blocker to become clinically available. It blocks both $beta_1$ and $beta_2$ receptors; $beta_1$ receptors are more responsive to norepinephrine, while $beta_2$ receptors are more responsive to epinephrine. $Beta_2$ receptor blockage inhibits thermogenesis, bronchodilation and skeletal muscle tone. Beta-blockers developed later, such as metoprolol (Lopressor) and atenolol (Tenormin), are selective for $beta_1$ receptors; they have the important advantage of causing less fatigue than propranolol. However, due to its more effective inhibition of epinephrine responses that mediate stress, nervousness, tremor, and other sympathetic reactions, propranolol is a popular drug for the treatment of stage fright and other transient anxiety states. Propranolol has a high affinity for serotonin and for sigma receptors, so that it now appears to have effects far beyond those of beta adrenergic inhibition. Pindolol (Visken), another beta-blocker with strong affinity for serotonin neurons, avoids the typical beta-blocker reduction of cardiac output and force, so there is less probability of heart failure. However, pindolol appears to generate more anxiety and fatigue than other beta-blockers, possibly due to its serotonergic actions.

The serotonergic action of propranolol and pindolol is complicated by their complex action on different serotonin nerve receptors. For instance, they have been found to inhibit 5-HT_{1A} serotonin receptors (Oksenberg & Peroutka, 1988). However 5-HT_{1A} receptor activation can have a positive sexual effect, given that 5-HT_{1A} receptors may function as autoreceptors that decrease the activity of other serotonin receptors (see section on buspirone in this chapter). Consequently, it may be more correct to say that propranolol and pindolol may affect serotonin activity in a characteristically negative sexual direction by reducing sex drive and inhibiting orgasm. With the complexity introduced by the recent discovery of a multitude of receptors that have different actions within the same chemical class (e.g., serotonin), simple heuristic statements of a given neurotransmitter's action will be increasingly subject to contradiction and paradox. Table 16.1 summarizes the characteristics and side effects of beta-blockers.

Propranolol

Despite the availability of newer drugs with fewer side effects, propranolol (Inderal) is still a widely used antihypertensive that was in clinical use for over 20 years before some of its more troublesome side effects were recognized. It is now known that 5–15% of patients taking propranolol may experience such severe depression that they may require antidepressant medication (Avorn, Everitt, & Weiss, 1986). While some recent studies evaluating the incidence of depression in patients on propranolol have failed to find a higher incidence than in patients on other medications (Bartels, Glasser, Wang, & Swanson, 1988; Carney et al., 1987), a recent literature review and meta-analysis has shown that propranolol causes significantly more depression than various control medications (Patten, 1990).

Sexual Side Effects Although propranolol was introduced as an antihypertensive with fewer side effects than its predecessors, reserpine and methyldopa, comprehensive studies of antihypertensive treatment have shown it to have similar or more severe sexual side effects than both drugs it was intended to replace. Impotence frequently has been reported in patients treated with propranolol (Knarr, 1976; Forsberg, Gustavii, Hojerback, & Olsson, 1979; Miller, 1976; Warren & Warren, 1977). (Unfortunately, deficits in sex drive have rarely been investigated.) In a 1977 Veterans Administration Cooperative Study (VA, 1977), a 14.3% rate of impotence was reported for propranolol and thiazide, compared with a 10.7% rate of impotence for reserpine and thiazide. Hogan et al. (1980) have been widely cited for reporting a 23% impotence figure for propranolol. Employing a four-question definition of impotence that included loss of sexual interest, inability to achieve or maintain erection, or inability to ejaculate, these researchers questioned men prior to and during treatment. Questions included whether symptoms had improved, worsened, stayed the same, or were no longer a problem.

The control group in Hogan's sample showed a 4% impotence rate compared to 9% on diuretic, 13% on methyldopa, 15% on clonidine, and 23% on a combination of high-dose propranolol (160–320 mg) and hydralazine (100 mg). Patients on the propranolol-hydralazine combination

Table 16.1 *Profile of Beta-Blockers*

	Daily Dose
Acebutolol (Secral)	200–1,200 mg
Atenolol (Tenormin)	25–100 mg
Betaxolol (Kerlone; Betoptic)	10–40 mg
Bisoprolol (Zebeta)	5–20 mg
Labetalol (Normodyne, Trandate)*	100–1,200 mg
Metoprolol (Lopressor)	50–200 mg
Nadolol (Corgard)	20–160 mg
Penbutolol (Levatol)	20 mg
Pindolol (Visken)	10–40 mg
Propranolol (Inderal)	40–320 mg
Betaxolol (Betoptic)	0.25% soln, 1–2 drops b.i.d.
Timolol (Timoptic, Blocadren)	0.25% soln, 1–2 drops b.i.d.

COMMON INDICATIONS

- Hypertension
- Arrhythmia
- Angina
- Acute myocardial infarction
- Migraine

MECHANISMS OF ACTION (GENERAL)

- Reduces cardiac output and contractibility
- Decreases sympathetic overactivity
- Modulates cardiovascular pacemaker sinus rate
- Regularizes heartbeat
- Prevents fibrillation and arrhythmia
- Reduces renin activity
- Blocks skeletal muscle receptors
- Enhances peripheral vasoconstriction

MECHANISMS OF ACTION (SEXUAL)

Negative

- Decreased beta-adrenergic activity
- Increased serotonin (5-HT)

DIRECT SEXUAL SIDE EFFECTS

- Desire disorders (in both sexes)
- Infertility
  - Decreased sperm motility
- Erection difficulties
  - Decreased quality of erection
  - Peyronie's disease

INDIRECT SEXUAL SIDE EFFECTS

Discomfort caused by hypothermia, nausea, rash/itching, weight gain, shortness of breath

Mood disorders resulting in anhedonia, depression

Neurological disturbances resulting in cognitive deficits, dizziness, fatigue, neuropathy, paresthesia, sedation, sleep disturbances, muscular weakness, decreases pelvic muscle responses

Vascular disturbances resulting in orthostatic hypotension, peripheral vasoconstriction

Endocrine disturbances precipitating or aggravating diabetes

SEXUAL CONTRAINDICATIONS/BENEFITS

Avoid with prior condition of

- Desire disorders
- Impotence
- Ejaculatory problems
- Peyronie's disease
- Infertility
- Depression

May be useful for

- Psychogenic impotence
- Premature ejaculation

ALTERNATIVES

- ACE inhibitors
- $Alpha_1$ blockers
- Calcium channel blockers

*Reviewed under $alpha_1$ blockers

may have had more severe hypertensive conditions than the other groups. All patients were also on diuretic. The study was not blind and subjects were not randomized to treatment. The 9% impotence reported in the diuretic-only group could have been higher than in the normal control group due to hypertension, the diuretic treatment itself, or both factors. It has been shown that impotence complaints more than double when normotensives are told they are hypertensive (Robbins, Elias, & Schultz, 1990). Apparently, patients assume the sick role and exaggerate other indications of disease.

While it appeared that the incidence of impotence in Hogan's study represented a change from baseline figures, it was not clear that the change necessarily indicated a higher rate. Hogan stated that his figures represented overall incidence of sexual dysfunction, which would include reports from all patients except those who no longer had a problem while on the study drug. Those who had improved or stayed the same would still be counted as impotent while on drug. Thus, if one perseveres in sorting through the statistical subtleties, one finds that the impotence rates for diuretic (9%), methyldopa/diuretic (13%), or clonidine/diuretic (15%) were not significantly different, despite the fact that they have been cited as meaningful differences in several reviews. The 23% impotence figure frequently cited for propranolol actually represented reactions to the combined effects of propranolol, hydralazine, and diuretic.

All in all, the sexual side effects of propranolol seem to be comparable to diuretics. The 1981 MRC side-effect questionnaires showed 22% impotence on diuretic versus 13.8% on propranolol and 8.9% on placebo. For diuretics, other side-effect figures were as high as 13–16% for symptoms such as dizziness, muscle pain, exertional dyspnea, and runny/blocked nose. Few were significant compared to placebo. However, after two years the rate of impotence due to propranolol remained the same, but diuretic-induced impotence increased with time (16.2% at three months to 22% at two years). These figures indicated that drug-induced sexual dysfunction may increase the longer the patient remains on diuretics.

Male/Female Differences No studies of male and female sexual side-effect differences have been performed on propranolol. Certain inferences, however, can be drawn. The high incidence of depression associated with propranolol in conjunction with the higher susceptibility of women to depression suggests that women would be more vulnerable to aggravation of depression by this drug than men. However, propranolol is capable of causing emotional problems in men they might otherwise not experience. Depression can be caused directly by the drug or indirectly as a result of impotence. In addition, depression can result in decreased libido and other manifestations of sexual dysfunction.

Because propranolol is used in young women for the treatment of migraine headaches (sometimes on a continual basis), sex drive disorders and depression may be induced at a relatively young age. Generally, though, women do not become candidates for hypertensive medication until menopause, when they become almost as susceptible to heart disease and hypertension as men. However, the vascular effects of beta-blockers are not as damaging to female sexual response as they are to erectile function. Nonetheless, the potential for depression is sufficiently great to recommend against the use of propranolol in women, unless other drugs are not effective.

Sexual Benefits No studies suggesting a direct sexual value for propranolol exist. However, due to its ability to decrease serotonin 5-HT_{1A} activity and decrease adrenergic activity, some clinicians have proposed that it might be valuable in the treatment of premature ejaculation by reducing anxiety and sex drive and by diminishing the sympathetic trigger for ejaculation. There is also the theoretical possibility that propranolol (or some version of a beta-blocker) might be valuable in the treatment of anxiety-induced impotence. Psychogenic impotence typically triggers an epinephrine response associated with fears of sexual performance not unlike stage fright. Since propranolol has been used widely to treat the peripheral manifestations of stage fright (Clark & Agras, 1991), it may have some limited value in helping intact, virile men, who become psychogenically impotent due to anxiety. However, lowering adrenergic excitation for one purpose—reducing anxiety—may compromise the excitation necessary for sexual anticipation and response.

Alternatives Newer, more specific beta-blockers such as atenolol or bisoprolol are recommended, as are ACE inhibitors, calcium channel-blockers, or alpha$_1$ blockers such as prazosin.

Atenolol

From our clinical experience and the reports of colleagues, it is clear that the specific beta-blocker atenolol (Tenormin) causes sexual dysfunction. The chief sexual side effect of atenolol is usually impotence, but decreased sex drive is also a problem. In clinical studies showing a reduction of sexual side effects by switching to a newly available antihypertensive, atenolol is often the prior drug that generated the sexual side effect. Even though sexual dysfunction is evident with atenolol, however, questionnaires have generally failed to identify the problem. Furthermore, atenolol compares well with the low sexual side-effect profile of ACE inhibitors in most studies (see Table 16.2). When there is a noticeable discrepancy between clinical experience and research reports, we would recommend that you trust your clinical judgment.

Sexual Side Effects Sexual dysfunction associated with atenolol is the result of both direct and indirect side effects. Though not often cited in reviews as evidence that atenolol has major adverse sexual effects, a 1989 article by Antonicelli, Piani, and Paciaroni reported that atenolol (100 mg) caused impotence in six middle-aged patients. In most cases, impotence was reversed when these patients were switched to captopril (50–100 mg). Weakness and fatigue due to atenolol also may have contributed indirectly to sexual dysfunction. Atenolol's specificity and lack of entry into the brain are assumed to prevent adverse sexual effects typical of beta-blockers. Consequently, atenolol has been suggested as a better alternative to older beta-blockers, a reputation which may not be entirely deserved.

Alternatives If a beta-blocker is necessary, the most sexually benign choice may be the recently marketed bisoprolol (Zebeta), which has not yet been shown to have negative sexual effects (Broekman, Haensel, Van de Ven, & Slob, 1992). To avoid the depression, fatigue, and sexual dysfunction associated with beta-blockers, ACE inhibitors and certain calcium channel blockers are the best alternatives.

Topical Ophthalmic Solutions

Until recently, eyedrops were not considered as a cause of sexual dysfunction. However, it has become apparent that some solutions can cause sexual effects equal to, or greater than, many oral medications. Timolol (Timoptic, Blocadren), for example, is a beta-blocker used in eyedrop form in the treatment of glaucoma. In retrospect, it is predictable that this medication could cause sexual dysfunction, as do other beta-blockers. Nonetheless, the first reports came as a surprise to the medical community and taught us that assumptions about the presence or absence of sexual side effects should not be based on the method of drug delivery.

Sexual Side Effects Fraunfelder and Meyer (1985) reported that the National Registry of Drug-Induced Ocular Side Effects had received complaints of sexual dysfunction from 25 patients treated with normal doses of the topical ocular beta-blocker, timolol. Twenty-three of the patients were male; two, female. Impotence was reported by 18 patients and decreased sex drive by nine. In most cases, sexual dysfunction was reversed upon discontinuance of the drug.

Fraunfelder and Meyer regarded this high number of sexual complaints as quite unusual, since no other eyedrop had ever been associated with sexual dysfunction. Their registry had never before received a report of sexual dysfunction on any other eyedrop. Ophthalmological patients are not usually questioned about sexual side effects, so the independent report of sexual dysfunction from 25 patients was actually quite impressive.

Timoptic was the 34th most prescribed drug

Table 16.2 *Quality-of-life Assessment: Atenolol vs. Ace Inhibitors*

Comparison Drugs	*Dose*	*Trial N*	*Trial Length*	*Differential Findings QL, SSE, SE*	*Reference*
Atenolol Captopril	50–100 mg 25–100 mg	125 M/F	8 weeks	No QL difference	Dahlöf, 1991
Atenolol Captopril Enalapril Propranolol	50–100 mg 94 mg 12 mg 132 mg	360 M	4 weeks	All drugs improved QL except propranolol	Steiner, Freidhoff, Wilson, Wecker, & Santo, 1990
Atenolol Captopril	50–100 mg 50–100 mg	306 M/F	8 weeks	Male sex index: Atenolol −0.20 ns Captopril +1.34 P < .05 Female sex index: Atenolol +1.75 ns Captopril +2.04 ns	Croog et al., 1990
Atenolol Captopril	50 mg 50 mg	125 M/F	8 weeks	No QL differences; improvement on some scales for both drugs	Fletcher et al., 1990
Atenolol Enalapril	50–100 mg 20–40 mg	162 M/F	12 weeks	No QL differences	Herrick et al., 1989
Atenolol Captopril Nifedipine Diuretic	50–100 mg 37.5–75 mg 40–80 mg	156 M	24 weeks	Atenolol: 26% decreased desire/erection; small decrease in sex index Captropril: no change	Suzuki, Tominaga, Kumagai, & Saruta, 1988
Atenolol Enalapril	50–100 mg 20–40 mg	58 M/F	4 weeks	No QL or SSE differences	Edmonds, Vetter, & Vetter, 1987
Atenolol Enalapril HCTZ	50–100 mg 20–40 mg 25–50 mg	436 M/F	16 weeks	Impotence: Atenolol +1.0 Enalapril +2.3 HCTZ +1.7 Atenolol: increased fatigue, muscular weakness, shortness of breath	Helgeland, Hagelund, Strommen, & Tretli, 1986
Atenolol Lisinopril	50–100 mg 10–20 mg	144 M/F	86 weeks	No SSE	Beevers et al., 1991

M = male; M/F = male/female; QL = quality of life; SE = side effect; SSE = sexual side effect

in the United States in 1983. Its manufacturer estimated that 1.4 million patients received glaucoma treatment during 1985, and 74% of these were being treated with Timoptic (Katz, 1986). While the manufacturer used these figures to minimize the reports of sexual dysfunction as insignificant, the same figures could be used to indicate how many patients were at risk for sexual dysfunction from Timoptic without knowing it.

Munroe, Rindone, and Kershner (1985) reviewed systemic side effects due to Timoptic. Until 1979, clinical trials with Timoptic had not reported central nervous system (CNS) side effects. In 1979, McMahon, Shaffer, Hoskins, and Hetherington reported a 10% rate of possible CNS side effects in 165 patients. By 1985, only three case reports of CNS effects secondary to Timoptic had been published, two involving hallucinations and one involving suicidal depression. However, during this same period—between 1978 and 1984—300 CNS side-effect reports of depression, confusion, hallucinations, fatigue, and decreased sex drive had been made to the National Registry. Shore, Fraunfelder, and Meyer (1987) analyzed 369 CNS reports given to the National Registry and reported 17% depression, 13% confusion, 11% fatigue, 10% dizziness, and 4% impotence. Most of these effects were reversible when Timoptic was discontinued. Other systemic side effects reported to the National Registry included bradycardia (72 reports) and various heart ailments (140 reports) such as heart failure, infarction, and angina. Pulmonary problems such as asthma, dyspnea, and respiratory distress were especially prevalent (200 reports). These breathing problems often occur with beta-blockers and can, in turn, cause sexual dysfunction.

Alternatives A new, topical ophthalmic beta-blocker called Betoptic (betaxolol) was introduced in 1985. This is an ophthalmic formulation of the beta-blocker betaxolol. Lynch, Whitson, Reay, Nguyen, and Drake (1988) contacted 18 patients who had experienced depression, sexual dysfunction, or emotional changes during Timoptic treatment. When switched to Betoptic, improvement was noted in 16 of the 18. Six of seven patients who had experienced impotence or decreased sex drive on Timoptic improved. De Vries, Van de Merwe, and Jan de Heer (1989) reported on many patients on Timoptic, whose symptoms (pulmonary effects, cardiac symptoms, headache and dizziness) resolved when switched to Betoptic. However, Betoptic was somewhat less effective in decreasing intraocular pressure. Duch, Duch, Pasto, and Ferrer (1992) studied eight glaucoma patients diagnosed with depression during chronic timolol treatment in a double-blind, crossover study with treatment by either timolol (Timoptic) or betatolol (Betoptic). Patients showed significantly higher depression scores on timolol than on betaxolol. In general, Betoptic has fewer peripheral effects than Timoptic and consequently a lower side-effect profile. For both quality of life and sexual function, Betoptic is preferable to Timoptic as long as it controls intraocular pressure equally well. A new, longer-acting formulation of ophthalmic timolol, Timoptic-XE, may be an improvement over Timoptic both in effectiveness and side effects.

ALPHA$_1$ BLOCKERS

Prazosin

Prazosin (Minipress) has many advantages due to its low side-effect profile. Its use avoids the adverse metabolic and inotropic changes of diuretics and beta-blockers. However, although prazosin can be helpful (at high doses) in the treatment of congestive heart failure, its therapeutic value diminishes with time. It is particularly useful in the treatment of asthma, since it does not block beta-adrenergic receptors and can aid bronchodilation through phosphodiesterase inhibition similar to theophylline. There is disagreement over whether prazosin causes dizziness and chronic susceptibility to orthostatic hypotension. It appears that these symptoms are more likely to occur when patients take their medication erratically.

Some of the newer alpha$_1$ blockers appear to cause more side effects than prazosin. However, this greater incidence of side effects may be due to the greater appreciation of the presence of side effects in the late 1980s. In a placebo-controlled study, doxazosin (Cardura) caused asthenia/weakness in 41% of the 17 patients (Young & Brogden, 1988). Other side effects were also frequent: palpitations (29%), dizziness (24%) and headache (24%). The labeling on doxazosin (*Physicians Desk Reference*, 1991a) warns that dizziness (19% on doxazosin versus 9% on placebo) and fatigue/malaise (12% on doxazosin versus 6% on placebo) are frequent, and that weight gain and somnolence occur significantly more than on placebo. Sexual dysfunction is noted for 2% of patients versus 1% on placebo. Terazosin (Hytrin) has also shown significant side effects compared to placebo (*PDR*, 1991a; Sperzel, Glassman, Jordon, & Luther, 1986):

dizziness (19.3% versus 7.5%), asthenia (11.3% versus 4.3%), somnolence (5.9% versus 2.6%), and palpitations (4.3% versus 1.2%). However, the labeling notes less impotence on terazosin (1.6%) than on placebo (1.9%).

Although side effects from doxazosin and terazosin are more frequent than usually shown with prazosin, studies directly comparing terazosin with prazosin have shown no differences. Evidently, prazosin must also cause such effects, since these drugs have the same pharmacological action. It is safe to assume that when dizziness, fatigue, asthenia, and somnolence are present, some degree of sexual dysfunction is also probable. A recent 29-week study of doxazosin treatment of symptomatic benign prostatic hyperplasia showed no decrease in sexual function in any patient (Holme et al., 1994).

Sexual Side Effects Prazosin has maintained its reputation for minimal or no sexual side effects for many years. Although some sexual side effects do occur during prazosin treatment, with the exception of retarded ejaculation, which is occasionally reported, they appear to be infrequent. A large, six-month study by the Veterans Administration (VA, 1981) compared hydrochlorothiazide (HCTZ) in combination with prazosin (10mg/day) or hydralazine in male patients. Patients with pre-existing sexual dysfunction were excluded from the calculations regarding sexual side effects. Considerable sexual dysfunction was noted for prazosin in combination with diuretic (27.7%) compared to 17.8% on hydralazine plus diuretic. This sexual dysfunction continued for at least two months in 16.3% of patients on prazosin and 8.5% on hydralazine. Prazosin patients also showed significantly more lethargy, dizziness, and orthostatic hypotension. Perhaps due to the high prevalence of these side effects, compliance was 70% or less. It is unclear whether the high rate of sexual dysfunction was due to diuretic or prazosin. Strangely, this 1981 trial showing substantial sexual dysfunction (16–28%) on prazosin is rarely cited in the literature. Instead, a 1975 low surveillance figure of 0.6% is repeatedly given.

The chief adverse sexual effect noted for prazosin has been priapism (Stevenson & Umstead, 1984). Many cases of priapism have been reported under a variety of circumstances, sometimes with concurrent disease such as renal failure. Prazosin may cause priapism by adrenergic blockade of the sympathetic system, which mediates detumescence through adrenergic-induced vasoconstriction. Drug-induced priapism is not accompanied by pleasurable sensations. On the contrary, it is often painful and can cause permanent penile tissue damage if not reversed promptly. In addition, drugs that cause priapism often have other negative effects on sexual functioning.

Sexual Benefits Possible therapeutic uses of antihypertensive adrenergic blockers in the treatment of premature ejaculation are yet to be investigated. A relative of this class, phenoxybenzamine, is a powerful adrenergic inhibitor, well known in clinical circles to inhibit ejaculation. Through its effect on adrenergic-sympathetic responses, prazosin might be helpful in treating premature ejaculation. However, even with labetalol, which has been shown to inhibit ejaculation at high doses, this potential has not been realized. If prazosin is strong enough to block orgasm and ejaculation, it may also be potent enough to undermine arousal. The combination of prazosin with one of the new SSRIs could work synergistically to delay orgasm/ejaculation in premature ejaculators. Whether this drug combination would result in better sympathetic control or in increased depression of arousal, however, remains open to question. Both doxazosin and terazosin have been shown to successfully treat the symptoms of benign prostatic hypertrophy without apparent negative effects on sexual function (Holme et al., 1994).

Labetalol

Labetalol (Trandate, Normodyne) is an efficient and potent antihypertensive with few toxic metabolic effects when used at moderate dosages. Although it is generally categorized as an $alpha_1$ antagonist, labetalol has both alpha- and beta-blocking properties. The combination of these properties serves to minimize beta-blocking effects such as fatigue, depression, bradycardia, cold hands and feet, diabetic complications, and sleep disruption. When prazosin is not sufficient to control blood pressure, labetalol is a potent alternative. Combinations of alpha- and beta-blockers such as prazosin with atenolol are rarely used but deserve investigation.

Sexual Side Effects In our experience, doctors sometimes try to use labetalol at low doses (200–400 mg) to avoid sexual problems. Unfortunately, addition of a diuretic is often needed for efficacy. Since diuretics can cause sexual and metabolic problems, any advantage of a lower labetalol dose is lost by adding diuretics. Decreased desire, impotence, and ejaculation failure have been noted in about 10% of labetalol patients in smaller studies.

In a long-term open study of 337 labetalol patients, 14% experienced sexual dysfunction, usually failed ejaculation or impotence, and 7% withdrew due to these symptoms (Michelson et al., 1983). Ohman and Asplund (1984) found blocked ejaculation in four of 27 subjects on labetalol (300–1200 mg). One patient considered it a "good male contraceptive drug," because it prevented ejaculation. However, at doses strong enough to block ejaculation, labetalol also causes fatigue, muscle weakness, dizziness, blurred vision, and even heart failure. Dux, Grosskopf, Boner, and Rosenfeld (1986) closely monitored the side effects of labetalol in patients with moderate hypertension (diastolic over 100 mm). Doses between 600 and 800 mg were used. Impotence and muscle weakness were found in six of 29 patients; weight gain also occurred (mean increase of 4.3 kg overall); intermittent claudication was noted in three patients; dizziness, in four; and five patients chose to withdraw due to impotence. O'Meara and White (1988) described three cases of failed ejaculation on labetalol. One patient reported a time-sensitive effect: no ejaculate three hours after labetalol; decreased and thin ejaculate six hours afterward; and normal ejaculate eight to ten hours afterward. None of the men experienced ejaculatory failure on other antihypertensives.

In a study comparing labetalol (up to 600 mg) and propranolol, sexual side effects occurred in 10 of (8/81) of labetalol patients versus 7% (6/84) on propranolol (Flamenbaum et al., 1985). Ejaculation failure occurred in four labetalol patients but in none of the propranolol patients. Greater fatigue was noted on propranolol than on labetalol (13% versus 5%), but more dizziness was reported on labetalol (12% versus 3%). Frishman, Shapiro, and Charlap (1989) noted ejaculation failure in two of 21 and impotence in three of 21 labetalol patients compared to a single ejaculation failure and no impotence on propranolol.

Stokes, Mennie, Gellatly, and Hill (1983) compared labetalol to an alpha-blocker (prazosin) and beta-blocker (metoprolol) given together. Among 19 labetalol patients, impotence occurred in four and failed ejaculation in three. With the prazosin and metoprolol combination, no impotence or failed ejaculation was reported (0/8).

In contrast to the notable sexual side effects of labetolol found in the smaller studies, larger surveillance studies have failed to identify sexual problems. Gomez and Philips (1980) found only five instances of sexual dysfunction and nine instances of fatigue or lethargy among 1,286 patients treated with labetalol for up to two years. Sexual dysfunction was reported in less than 1% of patients. However, surveillance study figures may not be the best indicators of the presence of drug side effects.

Male/Female Differences The only study of labetalol's effects on female sexual response was conducted by Riley and Riley (1981), who administered 100 mg labetalol, 80 mg propranolol, or placebo to six normal subjects. The women stimulated themselves to orgasm after ingesting each drug, and blood pressure at orgasm was recorded. Labetalol caused a reduction in the blood pressure spike that typically occurs during orgasm. In subjective ratings, labetalol caused a reduction in lubrication. No differences were noticed on propranolol or placebo. (Labetalol might prove helpful for women who experience hypertensive vascular headaches during orgasm.) No other adverse sexual side effects have been noted in female patients. Given the effects on males, however, it is probable that additional female sexual dysfunction eventually will be associated with labetalol.

Sexual Benefits Riley, Riley and Davies (1982) have suggested that labetalol could be used to treat premature ejaculation. Measuring erection and time to ejaculation in six normal subjects on labetalol, they found that, compared to placebo, ejaculation was delayed minimally with 100 mg of labetalol and clearly evident at 300 mg. Erection and subjective arousal were not affected with this acute treatment. They then administered 200 mg labetalol to premature ejaculators prior to intercourse. No improvement was noted, but the researchers noticed that labetalol extended erection beyond ejaculation in some of their subjects, suggesting that labetalol might cause priapism.

Indoramin

Indoramin (Wypress) is an $alpha_1$ blocker widely used in Europe but not available in the United States. Fatigue, sedation, and weight gain are common side effects. The sexual side effects of indoramin resemble those of older, peripheral $alpha_1$ blockers such as guanethidine more than those of prazosin. Holmes and Sorkin (1986) have reviewed the incidence of ejaculatory failure in patients on indoramin, citing a pilot trial examining patients with migraine which reported 55% (6/11) ejaculation failure. However, multi-center surveillance trials found only 2.5% ejaculation failures in 569 male patients treated up to 24 months. Indoramin is usually given in conjunction with a diuretic, which would compound its negative effects on sexual functioning. Though said to be rare, erection difficulties could develop with prolonged use secondary to impairment of ejaculation. Ejaculation failure figures range from 8% to 40%. Indoramin can also decrease sperm motility. Table 16.3 summarizes the characteristics and side effects of $alpha_1$ blockers.

Alternatives The best alternatives to $alpha_1$ blockers are ACE inhibitors and newer calcium channel blockers. In summary, most $alpha_1$-blocker studies have concentrated on prazosin and labetalol; less is known about the other drugs in this class. Prazosin is relatively free of sexual side effects, but is often used with diuretics that cause sexual problems. Labetalol, a stronger adrenergic blocker that has some beta-blocker activity, has dose-dependent effects inhibiting ejaculation. Sexual side effects appear minimal with the newer $alpha_1$ blockers, terazosin and doxazosin. However, symptoms may become more apparent in time. Other side effects such as dizziness and fatigue may be more frequent with indoramin than with prazosin and indirectly cause sexual problems.

$ALPHA_2$ AGONISTS (CLONIDINE)

$Alpha_2$ agonists reduce sympathetic activity by stimulating $alpha_2$ receptors, which decrease adrenergic activity through the inhibition of $alpha_1$ receptor adrenergic transmission. Clonidine (Catapres) is the representative $alpha_2$ agonist usually employed for research involving adrenergic/sympathetic activity. It is also the most common $alpha_2$ agonist used in the treatment of hypertension.

Sexual Side Effects Clonidine has negative effects on neurotransmitters related to sexual function: It reduces activation (hyperpolarizes) of neurotransmitters that promote sexual activation (dopamine, acetylcholine, epinephrine), and it reinforces neurotransmitters that reduce sexual activation (opiates, serotonin). Through reduction of cortisol and adrenergic excess, clonidine may have a tranquilizing effect that could be helpful for sexual dysfunction due to persistent nervousness and anxiety. When clonidine was first introduced, it had a low sexual side-effect profile, which encouraged its use in large doses (over 1 mg/day). At these doses, however, clinicians soon discovered that clonidine caused adverse sexual effects comparable to those of methyldopa. Despite the fact that subsequent use of clonidine at doses below 1 mg (0.2 to 0.8 mg/day) demonstrated fewer adverse sexual effects, its reputation has persisted. Doctors often assume, incorrectly, that sexual effects due to clonidine are inevitable and, when sexual problems are encountered, switch to alternative antihypertensives, rather than first trying a lower dosage.

Studies have shown increased eating and weight gain with clonidine treatment. It is possible that the adrenergic stimulation of $alpha_2$ receptors

Table 16.3 *Profile of Alpha$_1$ Blockers*

	Daily Dose
Doxazosin (Cardura)	1–16 mg
Indoramin (Wypress*)	50–200 mg
Labetalol (Trandate, Normodyne)	400–800 mg
Prazosin (Minipress)	1–20 mg
Terazosin (Hytrin)	1–20 mg

COMMON INDICATIONS
Hypertension

MECHANISMS OF ACTION (GENERAL)
Decreases peripheral vascular resistance
Blocks adrenergic alpha$_1$ receptors
Inhibits phosphodiesterase enzyme activity (prazosin)
Blocks both alpha$_1$ and beta-adrenergic receptors

MECHANISMS OF ACTION (SEXUAL)
Negative
Decreased adrenergic (alpha$_1$) activity

DIRECT SEXUAL SIDE EFFECTS
Erection difficulties
- Priapism
- Impotence

Ejaculation retarded

INDIRECT SEXUAL SIDE EFFECTS
Discomfort caused by dryness of skin, mouth, mucous membranes, edema, nasal congestion, nausea, rash/itching, urinary problems (incontinence), weight gain, shortness of breath

Mood disorders resulting in depression, nervousness

Neurological disturbances resulting in dizziness, fatigue, headache, pain, paresthesia, sedation, muscular weakness

Vascular disturbances resulting in arrhythmias, headache, orthostatic hypotension

SEXUAL CONTRAINDICATIONS/BENEFITS

Avoid with prior condition of	*May be useful for*
Impotence	Orgasmic headaches (labetalol)
Ejaculatory problems	Premature ejaculation
Priapism	
Anorgasmia	

ALTERNATIVES
ACE Inhibitors
Calcium channel blockers
Indapamide (Lozol)

*Not available in the United States.

by clonidine facilitates neuropeptide Y, a peptide that can inhibit sexual activity. Stimulation of alpha$_2$ receptors can also decrease insulin, causing other metabolic effects that promote diabetes and decrease fat breakdown (Vidal & Riou, 1989). All of these factors can contribute indirectly to sexual dysfunction.

Large, well-controlled longitudinal studies have not been conducted to investigate the sexual effects of clonidine. Recent studies in which low doses of clonidine or clonidine patches were used have shown little sexual dysfunction. However, as we have seen, diuretics also registered few sexual side effects originally, until investigated in controlled, longitudinal trials.

An early trial of clonidine treatment with moderate doses (0.6 to 1.0 mg/day) showed a 24% (14/59) incidence of impotence, which was persistent in 22% of the subjects (Onesti, Bock, Heimsoth, Kim, & Merguet, 1971). However, other trials of clonidine treatment have shown little or no sexual dysfunction: Mrozek, Leibl, and Finnerty (1972) reported 9.0% (1/11) impotence; Jerie (1986) noted impotence in 6 of 126 clonidine patients (5%) versus 2 of 123 placebo patients (2%). Ferder, Inserra, and Medina (1987) reported 3.3% (2/60) impotence; Planitz (1987) reported 0% (0/30) sexual dysfunction; and Schmidt, Schuna, and Goodfriend (1989) reported 9% (2/22) impotence in elderly patients over 60.

Langley and Heel (1988) reported a 6% impotence rate with transdermal clonidine in an extensive review article. Previously, Popli et al. (1986) had reported no incidence of sexual dysfunction in 15 patients on transdermal clonidine and, further, found that the incidence of drowsiness was no different between clonidine and placebo patients (13% versus 13%). A quality-of-life study by McMahon, Jain, Vargas, and Fillingim (1990) comparing transdermal clonidine to oral captopril treatment for eight weeks, showed impotence in 1 of 33 patients on clonidine and 0 of 35 on captopril. A slight decrease in satisfaction with sex life and energy/vitality was found in transdermal clonidine patients.

Clonidine has actions opposite to yohimbine, which blocks alpha$_2$ receptors. Since yohimbine is considered a selective sexual stimulant, it has been hypothesized that clonidine prevents sexual stimulation or acts as a sexual depressant (see Chapter 31). It is difficult to distinguish specific sexual depressant effects due to clonidine from its overall sedative properties. Animal research has shown that yohimbine directly stimulates areas of the brain that govern sexual activity, such as the anterior hypothalamus and, in particular, receptors stimulated by testosterone. It is possible that clonidine (particularly at high doses) inhibits stimulation in these brain regions and at these receptor sites. The clinical effect would range from a specific reduction of blood flow to the genitals to a general decrease in attention and alertness needed for sexual activation. In addition, clonidine has been found to reduce the arousal peptide vasopressin (Peskind et al., 1987). Alpha$_2$ agonists also inhibit other peptides that contribute to genital excitement, including VIP, prostaglandins, and substance P (Cox & Cuthbert, 1989).

It is possible that some of the negative effects of alpha$_2$ agonists are balanced by their positive effects as imidazole agonists, resulting in fewer sexual and metabolic problems with clonidine than might be otherwise expected. Clonidine, which is itself an imidazole drug, may stimulate imidazole receptors (Lehmann, Koenig-Berard, & Vitou, 1989). Drugs active at imidazole receptors can stimulate sexual activity (Ferrari, Baggio, & Martinelli, 1986). However, such a sex-facilitating effect of clonidine through imidazole receptors is contradicted by the finding that clonidine antagonizes both yohimbine and imidazole stimulation of copulation (Ferrari et al., 1986). Downie, Espey, and Gajewski (1991) showed that clonidine acted in the spinal cord of the cat to depress pudendal nerve reflexes, an action that could interfere with erectile and urinary function. Previously, Downie and Bialik (1988) had shown that clonidine depressed the bulbocavernosus reflex. The bulbocavernosus muscle is involved in orgasm and maintenance of penile rigidity (McKenna & Nadelhaft, 1989). Depression of the bulbocavernosus reflex may reflect interference. Depression of the bulbocavernosus reflex in cats by clonidine was also shown by Galeano, Corcos, Carmel and Jubelin (1989).

Male/Female Differences There is persuasive evidence from the study of animals that clonidine reduces active sexual activity (Clark & Smith, 1990). Its facilitation of lordosis in some animals is typical of drugs that promote passive reception of sexual advances, such as GABA agonists and serotonergic agents, and may involve a tranquilizing action similar to benzodiazepines.

Since men seem to be more vulnerable to peripheral vasoconstriction than women, there is

Table 16.4 *Profile of Alpha$_2$ Agonists*

	Daily dose
Clonidine (Catapres)	0.1–0.15 mg
(Catapres TTS transdermal patch – one weekly)	0.1 to 0.3 mg/day
Guanfacine (Tenex)	1–3 mg

COMMON INDICATIONS

Hypertension
Opiate/alcohol withdrawal

MECHANISMS OF ACTION (GENERAL)

Stimulates alpha$_2$ adrenergic receptors
Inhibits presynaptic release of catecholamines at synapse
Decreases activity at alpha$_1$ adrenergic receptors
Decreases sympathetic/adrenergic transmission

MECHANISMS OF ACTION (SEXUAL)

Positive

Decreased cortisol
Increased growth hormone

Negative

Decreased adrenergic (alpha$_1$) activity
Increased adrenergic (alpha$_2$) activity
Decreased cholinergic activity
Increased opioids
Decreased prostaglandins
Decreased substance P
Decreased vasoactive intestinal peptide
Decreased vasopressin

DIRECT SEXUAL SIDE EFFECTS

Desire disorders (in both sexes)
Erection difficulties
Ejaculation retarded

INDIRECT SEXUAL SIDE EFFECTS

Discomfort caused by constipation, dryness of skin, mouth, mucous membranes, nausea, rash/itching (local rash experienced at site of TTS transdermal patch), urinary problems (retention)

Mood disorders resulting in depression, nervousness

Neurological disturbances resulting in analgesia, cognitive deficits, dizziness, fatigue, sedation, sensory loss, asthenia – a feeling of weakness

Vascular disturbances resulting in orthostatic hypotension, peripheral vasoconstriction

Endocrine disturbances precipitating or aggravating diabetes

SEXUAL CONTRAINDICATIONS/BENEFITS

Avoid with prior condition of

Desire disorders
Impotence
Ejaculatory problems

May be useful for

Premature ejaculation?

ALTERNATIVES

ACE Inhibitors
Alpha$_1$ blockers
Calcium channel blockers
Indapamide (Lozol)

some possibility that men are more sensitive to the sympathetic/adrenergic changes that occur with clonidine. Freedman, Sabharwal, and Desai (1986) found that men, but not women, experienced peripheral dose-related vasoconstriction in response to clonidine infusions. However, no male/female differences were found for vasodilating and vasoconstricting substances (nitroglycerin and digoxin), which act directly on vascular smooth muscle rather than through adrenergic receptors.

In summary, $alpha_2$ agonists have the potential to cause sex-drive disorders in both sexes via their sedative effects and impotence in the male secondary to peripheral vasoconstriction. Among the older blood-pressure medications, clonidine given at low doses is probably kinder to sexual function than most, although it, too, should be avoided in patients with preexisting sex-drive or erection deficiencies. Table 16.4 summarizes the characteristics and side effect of $alpha_2$ agonists.

Alternatives The transdermal clonidine patch is preferable to oral clonidine due to the lower dose required for equal therapeutic effect. $Alpha_1$ antagonists, such as prazosin or terazosin, are alternatives that also decrease sympathetic/adrenergic activity. Although newer calcium channel-blockers (e.g., felodipine, amlodipine) or diltiazem (Cardizem) achieve similar effects, ACE inhibitors are the antihypertensive drugs of choice at this time.

17

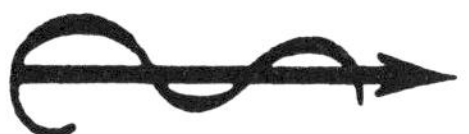

Ace Inhibitors and Calcium Channel Blockers

OBJECTIVES

- To define the sexual advantages and drawbacks
- To identify previously unidentified sexual problems with calcium channel blockers

Angiotensin-converting enzyme (ACE) inhibitors and calcium channel blockers are currently the most effective antihypertensive medications for patients who wish to avoid sexual dysfunction. Thus far, ACE inhibitors appear to be the most benign and may have additional advantages for quality of life and, perhaps, even longevity. Calcium channel blockers, perhaps due to their peripheral vasodilating properties (which may have the potential to facilitate erection), quickly developed a reputation as sexually benign antihypertensives. However, in time it became clear that calcium channel blockers, such as nifedipine and verapamil, could decrease sex drive and orgasmic responsiveness/intensity in both sexes. Nonetheless, in comparison to antihypertensives like beta-blockers, reserpine, guanethidine, and diuretics, calcium channel blockers are still a tremendous improvement.

The marketing of ACE inhibitors and calcium channel blockers has had a profound historical impact on the direction of drug development and research. The manufacturer of the first ACE inhibitor, captopril, used the low incidence of sexual side effects associated with this novel antihypertensive as a formidable marketing tool. Patients' responses to these particular drugs have demonstrated to physicians and pharmaceutical companies alike that there is a tremendous demand for drugs that preserve sexual function. Attitudes are indeed changing. A few decades ago, sexual dysfunction was assumed to be a necessary price to pay for health when illness required drug therapy. Today, the industry has discovered the commercial value of protecting the sexual lives of patients. Hopefully, this new direction in drug research will accelerate research and development in this area.

ACE INHIBITORS

Captopril, the first ACE inhibitor, was derived from snake venom (Ferreira, 1985). Similar to Gila monster venom, it stimulates potent vasodilating sensory peptides in the genitals, skin, and mouth. Captopril was subsequently successfully synthesized by chemists at Squibb Pharmaceuticals, eliminating the need for a large source of snake venom and allowing oral dosing. Most of the literature on ACE inhibitors pertains to captopril (see also Chapter 14), since enalapril and lisinopril have been marketed relatively recently. Captopril was approved by the Federal Drug Administration in 1981 for the treatment of heart failure and severe hypertension. The initial Federal Drug Administration labeling approved its use only for "patients who have failed on multi-drug therapy (including triple therapy)," with the warning that "adverse effects have occurred (proteinuria, membranous glomerulopathy, neutropenia, agranulocytosis, hypotension, and impaired renal functions)."

Consequently, captopril was used to treat only high-risk cardiovascular patients with compromised immune systems or renal insufficiency, who had been unresponsive to other antihypertensives. Because of the high dosage used (over 400 mg/day), there was a 7.2% incidence of neutropenia. However, in patients without renal insufficiency, the incidence of neutropenia was only 0.2%. In fact, captopril has been shown to have a protective effect on the renal system, which can prevent such deterioration from occurring (Schersten, 1988).

Captopril's advantages and side-effect profile became apparent as lower doses were used in more typical cardiovascular patients. (Williams, 1988, has written a comprehensive review of ACE-inhibitor development, clinical use, and chemical actions, summarizing the previous information in far greater detail.) Captopril also produces an inotropic action (increased force of cardiac output), which is an advantage over antihypertensives (e.g., some calcium channel blockers) that result in negative inotropy. A mild weight-loss feature is also attractive. Some articles have suggested that captopril may also function as an antidepressant through mood improvement (e.g., Cohen & Zubenko, 1988; Deicken, 1986; Germain & Chouinard, 1989).

All ACE inhibitors have secondary actions, both positive and negative, due to the fact that the angiotensin enzyme is also involved in the breakdown of prostaglandins, bradykinin, and enkephalin. Captopril appears to have a particularly strong effect on these peptides (Zusman, 1984). Positive secondary actions include potentiation of sensation and blood flow in peripheral tissues, including the genitals (see Chapter 30), and unique antioxidant and free radical scavenging properties. However, some peptides stimulated by ACE inhibitors can cause negative side effects as well. Bradykinin is associated with pain and aches due to colds, and prostaglandin inhibition is the chief mechanism by which aspirin or ibuprofen reduces pain, fever, and inflammation. Severe rash (rare but serious), autoimmune reactions, and loss of taste have also been associated with captopril. These unusual effects are thought to be the result of captopril's sulfhydryl chemical structure (common to other drugs such as penicillamine) (Przyklenk & Kloner, 1991). Subsequent ACE inhibitors such as enalapril have been considered safer because they lack this sulfhydryl structure.

Although captopril was initially targeted for use with congestive heart-failure patients, it was approved by the Federal Drug Administration for treatment of all levels of hypertension in 1985 and is now widely used as an antihypertensive. The influential study report (Croog et al., 1986) on quality-of-life benefits helped it to become a part of routine clinical practice. This study, which set standards for many to follow, concluded that captopril had no adverse effects on the quality of sex. A subsequent analysis of the 1986 study (Croog et al., 1988) focused entirely on the differential sexual effects of captopril and remains a model for evaluative surveillance research on the sexual side effects of antihypertensive drugs. The results indicated that captopril had significantly fewer negative effects on sexual functioning than several other antihypertensive drugs.

It should be noted, however, that captopril was not compared to some of the newer antihypertensive drugs that have different mechanisms of action. A 22-week antihypertensive quality-of-life study on 309 women aged 60 to 80 years showed no significant sexual or quality-of-life differences between the ACE inhibitor enalapril (Vasotec), the beta-blocker atenolol (Tenormin), or the newer calcium channel blocker isradipine (DynaCirc) (Croog et al., 1994). An influential and favorable review of ACE-inhibitor use in the *New England Journal of Medicine* (Williams, 1988) provided a comparison of ACE inhibitors and asserted that the long-acting drugs such as enalapril and lisinopril had "more frequent and more serious" side effects than the short-acting captopril, an assertion subject to dispute. However, a 24-week double-blind quality-of-life study on 379 hypertensive men by Testa et al. (1993) showed no differences in sexual drive or function between captopril and enalapril (both groups showed a slight decline, possibly due to the use of diuretics by some patients).

By 1989, United States doctors were prescribing ACE inhibitors as often as diuretics and beta-blockers for initial antihypertensive treatment, particularly for patients under 60 years old (Bostick et al., 1991). Of the 20 most frequently prescribed drugs in the United States, enalapril ranked eleventh and captopril, fifteenth (*American Medical News*, 1991). However, beta-blockers and diuretics were preferred in other industrial nations (e.g., Germany) during 1988, with calcium channel blockers as the chief alternative (Weiland et al., 1991). Table 17.1 summarizes the characteristics and side effects of ACE inhibitors.

Sexual Side Effects

Drug-related impotence is occasionally reported with captopril and other ACE inhibitors. However, the percentages for impotence recorded for both placebo and drug are lower than the estimated percentage in the general population. For example, a Veterans Administration study (VA, 1984) compared captopril, hydrochlorothiazide, and both in combination. With long-term treatment, 4% impotence was reported with hydrochlorothiazide, 0.8% impotence with captopril (the minimum placebo rate expected would be 1%), and 2.3% impotence for the combination of both drugs used together. Weakness and fatigue occurred in 8.8% of the hydrochlorothiazide group, 4.6% of the captopril group (3.4% expected on placebo), and 14.3% for the combination. Apparently, the addition of thiazide increases the incidence of impotence. In the quality-of-life measurements, captopril appeared to have few negative sexual effects, unless it was used in conjunction with diuretics. Indirect sexual side effects secondary to weakness and fatigue are not common with captopril, but should be recognized as such when they occur.

Although the assumption that ACE inhibitors do not have adverse sexual side effects is derived from research, it should be recalled that in the captopril quality-of-life study (Croog et al., 1986) physicians discontinued the use of the drug with five patients because of sexual symptoms; in addition, six were withdrawn from propranolol and six from methyldopa. Therefore, the claim that ACE inhibitors produce no adverse sexual effects is exaggerated and potentially misleading. Nonetheless, it *is* encouraging that, in spite of wider use, there have been few reports of negative sexual effects, either direct or indirect, due to ACE inhibitors. However, it would be premature to draw absolute conclusions; more problems may become apparent with additional years of clinical use. One example of this point has been demonstrated recently. The incidence of cough was originally listed as 0.5% for captopril versus 1.33% for enalapril (Federal Drug Administration reviewed *PDR* labeling). Subsequent experience has shown that the true incidence of cough for all ACE inhibitors appears to be nearly 6% (Sebastian, McKinney, Kaufman, & Young, 1991; Yeo, MacLean, Richardson, & Ramsay, 1991). These figures strongly suggest previously unreliable data and underreporting of side effects. Therefore, until long-term studies provide verification, we cannot be certain how ACE inhibitors affect sexual functioning.

Negative sexual and psychological effects appear to be less frequent with captopril than with enalapril or lisinopril (Warner & Rush, 1988). Although the incidence of sexual dysfunction is still negligible with this class of drug, impotence seems to occur more often with the newer ACE inhibitors than with captopril. There seems to be more fatigue, lassitude, and dizziness with enalapril and lisinopril—approximately twice that of captopril and sometimes equal to the beta-blocker atenolol (Frcka & Lader, 1988). Enalapril may have more psychological side effects, such as depression and fatigue, whereas captopril has more pronounced physical side effects, such as rashes and allergic reactions (Warner & Rush, 1988). While beta-blockers and some ACE inhibitors cause varying degrees of depression, captopril does not appear to have this effect. In fact, there is some evidence to suggest that ACE inhibitors positively affect mood. Hodsman et al. (1983) reported that several patients on enalapril felt increased well-being. Frcka and Lader surveyed normal subjects after eight days of enalapril treatment. Increased calmness as

Table 17.1 *Profile of Angiotensin-Converting Enzyme (Ace) Inhibitors*

	Daily Dose
Benazepril (Lotensin)	20–40 mg
Captopril (Capoten)	25–100 mg
Enalapril (Vasotec)	5–40 mg
Fosinoprol (Monopril)	20–80 mg
Lisinopril (Zestril, Prinivil)	5–40 mg
Quinapril (Accupril)	10–80 mg
Ramipril (Altace)	5–40 mg

COMMON INDICATIONS
- Hypertension
- Congestive heart failure

MECHANISMS OF ACTION (GENERAL)
- Inhibits angiotensin-induced vasoconstriction
- Reduces peripheral vascular resistance
- Inhibits the angiotensin-converting enzyme
- Decreases conversion of angiotensin I into angiotensin II
- Deceases aldosterone
- Increases plasma renin activity
- Increases potassium

MECHANISMS OF ACTION (SEXUAL)

Positive
- Decreased angiotensin II
- Increased calcitonin-gene-related-peptide
- Increased cholinergic activity
- Increased prostaglandins
- Increased substance P

Negative
- Decreased adrenergic ($alpha_1$) activity
- Decreased luteinizing hormone releasing hormone
- Increased opioids
- Decreased vasopressin

DIRECT SEXUAL SIDE EFFECTS
- Erection difficulties
- Birth defects

INDIRECT SEXUAL SIDE EFFECTS

Discomfort caused by persistent cough, edema, indigestion, nausea, pain, rash/itching, weight loss

Mood disorder resulting in depression

Neurological disturbances resulting in dizziness, fatigue, headache, loss of taste, muscular weakness

Vascular disturbances resulting in headache, peripheral vasodilation, hypotension

SEXUAL CONTRAINDICATIONS/BENEFITS

Avoid with prior condition of
- Erectile disorders (psychogenic)

May be useful for
- Erectile disorders (vascular)
- Premature ejaculation

ALTERNATIVES
- Amlodipine (Norvasc)
- Felodipine (Plendil)
- Isradipine (DynaCirc)
- Bisoprolol (Zebeta)
- Indapamide (Lozol)
- Prazosin (Minipress)

well as increased headaches were reported. Olajide and Lader (1985) observed hypertensive patients and medical student controls on enalapril. On the Profile of Mood States (POMS) mood scale, high levels of energy and even clinical euphoria were reported. Subjects felt "nervous and restless, but also alert, happy, and energetic." Similar mood-elevating effects have occasionally been noted with captopril (Zubenko & Nixon, 1984). Cohen and Zubenko (1988) successfully treated one woman for depression with captopril and four patients with co-existing depression and hypertension. Germain and Chouinard (1989) successfully treated seven depressed patients with captopril and showed an antidepressant effect for captopril versus placebo in a small study (n = 14).

Male/Female Differences

Since women are more susceptible to immune disregulation (Schuurs & Verheul, 1990), skin reactions induced by ACE inhibitors can be expected to be more frequent and severe in women and should be monitored closely. Also, the incidence of severe and persistent cough is greater in women than in men (Yeo et al., 1991) and may precipitate stress incontinence as well as associated sexual inhibitions. Although ACE inhibitors appear to be relatively free of sexual side effects, the few reported cases target male erection and ejaculation. There is no indication of problems with sex drive in either sex.

Sexual Benefits

A major marketing attraction of ACE inhibitors is their apparent lack of sexual side effects. Given that negative sexual effects with captopril have rarely been reported in the literature, we have the luxury of speculating on the possible sexual properties of captopril compared to other old, new, and still investigatory antihypertensives.

For possible beneficial effects on sexuality, ACE inhibitors are the only class of antihypertensives recommended. Resolution of drug-induced impotence has been reported once patients have been switched to ACE inhibitors. For example, Antonicelli et al. (1989) studied nine men between the ages of 36 and 57 who had been treated successfully with beta-blockers but were complaining of impotence. Six of these men were being treated with 100 mg atenolol. When captopril was substituted for atenolol at doses of 50 to 100 mg, blood pressure was adequately controlled and resolution of impotence was reported by all six men within three months. Another patient showed improvement, but two patients remained impotent.

Captopril may also be efficacious in treating psychogenic sexual dysfunction resulting from anxiety reactions (e.g., the epinephrine reflex) by interfering with the production of angiotensin II, which potentiates adrenergic vasoconstriction. With long-term ACE-inhibitor treatment, adrenergic activity might decrease to a lower set-point, so that fight-or-flight adrenergic reactions have less physiological impact. If such were the case, sex therapy could be used to take advantage of captopril-induced changes, and captopril could become a resource in the treatment of psychogenic impotence.

Since ACE inhibitors lower adrenergic reaction potential, it is conceivable that they could also delay the ejaculatory response, which works through an adrenergic mechanism. Further investigation of captopril as an adjunct to the treatment of premature ejaculation is warranted, despite the fact that no reports of decreased or inhibited ejaculation with any ACE inhibitor have been published to date.

ACE inhibitors can increase blood-flow by two mechanisms—vasodilation and inhibition of vasoconstriction, thereby creating a favorable internal "environment" for achieving erection. Comparable to their beneficial effects on heart tissue, ACE inhibitors can decrease pathological smooth muscle hypertrophy and improve circulation in blood vessel walls (Clozel, Kuhn, & Hefti, 1990). Substance P, prostaglandins, and CGRP peptides are involved in sensation and blood flow and are highly concentrated in the genitals; captopril stimulates the activity of these peptides (Zusman, 1984).

As noted, captopril stimulates a range of peptides, such as prostaglandin E2 and substance

P, which can have major sexual arousal benefits, particularly in the genitals where these peptides have vasodilating and sensory properties. The physical sexual response benefits of some of these peptides will be covered in Part VII, which examines sexually effective drugs. Captopril's sulfhydryl structure could give it special therapeutic benefits, since the range of peptide and enzyme functions affected are more extensive. The rash-inducing feature of captopril may also be a unique property of this drug, involving peptides that may play a role in the flushing response and aspects of sexual sensation. However, whereas the rash has been observed, these positive sexual effects have not been reported, observed, or investigated.

Quality-of-Life Benefits

An exciting aspect of ACE inhibitors is the possibility of a longevity effect through healthier body tissue. As noted, other antihypertensives lack such therapeutic actions and indeed may contribute to further weakening and deterioration. The ability of captopril to improve the quality of life beyond the benefits attributed to the treatment of hypertension remains an unexplored possibility. While it is theoretically possible that improvement would occur on captopril in a comprehensive "wellness" program, this effect has not yet been studied or demonstrated. In prospective trials of maintenance therapy, most antihypertensive drugs have failed to prolong life, in spite of their cardiovascular benefits. ACE inhibitors, however, may be able to extend both life and health through their inotropic and tissue repair actions (Clozel et al., 1990; Gavras & Gavras, 1991). Recognition and use of ACE inhibitors are already generating a search for other molecular drugs based on their intricate and peculiar mix of peptide and enzyme mechanisms.

Beneficial mood effects of captopril have been observed in both depressed and aging patients (Cohen & Zubenko, 1988; Germain & Chouinard, 1989). It remains unclear to what extent such beneficial effects occur in patients treated for hypertension, but the fact that ACE inhibitors do not appear to cause depression is of great benefit in the treatment of the elderly, who are prone to this disorder for a variety of other reasons. In addition, captopril can generate mild weight loss and can increase exercise tolerance through its inotropic action—both of which are conducive to longevity.

Enalapril (Vasotec) and lisinopril (Zestril, Prinivil) are more recently marketed ACE inhibitors, but they do not seem to have as much potential for supplemental benefits as captopril.

Alternatives

The newer calcium channel blockers—amlodipine (Norvasc), felodipine (Plendil), and isradipine (DynaCirc)—are discussed in the following section and are possible alternatives to captopril and other ACE inhibitors.

CALCIUM CHANNEL BLOCKERS

Calcium channel blockers (CCBs) are relatively new resources in the treatment of hypertension. In general, their sexual side-effect profile is benign compared to most other antihypertensive drugs. They also have fewer psychological side effects than other antihypertensives, although there have been infrequent reports of depression. Case reports of CCB-induced depression have been published (Biriell, McEwen, & Sanz, 1989; Eccleston & Cole, 1990). However, calcium channel blockers have also been used to treat depression (Hoschl, 1983; Lancon, Valle, & Jadot, 1990). Troublesome physical side effects include peripheral vasodilation associated with flushing, dizziness, constipation, and orthostatic hypotension. Effects on quality of life, however subtle, can include diminished energy and stamina (factors which become increasingly important in the treatment of the elderly). Table 17.2 summarizes the characteristics and side effects of calcium channel blockers.

Sexual Side Effects

Controlled clinical test trials and general practice reports of calcium channel blockers indicate

Table 17.2 *Profile of Calcium Channel Blockers*

	Daily Dose
Amlodipine (Norvasc)	60–360 mg
Bepridil (Vascor)	300 mg
Diltiazem (Cardizem)	120–360 mg
Felodipine (Plendil)	5–20 mg
Flunarizine (Sibelium*)	
Isradipine (DynaCirc)	2.5–10 mg
Nicardipine (Cardene)	20–40 mg
Nifedipine (Adalat, Procardia)	30–120 mg
Nimodipine (Nimotop) (not approved for hypertension)	30–60 mg
Nitrendipine (Baypress*)	10–80 mg
Verapamil (Calan, Isoptin)	120–480 mg

COMMON INDICATIONS

Hypertension
Angina
Congestive heart failure
Arrhythmia

MECHANISMS OF ACTION (GENERAL)

Decreases vascular resistance
Blocks cardiac/smooth muscle calcium transmission action

MECHANISMS OF ACTION (SEXUAL)

Positive

Increased DHEA
Decreased serotonin (5-HT)

Negative

Decreased adrenergic ($alpha_1$) activity
Decreased dopamine
Decreased oxytocin
Increased prolactin
Decreased substance P
Decreased vasopressin

DIRECT SEXUAL SIDE EFFECTS

Desire disorders (in both sexes)
Erection difficulties
- Impotence (occasional)

Ejaculation retarded

Menstrual disorders
- Menorrhagia

Infertility
- Decreased sperm motility

Breast Disorders
- Gynecomastia
- Galactorrhea

INDIRECT SEXUAL SIDE EFFECTS

Discomfort caused by constipation, edema, weight gain, nausea, urinary problems (nocturia)

Mood disorders resulting in depression

Neurological disturbances resulting in cognitive deficit, dizziness, fatigue, headache, sleep disturbances, muscular weakness

Vascular disturbances resuling in arrhythmias, headache, orthostatic hypotension, peripheral vasodilation

SEXUAL CONTRAINDICATIONS/BENEFITS

Avoid with prior condition of

Desire disorders
Ejaculation problems
Anorgasmia
Menstrual disorders

May be useful for

Impotence (secondary)

ALTERNATIVES

ACE Inhibitors
Alpha_1 blockers
Indapamide (Lozol)

*Not marketed in the United States.

few negative effects on sexual function or desire. Indeed, they are routinely and widely recommended for their lack of sexual toxicity. However, this perception is misleading, and while they have some advantages, their negative impact on sex may be far greater than has been appreciated by clinicians. Their mild diuretic properties often eliminate the need to use a second drug, which avoids the additional negative sexual effects and gives a certain advantage in some cases. Nonetheless, a close look at the literature suggests that calcium channel blockers have some significant sexual drawbacks. Though it is rarely noted, they can decrease dopamine activity (Gaggi & Gianni, 1990), thus reducing sexual drive. By interfering with dopamine, they may also inhibit the reinforcing properties of other dopamine stimulants (e.g., bupropion, deprenyl, cocaine) as well as direct brain stimulation reward (Pani, Kuzmin, Martellotta, Gessa, & Fratta, 1991). Without reinforcement, there is less anticipation, less incentive, less initiative, less sensation, less pleasure, and less satisfaction. Furthermore, dopaminergic inhibition in elderly (over 70 years old) patients treated with calcium channel blockers can cause Parkinsonism and depression, which may not be reversed even after discontinuing these blockers for more than a year (Garcia-Ruiz et al., 1992). While such severe toxicity was noted mainly for calcium channel blockers *not* used to treat hypertension (e.g., cinnarizine, flunarizine), milder toxicity may occur with calcium channel blockers used as antihypertensive drugs.

If dopamine is inhibited by calcium channel blockers, there may be an increase of prolactin, which could occasionally lead to gynecomastia (Clone, 1986). According to the general literature on the effects of prolactin on male sexuality, one can infer the potential for reduced sex drive and impotence (Clone, 1986). In 1988 the Federal Drug Administration issued an alert to physicians that it had received 31 reports of gynecomastia occurring during CCB treatment (Tanner & Bosco, 1988). Eleven cases were attributed to nifedipine, 18 to verapamil, and only one to diltiazem. Doctors were warned against pursuing unnecessary tests or surgery or both. The increase in prolactin with CCB use can cause fertility problems as well as gynecomastia and galactorrhea. A report from the University of Munich has shown that nifedipine, verapamil, and diltiazem all inhibited the motility and velocity of sperm (Placzek, Ohling, Waller, Krassnigg, & Schill, 1987).

While few sexual effects have been reported regarding calcium channel blockers, mild or moderate decreases in drive and response are likely to be overlooked. Even a marked sexual problem may be ignored if the physician considers calcium blockers free from sexual side effects. For example, Fogelman (1988) described the case of a 45-year-old man treated with verapamil who became impotent. Calls to his doctor complaining that verapamil was causing this problem without lowering his blood pressure brought an instruction from the doctor to increase the dose. The man became increasingly confused and depressed, until he had to be hospitalized for suicidal depression. Despite his wife's support, he feared she would leave him. Within 36 hours of discontinuing verapamil, the man had four erections and his depression was gone. When the doctor who had kept the patient on the verapamil was asked why he continued prescribing the drug, he responded that the drug-company representative had assured him the verapamil was free of sexual and depressive side effects.

In a large and extended quality-of-life study, Suzuki et al. (1988) found a substantial increase in ejaculation problems in patients treated with nifedipine (40–80 mg, slow release). They treated 156 male patients for one year. Four treatment groups (39 patients each) were compared: nifedipine, atenolol, captopril, and thiazide diuretic. A self-report questionnaire showed that only captopril was free of sexual side effects (the study was reported in a journal supplement sponsored by the maker of captopril). Ejaculation problems on nifedipine were more than double those found with atenolol or the diuretic; however, the nature of the ejaculation problems and the number of patients affected were not reported. A smaller increase in erection difficulties was found comparable to those found on atenolol and diuretic. In a general review of the relation of hypertension to impotence, Müller,

El-Damanhoury, Rüth, and Lue (1991) specifically noted that, in their own clinical practice, two hypertensive, impotent patients became potent after withdrawal of nifedipine.

Morrissette, Skinner, Hoffman, Levine, and Davidson (1993) closely monitored the sexual effects of slow-release nifedipine compared to atenolol or placebo in 16 older men (60 to 75 years old) treated for mild or moderate hypertension. Patients were treated for four weeks on either nifedipine of atenolol and then for four weeks on the alternative antihypertensive after a two-week washout period. Daily self-report diaries were used to follow all aspects of sexual activity and function. No significant differences were found between nifedipine, atenolol, or placebo, except for decreased erectile firmness with nifedipine compared to atenolol or placebo.

Using a similar design of successive four-week treatment periods for 13 men who had experienced antihypertensive-related sexual dysfunction, Rosen, Kostis, Jekelis, and Taska (1994) found no significant differences compared to placebo in self-report measures for atenolol, propranolol, dyazide, or even methyldopa. However, methyldopa caused decreased erectile firmness and sexual confidence compared to atenolol, propranolol, or dyazide. In both of these recent studies, the sample was too small and the four-week length of treatment too short (at least four months treatment should be used). With such inadequate testing, it is unlikely that significant, reliable, and definitive negative sexual side effects of calcium channel blockers will be found.

Calcium channel blockers also block the actions of excitatory sensory peptides, which are activated through calcium transmission. There is extensive evidence that calcium channel blockers decrease oxytocin, substance P, prostaglandins, and met-enkephalins (Andersson, 1988; Govoni, Goss, DiGiovine, Battaini, & Trabucchi, 1990; Spedding, 1987). These peptides are intimately involved in the perception and experience of genital sensation. (It is interesting to note that calcium channel blockers decrease the very peptides that ACE inhibitors increase.) When excitatory reactions are undesirable, as in migraine, mania, or drug withdrawal, such interference is welcome. However, blocking calcium is indiscriminate. A drug intended to prevent toxic calcium overload may prevent the normal expansion of activity required for maximum performance in exercise and sex as well. In addition, with calcium action blocked, sensation and cognition can both be reduced, leaving the brain and body less reactive and less active. Noticeable sexual dysfunction may not occur, but reduced sexual drive, sensation, responsiveness, and function could result.

Blocking calcium activity can decrease constriction of blood vessels associated with the epinephrine response. However, this block can also decrease bulbocavernosus/ischiocavernosus contractions essential for penile rigidity and orgasmic sensation. In addition, calcium blocker antagonism of dopamine and oxytocin can inhibit the triggers of the sexual response. Rat yawning and penile erections due to dopamine or oxytocin administration are eliminated by calcium channel blockers (Argiolas & Melis, 1989). Even the body's own endogenous vasodilator, endothelium-derived relaxing factor (EDRF), is decreased by the calcium blockers (Godfraind & Govoni, 1989). Orgasmic intensity can be decreased, since its muscular contractions are calcium-mediated.

In laboratory studies of animals, calcium channel blockers have been found to potentiate alcohol, opiates, and benzodiazepines (Deutsch, Kaushik, Huntzinger, Novitzki, & Mastropaolo, 1991; Kavaliers, 1987). It is possible that a few social drinks combined with calcium channel blockers could adversely impact sexual desire and function in both sexes. These drugs may also blunt physical sensitivity and orgasmic intensity by their potentiation of opioid analgesia, which has been shown in mice (Del Pozo, Caro, & Baeyens, 1987).

The possibility that calcium channel blockers have negative effects on physical aspects of the sex response is suggested by their similarity to thioridazine (Mellaril), a potent inhibitor of orgasm and ejaculation. The conspicuous inhibition of ejaculation and the prevalence of cardiovascular effects that occur with thioridazine have been attributed by Solomon Snyder (1989) to its calcium antagonist action, equivalent in kind to that which occurs with calcium channel blockers like nifedipine. Snyder and Reynolds (1985) theorized: "If thioridazine interferes with ejaculation because of calcium blockade, one wonders whether treatment with calcium antagonist drugs elicits this side effect. We are unaware of published report of such effects. [However,] *our findings with thioridazine suggest that cardiologists should be alert to the possibility of such effects in patients treated with calcium antagonist drugs*" [italics added].

Male/Female Differences

Through increased peripheral blood flow, calcium channel blockers may improve erectile function from a mechanical point of view. However, they may simultaneously decrease sex drive through inhibition of dopamine and adrenergic activation. A decrease in sex drive could eliminate the opportunity for sex and/or make erection difficult to achieve. Sex drive is often related to performance, so that decreased erection may be a reflection of decreased drive. Male drive, erection, orgasm, and ejaculation may change independently of each other and sometimes in different directions.

Few sexual effects due to calcium channel blockers have been reported in women. For women who have experienced no problems with initiative, sensation, assertiveness, or orgasm prior to taking the medication, calcium channel blockers may pose few problems. However, side effects that can indirectly affect sexual functioning may cause problems for women who already have sexual issues. Headache, flushing, edema, dizziness, and weakness can effectively dampen sexual desire and response for many women. The fact that calcium channel blockers have shown no negative effects on women's sexual function to date is unfortunately consistent with the fact that the effects of drugs on women's sexuality are often overlooked by researchers.

Sexual Benefits

As noted, calcium channel blockers may have some positive value for male sexual function by enhancing peripheral circulation and promoting blood flow to the erection. Due to the inhibition of muscle fiber irritability and adrenergic blocking, there is the theoretical possibility that calcium channel blockers could help reduce premature ejaculation. In women, the vasodilating and calming physical effects of calcium antagonists may be sexually positive; however, there is a possibility that genital contractions may be reduced. The increase in DHEA and decrease in insulin resistance shown for amlodipine, nitrendipine, and diltiazem (Beer et al., 1993a, 1993b, 1994) suggest a positive sexual effect, but the relation of calcium channel blocker induction of DHEA to sexual drive and function has yet to be studied. In open trials nifedipine treatment has been shown to be effective in treating dysmenorrhea and bladder instability (reviewed by Childress & Katz, 1994), apparently through reducing genital tissue hypercontractive activity, as well as in the treatment of interstitial cystitis through an immunosuppressive action (Fleischmann, Huntley, Shingleton, & Wentworth, 1991).

Quality-of-Life Concerns

Calcium channel blockers are recommended as the drug of choice for the elderly, but they can shorten a patient's life span due to their negative inotropic effect. In addition, quality of life may be compromised by adverse cognitive effects. A number of studies have shown cognitive deficits due to nifedipine. For instance, the Bulpitt-Fletcher group (Palmer, Fletcher, Hamilton, Muriss, & Bulpitt, 1990) found a 31% decrease in cognitive scores during nifedipine treatment (compared to a 22% increase on verapamil). Skinner et al. (1992) noted a substantial deficit in word-recall tasks in 31 elderly (aged 60 to 81) men and women treated with nifedipine compared to either placebo or atenolol treatment. Turkkan and Heinz (1991) have shown similar cognitive and sensory deficits in baboons treated with nifedipine or verapamil. On the other hand, cognitive ability has been increased in old animals and Alzheimer patients by calcium antagonists (chiefly nimodipine, which is not indicated for treatment of hypertension) (Baumel, Eisner, Karukin, MacNamara, & Raphan, 1989; Sandin, Jasmin, & Levere, 1990). Cognitive benefits that occur with newer and more specific calcium antagonists like nimodipine may not occur with currently available calcium channel blocker antihypertensive drugs. Van Zweiten (1986) labeled these new selective calcium antagonists with the term *calcium overload blocker,* to indicate their more specific action.

Dizziness caused by calcium channel blocker vasodilation can cause falls in the elderly, with serious consequences (including premature death). Le Jeunne, Hugues, Munera, and Ozanne (1991) observed orthostatic weakness, dizziness, and fainting among elderly patients treated with calcium blockers. Perhaps the most serious danger of using older calcium channel blockers (e.g., nifedipine, verapamil, diltiazem) as treatment for elderly patients with hypertension is that these drugs can cause death due to heart failure brought on by their negative inotropic action (Held & Yusuf, 1994; Packer, 1992). Significant negative inotropic effects from most calcium channel blockers have been shown in laboratory studies of diseased human myocardium and in animals (Ezzaher, Bouanani, Su, Hittinger, & Crozatier, 1991; Schwinger, Bohm, & Erdmann, 1991). In a large calcium channel blocker trial, Elkayam et al. (1990) found increased hospitalization due to heart failure exacerbation and premature discontinuation due to disease progression or premature death. Increased heart failure has also been found with diltiazem.

In summary, calcium channel blockers, previously considered sexually benign, have the potential to inhibit sexual desire in both sexes, perhaps to a significant degree. They may also have a mild, inhibiting effect on ejaculation and orgasm and decrease erectile rigidity. However, because of their peripheral vasodilating properties, they do not critically impede erectile function (except through diminished desire). Indeed, they may even have sexual value by enhancing blood flow to the erection and by decreasing premature ejaculation. Quality-of-life issues remain a drawback, however. Calcium channel blockers may cause dizziness, cognitive impairment, and premature death due to heart failure in the elderly.

Alternatives

When complications do not occur, calcium channel blockers can serve patients well, with fewer adverse side effects than some of the older cardiac drugs. Nonetheless, the potential for cognitive impairment and depression as well as sex drive disorders should be carefully considered. Fortunately, the variety of calcium channel blockers, including many newly available, allows the choice of one with minimal inotropic compromise. For instance, amlodipine (Norvasc), felodipine (Plendil), isradipine (DynaCirc), and nicardipine (Cardene) are thought to lack negative inotropic properties. (Although nifedipine was believed to be the least negative, its strong vasodilator properties limit contraction-expansion action of the cardiovascular system.) Calcium overload blockers, which limit only excess, harmful calcium activity, may be available soon.

Calcium channel blockers also do not appear to cause or worsen insulin resistance (i.e., do not have a diabetogenic effect) (Zanetti-Elshater, Pingatore, Beretta-Piccoli, Riesen, & Heinen, 1994). Possibly due to an increase in DHEA and/or a decrease in insulin, they may be particularly beneficial in hypertension associated with obesity.

Since calcium channel blockers and ACE inhibitors are both vasodilators, ACE inhibitors can usually be used in place of calcium channel blockers. However, the use of ACE inhibitors may require a concurrent diuretic, thereby eliminating the sexual advantage. In the elderly, both prazosin and ACE inhibitors can cause acute hypotension, which can be avoided if patients are started at very low doses at bedtime and only gradually increased to efficacious doses. However, if patients are noncompliant or forget to take their pills, first-dose hypotension will continue to be a possibility.

With the current availability of new calcium channel blockers, and the recognition of negative diuretic actions, calcium channel blocker use can be expected to increase. When a diuretic is necessary, particularly in women, it is not clear whether low-dose HCTZ or indapamide is preferable to calcium channel blockers. When medically appropriate, monotherapy with prazosin or ACE inhibitors is strongly recommended. Since ACE inhibitors have definite cardioprotective actions that mitigate against heart failure, they are clearly the drugs of choice for long-term use after myocardial infarction (Sambhi, Gavras, Robertson, & Smith, 1993; Simoons, 1994). Because function of the heart and blood vessels is extended by ACE inhibitor treatment after myocardial infarction, it is possible that there is a similar benefit for penile/genital tissue and blood flow.

Part V

PSYCHOTROPICS

18

Antianxiety Agents/Tranquilizers: 5-HT$_{1A}$ Agonists and Benzodiazepines

OBJECTIVES

- To distinguish antianxiety and sedative applications
- To examine unique characteristics of buspirone
- To examine amnesic and addictive properties of benzodiazepines, as well as effects on sexual functioning

Although antianxiety agents, tranquilizers, sedatives, and hypnotics are distinct categories, typically the "lines" between them become blurred in clinical practice. A mild tranquilizer might be used at night for sleep instead of a hypnotic; sleeping pills are often used to quell the anxiety and stress of everyday living or relationship problems. Most drugs in these categories have the potential for abuse: dependence and addiction are the most typical categories that come to mind. However, additional forms of abuse also occur with these particular classes of drugs. Some of the benzodiazepines, which have powerful amnesiac effects, have been used by unscrupulous professionals to sexually abuse patients because of the high probability that the patients will not remember the event. Another form of sexual abuse is inadvertent. A woman who takes benzodiazepines may not realize that one of the effects is to reduce certain sexual inhibitions. While chronic use of benzodiazepines tends to decrease the active sexual response, it may increase the passive receptive sexual response, making the woman more compliant sexually and less apt to reject sexual advances that, without the drug, would be unwelcome. Paradoxically, the disinhibition associated with benzodiazepines can also cause uncharacteristic aggression and irritability in both men and women. Associated with the amnesia that may occur, individuals taking heavy doses of Xanax, for example, may become aggressive, perhaps even physically abusive, and have no recall of their offensive behavior the following day.

There are basically two major classes of benzodiazepines: antianxiety drugs/tranquilizers and sedative/hypnotics. The drugs used for anxiety and those used for sleep are generally different. Alprazolam (Xanax), for example, is more typically used for antianxiety, while the short-acting triazolam (Halcion) is more common for the treatment of insomnia. Benzodiazepines used as sedative-hypnotics are shorter-acting than those used as antianxiety medications. We will be addressing the sedative hypnotic aspect of benzodiazepines in the next chapter; because of their discrete action on sleep and their specific indications and prescription for this purpose, they are being treated separately. Buspirone (BuSpar), an antianxiety medication in the 5-HT$_{1A}$ agonists group, is a departure from the others. Chemically, its mechanism of action is entirely different from benzodiazepines, since it does not have an impact on GABA; instead, it somehow balances serotonin activity by stimulating the serotonin 5-HT$_{1A}$ receptor. It appears to treat anxiety without the tranquilizing and sedating effects characteristic of the benzodiazepines. (It may also have mild antidepressant properties as well.) Most importantly, buspirone is non-addictive and has only a minimum of adverse sexual properties. It may even enhance sex drive in men and women, improve orgasmic responsiveness in women, and offer an effective treatment for ejaculatory inhibition in men. Buspirone and benzodiazepines primarily used as antianxiety agents/tranquilizers are discussed in this chapter; those benzodiazepines that act as sedative/hypnotics are examined in the following chapter.

5-HT$_{1A}$ AGONISTS

Buspirone is currently the sole medication in a new class of antianxiety medications. Introduced in the mid-1980s, buspirone does not have the tranquilizing effect of benzodiazepines. For this reason, many doctors doubt that it can be an effective antianxiety agent, despite the evidence of controlled trials and Federal Drug Administration approval for this indication. The antidepressant effect of buspirone and the related 5-HT$_{1A}$ agonist gepirone have also been investigated; their efficacy appears to be somewhat less than currently approved antidepressants, and they have not received FDA approval for treatment of depression. A 12-week placebo-controlled trial of buspirone treatment of 61 anxious alcoholics showed that buspirone decreased relapse and reduced anxiety that would likely contribute to relapse (Kranzler et al., 1994). In an open six-week trial, Gawin, Compton, and Byck (1989) found that buspirone reduced smoking and craving to smoke in eight smokers trying to quit.

As more is learned about the various types of serotonin receptors, the appropriateness of buspirone treatment for differing kinds of anxiety should add specificity and confidence to its clinical use. Its efficacy as an antianxiety drug clearly indicates that a CNS-depressant is not the only means to soothe anxiety. Indeed, buspirone stimulates the locus coeruleus area of the brain, which has been associated with anxiety, withdrawal effects, and the epinephrine response, thus opening a new arena of antianxiety investigation. Table 18.1 summarizes the properties and side effects of 5-HT$_{1A}$ agonists.

Sexual Dysfunction

No adverse sexual side effects have been reported for buspirone. However, it has only been available since 1987, not long enough for a clear sexual profile to emerge. Since it has no specific relaxing or sedating effects, sex drive and arousal are likely to be unaffected. Furthermore, buspirone causes no immediate mood change that could generate abuse or dependence. It generally requires about one or two weeks to begin reducing anxiety, and there are no withdrawal symptoms when treatment is discontinued. It does not potentiate alcohol, does not decrease pain, and has no apparent cognitive effects in humans (in rats, some adverse effects on learning have been reported). All of these factors reinforce the likelihood that buspirone does not affect sexual desire or drive and is not addicting. At present, there is little published research on the sexual effects of buspirone in humans; a single case report of buspirone treatment noted that it reduced paraphilia fantasies and transvestic fetishism (Fedoroff, 1992).

In contrast to the lack of information on 5-HT$_{1A}$ drugs on humans, there is fascinating animal research on the sexual effects of buspirone and 5-HT$_{1A}$ by researchers at Stanford and by several European groups is available. These groups have shown that the 5-HT$_{1A}$ agonists 8-OH-DPAT and buspirone reduce the amount of copulatory stimulation required for ejaculatory behavior in rats and increase copulatory rate (Ahlenius & Larsson, 1984a, 1984b; Kwong, Smith, Davdison, & Peroutka, 1986; Mathes, Smith, Popa, & Davidson, 1990; Schnur, Smith, Lee, Mas, & Davidson, 1989). This excellent research will hopefully inspire further studies in humans.

Male/Female Differences

5-HT$_{1A}$ drugs affect characteristic male sexual behavior differently from female sexual behavior. Buspirone increases sexual desire and activ-

Table 18.1 *Profile of 5-HT_{1A} Agonists*

	Daily Dose
Buspirone (BuSpar)	10–40 mg
Gepirone (in clinical trials for depression)	
Ipsapirone (in clinical trials)	

COMMON INDICATIONS
- Anxiety
- Depression

MECHANISMS OF ACTION (GENERAL)
- Stimulates 5-HT_{1A} receptors on neurons
- Decreases release of 5-HT at some synapses

MECHANISMS OF ACTION (SEXUAL)

Positive	*Negative*
Increased adrenergic $alpha_1$ activity	Decreased dopamine
Decreased cortisol	
Decreased serotonin	

DIRECT SEXUAL SIDE EFFECTS

Desire enhanced (in both sexes)	Ejaculation disorders
Orgasm enhanced	• Premature ejaculation (worsened)
	• Ejaculatory inhibition (improved)

INDIRECT SEXUAL SIDE EFFECTS
- *Discomfort* caused by nausea, weight loss
- *Mood disorders* resulting in nervousness
- *Neurological disturbances* resulting in dizziness, fatigue, headache (buzzing in the head), insomnia
- *Vascular disturbances* resulting in headache

SEXUAL CONTRAINDICATIONS/BENEFITS

Avoid with prior condition of	*May be useful for*
Premature ejaculation	Desire disorders
Erection disorders (physical or medical)	Inhibited ejaculation
	Female orgasmic disorders
	Erection disorders

ALTERNATIVES
- Alprazolam (Xanax)
- Clonazepam (Klonopin)
- Fluoxetine (Prozac)

ity in male animals, causes quicker ejaculation, and possibly weakens erection. In female rats, buspirone can promote *active* sexual responses and decrease lordosis (passive receptive sex). Such a combination may be desirable for women to the degree that female sexual problems involve desire disorders and inhibited orgasm (orgasm cannot be identified or measured in female rats). For men, a drug that quickens ejaculation could contribute to real or perceived problems of premature ejaculation in some cases; in other cases, with prior conditions of ejaculatory inhibition (retarded ejaculation or lack of ejaculation), buspirone could be helpful. It should also be noted that, while buspirone may make orgasm occur more quickly in both men and women, there is no evidence that it increases physical intensity.

In male rats allowed to copulate and ejaculate to exhaustion, administration of the 5-HT_{1A} agonist 8-OH-DPAT revived these rats to again copulate and ejaculate (Rodríguez-Manzo & Fernandez-Guasti, 1994). Buspirone administered to male rats prior to sexual tests shortened the time to ejaculation and to renewed copulation after ejaculation (Mathes et al., 1990). However, Choi, Maayani, and Melman (1988) found that buspirone decreased penile reflex erections to stimulation, despite enhancing copulatory behavior to ejaculation. Buspirone administered to female rats prior to sexual tests reduced receptive sexual behavior (lordosis) (Johansson & Meyerson, 1991; Mendelson & Gorzalka, 1986).

Sexual Benefits

The complexity and unpredictability of buspirone's effects may make controlled trials intended to identify sexual side effects difficult. A more serious obstacle, however, is financial. The maker of buspirone, Bristol-Myers Squibb, does not own the sexual dysfunction "use patent" and is therefore unlikely to invest in efficacy studies for the treatment of sexual dysfunction. Instead one enterprising researcher filed his own "use patent" for buspirone treatment of sexual dysfunction and conducted a small (n = 10), short (four-week) open trial (Othmer & Othmer, 1987). The results indicated that buspirone had a beneficial effect on the patients, who also had severe anxiety disorders. After four weeks, sexual function was self-rated as returned to normal, even when anxiety persisted. The sexual improvement (in desire, response, and orgasm) may have been indirect, an early byproduct of incompletely reduced anxiety, or may have reflected a simple regression to the mean, which is to be expected with the effective treatment of anxiety. When anxiety is reduced to a critical level, normal pleasurable activities are resumed. After that threshold is reached, however, further reductions in anxiety do not increase sexuality proportionally. Perhaps this critical threshold phenomenon explains the low correlations reported by the authors in their small study between anxiety reduction and sexual improvement. When the results of this study are considered in the context of the sexual findings in animal research, it is also conceivable that the sexual improvements are a direct effect of the drug. Unfortunately, this interesting but preliminary open trial has not been replicated or expanded into a meaningful double-blind study.

Our own clinical experience with buspirone is somewhat consonant with the Othmers' finding of a beneficial sexual effect. The sexual depression experienced on benzodiazepines can be relieved by switching to buspirone. However, some doctors avoid prescribing buspirone because it does not seem to be as effective as benzodiazepines during initial treatment. Also, when first taken, buspirone may cause a buzzing in the head, more like a tingle than a headache. Patients may reject buspirone prematurely because of this initial, bothersome symptom and doctors may assume incorrectly that buspirone increases rather than decreases anxiety.

Alternatives

Due to buspirone's apparent lack of sexual side effects, alternatives are generally not necessary. One exception occurs when treating men: if symptoms of premature ejaculation appear (or if premature ejaculation is a preexisting condition). In such cases, benzodiazepines such as alprazolam (Xanax) may be preferable. 5-HT uptake inhibitor antidepressants (e.g., fluoxetine, paroxetine, nefazodone) are another useful alternative in select circumstances in which buspirone is ineffective or inadequate in treating anxiety. Gepirone, currently in clinical trials for treatment of depression, is a drug similar to buspirone but without buspirone's slight antidopaminergic effect. Other buspirone-like drugs are also being developed and tested by various drug companies. With no patent problems and much competition, companies can be expected to conduct sexual side-effect trials with these new antianxiety drugs. Studies of sexual side effects will probably show that buspirone and its relatives are less disruptive to sex than SSRIs or benzodiazepines.

Because of buspirone's benign profile, physicians may switch patients on benzodiazepines to buspirone; however, buspirone is often without sufficient effect for these patients, so making the change may be difficult. A gradual shift from benzodiazepines to buspirone can usually be effective in conjunction with appropriate psychotherapy.

BENZODIAZEPINES

Benzodiazepines can release behavior ordinarily inhibited by pain (e.g., shock, food poisoning) or lack of experience (e.g., novelty). An ideal method for testing this releasing effect is the conditioned emotional response (CER) paradigm. Geller and Seifter (1960) trained hungry rats to press a lever for milk. After this response pattern was established, every 15 minutes a tone was emitted and a shock was delivered if the rat pressed for milk. Responding stopped whenever the tone came on. After a number of these experiences with the tone/shock sequence, shock was no longer necessary; the tone was sufficient to suppress responding (CER). However, when the rats were treated with a benzodiazepine, they resumed responding in spite of the punishing tone. Apparently, benzodiazepines inhibit the effect of the conditioned emotional response stimulus as though the subject "forgets" that it signaled pain. Lack of memory and attention occurs for positive conditioned emotional reactions as well. At relatively lower doses, cognitive deficits can occur for memory of past conditioning, attention to present emotional signals, and learning for the future. At higher doses, there may be no response to either pain or pleasure due to sedation.

The anxiolytic efficacy of benzodiazepines is measured in animal experiments by their capacity to disinhibit punished behavior or to disinhibit the suppression of behavior in the presence of a negatively conditioned stimuli. Since the animal is placed in the conflicted position of responding for reward and receiving punishment, this situation may be defined as neurotic. Benzodiazepines decrease the influence of pain and other distress signals that would ordinarily suppress responding; in essence, they temporarily reduce neurotic tendencies, which return when the drug is discontinued. Similarly, benzodiazepines facilitate response to novel situations that would normally elicit fear, wariness, trepidation, or caution. Benzodiazepines are particularly efficacious when used to relieve neophobias (i.e., when foods are avoided due to a negative association with illness or transient nausea). Unpredictable and inappropriate outbursts of anger can also result from the general disinhibitory effect of benzodiazepines. The usual restraints are not intact and uncharacteristic aggressive behavior can occur in both sexes. Table 18.2 summarizes the characteristics and side effects of benzodiazepines.

Sexual Dysfunction

Many clinicians are under the impression that benzodiazepines do not have negative effects on sexual functioning and can even improve dysfunction that is caused by anxiety. This conclusion is misleading. Benzodiazepines can cause or aggravate sexual dysfunction in both men and women, but they affect the sexes in distinctly different ways (described later in this chapter). Only in select circumstances do benzodiazepines improve anxiety-related sexual dysfunction.

Benzodiazepines appear to have paradoxical effects on sexual functioning; they (and GABA) appear to reduce serotonin activity and inhibit the firing rate of serotonergic neurons in the spinal cord, dorsal raphe nucleus, and various other brain areas (Rex, Marsden, & Fink, 1993; Van de Kar et al., 1985). Consequently, negative effects of benzodiazepines on arousal and orgasm may be balanced by a positive effect caused by decreased serotonin activity. Since benzodiazepines can increase relaxation and decrease excitement, effects on male sexuality are unpredictable. While decreasing anxiety can facilitate erection, lessened excitement and sensation can undermine interest and concentration during sexual activity. Chlordiazepoxide (Librium) can extend the time to ejaculation and even strengthen erection, but it can also have a pronounced negative effect on sexual desire.

Few case reports of ejaculatory inhibition associated with antianxiety benzodiazepines such

Table 18.2 *Profile of Benzodiazepines*

	Daily Dose
Alprazolam (Xanax)	0.25–4 mg/day
Chlordiazepoxide (Librium)	15–100 mg/day
Clonazepam (Klonopin)	1–5 mg/day
Clorazepate (Tranxene)	7.5–60 mg/day
Diazepam (Valium)	4–40 mg/day
Flurazepam (Dalmane)	15–30 mg/day
Lorazepam (Ativan)	0.5–4 mg/day
Oxazepam (Serax)	30–120 mg/day
Prazepam (Centrax)	15–30 mg/day
Temazepam (Restoril)	15–30 mg/day

COMMON INDICATIONS

Anxiety, panic/phobic disorder, obsessive/compulsive disorder, pain (chronic, back, muscle spasm), insomnia, alcohol withdrawal, jet lag

MECHANISMS OF ACTION (GENERAL)

Stimulates endogenous benzodiazepine receptors
Increases GABA transmission
GABA inhibits (hyperpolarizes) the firing of neurons

MECHANISMS OF ACTION (SEXUAL)

Positive
- Increased cholinergic activity
- Decreased cortisol
- Decreased serotonin

Negative
- Increased GABA/benzodiazepine
- Increased progesterone
- Decreased adrenergic $alpha_1$ activity
- Decreased LHRH
- Decreased substance P
- Decreased testosterone

DIRECT SEXUAL SIDE EFFECTS

Desire disorders (in both sexes)
- Hyposexuality (decreases)
- Sexual aversion (decreases)
- Hypersexuality

Orgasm disorders
Paraphilia
Dyspareunia
Erection disorders
Ejaculation disorders
- Retarded ejaculation (helps/hurts?)
- Premature ejaculation (improves)
- Painful ejaculation (improves)

INDIRECT SEXUAL SIDE EFFECTS

Discomfort caused by constipation, nausea, weight gain, rash/itching, urinary problems (incontinence)

Mood disorders resulting in aggression, anhedonia, depression, detachment, irritability, manic behavior

Neurological disturbances resulting in addiction-withdrawal, analgesia, cognitive deficits, dizziness, fatigue, movement disorder (ataxia, dyskinesia), sedation, sensory loss, tremor, muscular weakness

Vascular disturbances resulting in headache

SEXUAL CONTRAINDICATIONS/BENEFITS

Avoid with prior condition of
- Desire disorders
- Erection disorders
- Anorgasmia
- Retarded ejaculation

May be useful for
- Desire disorders (anxiety)
- Erection disorders (anxiety)
- Premature ejaculation (anxiety)
- Vaginismus

Table 18.2 *Continued*

ALTERNATIVES
Buspirone (BuSpar) for anxiety
Fluoxetine (Prozac), fluvoxamine (Luvox), paroxetine (Paxil) for panic/phobia and obsessive-compulsive disorders
Trazodone (Desyrel) for nocturnal sedative, dyspareunia

as chlordiazepoxide (Hughes, 1964) or valium (Munjack & Oziel, 1980) have been reported in the last 30 years. Decreased sexual interest or responsivity with antianxiety/antipanic benzodiazepines such as alprazolam (Xanax) has also been reported only infrequently and usually at high doses (for example, alprazolam, 3–10 mg/day). Nevertheless, several cases of ejaculatory difficulties and decreased sexual desire have been reported with benzodiazepines. As noted, Hughes (1964) reported ejaculatory inhibition due to 30 mg chlordiazepoxide (Librium). In 1980, Munjack and Oziel reported that several patients developed retarded ejaculation and decreased sexual desire on diazepam (Valium), and in a 1986 case study, Munjack and Crocker noted that ejaculatory inhibition in conjunction with alprazolam (Xanax). It may be expected that more reports of sexual dysfunction will occur on the high daily benzodiazepine doses recently approved for treatment of panic and phobia.

Effects on female orgasm have rarely been studied. However, anecdotal reports have suggested decreased sexual desire and anorgasmia. For example, Sangal (1985) reported a case of a depressed 44-year-old woman with a prior history of sexual abuse, neuroleptic treatment, and tricyclic treatment. Within a few months of treatment with 7 mg of alprazolam, she developed complete anorgasmia and decreased sexual desire. Orgasm was restored when alprazolam was discontinued, but anorgasmia recurred when she resumed treatment with 5 mg alprazolam. Uhde, Tancer, and Shea (1988) reported the case of a 47-year-old woman who suffered decreased libido and anorgasmia during 4.2 mg/day alprazolam treatment of social phobia. Her desire and ability to achieve orgasm returned when the dose was lowered to 1.4 mg/day; but normal sexual functioning did not return until alprazolam was discontinued for two months.

While alprazolam most frequently appears to be the cause of sexual dysfunction, this is probably due to its widespread use. In our clinical practice, sexual dysfunction seems most frequent on clonazepam (Klonopin) and chlordiazepoxide (Librium), particularly in men.

The most impressive report on the sexual effects of benzodiazepines that included women was written by Lydiard, Howell, Laraia, and Balenger (1987) in a letter to the editor. Thirty-two patients (9 men, 25 women) answered an open questionnaire on changes in sexual function during alprazolam treatment for panic disorder. Predictably, this short but specific patient questionnaire revealed far more extensive sexual problems than those reported in literature based primarily on anecdotal reports or large surveys. Ratings on drive, erection, and orgasm were made on a scale of 0 to 10, with 5 representing no change. Fifteen patients (47%) indicated decreased sex drive (with ratings as low as 0 or 1 reported by eight patients); four patients (25%) reported increased drive (including two patients who gave a 10 rating). Sixteen patients (50%) rated their ability to have orgasm as decreased (with a 0 or 1 rating given by 12 of the 16); three (9%) reported improved orgasm (including one rating of 10). Four men (44%) indicated that erection was diminished, and one man reported a complete loss of erection and orgasm.

Ghadirian, Annable, and Belanger (1992) successfully treated a sample of 104 bipolar patients (45 men, 59 women) with lithium alone (35%) or lithium and benzodiazepines (49%). Sexual dysfunction was present in 14% of patients on lithium alone, but in 49% of patients on lithium and benzodiazepines. About 20% of both male and female patients experienced moderate to severe decrease in sexual desire, orgasm, and, for men, erection. When patients treated with additional drugs were excluded, it was found that 60% of patients on lithium and benzodiazepines had experienced a negative change in sexual desire or function.

Our own clinical experience has revealed adverse effects on erection. During a placebo-controlled panic treatment trial, loss of erection was noted in a healthy 40-year-old man treated for panic when alprazolam dose was increased to 7 mg; erection was restored when the dosage was reduced to 6 mg (J. P. Goldberg, unpublished observation, 1989). It should be noted that prophylactic treatment of panic disorders requires very high doses of alprazolam (3 to 10 mg per day). Perhaps at lower doses the sexual effects are less severe. In animals, benzodiazepines do not appear to weaken erection. In fact, in some animals chlordiazepoxide (Librium) has been shown to both increase and decrease sex drive, improve erection, and inhibit orgasm/ejaculation (Martino, Mas, & Davidson, 1987).

Male/Female Differences

Differentiation between male and female sexual responses is central to an evaluation of the degree to which benzodiazepines affect sexual function. The active "masculine" sexual response (copulation) is affected differently from the passive receptive female response (lordosis). These responses are separately innervated and are affected in opposite ways by particular neurotransmitters and hypothalamic brain nuclei. Benzodiazepines inhibit locomotion and diminish physical fear and pain reflexes that would ordinarily protect animals (and perhaps women) from undesirable sexual activity. While benzodiazepines (and GABA neurotransmission which is increased by benzodiazepines) generally dampen active sexual behavior in animals, they facilitate the passive, receptive lordosis response. Estrogen given to animals in combination with benzodiazepines also facilitates lordosis in response to rectal stimulation and probing. It can even induce lordosis in males. Interestingly, reflex genital anesthesia associated with lordosis can be potentiated by benzodiazepine treatment (Whipple & Komisaruk, 1988).

Because benzodiazepines have a disinhibitory effect on sex, mild sexual anxieties may be removed, resulting in reduction of inhibition similar to that experienced with alcohol. The apparently indiscriminate sexual behavior of some women treated with benzodiazepines may reflect impaired judgment specifically due to these drugs. Fava and Borofsky (1991) treated a 22-year-old woman experiencing anxiety, depression, and panic attacks, particularly when in physical proximity to men. She had quit her clerical job that required her to be close to men and she could no longer go dancing due to panic in response to male partners. Treatment over three months with 2 mg/day alprazolam and 75 mg nortriptyline (an antidepressant) allowed her to return to work and enjoy dancing again. Due to residual anxiety, she was switched from alprazolam to 1.5 mg/day clonazepam (Klonopin). After a few days on clonazepam, she quit her job and, with no apparent sense of guilt or remorse, became a strip-tease dancer, returning to the sexually promiscuous lifestyle that typified her teen years. However, upon discontinuing clonazepam, she quit her strip-tease job and felt tremendous guilt and remorse over her promiscuous behavior.

While women may reject the notion that such a natural female submissive response tendency exists, it may nonetheless be a biochemical fact (mediated by chemicals such as estrogen, progesterone, and GABA), and could be as inherent to female biochemistry and brain functioning as aggressive, violent responses are for men. Benzodiazepines can also decrease sexual aversion and avoidance by blunting self-protective escape reflexes. Depending on the circumstances, benzodiazepines can be therapeutic (reducing anxiety) or toxic (masking symptoms rather than treating them). Many of their effects are similar to those of alcohol and other substances used to reduce inhibitions.

Sexual Benefits

Kaplan (1987) has shown that many cases of inhibited sexual desire, sexual aversion, or avoidance of sex involve phobic or panic reactions. In selected patients with anxiety-related sexual disorders, benzodiazepines may have some value, although reports are typically mixed. In 1975, Maneksha and Harry showed that a group of sexually dysfunctional patients with anxiety disorders (including an impotent man and a woman with vaginismus and sexual aversion) benefited from four weeks of lorazepam (Ativan) treatment (3–6 mg). These patients also participated in brief psychotherapy. A subsequent comparison of Masters and Johnson therapy to oxazepam (Serax) treatment of sexual dysfunction showed no difference when compared with an untreated control group (Ansari, 1976).

Because of their antianxiety and muscle relaxant properties, benzodiazepines may be useful in the treatment of dyspareunia due to vaginismus. However, patients must be closely monitored for chemical dependence. Chlordiazepoxide (Librium) and diazepam (Valium) have been misused for many years as self-treatment for anxiety-related sexual disorders. The ease and danger of this abuse should caution doctors to prescribe this class of drugs for sexual dysfunction only when other resources have been ineffective. For premature ejaculators with associated anxiety, low doses might be sufficient for a transient beneficial effect.

Unfortunately, most of the cases of sexual dysfunction due to benzodiazepines involve patients who required high doses of the drug for other reasons; treatment with higher doses may reveal negative effects that are too subtle to be appreciated at lower doses. On the other hand, alprazolam at lower doses often has been noted to enhance both sexual desire, receptivity, and orgasm (Ghadirian et al., 1992; Post, 1994).

Because benzodiazepines also can undermine sexual desire, cause drowsiness, and have inconsistent effects on ejaculation, they have not been used widely for the treatment of premature ejaculation. Those with the least sedating effects, such as prazepam (Centrax), may be best for sexual considerations. Clearly, more study is necessary to better comprehend the potential sexual value of benzodiazepines.

Alternatives

In our clinical practice, we have often noted mild improvement in sexual desire and response when benzodiazepine-dependent patients are weaned off diazepam (Valium), lorazepam (Ativan), or alprazolam (Xanax) through gradual replacement with buspirone (BuSpar). Additional dividends include slight weight loss, improved alertness, and attentiveness.

Even though MAOI or SSRI treatments of panic/phobia disorders can create serious sexual problems by blocking orgasm and reducing sexual desire, this negative effect is usually less formidable than the dependency-withdrawal problems associated with benzodiazepines. Sexual problems are usually more amenable to therapy than drug addiction, so the overall prognosis when SSRIs are used is more favorable.

Sexual side effects of benzodiazepines and MAOIs or SSRIs have not been compared in anxiety or panic/phobia treatment trials. For panic/phobia and obsessive-compulsive disorders, fluvoxamine (Luvox), fluoxetine (Prozac), or paroxetine (Paxil) can be used, but they should be carefully monitored for sexual side effects of their own. For treatment of anxiety, buspirone (BuSpar) is an effective alternative, but because it is not as strong as benzodiazepines, it may not be as effective. An important difference between buspirone and benzodiazepines is that buspirone takes one to three weeks to achieve its antianxiety effect; hence, anxious patients do not get immediate relief. Also, buspirone is not useful for short-term treatment of acute anxiety or panic, such as may occur during trauma or emergencies.

Weight gain and sedation that occur on benzodiazepines may be decreased by switching to buspirone or fluoxetine (though with extended use, increased appetite and weight gain sometimes occur on buspirone). Lithium may be helpful when the anxiety diagnosis is uncertain due to mood swings between manic and depressive periods. However, major weight gain can occur with lithium treatment. For treatment of pain, benzodiazepines cause fewer negative sexual effects and less weight gain than tricyclic antidepressants such as amitriptyline (Elavil) or doxepin (Sinequan). Trazodone (Desyrel) can also decrease pain and serve as a nightly sedative for mild sleep disorders.

CONCLUSIONS

Most of the antianxiety drugs are sedating, with the notable exception of buspirone. In spite of their potential for abuse and misuse, they have been of great value in the treatment of anxiety and panic disorders. The potential for addiction and withdrawal, however, is real.

As with most hypnotics, these drugs can be sexually disinhibiting but essentially disabling. In addition, the danger of aggressive behavior patterns emerging as a side effect must be carefully monitored. With extended use, the adverse physiological sexual results of these drugs become evident. Unfortunately, clinical studies are rarely long enough to show the progression of sexual effects, which, although initially positive, may become distinctly negative. Retrospective evaluations of drugs also miss this dynamic process, often noting the negative with dismissal of the positive.

19

Sedatives/Hypnotics: Benzodiazepines and Methaqualone

OBJECTIVES

- To briefly explore the history of hypnotic drugs from ancient to present times
- To examine the physiological side effects of acute and chronic use of benzodiazepines
- To examine the sexual side effects of the "street drug" methaqualone

A recent nationwide audit of physician prescriptions has shown that since 1970 barbiturate prescriptions have dropped 24-fold, from 42.4 million to 1.8 million, compared to a rise in benzodiazepine sedative/hypnotic prescriptions from 0.7 million to 17.9 million (Wysowski & Baum, 1991). Prescriptions for other types of sedative/hypnotics (chloral hydrate, ethchlorvynol, and glutethimide) have dropped from 19.4 million in 1970 to 1.1 million in 1989. Overall, total sedative/hypnotic prescriptions have dropped from 62.5 million in 1970 to 20.8 million in 1989. Barbiturates were even less likely to be prescribed by psychiatrists than by general practitioners. Consequently, side-effect reports of psychiatric changes due to sedative/hypnotic use have been limited mainly to benzodiazepines. However, it should be noted that both barbiturates and benzodiazepines increase GABA activity. Discussion of GABA and limbic sexual effects of sedative/hypnotics is essential to an understanding of both barbiturates and benzodiazepines (see Chapter 4).

The class of drugs we now call *sedative/hypnotics* has a colorful past steeped in mythology. Ancient sleeping potions were associated with darkness, death, evil, and feminine mystery. Alcohol and the poppy opiate derivatives (opium) were the sleep inducing potions brought by the gods. The Greek god of sleep was Hypnos, often pictured with a poppy branch in his left hand and a wine horn in his right. The Roman god of sleep and dreams was Morpheus (morphine). Other ancient narcotic hypnotics were belladonna-like anticholinergics (hyoscyamine/scopolamine, atropine from mandrake root, henbane, and thorn-apple/jimsonweed). Belladonna (beautiful lady) was named for its seductive, pupil-dilating property; the herbal name for belladonna is *deadly nightshade.* Atropine was named after Atropos, the Greek god of fate, associated with delirium and death. In Greek mythology, Circe used a mandrake potion to seduce and sedate Odysseus and his crew. During the Middle Ages, *spongio seminiferal* was the ultimate sleep potion: a mixture of wine, opium, hyoscyamus, mandrigora, hemlock, and lettuce mild (Hartman, 1978).

In the late 1800s, the aura surrounding hypnotics shifted; the ancient cloak of feminine mystery was replaced by a practical, scientific (masculine) approach, cloaked in medical respectability. The calm, peaceful, but sometimes sinister female ambiance surrounding sleeping potions was replaced by an aggressive, no-nonsense, goal-oriented atmosphere. In succession, bromides, chloral hydrate, barbiturates, antihistamines, and meprobamate (Miltown) were introduced as appropriate hypnotic alternatives that could be dispensed by responsible physicians. The rarity of any mention in the clinical literature of sexual side effects due to hypnotics is a striking contrast to the popular association of sedatives with sexual disinhibition and romance.

Studies in the United States and other countries have shown a general prevalence of insomnia of about 35% (Weyerer & Dilling, 1991). Insomnia is greater in women than in men at all ages, but the difference is most obvious over the age of 50, when 40–50% of females have insomnia compared to about 30% in the men. For both sexes, insomnia increases with age. Mild insomnia is not usually related to psychiatric illness. However, moderate to severe insomnia occurs in 30–50% of persons with psychiatric illness (e.g., anxiety, depression). Nonetheless, the higher incidence of insomnia in women was not due to an excess of psychiatric or physical illness. Hypnotic drugs were used by 32.5% of those with moderate/severe insomnia and 8.3% with mild insomnia. Other studies have shown that about 10% of insomniacs use prescription hypnotics on a regular basis (Weyerer & Dilling, 1991). French studies have shown that about 16% of retired persons over 65 use hypnotics occasionally and 10–30% use tranquilizers (Colomes, Rispail, Berlan, Pous, & Montastruc, 1990).

In an American survey by Everitt, Avorn, and Baker (1990), physicians and nurse practitioners were asked to respond to patients with a history of "chronic insomnia," fabricated for the purpose of the study. Nearly two-thirds of physicians suggested a prescription sedative/hypnotic as treatment for insomnia and nearly 50% considered such a prescription as the single most effective therapy. The older the hypothetical patient, the more likely (60%) a prescription hypnotic was suggested. In contrast, nurse practitioners asked more questions about patients' sleep patterns and suggested lifestyle changes more frequently (55%) than prescription sedative/hypnotics (17%). Among physicians who suggested a prescription as the single most effective therapy, 19% considered triazolam (Halcion) as the drug of choice, 13% suggested flurazepam (Dalmane), 12% suggested temazepam (Restoril), and 10% suggested the antidepressant amitriptyline (Elavil).

Benzodiazepines and other sedative/hypnotics are Federal Drug Administration-approved for very limited use: occasionally or nightly for no more than one month. Over half of the hypnotics prescribed are consumed by people who use them nightly for more than four months and often for years (Kripke, 1985), in direct conflict with Federal Drug Administration protocols. Stricter regulation under present "safe and effective" limitations would, by law, result in more than a 50% reduction in prescription for benzodiazepine sedative/hypnotics.

A large Italian study of medication histories given by elderly patients to their physicians showed that 19.3% of the drugs prescribed had gone unreported (Spagnoli et al., 1989). Benzodiazepines prescribed for either insomnia or anxiety were the most frequent omissions. Kripke (1985) stated that, although no prescription hypnotic is recommended for long-term use and few have been shown to be effective beyond three to four weeks in controlled trials, use of hypnotics beyond four months accounts for about 75% of all hypnotic drug consumption. The extent of hypnotic drug use is seriously underestimated in general surveys when compared to prescription sales figures (Kripke, 1985).

Recently, the state of New York attempted to restrict benzodiazepine sedative/hypnotic use by requiring triplicate prescription (Freishtat, 1988). However, many physicians remain concerned that, when benzodiazepines are restricted, barbiturates and other more dangerous drugs will be used instead. Negative publicity has centered predominantly on the dangers of triazolam. The concern with the hazards of abuse and withdrawal of benzodiazepines has overshadowed serious study of insomnia treatments where these problems are not at issue. Since insomniac patients are often ill and aging, sexual function may be ignored or assumed to be in decline regardless of hypnotic use. Patients themselves may assume that sexual dysfunction is normal for their age and health status. While illness associated with age often compromises sexual function, many patients prefer relief from severe insomnia to optimal sexual function, if they must choose.

BENZODIAZEPINES (SEDATIVES/HYPNOTICS)

Benzodiazepine receptors are present in the body, although no natural benzodiazepine has yet been identified. However, benzodiazepine substances have been found in human mother's milk (Dencker & Johansson, 1990; Dencker, Johansson, & Milsom, 1992), suggesting a kind of "primary conditioning" to the contentment and drowsiness of the baby after feeding. Although benzodiazepines increase GABA activity, they do not force such activity beyond its normal limits. Consequently, benzodiazepines can induce sleep, but do not shut down the nervous system. Death solely through benzodiazepine overdose is rare, unless there are other pathological disease processes present. For instance, benzodiazepines can stop a weakened heart or labored breathing (sleep apnea) long enough to kill or cause coma. Similarly, benzodiazepines can increase the lethal potential of alcohol, barbiturates, and other inhibitory drugs.

Sexual effects found in research with two-ring benzodiazepines (tranquilizers) such as diazepam (Valium), chlordiazepoxide (Librium), oxazepam (Serax), clorazepate (Tranxene), and nitrazepam (Mogadon) are distinct from the newer three-ring structure benzodiazepines (sedatives/hypnotics) such as flurazepam (Dalmane) or temazepam (Restoril). Indeed, there is little evidence of any negative sexual effects in three-ring structure benzodiazepines. Similarly, sexual problems encountered with the triazolobenzodiazepines triazolam and alprazolam (Xanax) could be attributed to individual properties not shared by three-ring benzodiazepines.

Substantial indirect effects of benzodiazepines on sexual functioning may occur as a result of other side effects such as sedation, muscle relaxation, analgesia, lack of attention, and mood disorders. Hall and Joffe (1972) identified an "ego-alien" depressive syndrome in diazepam patients complaining of suicidal ideation, confusion, and depression. Weight gain and an emotional detachment characteristic of benzodiazepine use are important warning signals of overdosage. Patients themselves may be unaware of these symptoms until their partners point out that they are "just not here anymore" or their physicians confront the issue.

Often, only one's spouse may recognize that the drug is dampening sexual contact, expression, and satisfaction. In situations in which expression and reaction normally would be expected, none occurs. Even though the sleeping pills may not directly impede sexual functioning, their preemptory effect on personality can subvert sexual relations. Benzodiazepines suspend the active exercise of limbic activity, which mediates interpersonal intimacy. Their chronic use may undermine sexual desire and responsiveness.

In clinical practice, patients prescribed benzodiazepines as sedative/hypnotics rather than as tranquilizers are typically older, suffer from more illnesses, and are prescribed more concurrent medications (Smith, M., 1985). These concurrent medications, which often include antihypertensives and pain relievers, may have sexual effects themselves. Table 19.1 summarizes the properties and side effects of sedative benzodiazepines.

Sexual Dysfunction

Despite the inhibitory action of benzodiazepines, there are few reports in the literature of negative sexual side effects (Abel, 1985). Those that do occur may be a result of direct drug action, sedation, and/or disruption of normal sleep patterns. All sleeping medications interfere with attentional and emotional processes and can desynchronize natural body cycles. Such interference can generate undesirable personality and sexual effects. Sedatives/hypnotics undermine critical emotional development and interpersonal exchange that is intrinsic to good sex; at the same time, they may trigger neutral or negative emotional reactions resulting in bland sex, aversive sex, or no sex at all. Once endogenous sleep-inducing substances have been identi-

Table 19.1 *Benzodiazepines, Methaqualone, and Other Sedatives/Hypnotics*

	Daily Dose
Benzodiazepines	
Estrazolam (Prosom)	1–2 mg
Flurazepam (Dalmane)	15–30 mg
Midazolam (Versed)	1–2 mg
Quazepam (Doral)	15–30 mg
Temazepam (Restoril)	15–30 mg
Triazolam (Halcion)	0.25–0.5 mg
Miscellaneous	
Chloral hydrate (Noctec, etc.)	500–1000 mg
Ethchlorvynol (Placidyl)	500 mg
Glutethimide (Doriden)	250–500 mg
Hydroxyzine (Atarax, Vistaril)	50–100 mg
Methaqualone (Quaalude, Mequin)	discontinued in U.S.
Zolpidem (Ambien)	5–10 mg
Over-the-counter	
Diphenhydramine (Compoz, Nytol, Sominex)	
Doxylamine (Unisom)	

The sexual effects of sedatives/hypnotics are not usually of clinical concern because any direct sexual effects during sleep are not of concern when awake; however, chronic sleeping pill use typically masks waking anxieties and relationship disorders that are perpetuated by neglect/avoidance and chemical "anaesthesia." Disinhibition and promotion of aggression are side effects of long-term and short-term use. "Blackouts" and amnesia have been a problem, sometimes exploited for sexual abuse.

fied, it might be possible to develop drugs that are purely hypnotic and lack even indirect sexual effects. These drugs would have to work without suppressing limbic areas of the brain that govern attention and emotional reactivity, and they would have to be assimilated naturally into body rhythms.

Because benzodiazepines depress respiration, they are usually contraindicated in sleep apnea patients. Unfortunately, patients often report only the insomnia involved in sleep apnea without directly indicating the apnea itself, and therefore physicians typically prescribe a benzodiazepine sedative/hypnotic. As a result, sleep apnea is worsened along with sexual dysfunction. When breathing temporarily ceases and reactive arousal is decreased by hypnotics, death can occur. Guilleminault (1985) found that 30 mg flurazepam (Dalmane) increased sleep apnea and decreased oxygen saturation in sleep apnea patients. Recently, W. Mendelson (1991) and Bonnet, Dexter, and Arand (1990) have shown that 0.25 mg triazolam does not cause respiratory depression or increase apnea during sleep. Bonnet et al. (1990) successfully used 0.125 mg or 0.25 mg triazolam to treat sleep apnea, assumedly by reducing light stage one sleep and arousals during sleep. The frequent problems associated with triazolam must be weighted against the benefits it may have for this disorder. Sleep apnea worsens during middle age. Smoking, obesity, alcohol, and hypertension are commonly associated with sexual dysfunction as well as sleep apnea.

"Benzodiazepine Blackouts" Perhaps more sinister is the possibile disinhibition that can occur with benzodiazepine sedative/hypnotic use, similar to that which occurs with alcohol. The well-known amnesic, cognitive effects of benzodiazepines are an evident, disruptive factor (Curran, 1986). Though awake and functioning, patients may compromise attention so that they do not remember activities that occur on the day fol-

lowing benzodiazepine use (Scharf, Fletcher, & Graham, 1988). Triazolam is a frequent offender in this regard (Scharf et al., 1988).

Some patients treated with benzodiazepine sedative/hypnotics do not realize that they are taking a tranquilizing antianxiety medication and are not prepared for the possibility of a release from inhibitions. From their perspective, they are merely taking a sleeping pill. From a drug-abuse perspective, however, they are "nodding off." Explanatory inserts are usually not provided for patients along with their prescriptions. There is no informed consent which explains the nature, extent, and dangers of hypnotics, except for a warning not to drink alcohol and drive.

Benzodiazepine hypnotics can undermine judgment and release aggression and hostility; they can also destroy memory of such behavior. An individual might take a drug such as triazolam to aid sleep, quarrel with and hit his/her spouse or children, and have no memory of this episode the next morning. Rage and aggression have even been reported during sleepwalking that first occurred after the patient took a benzodiazepine hypnotic (Regestein & Reich, 1985).

Hindmarch, Sherwood, and Kerr (1993) found that triazolam was no worse than other benzodiazepine sedative/hypnotics when cognitive impairment was measured on perception and short-term memory tasks; rather, impairment was correlated to the sedative effect itself. Considerably more cognitive impairment and sedation occurred on 0.5 mg triazolam than on 0.25 mg triazolam.

A number of physicians have been accused of sexually assaulting patients under the influence of benzodiazepines. Sexual charges have also been made against dentists by female patients treated with benzodiazepine sedatives (Brahams, 1990; Dundee, 1990). A small dose of triazolam can render a woman unconscious and therefore sexually compliant. Triazolam is especially suited for this abuse because of its rapid effect and short action (two to four hours). It clears the system quickly, so that a drug test the next day is unlikely to show its presence. The antegrade amnesia aspect of benzodiazepine is exploited to avoid detection.

Benzodiazepine Disinhibition When benzodiazepines are taken regularly for insomnia, there may be many instances in which inhibitions are released and mental or physical harm committed with no remorse, realization, or recollection. Dietch and Jennings (1988) have used the term *aggressive dyscontrol* to describe the symptoms of benzodiazepine disinhibition such as hostility, aggressiveness, rage reaction. Aggressive dyscontrol with benzodiazepines was noted when they were first released for therapeutic use. Ingram and Timbury (1960) reported a man who physically assaulted his wife for the first time in 20 years of marriage after taking chlordiazepoxide (Librium). Since this time, there have been more than 56 case reports of increased hostility or aggressiveness in patients treated with benzodiazepines.

Early studies reviewed by Delgado (1973) indicated that benzodiazepines could be used to tame monkeys and various wild zoo animals. Subsequent observation, however, has shown that treatment with benzodiazepines can increase aggression unpredictably, resulting in sometimes fatal disruption of established dominance-submission hierarchies in animal colonies (File & Pellow, 1987). McNair et al. (1965) noted that an initial reduction in hostility due to benzodiazepine treatment may disappear after many weeks and, with extended use over many months, hostility may become more noticeable. DiMascio (1973) noted that a number of studies in the late 1960s showed that spontaneous, naturally occurring aggression (attack behavior) increased when benzodiazepines were administered chronically (e.g., for a week) and that aggressive, fear-induced, defensive behavior decreased. Similarly, DiMascio found that one week of treatment with chlordiazepoxide increased scores on animal tests measuring assaultiveness, direct hostility, and irritability.

Inappropriate anger and hostility reactions have also been associated with alprazolam (Xanax). Rosenbaum, Woods, Groves, and Klerman (1984) found such behavior in 10 of 80 panic/phobia patients treated with this drug. Most of these patients had no history of extreme anger or hostility and did not show these rage reactions when treated with other benzodiazepines. Hostility appeared within a week in all patients and after only a single dose in two. The authors of this 1984 report from Massachusetts General Hospital noted that "no mention has been made of hostility in the published reports of the clinical trials of alprazolam which involved more than 1,100 patients." In 1985 the manufacturer of alprazolam noted only four hostile reactions and 13 irritability reactions among 1,717 patients treated in studies submitted to the Federal Drug Administration. In the placebo groups, nine of 1,199 patients showed irritability reactions (Dietch & Jennings, 1988). Alprazolam was incorrectly believed to cause no more hostile or irritable reactions than placebo.

Patients with pre-existing behavior dyscontrol are especially prone to violent reactions with alprazolam use. Cowdry and Gardner (1988) characterized borderline personality disorder by the presence of labile mood states, tumultuous interpersonal relationships, and behavior dyscontrol. In 16 female borderline patients with severe pre-existing behavior dyscontrol, alprazolam was associated with increased assaultive behavior, self-mutilation, and suicidal tendencies. Pyke and Krause (1988) found that hostile reactions to alprazolam occurred in three of five panic patients with depression, but in none of 11 panic patients without depression.

Feldman (1962) found that many diazepam patients displayed a progressive development of dislikes or "hates," initially involving nonsignificant figures in the patients' environment, but progressing to key healthcare providers (such as aides, nurses, and physicians) and eventually encompassing parents and spouses. Overt acts of violence occurred in some cases. Petty, Kramer, and Speece (1991) have shown that there is a transient increase of serotonin during withdrawal form 21 days of diazepam treatment in rats. A decrease in serotonin may contribute to the paradoxical aggression often noted with benzodiazepines. For instance, lesions in the dorsal raphe, which may effect an analogous reduction of dorsal raphe serotonergic firing, facilitate miracidia (mouse-killing in rats) and defensive aggression (Potegal et al., 1988).

Despite these reports of aggressive dyscontrol on benzodiazepines, Dietch and Jennings (1988) noted that the undesirable behavior occurred in less than 1% of patients, which is no greater than on placebo. Overt rage reactions were noted to be extremely rare.

Anxiety and hostile reactions seem to occur much more often on the triazolobenzodiazepine triazolam than on other benzodiazepine hypnotics. In a controlled comparison study, triazolam (0.5 mg), lorazepam (2 mg), or placebo was given to 40 subjects (who were poor sleepers) for 25 consecutive nights (Adam & Oswald, 1989). Both drugs facilitated sleep. However, whereas no increase in distress was noted for lorazepam patients, complaints from triazalom patients increased from 14 at baseline to 59 within days 21 through 25. Reports of depersonalization, despair, and paranoia began about 10 days after beginning treatment with triazolam. In contrast, Rothschild, Bessette, Carter-Campbell, and Murray (1993) found hostile reactions or dyscontrol to be rare among 184 high-risk psychiatric patients treated between 1987 and 1990 with either triazolam or temazepam (about five in 100 for both). It should be noted that hostile dyscontrol frequently occurs when benzodiazepines are taken after or with alcohol (e.g., Terrell, 1988), which can be prevented in hospitalized patients.

Irritable reactions have occurred on 0.5 mg triazolam after only two weeks of nightly use. A small number of psychiatric inpatients were studied by Soldatos, Sakkas, Bergiannaki, and Stefanis (1986) in an alternating schedule of placebo for one week, triazolam for two weeks, and placebo again for one week. Four of the five patients showed irritability on triazolam, which persisted into the withdrawal week. Paranoid or hostile reactions occurred in three of the five patients. Similarly, Bixler, Kales, Brubaker, and Kales (1987) found a greater incidence of hyperexcitability and withdrawal reactions with triazolam than with flurazepam or temazepam. Hostility reactions were reported only on triazolam.

In a study sponsored by the manufacturer of triazolam the anger and tension ratings of the mood scale more than doubled for subjects on 0.5 triazolam nightly for five weeks, whereas almost no change was recorded for patients on placebo (Bliwise, Bliwise, Partinen, Pursley, & Dement, 1988). Since changes during withdrawal were not statistically significant, the report concluded that rebound anxiety did not occur on triazolam. (However, with only seven subjects in each group, the chance of finding a statistically significant effect was low.) Using frequent polysomnographic sleep recordings, the study reported no significant sleep benefit from triazolam beyond week 4 and rebound insomnia after discontinuing triazolam (but not placebo).

The marketing of triazolam was suspended in Great Britain, Norway, and Finland at the end of 1991; in France and Spain the sale of the 0.25 mg tablet, but not the 0.125 mg tablet, was suspended. Toxic effects cited were disinhibitory reactions, anxiety, depression, and anterograde amnesia (Rothschild, 1992). After the FDA review in the United States, continued sale was approved but with a strong warning against chronic use or doses above 0.25 mg. Rothschild (1992) conducted an extensive literature search and evaluation from 1975 to 1992. He found that behavioral disinhibition during use of triazolam was associated with higher doses (0.5 mg and above) and higher pretreatment levels of hostility. These reactions did not appear to occur more frequently on triazolam than on other benzodiazepines. An extensive review of the entire clinical trial database for triazolam by its manufacturer (Upjohn) similarly showed that infrequent hostile, depressive, or irritable reactions occur equally often on triazolam and other short-acting benzodiazepines (Jonas, Coleman, Sheridan, & Kalinske, 1992). While the debate continues, it seems clear that minimal doses of benzodiazepine sedative/hypnotics should be used as seldom as possible and should not be used by persons prone to depression, hostility, or even moderate use of alcohol.

Rebound Anxiety Although alprazolam (Xanax) has been designated as an antianxiety drug, it is often prescribed for sleep. If insomnia does not originally accompany anxiety, it may become a problem when a patient attempts to stop alprazolam. Such withdrawal-induced insomnia may be the chief impediment to discontinuing the drug, even when anxiety is no longer a problem.

Rebound anxiety reactions with hypnotic withdrawal (similar to rebound insomnia) may aggravate pre-existing tendencies or occur for the first time (Adam & Oswald, 1989). Panic, fear, depression, and derealization, which may occur following chronic benzodiazepine use, can lead to increased use. By definition, repetitive withdrawal occurs with hypnotic use each morning.

ALTERNATIVES

The alternative non-benzodiazepine medication, buspirone (BuSpar), does not induce sleep. Therefore, it relieves withdrawal-induced insomnia only to the extent that it treats the anxiety itself. Although buspirone is used quite successfully in patients not on benzodiazepines and may even have an antidepressant action, it is often insufficient for patients already on benzodiazepines. Trazodone (Desyrel) can be used as a nocturnal sedative at low doses of 50–100 mg nightly without dependence and with the advantage of a possible antidepressant effect in patients with mild depression or undiagnosed dependence.

Zolpidem (Ambien)

Zolpidem (Ambien) is a nonbenzodiazepine sedative/hypnotic recently approved in the United States, which stimulates a benzodiazepine subtype. It belongs to a new class of tranquilizer drugs, the *imidazopyridines* (Sauvenet et al., 1988). Zolpidem binds to a specific benzodiazepine/GABA site, the benzodiazepine-1 receptor (also called the omega-1 receptor), which differentiates it from drugs with exclusive benzodiazepine affinity (Langer, Arbilla, Scatton, Niddam, & Dubois, 1988). Action at this benzodiazepine-1 receptor has a strong hypnotic effect but only weak anticonvulsant and muscle-relaxant effects. Zolpidem has been described as rapid in onset (15 to 30 minutes), with an ideal duration of action (six to seven hours). It is reputed to produce natural physiological sleep with no decrease in deep slow-wave sleep or REM dream sleep (Kryger, Steljes, Pouliot, Neufeed, & Odynski, 1991; Medical Letter, 1993). It is also claimed to be free of residual effects such as daytime drowsiness, anxiety, rebound insomnia, tolerance, withdrawal, dependence or abuse potential, significant memory impairment, and respiratory depression (Sauvanet et al., 1988). The adverse side effects of zolpidem appear equal to or a bit more frequent than with currently available benzodiazepine hypnotics. These side effects include dizziness, drowsiness, fatigue, headache, memory disorders, confusion, and falls (Emeriau et al., 1988; Louvel et al., 1988; Palminteri & Narbonne, 1988). The suggested dose of zolpidem is 10 mg at bedtime, taken when needed for sleep.

In clinical trials, the effects of zolpidem on EEG and various aspects of sleep are no different from those of benzodiazepine hypnotics such as flunitrazepam and triazolam (Emeriau et al., 1988; Louvel et al., 1988). However, in contrast to benzodiazepine sedative/hypnotics, deep sleep stages (3 and 4) and REM sleep are not shortened (Kryger et al., 1991). Contrary to many studies (Kales, 1985) showing that tolerance develops to triazolam and other hypnotics within one to two months, a company-sponsored controlled trial found both zolpidem and triazolam to remain at full efficacy over three months of daily use (Louvel et al., 1988).

As yet, there is no evidence that zolpidem has any adverse sexual effects, although its mechanism of action suggests that it is likely to decrease sex drive and response. Agonists as well as inverse agonists of GABA have been shown to have positive sexual effects in animals. Beta-carbolines, which cause excitement and anxiety, appear to bind to the same benzodiazepine/omega-1 site as zolpidem. Since beta-carbolines have been shown to have positive excitatory sexual effects in animals, zolpidem may be expected to have the opposite effect, namely depressed sexual excitation. However, zolpidem may have far weaker anticonvulsant and muscle-relaxing properties than benzodiazepines. Since muscular excitement and muscle spasm are inherent components of orgasm and ejaculation, zolpidem may not have the significant adverse effects on sexual sensation and orgasm that can occur with stronger anticonvulsants.

Although zolpidem may have the important advantage of less dependence and withdrawal, there is no reliable clinical evidence that it is any safer or more effective than currently available benzodiazepine/hypnotics. The claim of preserving natural physiological slow-wave and REM sleep would be a major advantage over benzodiazepines. However, zolpidem is not a natural sleep factor and probably does not work through a natural endogenous sleep factors as do the benzodiazepines, which decrease slow-wave and REM sleep.

METHAQUALONE (QUAALUDE)

Methaqualone (Quaalude) was first synthesized in India in 1955 as an antimalarial drug, but was soon found to be an effective sedative/hypnotic alternative to barbiturates. It was approved in the United States in 1965 as a schedule V drug (minimal abuse potential); by 1971, it had become the sixth most popular sedative/hypnotic. In the 1960s and 1970s, methaqualone became a popular "yuppie drug." Like cocaine, it was considered nonaddicting and relatively safe, particularly when compared to barbiturates. In contrast to barbiturates, it was said to allow one to become "high" without excessive drowsiness. Due to its abuse by younger people, it was made a schedule II drug (high abuse potential) in 1984.

Chemically, methaqualone is a quinozoline derivative, but its mechanism of action is unknown. Quinozoline drugs are active at (newly discovered) excitatory amino acid glutamate receptors, but methaqualone does not appear to have any special affinity for these receptors. Unlike other hypnotics, it has minimal action on brainstem reticular arousing activity. Nevertheless, it has also been shown to have anticonvulsant, antitussive (cough), antispasmodic, and anesthetic (but not analgesic) efficacy. Methaqualone acts within 10 to 30 minutes and its effects may last for about four hours. In overdose, it differs from other sedative/hypnotics in that it sometimes can provoke seizure. Such convulsive effects occur more frequently with Mandrax, a combination of 250 mg methaqualone with 25 mg diphenhydramine. Like other barbiturates, methaqualone has depressive effects and seizures occur upon withdrawal.

When methaqualone was used as a hypnotic, mild side effects occurred in about 5–10% of patients, including headache, dizziness, nausea, diarrhea, tachycardia, and skin rashes (Blum, 1984). Paradoxical restlessness and anxiety were also frequently reported. Methaqualone is potentially lethal when used with alcohol or other depressant drugs. Although Yanagita and Miyasato (1976) found that methaqualone did not produce dependency in rhesus monkeys, it served as a reinforcer when self-administered intravenously and could be expected to be subject to abuse.

Sexual Effects

Methaqualone became a street drug early in its "life" and most scientists lost interest in it. It is unfortunate that we do not know more about it. Methaqualone appears to have definite sexual effects, facilitating libido, receptiveness, erection, and delaying orgasm/ejaculation. However, because it is a depressant drug, the sexual effects tend to decrease with continued use. The popular reputation of methaqualone as a love drug and "heroin for lovers" practically ensured its abuse, similar to labeling MDMA as ecstasy.

In a survey of college students, Kochansky, Salzman, Shader, Harmatz, and Ogeltree (1975) found that females preferred methaqualone even to marijuana as their "aphrodisiac of choice." Its libido-raising property was effective in women due to its sedating, relaxing, anxiety-reducing, and mildly euphoric effects. Males preferred the drug because of its ability to make them "last" longer. Gay and his Haight-Ashbury clinical colleagues (1982) noted that 33% of drug-user respondents considered methaqualone useful for enhancing and prolonging sex, indicating that it delays orgasm/ejaculation. In place of orgasm, the drug produced "tingling numbness in the extremities and a rubberiness of the skin that pleasantly modify the physical sensations of sex" (Blum, 1984). Buffum (1982) also noted that it caused ataxic weakness of the extremities and had "an inhibitory action on polysynaptic pathways, and produce[d] hind limb weakness in animals."

Much of the information on methaqualone's "aphrodisiac" properties as they affect humans comes from researchers in San Francisco. However, similar experiences have occurred with normal sedative doses of quaaludes (200–250 mg). At Harvard's McLean Hospital, Ionescu-Pioggia, Bird, and Cole (1988) noted that methaqualone produced euphoria in nonaddict men and women even at the low dose of 200 mg, and sexual feelings were reported more often than would be expected from placebo.

The failure of researchers to identify methaqualone's chemical actions indicates that the drug may affect unknown neural receptors and brain areas. The receptors may involve excitatory amino acid glutamate transmission, but these do not seem to be either sigma or PCP receptors. The brain area involved in mediating the sexual effects is surely the limbic system rather than lower areas such as the hypothalamus. Methaqualone has unexplained complex actions (neuronal underactivity or overactivity) that can be fatal. Discovering the chemical basis of methaqualone abuse may tell us much about the mechanisms of action that mediate obsessive-compulsive sexuality and/or sex addiction.

CONCLUSIONS

Hypnotics as a class are subject to a variety of abuses. The most common is chronic use at normal dosage. The second form of abuse is the use of these sedatives to induce sleep and, in effect, to mask unresolved, anxiety-provoking issues related to job, life style, parents, children, or relationships. The better known form of abuse involves nontherapeutic doses taken with other drugs and/or alcohol.

Disturbances in sleep and sex naturally involve limbic disturbances. An incomplete understanding of this phenomenon and the absence of a comprehensive approach remain as challenges for the fields of psychology, psychiatry, and medicine. Currently, the medical approach to pharmacological narcosis is giving way to sleep clinics that emphasize the rhythmic methods of influencing limbic system dynamics and integration. The degree to which these sleep disorder centers include "mind" issues such as thought and emotion determines the comprehensiveness of the approach.

None of the hypnotic drugs appears to act through natural sleep mechanisms. Because they depress or inhibit the nervous system, most have secondary effects responsible for the sedative action. As such, they are "insults" to normal physiological regulation, inducing changes for which the body is not prepared and may react against, as with rebounding insomnia or disruption of circadian rhythm and natural body cycles.

With the availability of more specific GABA and benzodiazepine drugs, there is a possibility of synthesizing substances that are sleep-inducing but without the associated anxiety, mental disablement, and sensation-reducing effects of currently available sedatives/hypnotics. Whether such drugs will be superior is questionable, since the antianxiety and relaxant properties of current benzodiazepine hypnotics may have positive psychological benefits that facilitate their hypnotic action.

20

Antidepressants I: Tricyclics and MAO Inhibitors

OBJECTIVES

- To examine the direct and indirect sexual side effects of tricyclic antidepressants
- To examine the direct and indirect sexual side effects of MAO inhibitor antidepressants

Antidepressants have improved dramatically in regard to sexual side effects over the course of their development. The first-generation antidepressants, represented by the monoamine oxidase inhibitors (MAOIs) and tricyclics, are associated with significant degrees of sexual dysfunction. With newer, synthetically engineered antidepressants such as bupropion and trazodone, not only have sexual side effects been minimized but, in some cases, sexual functioning has improved.

The MAOIs and tricyclics are discussed primarily in this chapter; the newer antidepressants (bupropion, trazodone, SSRIs) will be addressed here, in the following chapter, and in chapters on sexually effective drugs. As is the case with tranquilizers, sedatives, and hypnotics, women are the greatest consumers of antidepressant medications. Therefore, while the adverse sexual consequences addressed in this chapter pertain to both sexes, the impact is greater for women.

TRICYCLICS

Tricyclic antidepressants characteristically require two to four weeks to work. Their action appears to involve rebalancing NA and 5-HT neural transmission; such rebalancing may normalize other body rhythms, including sleep and circadian hormonal activity. Tricyclics do not directly affect levels of dopamine (DA), but they may restore dopaminergic sensitivity, which has been blunted due to the dysregulation intrinsic to depression. The best-known tricyclic side effects are sexual dysfunction and weight gain. Depression itself can cause sexual dysfunction (Nofzinger et al., 1993). However, for some depressed patients, sexual dysfunction occurs for the first time with tricyclic treatment. Tricyclics can cause sexual problems directly, or as an indirect result of sedation, weight gain, and other unpleasant side effects. Sexual dysfunction is a notable symptom of untreated clinical depression in at least 50% of cases (Casper et al., 1985; Nofzinger et al., 1993); this dysfunction is then further aggravated by medication. Hollister (1990) expressed the debilitating side effects of tricyclics when he noted:

> Some years ago, a nice controlled clinical trial showed that imipramine was equal to a benzodiazepine for treating anxiety. My first comment was "how did they manage to get the patients to take it [the tricyclic]? . . . " Unless you are depressed, these are noxious agents. It is not surprising, therefore, that patients went off tricyclics, which is why noncompliance is a major problem in treating depression with these drugs, let alone something else.

Table 20.1 summarizes the properties and side effects of tricyclic antidepressants.

Table 20.1 *Profile of Tricyclic Antidepressants*

	Daily Dose
Amitriptyline (Elavil)	25–300 mg
Clomipramine (Anafranil)	25–150 mg
Desipramine (Norpramin, Pertofrane)	50–300 mg
Dothiepin (Prothiapin*)	75–300 mg
Doxepin (Sinequan, Adapin)	50–300 mg
Imipramine (Tofranil)	50–300 mg
Nortriptyline (Pamelor, Aventyl)	20–150 mg
Protriptyline (Vivactil)	15–60 mg
Trimipramine (Surmontil)	25–300 mg

COMMON INDICATIONS

Depression, chronic pain, eating disorders/bulimia, panic/phobia, anxiety, post-traumatic stress disorder, enuresis, and attention deficit hyperactive disorder (usually in children)

MECHANISMS OF ACTION (GENERAL)

Inhibits the re-uptake of norepinephrine and serotonin (5-HT)

Modulates norephinephrine and 5-HT activity at the neural synapse

MECHANISMS OF ACTION (SEXUAL)

Positive

Increased adrenergic $alpha_1$ activity

Decreased cortisol

Negative

Decreased beta-adrenergic activity

Decreased cholinergic activity

Decreased histamine

Decreased oxytocin

Increased prolactin

Increased serotonin

DIRECT SEXUAL SIDE EFFECTS

Desire disorders (in both sexes)

Erection difficulties

Dyspareunia

Menstrual disorders (amenorrhea)

Infertility

Orgasm irregularities
- Orgasmic inhibition
- Anorgasmia
- Spontaneous orgasm

Ejaculation irregularities
- Retarded ejaculation
- Ejaculation without orgasm
- Anesthetic ejaculation

Breast disorders
- Pain/tenderness
- Galactorrhea
- Gynecomastia

INDIRECT SEXUAL SIDE EFFECTS

Discomfort caused by dryness of skin, mouth, and mucous membranes; constipation, edema, weight gain, indigestion, nausea, rash/itching, urinary problems (retention)

Mood disorders resulting in anhedonia, anxiety, nervousness, depression, detachment, irritability, mania, nervousness

Neurological disturbances resulting in analgesia, cognitive deficits, dizziness, fatigue, headache, movement disorder, pain, paresthesia, sleep disturbances, sensory loss, tremor, weakness

Vascular disturbances resulting in arrhythmias, headache, peripheral vasoconstriction, shortness of breath

SEXUAL CONTRAINDICATIONS/BENEFITS

Avoid with prior or current condition of

Desire disorders

Erection disorders

Anorgasmia

Lubrication disorders

May be useful for

Vaginismus

Dyspareunia

Hypersexuality

Inhibited ejaculation

Premature ejaculation

Table 20.1 *Continued*

ALTERNATIVES	EJACULATORY/ORGASMIC SUPPLEMENTS
Trazodone (Desyrel): depression with insomnia, chronic pain Bupropion (Wellbutrin): depression, attention deficit disorder Fluoxetine (Prozac): depression, panic/phobia, eating disorders/bulimia, post-traumatic stress disorder Nefazodone (Serzone): depression	These drugs can be used in conjunction with tricyclics to reverse some side effects: bethanechol, neostigmine, and cyproheptadine.

*Not available in the United States.

Sexual Dysfunction

Sex drive disorders are probably the most common sexual side effects of tricyclics, and the most frequently overlooked. Erection and orgasm/ejaculation difficulties are the most apparent. Tricyclics interfere with most body fluid secretions, including salivation, lubrication, precoital fluid, and ejaculatory volume. Dry mouth makes kissing difficult and promotes halitosis. Diminished vaginal lubrication can be corrected with artificial lubrication, and concern about diminished ejaculatory volume can be addressed with reassurance. If a patient is forewarned, these side effects are usually manageable. Many cases of ejaculatory delay are not reported because men do not consider it to be a problem. However, continued inhibition of orgasm and ejaculation is associated with diminished desire, which usually leads to decreased frequency.

Anorgasmia or delayed orgasm is now clinically recognized as a common tricyclic-induced sexual problem for women as well. While deficiencies in lubrication or genital feeling have not been reported in the literature, they are frequently mentioned by individual patients in clinical practice. Because of their antispasmodic and anesthetic properties, some patients are placed on tricyclics to treat genital pain and/or muscle spasm. Cases of female anorgasmia with tricyclics have been reported by:

- Couper-Smartt and Rodham, 1973: 100 mg imipramine
- Sovner, 1983: 150–200 mg imipramine
- Sovner, 1984: 60 mg nortriptyline
- Riley and Riley, 1986: 75–150 mg imipramine
- Steele and Howell, 1986: 150 mg imipramine
- Pontius, 1988: 225 mg desipramine

Harrison et al. (1986) conducted a six-week placebo-controlled antidepressant trial with imipramine (200–300 mg) and phenelzine, using a comprehensive sexual questionnaire for both men and women. Male subjects (36/82) reported no significant sexual differences between imipramine and placebo in desire, enjoyment, erection, nocturnal erection, or frequency of intercourse. However, orgasm and ejaculation were significantly more difficult with imipramine (mean dose = 289 mg) than with placebo. Female subjects (46/82) reported no significant sexual differences due to imipramine. Orgasm during masturbation was somewhat more difficult, but there was a small improvement in enjoyment, arousal, and orgasm during intercourse.

Sexual dysfunction and weight gain more commonly occur after the initial six weeks of antidepressant treatment (Harrison, 1987). Consequently, the relatively small number of sexual side effects found in the Harrison et al. (1986) six-week study probably under-represented those that occur with long-term treatment. No studies examining the development of these long-term side effects have been conducted thus far. Decreases in sexual desire, erection, orgasm, and ejaculation are probably more frequent than noted in the tricyclic literature, perhaps because the sexual dysfunction is automatically attributed to depression instead of drug treatment.

Several cases of ejaculation deficits with tricyclics were reported in a 1983 review by Mitchell and Popkin. Relying mainly on the cases reported to drug manufacturers, the researchers cited ejaculatory dysfunction with numerous tricyclics: amitriptyline (3 cases at 100 mg/day minimum dose), imipramine (4 cases at 75 mg/day minimum dose), trimipramine (3 cases), desipramine (1 case), doxepin (1 case). Other reports (mostly single case studies) of ejaculatory dysfunction associated with tricyclics include (beginning with most recent): Rosenbaum and Pollack, 1988; Segraves, 1987; Yager, 1986; Glass, 1981; Nininger, 1978; Couper-Smartt and Rodham, 1973; Simpson, Blair, and Amuso, 1965. Reports of desire and erection deficits due to tricyclics include (beginning with the most recent): Mitchell and Popkin, 1983; Clark, Schmidt, Schaal, Bondoulas, and Schuller, 1979; Hekimian, Friedhoff, and Deever, 1978; Everett, 1975; Guilleminault, Carskadon, and Dement, 1974; Greenberg, 1965; Simpson et al., 1965. In its surveillance program, the Federal Drug Administration reported erection problems due to tricyclics in only 14 patients between 1969 and 1977 (Petrie, 1980). In contrast to the minimal sexual side effects of antidepressants reported through surveillance monitoring, a high rate of sexual side effects may be found with careful questioning and detailed questionnaires. Balon, Yeragani, Pohl, and Ramesh (1993) interviewed 60 anxiety or depression patients (22 men, 38 women) treated with various antidepressants for an average of 5.8 months. Sixteen of 29 patients (eight of 16 women, eight of 13 men) reported sexual dysfunction on imipramine (usually, decreased libido and difficulty reaching orgasm), compared to six of 14 patients treated with fluoxetine. No sexual dysfunction was reported by five women treated with trazodone.

It appears that accurate reporting of sexual side effects associated with tricyclics has required two decades of lag time, and counting. Indeed, the authors of a text on major sexual therapy stated that they "have seen no cases of impotence secondary to antidepressant use" (Schmidt, 1983).

Clomipramine (Anafranil), amitriptyline (Elavil), and doxepin (Sinequan) appear to be the most sexually toxic tricyclics. While sexual dysfunction on doxepin and amitriptyline appears strongly dose-dependent, negative sexual effects may be quite frequent even at relatively low doses of clomipramine. (The sexual effects of clomipramine will be discussed in the next chapter because of its particularly strong serotonin uptake action.) Dothiepin (Prothiapin), which is widely used outside the United States, has sexual side effects equivalent to amitriptyline. Clomipramine, amitriptyline, and doxepin are commonly used in pain treatment clinics to treat chronic pain and diabetic neuropathy (Loldrup, Langemark, Hansen, Olesen, & Bech, 1989; Magni, 1991; Max et al., 1992; Wright, 1994). These combination norepinephrine and serotonin uptake inhibitor antidepressants have been shown to be more effective than selective SSRIs in pain treatment (Max et al., 1992; Sindrup et al., 1992). Imipramine (Tofranil) and protriptyline (Vivactil) have moderately severe sexual side effects. Although protriptyline has the same anticholinergic side effects as amitriptyline, it is more activating, sometimes causing jitteriness and insomnia, and causes fewer sexual problems. Little is known about the sexual side effects of trimipramine, but they are probably similar to those of imipramine, given their molecular relationship. Desipramine (Norpramin, Pertofrane) and nortriptyline (Pamelor, Aventyl) have the least bothersome side effects in general (less sedation, less anticholinergic activity, less postural hypotension, and less weight gain) and the fewest sexual side effects in particular. While they have sexual effects similar to all the other tricyclics, these effects occur much less frequently. However, desipramine can cause irritability, possibly due to its activating properties, and among clinicians is sometimes referred to as "the divorce drug." However, this aspect of desipramine has not been documented in the literature.

Tricyclics such as amitriptyline and clomipramine are notorious for causing weight gain, and sexual dysfunction can be a secondary effect. Recovery from depression is often not complete because of weight gain and sexual dysfunction. In addition to sexual dysfunction, weight gain is a serious cause of noncompliance and must be considered. In a three-year follow-up study of 107 panic/phobia patients treated with tricyclic antidepressants, Noyes, Garvey, Cook, and Samuelson (1989) found that 35% discontinued treatment due to side effects. (Thirty-four percent of patients gained five to 50 pounds.) Among the tricyclics, amitriptyline, doxepin, and clomipramine caused the most weight gain (five to 40 pounds), and desipramine the least (from zero to 10 pounds); imipramine and other tricyclics registered from zero to 30 pounds. These same tricyclics also caused the most and the least sedation, respectively, due in large part to their antihistamine effect.

As a result of intolerable weight gain, 35–48% of patients terminated otherwise necessary long-term tricyclic antidepressant treatment. Although weight often decreases with tricyclic withdrawal, depression usually increases. Persistent sexual dysfunction triggered by tricyclic treatment may cause a low-grade depression (dysthymia) for many years after the original depressive episode and treatment.

Male/Female Differences

Tricyclics have similar sexual effects in both men and women: inhibited desire, orgasm/ejaculation difficulties, and diminished sensation. Diminished lubrication can become a problem for women who are not receptive to using artificial lubrication and for menopausal women who are already experiencing decreased lubrication. Painful testicular swelling has been observed with desipramine (Deicken & Carr, 1987). Aizenberg, Zemishlany, Hermesh, Karp, and Weizman (1991) reported four case studies of patients experiencing painful ejaculation on either 125 or 150 mg of imipramine or clomipramine, which did not occur when medication was discontinued or reduced to 75 mg. Balon et al. (1993) reported painful "orgasm" (not differentiated from painful ejaculation) in four of 11 men treated with imipramine (dose assumed to be over 100 mg) but in none of 16 treated women.

Reduced nocturnal penile tumescence (NPT) has been demonstrated with tricyclics. Kowalski, Stanley, Dennerstein, Burrows, and Maguire (1985) measured NPT in six normal male volunteers (18 to 35 years old) after two weeks of treatment with 150 mg of amitriptyline. Compared to placebo, amitriptyline caused decreased amplitude and duration of nocturnal erections. Decreased NPT has not been found with trimipramine (200 mg), which also does not alter REM sleep (Wohrmann, Steiger, Benkert, & Holsboer, 1988). Karacan (1986) found decreased nocturnal erections in a narcoleptic man treated with 50–100 mg imipramine.

The full significance of these NPT deficits reported by Kowalski et al. (1985) is difficult to evaluate because two weeks of treatment is too short for adequate evaluation of sexual side effects, especially with tricyclics. These subjects did not report subjective changes in erection, enjoyment, orgasm, or ejaculation, which is not surprising considering the brief time interval. The NPT results were compelling objective evidence that adverse physiological sexual effects occur early in treatment. With the exception of the selective use of tricyclics as analgesic/antispasmodic treatment for painful intercourse, tricyclics other than desipramine or nortriptyline should not be prescribed if sexual function is a consideration.

Sexual Benefits

Tricyclics have occasionally been used in clinical practice to treat premature ejaculation, but their effectiveness is unpredictable and any value is usually complicated by diminished desire. In certain cases of dyspareunia and vaginismus, tricyclics have been used as an adjunct to therapy and other medical or surgical treatment. The tricyclics also may have limited value in the voluntary treatment of depressed patients who are also hypersexual.

Isolated cases of paradoxical sexual responses

occur occasionally with drugs that usually affect sexual function adversely. There have been a few reports of direct sexual stimulation by clomipramine and imipramine (spontaneous orgasm with yawning). Clomipramine has caused yawning accompanied by orgasm or "irresistible sexual urges" in two women and one man (McLean, Forsythe, & Kapkin, 1983). Semen emission occurred repeatedly during defecation in a 54-year-old man treated alternately with imipramine and desipramine (Brier, Ginsberg, & Charney, 1984). Sustained yawning (but not orgasm) was reported in a 30-year-old woman on imipramine (Goldberg, 1984).

Alternatives

The best approach for resolving tricyclic-induced sexual dysfunction is to substitute an alternative antidepressant (see Table 20.2). In some cases, supplementing tricyclic therapy with cholinergic or antiserotonin agents may reverse the dysfunction—but not without additional undesirable side effects. The alternative antidepressants with the least sexual side effects are bupropion (Wellbutrin), trazodone (Desyrel), and the recently marketed nefazodone (Serzone).

Table 20.2 *Best and Worst Tricyclic Antidepressants*

*Sexual Side Effects**		
Best	*Moderate*	*Worst*
Desipramine	Protriptyline	Clomipramine
Nortriptyline	Imipramine	Amitriptyline
		Dothiepin
		Doxepin
Weight Gain		
Best (0–10 pounds)	*Moderate (0–30 pounds)*	*Worst (5–40 pounds)*
Desipramine	Imipramine	Amitriptyline
	Nortriptyline	Doxepin
	Protriptyline	Clomipramine

*Decreased lubrication, decreased sex drive, impotence, anorgasmia, inhibited ejaculation.
Mitchell and Popkin, 1983; Noyes et al., 1989.

Cholinergic Agents The following research reported the favorable impact of bethanechol (Urecholine) on sexual function and/or other tricyclic side effects:

- reversed tricyclic-induced anorgasmia: Segraves, 1987; Yager, 1986; Gross, 1982
- relieved urinary retention and dry mouth but not loss of sexual desire and erection: Everett, 1975
- decreased erection difficulties: Pollack and Rosenbaum, 1987
- relieved constipation but did not reverse anorgasmia: Pontius, 1988
- facilitated urination and orgasm in men after prostate surgery: Segraves, 1987; Everett, 1975

Bethanechol can cause nausea and dysphoria that is more unpleasant than the lack of orgasm. Therefore, it is preferable to switch to an antidepressant without anticholinergic effects, when possible.

Antiserotonergic Agents Despite their notorious reputation, anticholinergic effects are probably less important than serotonergic effects in tricyclic-induced sexual dysfunction in general and in orgasm/ejaculatory deficits in particular. The following research on the antiserotonergic drug cyproheptadine (Periactin) was reported:

- reversed anorgasmia due to tricyclic or MAOI antidepressants: Riley and Riley, 1986; De Castro, 1985; Sovner, 1984
- reversed imipramine-induced anorgasmia: Steele and Howell, 1986
- eliminated anorgasmia when imipramine was replaced by desipramine: Steele and Howell, 1986
- failed to reverse imipramine anorgasmia: Riley and Riley, 1986

There are more undesirable side effects with cyproheptadine than with bethanechol. Cyproheptadine has caused anticholinergic reactions of fever, hypertension, dry mouth and eyes, tremor, and anxiety when used to reverse desipramine-induced anorgasmia (Pontius, 1988). When given to reverse phenelzine-induced anorgasmia, cyproheptadine has caused irritability and even visual hallucinations (Kahn, 1987). Because of its antiserotonin and antihistamine properties, this drug can also cause weight gain and sedation. Jenike (1990) noted that anorgasmia was common in obsessive-compulsive patients treated with clomipramine and fluoxetine. When cyproheptadine was prescribed to treat the sexual dysfunction, the majority of patients reported "intolerable fatigue" and one patient reported that his obsessive-compulsive traits had worsened. Similarly, Feder (1991) reported that cyproheptadine caused severe dysphoria and depression in three male patients who had developed loss of orgasm during fluoxetine (Prozac) treatment.

As noted, the most beneficial way to reverse antidepressant-induced anorgasmia is by reducing doses or shifting to a different antidepressant. Patients can also be encouraged to ask their partners for more touching and direct genital stimulation. Bethanechol (10–30 mg) or cyproheptadine (4–12 mg) can be taken about an hour prior to sexual activity but should be closely monitored for adverse reactions. Patients often find both drugs unpleasant and not worth the additional side effects.

Yohimbine has also been shown to reverse anorgasmia induced by the tricyclic clomipramine and by SSRI antidepressants such as fluoxetine. When taken 90 minutes before intercourse, a patient on 150 mg of clomipramine became orgasmic again (Price & Grunhaus, 1990). Unless there are disturbing side effects such as nausea or anxiety, yohimbine is a preferred supplement for reversing antidepressant-induced sexual dysfunction because it has antidepressant effects of its own. However, yohimbine may generate severe anxiety and cardiovascular side effects when combined with tricyclics. The danger of such side effects would normally preclude its use with tricyclics; this combination should be avoided.

Currently, there are excellent alternatives to tricyclic treatment. However, they may not always be as effective as tricyclics in treating depression. Trazodone (Desyrel) can be substituted when sleep is a major problem, because it is also an excellent sedative. Nefazodone (Serzone) is a new version of trazodone relatively free of sedation and sexual side effects. Bupropion (Wellbutrin) is an effective alternative antidepressant unless patients find it too stimulating. Fluoxetine (Prozac) is also an alternative antidepressant; however, it can cause inhibited orgasm and decreased sexual desire. Sertraline (Zoloft) is an SSRI, equal in antidepressant efficacy to fluoxetine but with less associated anxiety. Venlafaxine (Effexor) is both a norepinephrine and SSRI; it has negative sexual effects apparently equal to fluoxetine, but it is possibly more potent as an antidepressant. As noted, when tricyclics must be used, desipramine (Norpramin) and nortriptyline (Pamelor) are preferable in terms of sexual side effects.

MONOAMINE OXIDASE INHIBITORS

Monoamine neural activity is regulated by removal of synaptic amines either by re-uptake into the presynaptic nerve ending destruction by MAO enzymatic breakdown or activation of presynaptic autoreceptors. Supposedly, in depression monoamine levels are reduced, leading to depressed mood, which can be corrected by tricyclic or MAO antidepressants, resulting in increased monamine activity. (See Table 20.3 for the properties and side effects of MAOIs.) MAOIs are antidepressants that increase monoamine (norepinephrine and serotonin) activity by blocking enzymes that metabolize monoamines and removing them from synaptic nerve endings.

Sexual Dysfunction

Since the mid 1980s monoamine oxidase inhibitors (MAOIs) have been known to cause sexual problems fairly frequently (Harrison et al., 1985; Mitchell & Popkin, 1983). Reliable sources have suggested a 20–40% incidence of sexual dysfunction (Harrison et al., 1985, 1986; Buigues

Table 20.3 *Profile of MAO Inhibitors (MAOIs)*

	Daily Dose
Isocarboxazid (Marplan)	10–40 mg
Phenelzine (Nardil)	30–90 mg
Tranycypromine (Parnate)	10–40 mg
Moclobemide (Aurora*)	

COMMON INDICATIONS

Depression, atypical depression (hypersomnia, hyperphagia, mood reactive), panic/phobia, obsessive-compulsive disorder, eating disorder/bulimia

MECHANISMS OF ACTION (GENERAL)

Decreases the neural monoamine oxidase enzymatic metabolic breakdown of norepinephrine and serotonin
Increases norepinephrine and serotonin activity at the neural synapse

MECHANISMS OF ACTION (SEXUAL)

Positive
- Increased adrenergic $alpha_1$ activity
- Decreased monoamine oxidase

Negative
- Decreased beta adrenergic activity
- Decreased cholinergic activity
- Increased prolactin
- Increased serotonin
- Decreased testosterone

DIRECT SEXUAL SIDE EFFECTS

Desire disorders (in both sexes) Erection difficulties	Orgasm irregularities • Orgasmic inhibition • Diminished number of orgasms	Ejaculation disorders • Retarded, inhibited • Premature ejaculation diminished	Breast disorders • Gynecomastia • Galactorrhea • Pain/tenderness	Menstrual Disorders • Amenorrhea

INDIRECT SEXUAL SIDE EFFECTS

Discomfort caused by dryness of skin, mouth and mucous membranes; constipation, edema, indigestion, nausea, weight gain, rash/itching, urinary problems (retention)

Mood disorders resulting in anhedonia, depression, detachment, mania, nervousness

Neurological disturbances resulting in analgesia, dizziness, fatigue, headache, ataxia, paresthesia, sedation, tremor, muscular weakness

Vascular disturbances resulting in headache, shortness of breath

SEXUAL CONTRAINDICATIONS/BENEFITS

Avoid with prior condition of
- Desire disorders
- Erection disorders
- Inhibited orgasms/ejaculation
- Anorgasmia

May be useful for
- Premature ejaculation
- Hypersexuality

ALTERNATIVES

SSRIs: panic, phobia, obsession-compulsion, atypical depression, depression, bulimia
Alprazolam (Xanax): panic
Wellbutrin (Bupropion): atypical depression, depression
Nefazodone (Serzone): depression

*New reversible MAOI not yet available in United States.

& Vallejo, 1987). Information on the nature and extent of MAOI sexual side effects, however, has been meager. Decreased erection has been noted occasionally under the label of impotence, but sex drive and orgasmic dysfunction are usually not examined. Reports on sexual drive or arousal difficulties with MAOIs have been sporadic. Lubrication deficits have never been mentioned. Monoamine oxidase inhibitors retard orgasm and ejaculation chiefly through increasing serotonin levels. Reports of anorgasmia were frequent when MAOIs came back into popularity in the 1980s, after a decline in use during the 1970s. Numerous case studies of MAOI-induced anorgasmia appeared in psychiatry journals during this time period. Given that MAOIs had been in use for more than 20 years prior to these reports of anorgasmia, it is reasonable to conclude that sexual side-effect questions were rarely asked. Indeed, only rare reports had appeared describing anorgasmia (in small population) due to phenelzine (Barton, 1979; Friedman, Kantor, Sobel, & Miller, 1978; Rapp, 1979).

Despite these published reports, anorgasmia was not mentioned in a comprehensive review of sexual dysfunction associated with antidepressants and MAOIs (Mitchell & Popkin, 1983).

In 1982, two psychiatrists, Lynn Lesko and Nada Stotland, and a well-known sex therapist/researcher, Taylor Segraves, reported three cases of female anorgasmia induced by either phenelzine or isocarboxazid (Lesko, Stotland, & Segraves, 1982). These patients were being treated for atypical depression, panic, and phobia. Reducing the dosage below 50 mg restored orgasmic function but clinical effectiveness was jeopardized.

Additional reports of MAOI-induced anorgasmia have surfaced since 1983 (Buigues & Vallejo, 1987; Harrison et al., 1985, 1986). Anorgasmia has been identified as occurring in conjuction with all three available MAOIs, but mostly with phenelzine at doses above 45 mg. There was no mention of impaired drive, arousal, or lubrication, despite the absence of orgasmic climax. Fraser (1984) reported anorgasmia and again pointed out that patients usually did not report this dysfunction unless asked.

The sexual information on MAOIs was primarily anecdotal and by case report until 1985, when the first systematic study was performed by Wilma Harrison, Judith Rabkin and their colleagues at Columbia University (Harrison et al., 1985), who reviewed the charts of patients treated with imipramine, phenelzine, and tranylcypromine. Anorgasmia, retarded ejaculation, or decreased erection occurred in 31 patients (22%) treated with phenelzine. Only one of 41 patients (2%) reported anorgasmia/impotence on tranylcypromine (an amphetamine-like MAOI) and only three patients (5%) reported sexual dysfunction on imipramine. Sexual dysfunction usually occurred with 45 mg or more of phenelzine and became evident after four to 12 weeks of treatment. However, patients rarely discontinued phenelzine due to these sexual effects. For half of these patients, the dosage was not lowered, in spite of the adverse sexual side effects.

Harrison et al. (1986) followed their MAOI-antidepressant review with a controlled comparison trial of antidepressant-induced sexual dysfunction. They compared the MAOI phenelzine with the tricyclic imipramine and placebo. Eighty-two subjects were treated for depression over a six-week period. A comprehensive sexual function questionnaire was administered, which encompassed the areas of desire, arousal, erection, lubrication, orgasm/ejaculation, enjoyment and frequency. The results indicated that phenelzine and imipramine caused more sexual dysfunction than placebo in both women and men. There were no significant differences in erection or lubrication, but there was a trend toward a decline in erection. Decreases in desire, enjoyment, and orgasm/ejaculation were much more pronounced with phenelzine than with imipramine. Sexual dysfunction was reported by 40% of the phenelzine patients, 30% of the imipramine patients, and only 6% of those on placebo. Among women, the only significant sexual deficit due to imipramine was absence of orgasm during masturbation. Only women with "good" orgasmic response prior to drug treatment showed a decline; those with orgasmic difficulties at baseline showed little increased difficulty due to the drugs.

Subsequently, sexual dysfunction due to phenelzine was found in a six-month open trial of 35 panic disorder outpatients by Buigues and Vallejo (1987). Sexual dysfunction occurred in 27.3% of men and 16.7% of women.

Male/Female Differences

While men and women are *physically* affected similarly by MAOIs—both may lose desire and experience inhibition of orgasm/ejaculation—*psychologically*, the sexual side effects may be better tolerated by men, who often consider a delay of ejaculation an advantage. Women generally perceive inhibition of orgasm as undesirable. Tolerance of sexual side effects associated with MAOIs also varies among women. For a woman who was rarely or never orgasmic before MAOI treatment, there is little probability that decreases in physical and sensory arousal will be noted. In addition, the conditions treated with MAOIs, such as panic, phobia, obsession-compulsion, and atypical depression, interfere with normal activity, including sex. Consequently, patients may be willing to accept the sexual difficulties as much less bothersome than the problems that are eliminated.

Bulimic women are typically sexually active (Abraham et al., 1985) and are frequently placed on drugs that dampen their interest and responsiveness. From the Harrison and Rabkin (Rabkin, Quitkin, Harrison, Tricarno, & McGrath, 1984) MAOI studies, we know that about one-third of women treated with phenelzine report a major decrease in drive and/or orgasm, and that this sexual inhibition is more noticeable in women who are sexually active and responsive. Despite this special vulnerability of sexually active bulimic women to MAOI sexual side effects, there have been no studies investigating sexual side effects specifically in bulimic women treated with MAO inhibitors. (Some physicians do not use MAOIs with bulimics to avoid the danger of a chocolate binge, which could induce a hypertensive crisis. Perhaps sexual function will eventually receive the same priority!) Drug doses in bulimia studies are typically quite high (60–120 mg phenelzine), so that both weight gain and loss of sexual function would be expected. Yet bulimia reports mention only postural hypotension, insomnia, diarrhea, and hypomania. There are few studies of psychotherapeutic treatment of psychosexual dysfunction in bulimic or anorectic patients; and the few reports that discuss this problem in eating disorder female patients indicated that they are frequently resistant to sex therapy interventions (Simpson & Ramberg, 1992; Zerbe, 1992).

Sexual Benefits

Prolonged erection (priapism) has been reported in association with phenelzine (Yeragani & Gershon, 1987). On the first day of treatment, a patient had erections that "lasted all night and part of the early morning." These erections were not related to sexual desire and were described as uncomfortable. It is unlikely that phenelzine improves or prolongs normal or deficient erection. Phenelzine may inhibit orgasm/ejaculation by serotonin potentiation; however, MAOIs have not been evaluated for treatment of premature ejaculation. Heightened sexual desire has not been reported with phenelzine except in association with hypomania.

Alternatives

Until fluoxetine (Prozac) became available in 1988, MAOIs were often used to treat phobia and obsessive-compulsive disorders. Some doctors still prefer MAOIs, despite the need for rigid dietary regulation and predictable sexual complications. Although patients may tolerate adverse sexual side effects in exchange for other therapeutic benefits, presumably they would prefer an equally effective drug free of sexual complications.

MAOIs may be preferred for phobia and atypical depression due to their effectiveness. However, SSRIs should also be considered prior to using MAOIs due to their lower level of side effects. Alprazolam (Xanax) is typically used in place of MAOIs for the treatment of panic disorders.

The new "reversible" MAOIs developed in Europe (e.g., moclobemide) appear to require few, if any, dietary restrictions and seem to have comparatively low levels of side effects (Fairweather, Kerr, & Hindmarch, 1993; Versiani et al., 1992). Moclobemide is completing investigatory clinical trials in the United States for treatment of depression, panic, phobia, and obsessive-compulsive disorders, and can be expected to be approved by the Federal Drug Administration and marketed in 1996. In a double-blind controlled study of 78 patients with social phobia treated with moclobemide, phenelzine, or placebo over eight to 16 weeks, there was decreased libido and/or retarded ejaculation in 42.8% of patients treated with phenelzine, in 3.6% treated with moclobemide, and in none treated with placebo (Versiani et al., 1992). In a European double-blind parallel group study of 237 depressed patients treated with doxepin or moclobemide, Phillip, Kohnen, and Benkert (1994) found equivalent antidepressant efficacy but greater improvement of impaired libido, erection, orgasm, and ejaculation with moclobemide compared to doxepin. Additionally, there was one case of moclobemide-induced sexual hyperarousal. A recent open trial treating breast-cancer patients with moclobemide to reduce vasomotor symptoms (flush frequency and severity, night sweats) showed definite improvement in 11 of 15 women, though insomnia, tension, depression, irritability, and nausea showed no significant improvement (Menkes, Thomas, & Phipps, 1994).

Tranylcypromine (Parnate) causes far less weight gain and sexual dysfunction than phenelzine (Nardil) or isocarboxazid (Marplan). Though less powerful and consistently less efficacious than phenelzine in our clinical experience, tranylcypromine is much better tolerated, particularly for chronic use. Although it is commonly assumed that tranylcypromine is metabolized to amphetamine, accounting for occasional cases of tranylcypromine abuse (Brady, Lydiard, & Kellner, 1991; Lichtigfeld & Gillman, 1992), amphetamine has never been identified as a tranylcypromine metabolite (Jefferson, 1992); abuse is extremely rare and only reported in former substance abusers (Brady et al., 1991; Lichtigfeld & Gillman, 1992).

Bupropion (Wellbutrin) may be an excellent choice for treatment of atypical depression. It has a PEA-like stimulating effect (similar to PEA "endogenous amphetamine") and can reduce weight and chocolate bingeing as well as enhance sexual function. Patients with atypical depression and obsessive traits are often extremely sensitive and tend to withdraw when upset. The effects of bupropion can help these patients become more active and assertive without the considerable risk of hypomania that is always possible with MAOIs. Bupropion can also facilitate psychotherapy, but requires careful monitoring. If bupropion causes excessive nervousness, weight loss, or compulsive sexuality, it should be discontinued. A controlled-release long-acting form of bupropion should be marketed in the near future, which would lessen the possibility of nervousness or seizure.

21

Antidepressants II: Serotonin Uptake Inhibitors, Trazodone, Lithium

OBJECTIVES

- To identify the sexual and paradoxical effects of serotonergic antidepressants
- To explore the unique properties of trazodone
- To explore the sexual side effects of lithium in relation to the impact of bipolar disorder on sexual function

Animal research has indicated that serotonin has an inhibitory effect on sexual function, while dopamine is generally stimulatory. Due to this reciprocal action between serotonin and dopamine, sexual effects can occur as much through a shift in the dopamine-serotonin balance as through an increase or decrease of either one alone. Effects may fluctuate due to compensatory reactions involving changes in metabolism and sensitivity. Furthermore, excessive activity in a neurotransmitter can lead to exhaustion or a refractory period, during which time the characteristic effects of that transmitter are reversed. Because of its erratic nature, dopamine activity is more subject to such refractory or inverse reactions than is serotonin.

While serotonin activity is slower and more regular than that of dopamine, when serotonin is disrupted the result can be more acute emotionally and psychologically. Some people have (genetically or otherwise defective) unstable serotonin systems. For these individuals stability is rarely achieved; rather, they live with an internal "floating" thermostat subject to erratic reversals that are more characteristic of the dopamine system. These individuals therefore are more vulnerable to rapid mood shifts from depression into hypomania; also they are more likely to manifest paradoxical reactions to serotonin potentiation (such as hypersexuality and suicidal ideation).

From this perspective, fluoxetine (Prozac), a serotonin uptake inhibitor (SSRI), would reduce sexual excitement, and alprazolam (Xanax), a benzodiazepine, would have little direct effect; indeed, this is what has been verified in clinical practice. In addition, SSRIs should have a beneficial effect on premature ejaculation (i.e., delay orgasm/ejaculation), while benzodiazepines will be a little direct help; this has also been confirmed in clinical practice.

Trazodone has mild negative and positive sexual properties. Many of its effects in relation to serotonin are paradoxical. It has particularly unpredictable effects on erectile function. Lithium is a difficult drug to evaluate because it is used to treat an underlying disease with a wide range of sexual manifestations that can resolve spontaneously. Effective treatment can also alter sexual function from either extreme. In this complex sexual setting, it still appears that lithium has adverse sexual properties of its own.

SEROTONIN UPTAKE INHIBITOR ANTIDEPRESSANTS

The serotonin uptake inhibitors illustrate numerous principles simultaneously: that psychotropic medications can have dramatic effects on sex; that the effects on men and women can be dramatically different; and that these same drugs can be selectively used to treat sexual dysfunction. Drugs like clomipramine and fluoxetine have been among the most fascinating sexually significant antidepressants to date. Fluoxetine has been a controversial and public drug, but its notoriety has just begun. Recently it has been identified as a dependable treatment for premature ejaculation; in men and women, it inhibits orgasm and reduces desire.

With the success of *Listening to Prozac*, this drug has become even more public, yet with its *potent* sexual effects, sexual aspects are barely mentioned—which further illustrates the degree to which sexual consequences of the drugs physicians prescribe are not recognized. Peter Kramer (1993) describes a man who found his interest in pornographic literature distinctly diminished while taking Prozac. If this effect were studied further, and found to be consistent, together with the known effect Prozac has on diminishing sex drive and orgasm, it may have some selective clinical value in the treatment of sex offenders and pedophiles.

Clomipramine is generally disadvantageous to sex, but can also cause paradoxical responses such as inducing orgasm and yawning simultaneously. Table 21.1 summarizes the properties and side effects of serotonin uptake inhibitors.

Clomipramine (Anafranil)

In humans, clomipramine increases both ACTH and cortisol (Golden, Hsiao, et al., 1989). Many studies have also shown that clomipramine increases prolactin (Cole, Groom, Link, O'Flanagan, & Seldrup, 1976; Jones, Luscombe, & Groom, 1977; Langer et al., 1980) due to its serotonergic effect (Golden et al., 1989). Clomipramine is five times as potent as imipramine in blocking the dopamine DA-2 receptor that inhibits prolactin (Richelson & Nelson, 1984). Several case reports of clomipramine-induced lactation-galactorrhea have been linked to this increase in prolactin (Anand, 1985; Mills, 1979). Fowlie and Burton (1987) noted a three-month history of galactorrhea, breast engorgement, loss of libido, and sneezing in a 20-year-old woman treated with 50 mg/day clomipramine. Plasma prolactin was found to be grossly elevated. With discontinuance of the drug, all symptoms resolved and prolactin returned to normal levels. Clomipramine increases beta-endorphins in the rat hypothalamus, whereas other antidepressants (imipramine, desipramine, amoxapine, and mianserin) decrease beta-endorphins in this region (Kurumaji, Mitsushio, Ichikawa, & Shibuya, 1986). This increase appears to occur through stimulation of serotonin; serotonergic agents such as fluoxetine, L-tryptophan, 5-HTP, and quipazine also increase plasma beta-endorphins (Meltzer et al., 1982).

Sexual Dysfunction Sexual dysfunction due to clomipramine treatment is frequent and quite often severe. Perhaps the most comprehensive evaluation of the negative sexual side effects of this drug was published in a multicenter collaborative report of 520 patients treated over 10 weeks for obsessive-compulsive disorder (OCD) (DeVeaugh-Geiss, Landau, & Katz, 1989). The average clomipramine dose was 200 mg/day (100–300 mg/day range). The sexual side-effect findings for male patients are shown in Table 21.2 (information provided by the manufacturer included in clomipramine's labeling is also shown in Table 21.2). Note that ejaculation failure is between 41–42% and impotence between 15–20%. Apparently decreased female sexual function (orgasm or lubrication) was either not examined or not noted.

Other side effects noted in this report which could adversely affect sexual activity included fatigue (38% versus 13% on placebo), somnolence (49% versus 14% on placebo), constipation (44% versus 9% on placebo), dizziness (53% versus 11% on placebo), and tremor (53% versus 2% on placebo), as well as nausea, dyspepsia, dry mouth, and nervousness. Surprisingly, at the end of eight weeks, weight gain

Table 21.1 *Profile of Serotonin Uptake Inhibitors*

	Daily Dose
Clomipramine (Anafranil)	50–300 mg
Fluoxetine (Prozac)	10–80 mg
Fluvoxamine (Luvox)	50–300 mg
Paroxetine (Paxil)	10–50 mg
Sertraline (Zoloft)	50–200 mg
Venlafaxine (Effexor)	75–375 mg

COMMON INDICATIONS

Depression, obsessive-compulsive disorder, panic, and phobia

MECHANISMS OF ACTION (GENERAL)

Work through selective serotonin-uptake inhibition

MECHANISMS OF ACTION (SEXUAL)

Negative

Increased cortisol
Increased opioids
Increased prolactin
Increased serotonin (5-HT)

DIRECT SEXUAL SIDE EFFECTS

Desire disorders (in both sexes)
- Hyposexuality
- Hypersexuality

Erection difficulties
- Inability/difficulty obtaining erection
- Decreased quality of erection
- Decreased or absent nocturnal/morning erections

Orgasm irregularities
- Orgasmic inhibition
- Anorgasmia
- Spontaneous orgasm

Ejaculation irregularities
- Retarded ejaculation
- Ejaculatory inhibition
- Premature ejaculation (improved)
- Dyspareunia

Menstrual disorders
- Amenorrhea

Breast disorders
- Gynecomastia
- Galactorrhea

INDIRECT SEXUAL SIDE EFFECTS

Discomfort caused by constipation, indigestion, nausea, rash/itching

Mood disorders resulting in anhedonia, nervousness, anxiety, detachment, mania

Neurological disturbances resulting in dizziness, fatigue, movement disorder, sedation, sleep disturbances, sensory loss, tremor, muscular weakness

SEXUAL CONTRAINDICATIONS/BENEFITS

Avoid with prior condition of

Sex drive disorders
Impotence
Ejaculatory disorders
Anorgasmia

May be useful for

Premature ejaculation
Sex offenders?

ALTERNATIVES

Bupropion (Wellbutrin)
Nefazodone (Serzone)
Trazodone (Desyrel)

Table 21.2 *Clomipramine-Induced Sexual Dysfunction in Males*

	Clomipramine	*Placebo*
DATA FROM DEVEAUGH-GEISS ET AL., 1989		
Ejaculation Failure	41% (46/111 males)	2% (2/121 males)
Libido Change	18% (47/260)	7% (3/260)
Impotence	15% (17/111 males)	2% (2/121 males)
LABELING FOR CLOMIPRAMINE (Federal Drug Administration Approved)		
Ejaculation Failure	42%	2%
Libido Change	21%	3%
Impotence	20%	3%

on clomipramine (7% increase) was not much greater than on placebo (8% versus 7% in one study and 14% versus 3% in another). Over the long term, weight gain on clomipramine can be as great as on phenelzine (Nardil). Clomipramine's FDA-approved labeling indicates weight increase in 18% of patients (versus 1% on placebo). This weight-gain effect is apparently due to clomipramine's tricyclic properties (antihistamine) rather than to its selective serotonin reuptake inhibiting property.

An eight-week double-blind study by Monteiro, Noshirvani, Marks, and Lelliott (1987) found even greater sexual dysfunction due to clomipramine. OCD patients were not forewarned of possible sexual side effects and patient reports were obtained during routine assessments. (Other drugs were not permitted.) Mean clomipramine dose was 140 mg/day (25–200 mg/day range). Difficulty in achieving orgasm started within the first few days on 25–50 mg/day and anorgasmia typically occurred after 100–150 mg/day. Most patients found it "hard work" trying to reach orgasm and became frustrated with sex. Specific results included:

- Reduced or total absence of orgasm/ejaculation was reported by 22 of 24 (92%) previously orgasmic patients (17 men, 7 women); total lack of orgasm occurred in 70%.
- Among 7 women, orgasm was delayed in 1 and absent in 5.
- Among 17 men, orgasm/ejaculation was delayed in 3 and absent in 13.
- Orgasm was less intense in 13 of 24 patients and there was less satisfaction with orgasm in 13.
- Sexual desire was reduced in 9 of 24 patients (3 women, 6 men), but 8 of these 9 considered disinterest to be secondary to anorgasmia.
- Erection or lubrication was reduced (slightly) in only 4 of 24 patients (2 women, 2 men) and 2 of these 4 considered the reduction to be secondary to anorgasmia.
- Frequency of sexual activity decreased in 7 of 24 patients (3 women, 4 men), but 5 attributed this decrease to anorgasmia.
- Pain at orgasm was noted by 4 men and 3 reported pain during urination.
- Due to sexual side effects, 5 of 24 patients reduced or occasionally stopped taking clomipramine.
- No changes in sexual function or orgasm occurred in 9 patients on placebo (5 women, 4 men).
- Sexual difficulties remained throughout 6 months of treatment on clomipramine but disappeared within 3 days of discontinuing the drug.
- Of the 2 patients who did not experience delayed or absent orgasm, one women re-

fused to take more than 25 mg/day due to other side effects and the other was a transvestite who reduced masturbating from 20 to 2 times a week.

Interestingly, the high percentage of patients experiencing anorgasmia due to clomipramine reported in Monteiro el al.'s (1987) study was not evident from a physical symptoms questionnaire, which asked the patients to rate themselves for sexual difficulties on a four-point scale from "no problem" to "severe." Thirty-six percent of patients with clomipramine-induced anorgasmia checked "no problem," despite spontaneously reporting, or readily admitting to, anorgasmia during interviews with the investigators. (Some patients even admitted secretly reducing their drug dose because of the sexual side effects.) An earlier clomipramine-OCD trial using this same questionnaire failed to show a difference in sexual difficulties between clomipramine and placebo (Marks, Stern, Mawson, Cobb, & McDonald, 1980). During Monteiro's 1987 study, spontaneous reports of anorgasmia by about a third of the patients caused the investigators to interview all patients in detail. A possible reason for the better communication between patient and investigator in this study was that patients being tested on clomipramine were also receiving psychotherapy.

Despite the above findings of 40–90% orgasm/ejaculation delay or failure, clomipramine review articles generally cite a 15–20% rate of ejaculation failure (Kelly & Myers, 1990), possibly disregarding cases of less severe ejaculatory delay and cases where ejaculation failure is not reported by male patients who sometimes consider it a benefit. Nonetheless, research clearly indicates that orgasm and ejaculation are both delayed in men, and one may assume that orgasm is often delayed or may be eliminated in women, though orgasm deficits are seldom cited. Libido decreases are cited in 3–20% of patients, but the relation of these decreases to orgasm or ejaculation inhibition is seldom discussed. An early report from the manufacturer of clomipramine (Beaumont, 1979) cited adverse sexual effects in 26% of men and 1% of women on low doses of clomipramine (15–30 mg/day). Adverse effects included reduced libido, reduced activity, impotence, and delayed or absent orgasm/ejaculation. These effects were dose-related, even at low levels.

While the report of spontaneous orgasm or ejaculation in a few patients on clomipramine (McLean et al., 1983) gained notoriety, negative reports of clomipramine-induced sexual dysfunction quietly accumulated. Quirk and Einarson (1982) reported one man and two women who became anorgasmic within one month of starting clomipramine (50–100 mg/day). Anorgasmia disappeared when clomipramine was discontinued and did not recur when two of these patients were subsequently treated with desipramine.

Yassa (1982) described three men who complained of impotence within a week of starting clomipramine (50 mg/day or more). In two cases, sexual desire was also reduced. Fraser (1984) reported two women who became anorgasmic due to clomipramine (75–100 mg). Steiger, Holsboer, and Benkert (1988) showed severe reduction (about 75%) in the natural erections of a normal volunteer treated with 100 mg/day clomipramine, indicating that clomipramine can disturb erection as well as orgasm/ejaculation.

A recent study of 11 depressed men (mean age = 39.2 years) treated for three months with 75 mg/day clomipramine compared hormonal and ejaculate sperm parameters to those of an age-matched untreated group of non-depressed men with erectile dysfunction (Maier & Koinig, 1994). Though hormonal levels and functioning were within the normal range for both groups (FSH, LH, GnRH, testosterone, prolactin, estradiol), all sperm samples in the clomipramine-treated group were abnormal (reduced volume, motility, and abnormal morphology) compared to 37% in the untreated group, a normal figure for this age range.

Sexual side effects of clomipramine have been noted much less frequently when it has been used as an antidepressant than in obsessive-compulsive disorder studies, suggesting a particular susceptibility to these sexual effects in obsessive-compulsive patients. More likely, the discrepancy reflects the inadequate recognition of negative sexual effects by investigators conducting antidepressant research. Company data on clomipramine side effects distributed in 1988 to doctors participating in an open OCD treatment program showed 0–5% incidence of ejaculatory and orgasm delay, impotence, and decreased libido in antidepressant trials, but 10–20% in OCD trials. However, even the antidepressant treatment studies found high levels of weakness, drowsiness, somnolence, lethargy, dizziness, tremor, nausea, constipation, blurred vision, and dry mouth. Along with frequent weight gain, these various nonsexual side effects are bound to cause sexual dysfunction in many patients.

The higher rate of adverse sexual effects from clomipramine noted in OCD patients in these studies may be age-related: these patients are younger (usually the mean age is about 35) than in antidepressant trials. Unfortunately, older patients may be more tolerant of sexual deficits or expect them as a result of aging, and doctors, assuming that sexual responsivity is less important for the elderly, may not ask pertinent questions. Younger patients may be more sexually active, more bothered by decreased sexual response, and more likely to report sexual problems. However, because clomipramine is often prescribed for obsessive-compulsive disorder in children and adolescents, who may have no frame of reference for sexual function or who may pass through puberty on a drug that makes them dysfunctional, there is cause for concern.

In animal research, Everitt (1977) showed that clomipramine (10 mg/day) reduced both passive and active sexual behavior (lordosis and soliciting) in estrogen-primed receptive female rats. Particularly striking inhibitory sexual effects of clomipramine were shown in four female rhesus monkeys (Everitt, 1977, 1980). Sexual invitations (proceptive sexual behavior) to male monkeys decreased to near zero and refusals of male attempts to mount (receptive lordosis) increased dramatically. Negative sexual effects quickly disappeared when clomipramine was discontinued. These changes have not been observed in humans, largely because the effect of this drug on women has not been investigated sufficiently. Although the finding of animal studies cannot be automatically attributed to humans, these particular results suggest the need for further research.

Sexual Benefits Due to its apparent ability to inhibit orgasm, clomipramine has been used for many years in Europe as a treatment for premature ejaculation. (It was not available in the United States until 1989.) However, little formal research has been conducted on this application, and little is known about how often or how long clomipramine is effective for this purpose. In animal research, clomipramine has been shown to prolong ejaculation latency in rats (Ahlenius, Heimann, & Larsson, 1979). A greater effect was seen at the lowest dose (1.5 mg/kg) than at higher doses (3 and 6 mg/kg). Delayed ejaculation was also observed with the direct serotonin precursor 5-HTP but not with the selective SSRIs zimelidine and alaproclate. In human research, Eaton (1973), an English psychiatrist, noted benefit in 12 of 13 patients treated for premature ejaculation. Improvement occurred within two weeks to two months on doses of 30 to 75 mg/day. While some patients required 75 mg/day for satisfactory effect, others could not ejaculate at all at this dose.

A double-blind trial of clomipramine treatment of premature ejaculation was reported by Goodman (1980), a psychosexual therapist and general practitioner in England. All men were in steady sexual relationships, were free of affective disorders, and had not benefited from "squeeze" technique training. Twenty patients entered the trial, but four soon withdrew due to nervousness, side effects, or protocol violations. Consequently, only seven patients started on clomipramine and nine on placebo. In the first part of the study, which was double-blind, patients were treated for four weeks on 10–40 mg/day. Subsequently, they were treated openly on clomipramine for a further four weeks. Overall, this study was methodologically inadequate for a number of reasons: too few subjects, inadequate time in the double-blind, and possibly too low dosage. No difference was noted between clomipramine and placebo over one month at the maximum dose of 40 mg. Subsequent improvement on open clomipramine could have been a placebo response. Furthermore, the global evaluation did not define with precision to what extent premature ejaculation decreased. There is no evidence from this study of a reliable and usable action of clomipramine on premature ejaculation.

Another small double-blind study in France (Porto, 1980) showed significant ejaculatory improvement in 75% (6 of 8) of clomipramine-treated patients compared to none on placebo (0 of 10). Patients were self-treated for approximately five weeks with 30 mg/day (10 mg three times a day). However, since patients were given all their medication at the start of the study (bottle of 300, 10 mg tablets), protocol violations were likely; patients would be tempted to try a large enough dose to determine whether they had been given the real drug or placebo.

A more noteworthy double-blind study of 50 patients treated for premature ejaculation was reported by endocrinologists at Cairo University in Egypt (Girgis, El-Haggar, & El-Hermouzy, 1982). Patients were given either 20 mg/day clomipramine or placebo for six weeks and then crossed over to the other drug condition for six weeks. Measurement was based on responses to two questions, self-answered after each occasion of sexual intercourse: "Was the sex act satisfactory?" and "Did you suffer any inconvenience during treatment?" Eight of 25 (32%) patients initially assigned placebo and 3 of 25 (12%) assigned clomipramine dropped out after the first visit "for no apparent reason." During the initial six weeks, clomipramine-treated patients reported 50.8% "satisfactory" intercourse, significantly different from the 32% rate in the placebo group. During the crossover, clomipramine patients switched to placebo maintained their "satisfaction" rate (52%), while placebo patients switched to clomipramine improved significantly from 32% to 49% satisfactory intercourse. The continued benefit over six weeks shown by clomipramine patients switched to placebo indicated that at least some treatment carry-over effect exists. The major defect of this study was the inadequately refined measurement of improvement. The beneficial effect on only 20 mg/day clomipramine was surprising and suggested that, at least to some extent, premature ejaculation could be treated by this very low dose, thus avoiding serious side effects.

Five case studies of clomipramine as treatment for premature ejaculation have been reported by a Canadian psychiatrist (Assalian, 1988). Improved control of ejaculation occurred in all cases in two to seven days on a 20–25 mg/day. Two patients only took clomipramine when needed (i.e., when sexual activity was anticipated, such as on weekends). Continued improvement was noted by two patients on follow-up interviews 12 and 18 months later. Premature ejaculation returned in one patient who had decreased his dose from 25 to 10 mg/day due to sedation; ejaculatory control returned when the dose was increased to 25 mg/day.

In a double-blind, placebo-controlled trial of clomipramine treatment of premature ejaculation in 15 couples, Althof, Levine, Corty, Risen, and Stern (1994) noted a 500% increase in time to ejaculation on 50 mg clomipramine and 250% on 25 mg (both increases significantly greater than on placebo). Significant improvements were noted on men's and women's sexual satisfaction and men's psychological well-being and marital satisfaction scores. At a two-month follow-up after discontinuing clomipramine, all sexual gains were no longer present, except for men's marital satisfaction scores.

The results of these small studies indicate that clomipramine can either improve control in premature ejaculators or sufficiently delay orgasm/ejaculation. Since the effect often occurs in only a few days and at doses as low as 20 mg/day, it is not simply due to clomipramine's antidepressant, antipanic, or antiobsessive actions, which take longer (two weeks or more) to occur and require higher doses (50–250 mg/day). Furthermore, for some patients satisfactory response can be maintained without daily treatment.

In our clinical practice, many patients have experienced some degree of improvement in ejaculatory control with clomipramine. Some patients, however, have complained that the drowsiness and fatigue from the drug were worse than the premature ejaculation. With prolonged use, constipation and weight gain are likely, even at low doses (20–75 mg/day). Many premature ejaculators may be Type A personalities who cannot tolerate medications that decrease their vigor and alertness. Although published studies claim that erection is not decreased, the delay or absence of orgasm/ejaculation often undermines sexual desire and erectile function. For many patients, the ejaculatory delay effect may require as much time to occur as the antidepressant effect (two to five weeks). Moreover, doses higher than 25 mg/day are usually necessary, and ejaculatory delay usually disappears soon after stopping clomipramine (particularly if there is no concurrent therapy).

Although Assalian (1988) has attributed the inhibition of ejaculation to a blockade of adrenergic receptors, as is noted with phenoxybenzamine, the effect is actually quite different from phenoxybenzamine. Semen is ejaculated normally when orgasm occurs with clomipramine, in contrast to the dry orgasm occurring with phenoxybenzamine. Instead of blocking ejaculation, clomipramine reduces the buildup to orgasmic climax and orgasm itself. In our clinical practice, we have found that peripheral penile sensations are also blunted. The effect is identical to the orgasm/ejaculation delay we have found with much more selective and powerful SSRIs, such as paroxetine. Consequently, we suspect it is due to serotonin uptake inhibition (rather than adrenergic blockade), which potentiates the blunting action of serotonin over excitement and impulsive reactions. Colpi, Fanciullacci, Aydos, and Grugnetti (1991) measured sacral and dorsal nerve/cortical evoked responses and genital sensory thresholds in 15 premature ejaculators before and during successful treatment over 30 days with 20 mg/day clomipramine. They found that latency and amplitude of evoked responses were unchanged, but genital sensory thresholds increased significantly during clomipramine treatment (i.e., more intense stimulation was necessary to be sensed through the genitalia.)

Alternatives Bupropion (Wellbutrin) can be used in place of clomipramine for treating depression, but has not been determined to be efficacious as a treatment for obsessive-compulsive disorder. Other SSRIs may not be quite as effective as clomipramine for the treatment of obsessive-compulsive disorder (Tamini & Mavissakalian, 1991), but they have fewer and less severe side effects (though all have relatively frequent negative sexual side effects). Both fluoxetine and paroxetine have been shown to be effective treatments for obsessive-compulsive disorder (Kaye & Dancu, 1994; Tollefson et al., 1994), and fluoxetine was approved for this application in 1994. However, sertraline was not found to be efficacious in obsessive-compulsive treatment in a 10-week, double-blind placebo-controlled trial (Jenike et al., 1990).

The SSRI fluvoxamine (Luvox) was approved in the United States at the end of 1994 for marketing as a treatment for obsessive-compulsive disorder (it has been used for several years in England and Europe as an antidepressant). It may be more potent than other SSRIs for both obsessive-compulsive disorder and panic disorder with or without phobia. Freeman, Trimble, Deakin, Stokes, and Ashford (1994) found equal efficacy in the treatment of 64 obsessive-compulsive patients for fluvoxamine and clomipramine in a double-blind trial, with fewer treatment dropouts in the fluvoxamine group (6 of 34) compared to the clomipramine group (11 of 30). There were more cases of sexual dysfunction in the clomipramine group (10 of 30 = 33%) than in the fluvoxamine group (4 of 34 = 12%). In our clinical experience, we have found fluvoxamine to be a highly effective treatment for panic/phobia, with frequent but well-tolerated side effects (nausea and somnolence were most frequent). We have observed decreased libido and delayed orgasm in both men and women treated with fluvoxamine, but much less severe in men than we have previously observed with paroxetine (Paxil), which frequently makes orgasm/ejaculation impossible in men.

Fluoxetine (Prozac)

Sexual Dysfunction Negative sexual effects such as delay of orgasm/ejaculation and decreased sexual desire were noted in investigatory trials prior to Federal Drug Administration approval of fluoxetine (Prozac) in 1988, but were not generally discussed until the drug had been widely used for a few years. Since 1989, several reports, noted below, of adverse sexual effects have been published. Among many therapists who initially failed to notice any negative sexual effects in their patients prescribed fluoxetine, there may even now be an overreaction to these sexual effects which discourages fluoxetine use and encourages use of other antidepressants with much more toxic side effect profiles. The sexual deficits that occur on fluoxetine are evidently due to selective serotonin reuptake inhibition. However, it should be noted that the same effects may occur more often on other SSRIs more recently marketed in the United States (e.g., paroxetine [Paxil], sertraline [Zoloft]).

The first published report of delayed orgasm due to fluoxetine (Kline, 1989) included case studies of a 35-year-old woman treated for depression and obsessive-compulsive disorder and a 47-year-old man treated for depression. The woman reported increasing difficulty reaching orgasm after a month of 20 mg/day fluoxetine. When she could no longer reach orgasm at all, fluoxetine dose was reduced to 20 mg every other day. Her difficulty reaching orgasm partially resolved at this lower dose. The man reported difficulty attaining orgasm after five weeks on 40 mg/day fluoxetine. Retardation of orgasm was reduced by prescribing 20 mg and 40 mg on alternate days. The author noted that anorgasmia was not noted in the manufacturer's side effect information.

Herman et al. (1990) reported fluoxetine-induced delayed or absent orgasm in five of the first 60 (8.3%) patients treated at their clinic. Three men on 20 mg/day fluoxetine developed severely retarded orgasm (usually about one hour) and two women became anorgasmic on 20–80 mg/day. The men had previously experienced sexual dysfunction during MAO-inhibitor treatment, but were free of sexual dysfunction when fluoxetine was begun. Delayed orgasm/ejaculation occurred within the first week of treatment and persisted for at least six weeks in two of the men. Anorgasmia in the women was noted within three weeks and continued unabated for two to three months. When one of these women discontinued fluoxetine after three months, orgasmic response returned to normal within a week.

Musher (1990) noted anorgasmia in his fluoxetine patients at a much higher rate than the 1.9% percentage cited by the manufacturer. Reviewing his practice for the preceding 15 months, Musher found that, of the 32 patients for whom he had prescribed fluoxetine, five (16%) (four women, one man) had specifically complained of anorgasmia, whatever the form of sexual stimulation used. All but one remained anorgasmic over several months, yet only one wanted to stop treatment because of the sexual problem. The author believed that the actual rate of sexual dysfunction was higher than 16%, noting that some of the 32 patients were not sexually active and speculating that others might be embarrassed or unwilling to discuss their sex lives.

Vaginal and penile "anesthesias" have been reported during fluoxetine treatment. King and Horowitz (1993) reported the case of a 37-year-old women treated for depression with 20 mg/day fluoxetine. Within two weeks, she developed total anesthesia (lack of sensation) in her vagina and vulva, which was medically confirmed by a needle-prick test. After seven weeks, she had recovered from depression and stopped fluoxetine treatment. Genital sensation gradually returned to normal during the subsequent four weeks.

Neill (1991) described a 47-year-old man treated for severe depression with gradually increasing doses of fluoxetine over two months. During the second week on 60 mg/day, the man reported that he desired intercourse but could not become erect; instead he experienced numbness of the glans penis and had difficulty achieving orgasm/ejaculation. Since he experienced a remarkable recovery from depression, he remained on 60 mg/day fluoxetine for several months with continued penile numbness and retarded orgasm/ejaculation. Subsequently, fluoxetine was discontinued and depression recurred within two weeks, but the penile numbness and orgasm/ejaculation difficulty disappeared.

Measom (1992) reported on a 47-year-old man without prior sexual dysfunction other than loss of libido associated with his depression. When treated over four weeks with 20 mg/day fluoxetine, he recovered from depression but reported lack of sensation in his penis. At first, this lack of penile sensation was not a problem for the patient; but over three months of 20 mg/day treatment, orgasm/ejaculatory difficulties developed. A decrease in dose to 20 mg every other day eliminated ejaculatory difficulties, but penile anesthesia continued.

Zajecka, Fawcett, Schaff, Jeffries, and Guy (1991) noted six cases (five women, one man) of anorgasmia or delayed orgasm among 77 depressed patients (7.8%) treated with 20–80 mg/day fluoxetine in a non-double-blind open protocol. Physicians did not specifically inquire about sexual effects; therefore, the rate of orgasm difficulties was probably higher; all complaints of orgasmic dysfunction were spontaneously reported. Difficulties were noted within the first six weeks of treatment; in two patients the difficulties were reduced with the addition of 4–12 mg of the antiserotonergic drug cyproheptadine (Periactin) given one to two hours prior to sexual activity.

Jacobsen (1991, 1992) also noted sexual dysfunction in 54 of 160 (34%) patients successfully treated for depression over a three-year period of time. Sixteen patients reported decreased sexual desire, 21 reported decreased sexual response, and 17 reported decreases in both desire and response. Fifteen patients (six women, nine men) with fluoxetine-induced sexual dysfunction were treated with 16 mg/day yohimbine added to fluoxetine. Sexual dysfunction was completely or partially reversed in 11 of the 15.

Feder (1991) reported anorgasmia or severely retarded orgasm/ejaculation in three male patients on 20–80 mg/day fluoxetine. Cyproheptadine (2–6 mg) was administered to reduce the orgasmic difficulties, but instead caused dysphoric reactions and the return of depression while having no effect on orgasm. Nevertheless, the men preferred to continue treatment with fluoxetine; they continued to have difficulties with orgasm/ejaculation for at least eight to ten months.

Goldbloom and Kennedy (1991) reported two women who became anorgasmic within a few months of 40–60 mg/day fluoxetine treatment for bulimia. Given 4–8 mg/day cyproheptadine along with fluoxetine to treat the anorgasmia, within a few weeks their bulimia symptoms returned at full force, including bingeing, depression, chocolate craving, hypersomnia, and weight gain. The cyproheptadine was stopped and the women continued treatment on 60 mg/day fluoxetine with continuing anorgasmia.

Solyom, Solyom, and Ledwidge (1990) noted decreased sex drive and anorgasmia in four of 10 (40%) women treated with 80 mg/day fluoxetine in a three-month study of bulimia. Other fluoxetine side effects such as nausea, nervousness, and insomnia abated within four weeks, but sexual problems continued. At the end of the three months, two anorgasmic women still on fluoxetine were given 4–8 mg of cyproheptadine prior to intercourse with some benefit. During 1994, fluoxetine was approved by the Federal Drug Administration for treatment of bulimia, which typically requires large daily doses of 40–80 mg; decreased orgasm and/or libido will be a major negative side effect in such treatment.

Inhibited ejaculation or other sexual dysfunctions are usually noted in about 7% of patients treated with fluoxetine in OCD trials (Fontaine & Chouinard, 1989; Jenike, 1990). Often, no sexual side effects are noted (Liebowitz et al., 1989). Obsessive-compulsive patients frequently show preexisting sexual dysfunction, which is more severe and long-lasting than in cases of depression or panic disorder. For instance, 16 of 24 married agoraphobic women reported severe loss of sex drive with the onset of agoraphobia (Buglass, Clarke, Henderson, Kreitman, & Presley, 1977). For these patients, additional sexual difficulties during drug treatment were unlikely to be noted or reported. However, in a careful crossover OCD trial, Pigott et al. (1990) found that individual ratings of decreased sex drive and anorgasmia more than doubled from baseline in patients (six men, five women) treated over 10 weeks with either fluoxetine or clomipramine. While ratings were somewhat worse on clomipramine than on fluoxetine, the differences were slight and nonsignificant. The greatest increase in severity of side effects for either fluoxetine or clomipramine was noted for anorgasmia. In an understatement, the authors commented that "this study indicates that the initial optimism concerning a possible low incidence of sexual dysfunction with fluoxetine treatment may not be warranted."

Patterson (1993) noted that retarded or absent ejaculation was reported by 45 of 60 (75%) male patients treated with fluoxetine, even though most were treated with only 20 mg/day. The high number of reports was due to the fact that patients were specifically questioned about ejaculatory changes. Lowering the fluoxetine dose helped decrease ejaculatory difficulties in 50% of patients.

Given the above evidence of serious and continuing sexual dysfunction due to fluoxetine, it is remarkable that fluoxetine-induced anorgasmia was not noted in investigatory trial reports and was not noted as a side effect on the Federal Drug Administration-approved labeling of fluoxetine. The 1.9% sexual dysfunction rate noted in the labeling is an example of the failure of Federal Drug Administration to even consider sexual effects of drugs. As a partial excuse for the under-reporting of sexual dysfunction and the nonreporting of anorgasmia, the manufacturer pointed out that the official government side effect coding form (COSTART) did not include anorgasmia on its list. In a postmarketing surveillance study of 2,487 patients treated with fluoxetine (Fisher, Bryant, & Kent, 1993), only 16 cases of orgasm problems (0.64%) and 32 cases of loss of sex drive (1.2%) were reported, indicating the irrelevance of current postmarketing surveillance procedures for quality-of-life side-effect information.

Strategies for Treating SSRI-Induced Sexual Dysfunction

The serotonin antagonist and antihistamine cyproheptadine (Periactin) has continued to be used for reversing SSRI-induced retarded or absent orgasm and ejaculation. Modell (1989) reported a case of yawning, clitoral engorgement, and spontaneous orgasm on fluoxetine, while Cohen (1992) reported a case of fluoxetine-induced yawning and *anorgasmia* in a 48-year-old man treated for one month with 20 mg/day fluoxetine. Besides excessive daytime yawning, he reported difficulty experiencing orgasm/ejaculation despite a full erection. Cyproheptadine (4 mg three times a day) eliminated both yawning and difficulty experiencing orgasm/ejaculation. After six months of normal sexual functioning and no abnormal yawning, the patient discontinued the cyproheptadine use and yawning and anorgasmia returned within one week. Restarting daily cyproheptadine again eliminated yawning and anorgasmia. Typically, cyproheptadine treatment for orgasm/ejaculation difficulty consists of either 4 mg prior to sexual activity or daily 2–8 mg dosing (Feder, 1991; Goldbloom & Kennedy, 1991; McCormick, Olin, & Brotman, 1990; Zajecka et al., 1991). Arnott and Nutt (1994) reported the use of 4–6 mg cyproheptadine two hours prior to intercourse to reverse anorgasmia in a 63-year-old man treated for depression with 100–150 mg fluvoxamine. Unfortunately, negative interactions between cyproheptadine and fluoxetine have been reported, including return of depression (Feder, 1991), return of bulimic binge-eating and weight gain (Goldbloom & Kennedy, 1991), and the appearance of irritability, dysphoria, and suicidal thoughts (Katz & Rosenthal, 1994). Adverse effects, such as drowsiness, anxiety, weakness, hallucinations, and paranoid reactions, have also been noted when cyproheptadine has been added to tricyclic or MAOI antidepressant treatment (Kahn, 1987; Pontius, 1988; Riley & Riley, 1986).

Bethanechol has been used chiefly as a cholinergic drug to reverse anticholinergic tricyclic antidepressant-induced sexual dysfunction (e.g., Everett, 1975; Gross, 1982; Segraves, 1987a; Yager, 1986). Its efficacy with SSRIs, which lack anticholinergic action, is questionable. The dopaminergic drug amantadine (100–200 mg) has also been used to reverse fluoxetine-induced anorgasmia (Balogh, Hendricks, & Kang, 1992); and Gitlin (1994) has stated that dopaminergic stimulants, including dextroamphetamine and pemoline, can reverse anorgasmia induced by the SSRI sertraline or the MAOI phenelzine. The best pharmacological treatment for SSRI-induced orgasmic difficulties or other sexual dysfunctions is probably yohimbine 5.4 mg prior to intercourse or 5.4 mg yohimbine three times per day. However, yohimbine can induce nausea, anxiety, urinary frequency, excessive sweating, shakiness, and tension (Hollander & McCarley, 1992; Jacobsen, 1992; Price & Grunhaus, 1990). The first and preferred treatment of SSRI-induced sexual dysfunction is to lower the dose and reassure the patient that this is an expected and transient drug side effect. Mixing drugs has the danger of unexpected consequences.

Sexual Benefits Although fluoxetine adversely affects sex drive in both men and women, premature ejaculators appear to experience some benefits. Some men consider diminished drive as a "small price to pay" for enhanced endurance or, perhaps, the adverse effect on sex drive is not as noticeable in premature ejaculators as in normal ejaculators. Crenshaw (1992) conducted a research study on 46 men with premature ejaculation using fluoxetine. He provided no therapy and used the subjects as their own controls. There was no placebo group. Within one month, some of the patients reported an improvement in their degree of premature ejaculation. For the non-responders and those who had not reached their therapeutic goals, he increased the dosage until the desired effect was achieved. Most of his subjects experienced satisfactory clinical results at dosages of 20–40 mg; some required 60–80 mg. He reported that the desired effect was consistently achievable in patients, though dose-dependent. A particularly interesting facet of Crenshaw's study is that after three to six months of treatment patients could sustain the sexual results without continuing the medication. This sustained positive effect is similar to the experience we have had with bupropion, in which the sexual effect was maintained over time.

Fluoxetine appears to be a dependable treatment for premature ejaculation, which can be used by men with an acceptably low level of side effects. Newer serotonin uptake inhibitors (paroxetine, sertraline, fluvoxamine) may also prove to be useful treatments for premature ejaculation. However, the fluoxetine effect on premature ejaculation should be approached with caution. Because fluoxetine can have serious side effects in some patients, it should not be prescribed liberally for sexual dysfunction, regardless of patient demand.

While adverse sexual effects in women are also common—namely, diminished desire and inhibited orgasm or anorgasmia—many feel that the general sense of well-being they experience from treatment with fluoxetine is well worth the loss, at least in the short term. As with other drugs, not all women who take this drug experience adverse sexual consequences. For those who do, adjustments in dosage may be helpful; as always, the risk-benefit ratio must be carefully evaluated.

Paradoxical Effects Animal and human clinical research on SSRIs, MAOIs, the serotonin precursor 5-HTP, and the sexual effects of serotonin depletors such as PCPA indicates that serotonin is predominantly inhibitory to sex drive and response, particularly to active male sexuality. Nevertheless, unexplained paradoxical effects of serotonergic drugs are relatively common. Hypomania associated with hypersexuality frequently occurs, often requiring drug withdrawal. Reports of suicidal ideation have confounded fluoxetine treatment of depression, despite the fact that serotonin is considered to decrease suicidal behavior (Teicher, Glad, & Cole, 1990).* The assumption that a relatively nonspecific neurotransmitter is specifically inhibitory to sex (or suicidal ideation) is obviously simplistic, as shown by these many examples of clear sexual stimulation associated with serotonin potentiating drugs.

Modell (1989) presented the case of a 30-year-old woman treated with 40 mg fluoxetine who yawned repeatedly without drowsiness and experienced "multiple orgasms associated with clitoral engorgement in the absence of voluntary sexual stimulation." The patient was asked to take notes on these fluoxetine-induced sexual events. No spontaneous orgasms occurred on 20 mg fluoxetine for two weeks. However, when a 40 mg dose was first taken, remarkable changes occurred:

> Sixty minutes later, she began yawning at an approximate rate of four yawns a minute . . . the

*Some patients reported as becoming suicidal due to Prozac have subsequently been shown to be prone to unstable (and suicidal) reactions to other drugs.

> yawning gradually decreased in frequency and intensity over the following 30 minutes, and then disappeared. Five minutes after the yawning began, the patient experienced a feeling of sexual arousal and fullness in the genital region, associated with clitoral engorgement (verified visually by the patient). Three minutes later, she experienced an orgasm of intensity level 5 [on a 1-10 scale of mild to overwhelming], followed by seven spontaneous orgasms over the next 45 minutes that gradually decreased in intensity until they disappeared. Orgasms persisted for five minutes following the cessation of yawning, and the two symptoms did not appear to the patient to be causally linked.

The patient then discontinued fluoxetine for two weeks due to a sinus infection. When she resumed on a 40 mg dose, within 55 to 110 minutes she experienced 24 separate orgasms graded between one and three on the intensity scale. Over the next seven days, yawning occurred but no further sexual sensations. Increasing the dose to 60 mg on days eight and nine resulted in clitoral engorgement and 13 orgasms. However, no further spontaneous orgasms occurred.

We are not suggesting that orgasms precipitated by yawning are of sexual value. The point of this paradoxical effect is to illustrate that fluoxetine can have a biochemical impact (under very select circumstances) that triggers spontaneous orgasm in females. Investigating this phenomenon could lead to an understanding of the mechanism responsible for orgasm, which in turn could lead to the development of sexually effective drugs for anorgasmic women.

New Serotonin-Uptake Inhibitors

Recently, three new serotonin uptake inhibitors have been marketed in the United States, offering potentially effective alternatives to fluoxetine: sertraline (Zoloft), paroxetine (Paxil), and fluvoxamine (Luvox). The newer SSRIs may produce less initial anxiety than fluoxetine (Rickels & Schweizer, 1990), but their sexual side effects may be the same or worse. Additionally, they do not appear to have the weight-loss efficacy of fluoxetine.

Sertraline has a severely inhibitory effect on orgasm/ejaculation and its manufacturer has conducted a promising pilot trial of its efficacy in reducing premature ejaculation (Pfizer Pharmaceuticals, personal communication, 1991). Swartz (1994) has shown a consistently beneficial effect of sertraline in treatment of premature ejaculation. In addition to its selective serotonin reuptake inhibitory property, sertraline also appears to inhibit excitatory responses through blocking dopamine receptors and affecting excitatory amino acid sigma receptors (Koe, Lebel, Burkhart, & Schmidt, 1989). Company data indicated a 17.2% rate of sexual dysfunction compared to 8% on amitriptyline and 1.1% on placebo (Doogan & Caillard, 1988). Reimherr et al. (1990) found male sexual dysfunction in 21.4% of patients on sertraline compared to 7.7% on amitriptyline and 1.4% on placebo. Male sexual dysfunction due to sertraline occurred in seven of 81 (8.6%) elderly (over 65) patients treated for depression, but it was not noted whether several of the "unaffected" patients were already sexually inactive (Cohn et al., 1990).

Recently a case of galactorrhea lactation was reported in a woman treated with 100 mg/day sertraline (Bronzo & Stahl, 1993), and Hall (1994) reported breast swelling and discomfort in two menopausal women, 39 and a 68 years old, treated with 100 mg/day sertraline. Though an increase in prolactin might account for these effects, no measures of prolactin levels were taken.

Paroxetine (Paxil) has shown at least a 13% (5 of 40) rate of retarded ejaculation in a six-week double-blind trial compared to 0% on imipramine or placebo (Peselow, Filippi, Goodnick, Barouche, & Freve, 1989). The rate must be considerably higher in this trial because some of the patients on paroxetine must have been women who could not ejaculate. In a similar six-week study, Claghorn (1992) reported 17% retarded ejaculation on paroxetine versus 0% on placebo. A recent review article on paroxetine using accumulated company data showed 9% retarded ejaculation and 3% decreased sex drive (Dechant & Clissold, 1991).

In our limited clinical experience, paroxetine causes retarded or absent orgasm/ejaculation in about 50% of male patients. The effect is dose-related, mainly occurring above 20 mg (the recommended therapeutic dose is 20–50 mg/day but even 10 mg/day may be effective). The suppression of orgasm/ejaculation is clearly unlike that which occurs as a result of adrenergic blockers such as phenoxybenzamine (dry orgasm). With paroxetine (as with other SSRI antidepressants), ejaculation occurs normally with orgasm, but orgasm itself is often inhibited. Additionally, the sensory increase prior to climax is reduced; erection does not seem to be affected. However, after many months of a lack of orgasmic response, sex drive and erection may decrease. Paroxetine is perhaps the most potent SSRI in inhibiting orgasm in men and therefore can be used to treat premature ejaculation (R. Crenshaw, 1993, personal communication; Machalet Phanjoo, 1994; Waldinger, Hengeveld, & Zwinderman, 1994).

We were surprised at the relative lack of sexual inhibition in women patients compared to the powerful anorgasmia observed in men on this drug. A few women noticed delayed or absent orgasm when first engaging in sexual activity after a few weeks on paroxetine, but did not report continued sexual problems. Further clinical use may show no difference between women and men. Women who show intolerable anxiety reactions to fluoxetine do not experience these reactions on paroxetine. However, in our clinical experience, weight gain may occur on paroxetine during long-term use (over six months), in contrast to weight loss on fluoxetine.

Sexual side effects have only rarely been reported on fluvoxamine. However, the nervousness and severe nausea apparently induced by fluvoxamine in patients treated for depression could discourage sexual activity (Grimsley & Jann, 1992). Fluvoxamine has a less potent serotonin-uptake inhibitory effect than sertraline and paroxetine, which may account for a lesser impact on sexual function. Only clinical experience subsequent to marketing will show the extent of fluvoxamine's impact on sexual function. The negative sexual effects of fluoxetine were recognized only after it had been on the market in widespread use for two years.

In our clinical experience with panic/phobia and depressed patients treated with fluvoxamine, decreased libido and retarded orgasm has occurred in both men and women at doses of 100 mg/day or above. The incidence of these negative sexual effects is somewhere in the area of 10–30% and is clearly less than those seen with paroxetine. The first published case reports of fluvoxamine-induced sexual dysfunction were by Dorevitech and Davis (1994), who reported a 44-year-old woman treated for depression with 200 mg/day fluvoxamine. She developed difficulty achieving orgasm and also noted a decrease in her desire to masturbate. No sexual dysfunction had occurred during prior treatment with nortriptyline; in fact, prior to fluvoxamine, she had always experienced multiple orgasms. Additionally, they reported a 64-year-old man treated for depression who was unable to have an erection or orgasm/ejaculation on 100 mg/day of fluvoxamine. He had had no previous erectile or ejaculatory difficulties. Both patients regained normal sexual function one to three weeks after stopping fluvoxamine treatment and re-experienced the same sexual difficulties when again treated with fluvoxamine.

Venlafaxine (Effexor) is a combined serotonin and norepinephrine uptake inhibitor marketed in the United States early in 1994. From information on its labeling (*Physicians Desk Reference*, 1995), inhibited male orgasm/ejaculation and impotence are definite adverse sexual side effects (abnormal male orgasm/ejaculation 12% versus < 1% on placebo). Nausea (37% versus 11%), somnolence (23% versus 9%), dizziness (19% versus 7%), constipation (15% versus 7%), and asthenia (12% versus 6%) are also notable. However, various adverse effects—due to action at other receptors characteristic of tricyclic antidepressants (e.g., antihistamine, anticholinergic)—are avoided (Nierenberg, Feighner, Rudolph, Cole, & Sullivan, 1994). Pulse rate and blood pressure may be increased slightly, but weight gain is unlikely (Nierenberg et al., 1994). Schweizer, Feighner, Mandos, and Rickels (1994) assert that venlafaxine shows less sexual dysfunction self-reported by patients than other SSRIs, but such a difference in sexual effects is not indicated by venlafaxine's labeling or its chemical mechanisms.

TRAZODONE (DESYREL)

With the widespread use of SSRIs for everything from depression to chocolate craving, the sexual consequences of serotonin potentiation should be intensely scrutinized in the future. Trazodone (Desyrel) also increases serotonin, but does not behave exactly the way most drugs in this category do. Trazodone is a hybrid of sorts; it has been reported to increase sex drive, in contrast to most serotonin potentiators, which decrease drive. While increasing serotonin, it has the paradoxical effect of sustaining erections, sometimes to the point of priapism. While serving as an effective antidepressant, trazodone has been reported to improve sex drive. Although increased erections have also been reported as associated with trazodone, the incidence of penile priapism warrants caution regarding using trazodone as a treatment for impotence. Trazodone is one of the most fascinating drugs in regard to serotonin activity and poses numerous questions about the scope of its specific mechanism of action, which remains unknown. With further study, trazodone may provide insight into the dynamics of sexual neurochemistry that will add a valuable dimension to our understanding. Table 21.3 summarizes the properties and side effects of trazodone.

Sexual Benefits

Since trazodone has a predominant serotonergic effect, reduced desire and inhibited orgasm/ejaculation typical of other serotonin potentiators would be expected. However, it is not infrequently reported to increase sex drive (Gartrell, 1986; Sullivan, 1988). Because drive disorders as divergent as hypersexuality and sexual aversion may involve deficient serotonin regulation, serotonin potentiation may be used to treat both. The benefits and deficits that result from serotonin treatments will teach us much about the sexual dynamics involved. Unfortunately, monitoring of negative sexual effects of serotonergic drugs has been almost non-existent, but there have been interesting reports of positive sexual effects during treatment with many of these drugs—in particular, with trazodone but also with clomipramine, fluoxetine, fenfluramine, buspirone, and tryptophan. Positive sexual stimulation with serotonergic drugs has been shown predominantly in women, but also has occurred in both women and men, with no clear differentiation, despite the positive correlation between serotonin and estrogen and the negative correlation of serotonin with testosterone.

There are numerous small studies and case reports associating trazodone with sexual changes:

- Increased sex drive was reported in 6 of 13 (46%) women treated with trazodone for depression over three years (Gartrell, 1986). No sexual benefits occurred in those in whom depression was not improved. Of the eight women who became less depressed, six showed increased sex drive.
- A 26-year-old woman who had not masturbated for a year and had never been orgasmic reported decreased depression and greater sex drive on 150 mg/day trazodone. She masturbated daily and initiated new sexual relationships, but still continued to be anorgasmic (Gartrell, 1986).
- A 44-year-old post-mastectomy patient presented with low sex drive and withdrawal from sexual relationships, including masturbation. On 150 mg/day, she experienced obsessive sexual drive, resumed masturbation, and initiated contact with three former sex partners. After withdrawal from trazodone at six months, she noted reduction of sex drive back to a low level, but no return of depression (Gartrell, 1986).
- A third woman reported resumption of masturbation, a new sexual relationship, more frequent orgasm, and what she described as "the greatest sex drive she had ever experienced in her life" during seven months of treatment. Her sex drive decreased within a week after stopping trazodone and again increased within 11 days of resuming the drug (Gartrell, 1986).
- Sullivan (1988) reported sexual stimulation in three of 10 men treated for depression with trazodone, but the drug failed to relieve depression in any of the three. One man on 50 mg/day, formerly a passive sex partner, began initiating sex daily; another on 450 mg/day, who took trazodone (with lithium) for over two years, reported masturbation several times daily (Sullivan, 1988).

Table 21.3 *Profile of Trazodone (Desyrel)*

COMMON INDICATIONS
Depression
Pain

MECHANISMS OF ACTION (GENERAL)
Potentiates serotonin activity by blocking certain serotonin receptors, including the 5-HT_2 receptor
Stimulates other serotonin receptors
Inhibits serotonin reuptake

MECHANISMS OF ACTION (SEXUAL)

Positive	*Negative*
Blocks peripheral adrenergic $alpha_1$ activity	Decreased adrenergic ($alpha_1$) activity
Blocks serotonin 5-HT_2 receptor	Increased cortisol
	Increased serotonin

DIRECT SEXUAL SIDE EFFECTS

Desire enhanced (in both sexes)	Orgasm/ejaculation
Erection effects	• Inhibited
• Erection facilitated	• Dyspareunia helped
• Priapism	

INDIRECT SEXUAL SIDE EFFECTS
Discomfort caused by dryness of skin, mouth, mucous membranes, nausea, rash/itching
Mood fluctuations resulting in nervousness
Neurological disturbances resulting in analgesia, dizziness, fatigue, sedation, tremor, weakness
Vascular disturbances resulting in arrhythmias, orthostatic hypotension

SEXUAL CONTRAINDICATIONS/BENEFITS

Avoid with prior condition of	*May be useful for*
Hypersexuality	Sex drive disorders
Priapism	Impotence
Ejaculatory inhibition	Dyspareunia
Anorgasmia	

ALTERNATIVES

Fluoxetine (Prozac)	Paroxetine (Paxil)
Nefazodone (Serzone)	Sertraline (Zoloft)

- Cole and Bodkin (1990) reported that supplemental trazodone treatment relieved phenelzine-induced impotence in a man and phenelzine-induced anorgasmia in a woman.

During 1991 trazodone received media attention due to a urologist's report (Saenz de Tejada et al., 1991) that it generated extended nocturnal erections (NPT). The side effect of priapism was identified in 1983; priapism is often preceded by unusually prolonged nocturnal erections (Thompson, J. W., et al., 1990). The condition can be very painful, may require medical or surgical intervention, and can result in permanent impotence if allowed to continue. Patt (1985) reported a 50-year-old man who required surgical treatment for priapism after two months on trazodone. The patient had noted prolonged erections soon after starting the drug. Goldstein (1991) identified prolonged sleep erections with trazodone as a scientific demonstration that it is an aphrodisiac. The label of *aphrodisiac* seems grossly misapplied, however, when used to describe extended and sometimes painful erection devoid of sexual feeling or function. One of the authors of the sleep study suggested that "it [trazodone] may give patients an easier and less obtrusive option in dealing with their impotence" (Goldstein, 1991). However, the manifestation of erection would be unpredictable and not necessarily available for sex on demand.

Albo and Steers (1993) treated 33 psychogenically or organically impotent men (mean age = 46 years) with trazodone as initial therapy for impotence. Positive response was defined as an increase in frequency or quality of erections sufficient for intercourse within one to three weeks of treatment (50–150 mg/day). Sixty-four percent had a positive response, which was sustained from one month to two years of monitoring (cause of impotence, whether mental or physical, was not correlated with response). Lal, Rios, and Thavundayil (1990) reported a 50-year-old physician who was able to attain erection only if he took from 200–350 mg trazodone within a four-hour period prior to sexual activity. This case report indicates that trazodone can be used irresponsibly (abused), despite the fact that this doctor did not experience priapism. In our limited clinical experience, trazodone has not been an effective treatment of either psychogenic or organic impotence. However, some patients (both men and women) treated with trazodone for non-sexual reasons have reported marked, unexpected sexual improvements in both arousal and responsiveness.

Regardless of any possible benefit to erection, the risk of priapism should temper the thought of using trazodone for erectile dysfunction. Male patients treated with trazodone for depression or impotence should be warned of priapism and taught how to deal with it. There may be some potential use in patients with intractable impotence, for whom a penile prosthesis is the only alternative. The risk in normal patients may be unacceptable. The above study was conducted on healthy volunteers. No controlled studies have been conducted to investigate the effect of trazodone in organically impotent patients.

Trazodone was frequently noted to cause unusual erectile activity short of priapism in patients treated for pain and headaches (Aronoff, 1984; Seymour Diamond, personal communication, 1988). The Saenz de Tejada 1991 sleep study reported that subjects on trazodone exhibited 51% sleep erectile activity compared to 38% on placebo. Increased erection occurred in four of six subjects and was greatest at the highest dose of 200 mg given prior to sleep. One subject became erect one minute before sleep onset and remained erect all night (about six hours), except for a nine-minute respite. One case report of clitoral priapism and five cases of clitoral enlargement have been reported to the manufacturer (Thompson, Ware, & Blashfield, 1990). There have been a few additional reports of clitoral enlargement with concurrent use of trazodone and testosterone supplementation (Mead Johnson, 1991). Clitoral hypertrophy has not been related to increased sensation (Thompson et al., 1990). It is possible that trazodone may inhibit orgasm and pleasurable genital sensation in women, analogous to reports of inhibited ejaculation and uncomfortable prolonged erection due to trazodone (Erickson & Fisher, 1983; Jones, 1984).

NEFAZODONE (SERZONE)

Nefazodone (Serzone) is a phenylpiperazine compound similar to trazodone; however, it lacks the major sedative effect and the alpha$_1$ adrenergic property supposedly responsible for the priapism and increased nocturnal erections associated with trazodone. Nefazodone has potent 5-HT$_2$ receptor antagonist and serotonin uptake inhibition actions that are greater than trazodone (Eison, Eison, Torrente, Wright, & Yocca, 1990). This drug was approved by the Federal Drug Administration for treatment of depression at the end of 1994. During investigatory clinical testing as an antidepressant, it appeared to be free of sexual dysfunction side effects (Bristol-Myers Squibb, data on file, 1992). Additionally, its strong 5-HT$_2$ antagonism could directly enhance sexual desire and function; 5-HT$_2$ antagonists have been shown to facilitate male rate copulatory behavior (Foreman, Fuller, Nelson, et al., 1992; Watson & Gorzalka, 1994). In our own short clinical experience with nefazodone, we have noted a return to normal sexual desire which had been depressed during SSRI treatment.

LITHIUM

Untreated manic-depressive (bipolar) disorders have a wide range of associated sexual dysfunctions. The manic episodes are characterized by hypersexual drive and behavior; depressive episodes are associated with decreased libido and hyposexuality. When medications are added to this equation, the influences on sex become even more complex. Changes in sexuality may occur on two different levels. Increased or decreased sexuality reestablishing normal sexual function may occur due to spontaneous improvement or as a result of successful drug therapy of the bipolar condition. The second possibility is decreased sexual function due to the direct adverse effects of the treatment drug. It is often difficult to distinguish between these dynamics.

Lithium's most evident mechanism of action is to inhibit the breakdown of inositol-phosphate (IP) metabolism, which may ultimately decrease activation of protein kinase C (PKC). Both IP and PKC are molecular elements of neural transmission that have only recently been investigated. PKC is an enzyme that is activated by diacylglycerol (DAG). IP (or more correctly IP_3 + DAG) is a breakdown product of phosphatidylinositol-4, 5-bisphosphate. Change in modulation of IP metabolism also occurs with bupropion, which has been shown to treat manic-depressive disorders either alone or in combination with lithium (Haykal & Akiskal, 1990; Shopsin, 1983). Both lithium and bupropion can generate seizures, but bupropion has a clear dopaminergic stimulant effect not found with lithium. The efficacy of both drugs in treating manic-depression as well as the undesirable generation of seizures may be due to their interference with IP and PKC neuronal metabolism.

Weight gain commonly occurs with long-term lithium treatment, often resulting in patient withdrawal from treatment. Over two to six years, a weight gain of about 22 pounds has occurred in 64% of 70 patients in one study (Vendsborg & Rafelson, 1976), and 20% of 237 patients in another (Vestergaard, Amdisen, & Schon, 1980). The amount and predictability of weight gain as a side effect are serious detriments to extended use of lithium and result in noncompliance. Usually there is a large weight gain during the first year of treatment and weight remains higher for as long as the drug is taken (Vendsborg & Rafelson, 1976). With additional side effects of tremor, weakness, fatigue, dizziness and poor balance, it may be futile to ask some patients to increase their exercise. Given these problems, the rarity of reported sexual problems is surprising.

Slowed thinking and memory deficits have occasionally been reported in some studies of lithium, but have not been found in others (Glue, Nutt, Cowen, & Broadbent, 1987; Judd, 1979; Smiggan & Perris, 1983). In clinical practice, patients commonly complain of poor concentration, mental slowness, confusion, and memory problems, but the actual degree of cognitive disturbance is difficult to determine experimentally. Seizures, which occasionally occur on lithium, may be caused by increased cholinergic activity (Demers, Lukesh, & Prichard, 1970; Waldmeier, 1987). While this cholinergic effect conceivably could have beneficial effects on sexual response as well as cognition, the risk of seizure is not offset. Often seizure is a sign of toxicity and can occur when blood levels are not carefully monitored.

Lithium was found in the genital organs of rats injected with the drug (Gralla & McIlhenny, 1972). Testosterone initially decreased in rats or increased in mice due to lithium administration, but no change was found beyond the first week. Reduced fertility in rats or mice has been observed in a few studies. There have also been reports of reduced testosterone in humans, although acne eruptions associated with lithium treatment suggest increased androgen activity (Deandrea, Walker, Mehlmauer, & White, 1982). Women are more sensitive than men to cutaneous lithium reactions such as acne and body rash (Deandrea et al., 1982; Sarantidis & Waters, 1983). Hypothyroidism can occur in 1–30% of patients, requiring thyroxine supplementation (Schon, 1989). Undiagnosed hypothyroidism can lead to severe sexual dysfunction and weight gain. Table 21.4 summarizes the properties and side effects of lithium.

Sexual Dysfunction

Lithium has been reported to cause loss of desire and difficulties in erectile function, although there are few studies available and some reports show little difference compared with placebo. Vinarova, Uhlir, Stika, and Vinar (1972) found difficulties in obtaining and maintaining erection in two of 23 men on long-term lithium and in two of 10 men in a subsequent placebo-controlled trial. Blay, Ferraz, and Calil (1982) described two cases of decreased desire and erection due to lithium. In one patient, this sexual deficit was transient, but in the other it continued on lithium but not on placebo. Kristensen and Jorgensen (1987) conducted a retrospective interview review of sexual side effects in 24 patients on lithium for six months to two years. A comprehensive questionnaire that differentiated between male and female dysfunctions was used. Although two men and two women reported reduced sex drive, which they attributed to lithium, these difficulties were no greater than in the control group. The authors observed that male, but not female, sexual dysfunction sometimes occurred in their clinical practice when other psychotropic drugs were used in conjunction with lithium.

During the same year, an extensive British retrospective follow-up review of 59 patients on lithium for up to 17 years showed erectile dysfunctions as a side effect in five of 30 male patients (Page, Benaim, & Lappin, 1987). Weight gain occurred in 21 patients and 11 complained of loss of creativity. Over half of the patients were on concurrent tricyclic antidepressants, benzodiazepines, or neuroleptics. Because any of these drugs could have caused erection deficits, the results were inconclusive.

Ghadirian, Annable, and Belanger (1992) used a comprehensive sexual questionnaire to survey sexual changes in 104 bipolar outpatients on chronic lithium treatment (45 men and 59 women; mean age, 45; median length of treatment, six years and 90% on lithium for six months or longer). Sexual changes reported are shown in Table 21.5. Among the 36 (35%) patients on lithium alone, only one reported an adverse change in sexual function. In contrast, among the 50 (49%) patients on lithium combined with benzodiazepines (usually clonazepam), 11 (22%) reported a great decrease in sexual desire or function and six (12%) reported a moderate decrease.

Both men and women on lithium and benzodiazepines reported adverse sexual changes. Men chiefly reported decreased erection and/or orgasm and women reported decreased sexual desire and/or ability to have orgasm. Due to the sexual symptoms of the disease itself, it is difficult to determine to what extent lithium causes sexual dysfunction. However, sexual dysfunction clearly occurs when lithium and benzodiazepines are taken concurrently (see Table 21.5).

Sexual Benefits

Positive sexual effects with lithium are rare and seem to occur only in women. Ghadirian et al. (1992) found increased sexual desire and orgasm in over 20% of women treated with lithium alone or combined with other psychotropic drugs. Together with reports of the sexual benefits that can occur with trazodone, this finding may indicate that drugs like lithium or trazodone, which may increase serotonin activity, may also cause positive sexual changes in some women. Although the pronounced positive effects that occur with bupropion are not found with lithium, both bupropion and lithium may work through molecular actions that do not compromise sexual desire or response. While bupropion can act as a stimulant, the absence of stimulant or depressive effects is a key to lithium's unique therapeutic efficacy.

The infrequency of adverse sexual side effects reported with lithium compares favorably with the negative sexual effects associated with antidepressants, benzodiazepines, and neuroleptics. Given that lithium eliminates manic tendencies associated with increased sexuality, sexuality will sometimes decline due to this decrease in mania. Goodwin and Jamison (1986) have commented that women treated with lithium miss their height-

Table 21.4 *Profile of Lithium*

	Daily Dose
Eskalith	300–1200 mg/day
Lithobid	(serum concentration 0.6–1.2 mEq/L)

COMMON INDICATIONS

Manic-depressive (bipolar) disorder, alcoholism, cluster headache (prophylaxis)

MECHANISMS OF ACTION (GENERAL)

Limits excess monoamine activity

Balances molecular neural signal activity (adenylate cyclase versus phosphoinositide)

MECHANISMS OF ACTION (SEXUAL)

Positive

- Decreased adrenergic $alpha_2$ activity
- Increased cholinergic activity (uncertain)
- Decreased protein kinase C
- Increased negative serotonin receptor

Negative

- Increased serotonin (but decreased serotonin release)
- Increased cortisol
- Increased GABA/benzodiazepine
- Decreased testosterone
- Decreased thyroid hormone
- Decreased vasopressin

DIRECT SEXUAL SIDE EFFECTS

Desire disorders (in both sexes)

Erection difficulties

Infertility

- Decreased or malformed spermatogenesis
- Decreased male fertility
- Birth defects

INDIRECT SEXUAL SIDE EFFECTS

Discomfort caused by dryness of skin, mouth, mucous membranes, weight gain, edema, indigestion, nausea, diarrhea, rash/itching, acne, urinary problems (incontinence, polyuria)

Mood disorders resulting in anhedonia, detachment

Neurological disturbances resulting in cognitive deficits, dizziness, fatigue, movement disorder (ataxia, seizure), sedation, tremor, muscular weakness

Vascular disturbances resulting in arrhythmias

Endocrine disturbances precipitating or aggravating diabetes and hypothyroidism, insipidus due to excess urination

SEXUAL CONTRAINDICATIONS/BENEFITS

Avoid with prior condition of

- Desire disorders
- Erection problems
- Inhibited orgasms/ejaculation

May be useful for

- Hypersexuality

ALTERNATIVES

Bupropion (Wellbutrin) for manic-depression

Valproic acid (Depakene) for manic-depression

ened sexual intensity most, while men miss their social ease and elevated self-esteem. Doctors may not report sexual difficulties with lithium because they assume that any reduced sexuality is either a desirable therapeutic effect or a justifiable "price" for reduced or eliminated manic mood states. Lithium may have some value in treating hypersexuality unrelated to manic states, but no studies have addressed this possibility. In view of the potential for lithium to be used

Table 21.5 *Sexual Changes in 104 Bipolar Patients Treated with Lithium Alone or Lithium with Other Psychotropic Drugs*

Men on Lithium (n = 45)	
No sexual change	57% (25/45)
Mild difficulty in sexual function	23% (10/45)
Moderate or great difficulty in sexual function	18% (8/45)
Mild erectile difficulties	27% (12/45)
Moderate or great erectile difficulties	16% (7/45)
Mild decreased orgasm	18% (8/45)
Moderate or great decreased orgasm	18% (8/45)
Increased sexual desire or function	2% (1/45)
Women on Lithium (n = 59)	
No sexual change	61% (34/59)
Mild decreased sexual desire	20% (11/59)
Moderate or great decrease in sexual desire	20% (11/59)
Mild decreased orgasm	11% (6/59)
Moderate or great decrease in orgasm	19% (11/59)
Increased sexual desire	24% (14/59)
Increased quality of orgasm	21% (12/59)

Adapted from Ghadirian et al., 1992.

as a treatment for hypersexuality, we suspect that it also has potentially adverse effects on normal sexuality. However, no definitive conclusions can be drawn until further research is performed.

Paradoxical Effects

The effect of lithium has been hypothesized to involve increased serotonin transmission (Waldmeier, 1987), which should have some negative sexual impact. Increased serotonin should also cause weight loss, yet significant weight gain often occurs with lithium treatment. Despite the research showing that lithium increases serotonin, the nature and extent of this serotonergic activity and its relevance to lithium's therapeutic effect remain unclear. Numerous drugs affect serotonin in distinctly different ways: lithium, fluoxetine, phenelzine, trazodone, buspirone, sumatriptan, odansetron, ketanserin, and mianserin. The effects are diverse and difficult to interpret. Further research is needed to clarify the paradoxical effects of serotonin on sexuality. Conversely, sexual effects may serve to differentiate the serotonergic actions of these drugs.

Recent identification of multiple serotonin receptors with contradictory mechanisms of action may explain lithium's inconsistent effects on sexual function. For example, conventional symptoms in animals with increased serotonin levels (such as head shakes) are reduced by lithium instead of increased, as would be expected (Goodwin, De Souza, Wood, & Green, 1986). Serotonin synthesis and release seem to be increased in some parts of the brain and decreased in others (Glue, Cowen, Nutt, Kolakowska, & Grahame-Smith, 1986). However, total brain serotonin is generally increased (Waldmeier, 1987). Lithium can also increase unusual serotonin symptoms such as hyperlocomotion and the serotonin syndrome (forepaw-treading, stretching) that are characteristic of 5-HT_{1A} receptors (Glue et al., 1986).

Experimental research in animals has indicated that lithium stimulates 5-HT_{1A} receptors (Glue et al., 1986). Since these receptors are also stimulated by the anxiolytic buspirone, lithium and buspirone may have a common chemical effect. Specific stimulation of the 5-HT_{1A} receptor in animals causes increased sexual behavior (Mathes et al., 1990) and increased eating (Gilbert, Dourish, Brazell, McClue, & Stahl, 1988), which might be due to these recently discovered 5-HT_{1A} actions.

Alternatives

The anticonvulsant carbamazepine (Tegretol) is often used as an alternative to lithium, but it is toxic to sex and should be avoided. Valproic acid (Depakene) is preferable to carbamazepine, but it also has many anticonvulsant side effects (such as fatigue) that affect sexual function indirectly. If bupropion is appropriate and effective, it would be an ideal alternative. Supplementation of lithium with bupropion has been shown to be safe and effective in some clinic patients; however, bupropion could add to seizure risk already present with lithium. When fear of seizure would preclude the use of bupropion, valproic acid can be added to bupropion. Finally, since buspirone and lithium both stimulate the 5-HT_{1A} receptor, buspirone may be helpful in the treatment of manic-depressive disorder. However, it has not been evaluated for this purpose and bipolar disorder is not one of the approved indications of buspirone.

22

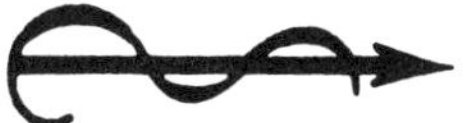

Antipsychotics/Neuroleptics

OBJECTIVES

- To compare and evaluate the sexual side effects and paradoxical effects of commonly used antipsychotic medications
- To identify the least sexually adverse alternatives

In spite of the well-recognized incidence of sexual dysfunction associated with antipsychotic medications, there are relatively few alternatives, and these alternatives are often inadequate for many patients. It is the prevailing view in medicine that the societal and personal benefits of controlling psychotic symptomatology far outweigh the individual sexual consequences of these medications. While this may be true, the limitations of this view become clear when the issue of outpatient compliance is considered: Patients often refuse to take their medications on a regular basis because of unacceptable sexual effects. It is therefore important for the successful management of psychotic disorders that medications be developed that have fewer side effects and, in particular, fewer sexual side effects. Until patients willingly consume their medication, perceiving its benefits to outweigh its drawbacks, the disease will continue to be a management challenge.

Neuroleptic, the original term used for antischizophrenia drugs, has been increasingly replaced by the more direct term *antipsychotic*. *Neuroleptic* was used in France in the 1950s, where chlorpromazine was first used in 1952 (Bailey & McKenna, 1990). The suffix *leptic* means "to hold or capture" in Greek; *neuroleptic* means a drug that holds or controls neurological/neuropsychiatric symptoms characteristic of schizophrenia and psychotic behavior (Bailey & McKenna, 1990). Delay and Deniker, who introduced the term, wanted to convey the notion of a calming effect, rather than the sedating effect characteristic of sedative tranquilizers (Bailey & McKenna, 1990). Increasingly since 1970, the chief function of these drugs has been viewed as an inhibition of excess dopaminergic activity. Recently, however, clinical and research work has centered on "atypical antipsychotics," which have prominent antiserotonergic actions.

The side-effect profile of antipsychotics, as a class of drugs, has not improved to the degree that antidepressants has. While the choices are limited, there are some distinctions among the medications that may be helpful concerning sexual function. However, sexual function is often sacrificed "for the sake of sanity" in psychotic disorders. Because antipsychotic drugs block dopamine and increase prolactin, they interfere with sexual desire and responsiveness. Given that dopamine is recognized as a critical factor in sex drive and sexual behavior, there is an obvious probability of negative sexual side effects with neuroleptics. The specific sexual characteristics vary, depending upon the individual drug and the dose. Table 22.1 summarizes the properties and side effects of antipsychotic/neuroleptic drugs.

SEXUAL DYSFUNCTION

Ejaculatory inhibition was first reported for thioridazine (Mellaril) in 1961, a few years after

Table 22.1 *Profile of Antipsychotics/Neuroleptics*

Class of Drug	**Daily Dose**
Phenothiazines	
Chlorpromazine (Thorazine)	100–600 mg
Fluphenazine (Prolixin)	10–60 mg
Mesoridazine (Serentil)	25–400 mg
Perphenazine (Trilafon)	8–64 mg
Thiordazine (Mellaril)	100–600 mg
Trifluoperazine (Stelazine)	10–60 mg
Butyrophenones	
Haloperidol (Haldol)	2–60 mg
Thioxanthenes	
Chlorprothixene (Taractan)	20–600 mg
Thiothixene (Navane)	5–60 mg
Fluphenthixol (Fluanxol – not marketed in United States)	
Miscellaneous	
Clozapine (Clozaril) – Dibenzodiazepine	100–800 mg
Loxapine (Loxitane) – Dibenzoxazepine	15–160 mg
Molindone (Moban) – Indolone	15–225 mg
Pimozide (Orap) – Diphenylbutylpiperidine	1–10 mg
Risperidone (Risperdal) – Benzisoxasde	4–10 mg

COMMON INDICATIONS

Psychoses, schizophrenia, schizoaffective disorder, mania, Tourette syndrome, agitated depression, psychotic dementia

MECHANISMS OF ACTION (GENERAL)

Block dopamine activity

Block sigma receptors and/or 5-HT_2 serotonin receptors

MECHANISMS OF ACTION (SEXUAL)

Negative

Decreased adrenergic $alpha_1$ activity

Decreased cholinergic activity

Decreased dopamine

Increased prolactin

Decreased testosterone

Decreased LHRH pulsatile activity

DIRECT SEXUAL SIDE EFFECTS

Desire disorders (in both sexes)
- Hyposexuality
- Hypersexuality (rare)

Erection difficulties
- Inability/difficulty obtaining/maintaining
- Decreased quality of erection
- Priapism

Orgasm irregularities
- Anorgasmia
- Diminished number of orgasms
- Orgasmic inhibition

Ejaculation irregularities
- Retarded ejaculation
- Ejaculatory inhibition
- Decreased ejaculatory volume
- Anesthetic ejaculation
- Orgasm without ejaculation
- Dyspareunia

Menstrual Disorders
- Amenorrhea
- Dysmenorrhea/menorrhagia

Infertility
- Hypogonadism
- Decreased or malformed spermatogenesis

Breast disorders
- Gynecomastia
- Galactorrhea
- Pain/tenderness

(*continued*)

Table 22.1 *Continued*

INDIRECT SEXUAL SIDE EFFECTS

Discomfort caused by dryness of skin, mouth, mucous membranes, constipation, fever (neuroleptic malignant syndrome), urinary problems (retention, painful urination)

Mood disorders resulting in anhedonia, depression, nervousness (akathesia, restlessness, hyperactive)

Neurological disturbances resulting in cognitive deficit, dizziness, fatigue, increased sensitivity to sun, movement disorder (akathesia, akinesia, dystonia, stiffness, tardive dyskinesia), sedation, seizure, sensory loss (blurred vision), tremor, muscular weakness

Vascular disturbances resulting in arrhythmias, hypotension

SEXUAL CONTRAINDICATIONS/BENEFITS

Avoid with prior condition of	*May be useful for*
Sexual aversion	Hypersexuality
Desire disorders	Premature ejaculation
Impotence	
Ejaculatory inhibition	
Anorgasmia	
Dyspareunia (male and female)	
Menstrual disorders	
Infertility	
Priapism	

ALTERNATIVES

Buspirone (Buspar) for schizoaffective disorder
Sertraline (Zoloft) for schizoaffective disorder

it was marketed. Subsequently, several cases of lack of ejaculation, delayed ejaculation, and erectile dysfunction have been reported (see Mitchell & Popkin, 1982, and Segraves, Madsen, Carter, & Davis, 1985, for reviews). The ability of thioridazine to block ejaculation was documented in a comprehensive study by Kotin, Wilbert, Verburg, and Soldinger (1976). Until this study, there had been isolated case study reports of ejaculatory failure, but only 31 such cases had been reported to its manufacturer, Sandoz, despite its use in over 10 million patients. The particular severity of ejaculatory disorders and higher prevalence of sexual dysfunction on thioridazine, as well as chlorpromazine (Thorazine), may be in large part due to their anticholinergic and sedative effects. Increased antidopaminergic potency of the low-dose neuroleptics and/or addition of anticholinergic medication can cause sexual dysfunction as severe as that on chlorpromazine or even thioridazine.

Kotin et al. (1976) reviewed the medical charts and interviewed 87 patients who had been on neuroleptics for over two weeks. The patients did not have other diseases which could affect sex, were not taking other drugs, and were sexually active. They were asked whether they had observed changes in erection, orgasm, ejaculation, or pain during sex since starting neuroleptics. Those taking thioridazine were compared to patients on other neuroleptics. Table 22.2 summarizes the results. Two thioridazine patients reported pain at orgasm; 19 complained of no ejaculation at orgasm; and nine complained of a decreased amount of ejaculate. The absence of any ejaculatory change in patients on other neuroleptics in this study is surprising, since this particular side effect has been reported with most neuroleptics in other studies and anecdotal reports (Mitchell & Popkin, 1982; Segraves et al., 1985).

Lack of ejaculate also occurs with the adrenergic blocker phenoxybenzamine (Dibenzyline), suggesting antagonism of adrenergic alpha$_1$ receptors by thioridazine. However, other neuroleptics also block adrenergic alpha$_1$ receptors

Table 22.2 *Review of Sexual Side Effects in 87 Patients Treated with Neuroleptics*

	Thioridazine	*Other Neuroleptics*
Sexual dysfunction	60%	25%
Difficulty achieving erection	44%	19%
Difficulty maintaining erection	35%	11%
Retarded ejaculation	49%	0%

Data from Kotin et al., 1976.

and most neuroleptics, including thioridazine, are anticholinergic and increase prolactin. Therefore, it is not clear why lack of ejaculation is so much more frequent with thioridazine. Gould, Murphy, Reynolds, and Snyder (1984) have suggested that lack of ejaculation on thioridazine is due to its strong calcium channel blocking property; however, the strongest available calcium channel blockers used to treat hypertension do not cause more than minor changes in ejaculation.

Although this particular effect of thioridazine is often referred to as retrograde ejaculation (failure of internal urinary bladder sphincter to close), there are no reports of significant amounts of semen recovered from post-coital urine. Ejaculation and emission evidently do not occur, so it appears that there is no semen to be diverted into the urinary bladder. When small amounts of semen have been found in the urine, it is thought to be due to slow leakage of excess accumulated semen from the seminal vesicles.

One of the authors in the Kotin study experienced a "tearing" pain and no ejaculation when he masturbated after taking 50 mg thioridazine, confirming the report of pain at orgasm by two of the patients on thioridazine. Only a few of the patients (4 of 57) in Kotin's sample who experienced sexual side effects requested any change in medication; apparently, only a few of the doctors suggested dose adjustments or a change to another neuroleptic. While this lack of reaction to drug-induced sexual dysfunction is puzzling, it is also typical.

Reports of priapism have been most frequent on thioridazine and chlorpromazine (e.g., Griffiths & Zil, 1984), which may be due to the fact that these two phenothiazine neuroleptics are the most widely prescribed. Priapism has also occurred with fluphenazine, mesoridazine, haloperidol, molindone, trifluoperazine, perphenazine, and chlorprothixene (Winter & McDonell, 1988). Men on neuroleptics should be warned to report unusual erections lasting more than two hours; physicians who prescribe neuroleptics should confirm a protocol with a hospital or a urologist for prompt treatment.

Priapism can occur at any dose and during any phase of treatment on neuroleptics. It can also occur at any age, but is most common between 30 to 50 years old. The cause of this condition has not been definitively determined; it may involve an adrenergic blocking property common to neuroleptics.

The most complete evaluation of neuroleptic side effects was presented as a supplement in *Acta Psychiatrica Scandinavia* (Lingjaerde, Ahlfors, Bech, Dencker, & Elgen, 1987). A large cross-section of psychiatrists in 50 Scandinavian hospitals used the comprehensive UKU side-effect rating scale to evaluate their patients on neuroleptics for at least one month. There were 2,391 patients in all (1,259 men and 1,132 women). Fifty-eight percent were being treated for schizophrenia; the rest, for various psychiatric disorders. Most patients had been on their current neuroleptic treatment between one and over 10 years; however, 19% were on their current neuroleptic for less than three months. Side effects were judged for severity (mild, moderate, severe) and supposed drug-relatedness (improbable, possible, probable). The side effect questions specified change due to medication. For instance, with ejaculatory delay a moderate side effect was described as "a distinct change in the patient's ability to control ejaculation, so that it becomes a problem for him." Results indicated:

- *Sexual desire increased* in 20% of women and men (24.4% of inpatients, but only 9.1% of outpatients).
- *Reduced sexual desire* was the most frequent sexual side effect in both male (36.6%) and female (36.9%) patients. (There was no difference between inpatients and outpatients.)
- Male patients reported 21.5% *erectile dysfunction* and 18.7% *ejaculatory dysfunction.*
- *Orgasmic dysfunction* was greater in female patients (19.3%) than in male patients (15.9%).
- *Amenorrhea* occurred in 21.7% of females.
- *Galactorrhea* occurred in 5.3% of females and 2.7% of males.
- *Gynecomastia* occurred in 3% of females and 6% of males.

The incidence of reduced sexual desire (about 36%) on neuroleptics was similar in patients from 20 to 60 years old, but rose sharply to 50% in patients between 60 and 70 years of age. The older patients might have been more vulnerable to negative sexual effects due to concurrent medications or other illnesses. Erectile, orgasmic, and ejaculatory dysfunctions were greatest (about 25%) among patients aged 50 to 70. Evidently, concern with sexual dysfunction was no less among older patients, since many of them complained about this side effect.

Negative sexual effects were most frequent (50%) between three and six months of treatment. After six months, medication may have been adjusted or terminated for many patients experiencing sexual dysfunction, so that fewer reports were filed. Sexual side effects on current neuroleptic medications did not change with duration of treatment, indicating that tolerance did not occur; as long as patients remained on their neuroleptic medications, most continued to experience negative sexual side effects.

Sexual effects were more frequent on high-dose (over 100 mg) neuroleptics than on low-dose ones. Those that require high doses, such as chlorpromazine, thioridazine, and chlorprothixene (Taractan), are generally more sedating. On these high-dose drugs, reduced desire occurred in 42.9% of patients. Erectile, ejaculatory, and orgastic dysfunctions occurred in 24.8%, 26%, and 28.5% of patients, respectively.

While this UKU study was not a placebo-controlled random clinical trial, it was nonetheless a remarkable example of how much useful data can be generated with a well written, comprehensive questionnaire. It is difficult and expensive to conduct a controlled trial for the extended time periods covered in this study, and studies should be at least six months long for a valid evaluation of sexual side effects. (The UKU side effects rating scale was included in its entirety in Lingjaerde et al.'s 1987 journal supplement.) The conclusions of the study in regard to sexual side effects were as follows:

- Reduced sexual desire was the most frequent effect of the neuroleptic drugs and occurred in about one of three patients.
- Orgasm, erection, and ejaculation deficits occurred in about one of four patients. Women experienced these sexual deficits as often as men.
- The sexual deficits occurred equally in young and old patients, perhaps slightly more in older patients.
- Sexual deficits increased up to six months after first starting neuroleptic treatment and remained as long as neuroleptics were continued.
- Sexual deficits were less with high potency, low-dose neuroleptics (under 100 mg). The authors speculated that fluphenazine (Prolixin) and flupenthixol (Fluanxol) might be the low-dose neuroleptics most free of side effects, such as weight gain and sedation that can cause sexual problems.

Neuroleptic-induced sexual dysfunction has been documented in both men and women in other studies as well. Degen (1982) reported two women with retarded orgasm due to neuroleptic treatment (one on trifluoperazine, the other on thioridazine). Ghadirian, Chouinard, and Annable (1982) studied 53 patients (26 men and 27 women) on long-term maintenance neuroleptic treatment for schizophrenia. The patients were first interviewed and then completed a sexual function rating scale. Changes in erection, orgasm, and ejaculation were compared to a prior time when patients were not receiving neuroleptics. (Since all patients had been on neuroleptics from one to 24 years, such a comparison may have been confounded by poor memory and age.) Females were asked to rate time to orgasm, quality of orgasm, and pain during orgasm; questions concerning arousal, lubrication, and sexual desire were not included. Most of the patients were treated with fluphenazine injections supplemented with procyclidine (Kemadrin), an antispasmodic anti-Parkinson medication with anticholinergic properties. Men experienced frequent erectile dysfunction (40%) and difficulty in orgasm/ejaculation (58%). Women noted orgasm difficulty (22%) and change in quality of orgasm (33%). A few women reported pain during orgasm (7%) and most women reported decreased menstruation (78%).

Despite the severity of psychotic symptomatology, patients have reported being equally disturbed by the sexual side effects of the drugs used to treat their conditions. Finn, Bailey, Schultz, and Faber (1990) questioned 41 neuroleptic-treated patients to determine how "bothered" they were by neuroleptic side effects compared to the symptoms of schizophrenia being treated. Then they asked a group of psychiatrists to rate how much they believed the schizophrenia symptoms and neuroleptic side effects bothered the patients. Ratings of bother ranged from 0 (no bother) to 5 (great bother).

Patients on neuroleptics experienced impotence (34%), inhibited/painful ejaculation (12%), and painful urination (12%); dizziness due to hypotension was experienced by 83%, movement problems by 73%, fatigue by 46%, and weight gain by 22%. Overall, 20 neuroleptic side effects and 19 schizophrenic symptoms (e.g., delusions, paranoia, hallucinations, thought reading by others) were rated. Of all the side effects and symptoms, the genital/sexual side effects were rated as the most bothersome by the patients and were the only side effects with a greater than "4" rating other than paranoid delusions. Impotence was rated by patients as worse than any of their schizophrenic disease symptoms.

MALE/FEMALE DIFFERENCES

Women on neuroleptics may experience normal sexual activity if partners/spouses take the initiative; in these cases, emotional satisfaction can compensate for decreased physical arousal and pleasure. Schizophrenic men often limit their sexual activity to masturbation, where diminished fantasy and physical response can be critical.

Because dopamine inhibits prolactin, and antipsychotics block dopamine, prolactin may increase to toxic levels. Abnormally high levels of prolactin can cause severely decreased sexual responses in men and amenorrhea and other menstrual irregularities in women. Elevated prolactin in women can also cause a syndrome of hostility, depression, and anxiety (Fava, G., Fava, Kellner, Serafini, & Mastrogiacomo, 1981; Fava, M., Kellner, Serafini, & Mastrogiacomo, 1982; Kellner, Buckman, Fava, & Pathak, 1984); hostility and anxiety can result in sexual aversion, and depression typically undermines sexual desire. Men do not seem to experience the negative psychological consequences of hyperprolactemia as frequently as women.

In men treated with neuroleptics, elevated prolactin can decrease testosterone (though not below normal) and pituitary LHRH function (Bartke, Suare, Doherty, Smith, & Klemke, 1983). The decrease in LHRH function appears to be important both in men's lack of sexual response and in women's lack of ovulation/menstruation. When hyperprolactinemic men were treated with bromocriptine, sexual desire and response returned before testosterone levels increased (Bartke et al., 1983).

Neuroleptic-induced hyperprolactinemia can cause a variety of sexual/endocrine problems in addition to decreased sexual activity. Galactorrhea (lactation) and decreased sperm are direct effects in males; osteoporosis and breast cancer may be indirect effects in females (Gammon, 1981). Gynecomastia may occur with neuroleptic treatment, but has not been correlated directly with excess prolactin. Breast discomfort and pain during orgasm may be specific instances of an increase in pain sensitivity due to neuroleptics (Decina, Caracci, Harrison, & Sandyk, 1990).

Prolactin levels over 40 mg/ml can directly cause sexual dysfunction; therefore, neuroleptic dosage should be adjusted to keep prolactin below 50 mg/ml whenever possible. Elevated prolactin levels between 25–50 mg/ml should be warning to monitor sexual function. Hyperprolactemia can also be avoided by switching to "atypical" neuroleptics such as clozapine (Clozaril) or risperidone (Hisperdal), which are less dependent upon dopamine blockade for their efficacy.

The movement disorders (akathesia, akinesia, dystonia, tardive dyskinesia) caused by neuroleptics can also directly impede sexual function. Yassa and Lal (1985) reported a man frequently unable to have intercourse because he was unable either to penetrate or maintain penetration due to involuntary movement spasms. As with hyperprolactemia, movement/motor disorders may be avoided by treatment with these newer, atypical neuroleptics.

SEXUAL BENEFITS

Several small studies have shown that certain neuroleptics can be used to treat premature ejaculation, but this finding has never been replicated in an adequate, placebo-controlled study. Singh (1963) and Mellgren (1967) reported successful use of thioridazine to treat premature ejaculation, and three reports of using either thioridazine or mesoridazine to treat premature ejaculation appeared in European journals during the 1960s (Petrie, 1980). In the last decade, the possibility of irreversible tardive dyskinesia as a neuroleptic side effect has discouraged further investigation of this drug class as a treatment for premature ejaculation in the United States.

In Europe, the haloperidol-like neuroleptic benperidol has been used since the 1960s to treat deviant hypersexuality. Tennant, Bancroft, and Cass (1974) studied the effects of benperidol and chlorpromazine on imprisoned male pedophiles in a placebo-controlled trial. They found a small but significant reduction in sexual thoughts, which they judged insufficient to prevent deviant sexual behavior. Bartova, Hajnova, Nahunek, and Svestka (1981) reported successful treatment of deviant sexual behavior with fluphenazine injections or injections of oxoprothepin, another European neuroleptic.

PARADOXICAL EFFECTS

Paradoxical effects of neuroleptics have been reported only rarely. Spontaneous ejaculation on neuroleptics was reported in 1983 by Keitner and Selub (1983). A 46-year-old man hospitalized for treatment of psychotic depression experienced spontaneous orgasm and ejaculation on two consecutive days after eight days of treatment with 20 mg trifluoperazine. A week later, he was shifted to 20 mg thiothixene and again experienced spontaneous orgasm/ejaculation on two consecutive days. All events occurred with women present, but in non-sexual contexts and without any observable stimulation.

Two reports of hypersexuality due to neuroleptics were recorded in the 1960s and 1970s. Seeman, Denber, and Goldner (1968) described the case of a 44-year-old paranoid schizophrenic woman who was tormented by obsessive sexual thoughts when treated with 150 mg chlorpromazine or 300 mg thioridazine. Varga, Haher, and Simpson (1975) reported hypersexual behavior in two men, one treated with fluphenazine and the other treated with 600 mg chlorpromazine.

ALTERNATIVES

Among all of the neuroleptics, fluphenazine (Prolixin) and flupenthixol (Fluanxol) seem to cause the least sedation, fatigue, weight gain and dizziness. One study examined neuroleptic patients concurrently treated with antidepressants, benzodiazepines, or lithium (Lingjaerde et al., 1987). Patients on antidepressants and benzodiazepines showed about a 10% higher incidence of sexual effects than those on neuroleptics alone. Patients concurrently on lithium showed about 10% lower incidence of sexual effects. Orgasm problems were also lower in patients on concurrent benzodiazepines (16.7%), but ejaculatory complaints were greater (35.3%) (indicating that the sexual effects of benzodiazepine can be worse in men than in women). The relative lack of negative sexual effects with concurrent neuroleptic and lithium treatment, though noteworthy, occurred only when high-dose neuroleptics were used, which can cause additional, severe problems.

Antipsychotics cause a myriad of sexual problems that significantly complicate effective clinical treatment. As long as patients are institutionalized, their medications can be monitored and noncompliance kept to a minimum. As outpatients, many abandon their medications because of intolerable sexual dysfunction as well as other undesirable side effects. If/when psychotropic medications that have fewer sexual complications are discovered, the overall treatment of psychotic symptoms will be vastly improved due to the compliance issue alone.

ATYPICAL ANTIPSYCHOTIC DRUGS

A recently introduced class of antipsychotic drugs in the United States achieves its therapeutic effect more by blocking 5-HT_2 receptors than dopamine receptors. The ratio of 5-HT_2 receptor blockade to conventional dopamine DA_2 receptor blockade for currently marketed atypical antipsychotics is 1.30 for clozapine (Clozaril) and 1.15 for risperidone (Risperdal) versus a ratio of 0.89 for the conventional antipsychotic haloperidol (Haldol) (Richelson, 1994). The term *atypical* was given to the prototypical antipsychotic clozapine more than 20 years ago in 1971, after the conclusions of investigatory clinical trials that began in 1962 (Coward, 1992). Unfortunately, clozapine use in the United States was delayed for many years after the discovery of an occasional but potentially lethal side effect of agranulocytosis (lowered white blood-cell count) (Krupp & Barnes, 1992). Due to the need for careful monitoring to avoid infrequent but severe toxicity, use of clozapine is somewhat complicated and very costly.

Atypical antipsychotics are generally characterized by minimal or no movement/motor/posture abnormalities (extrapyramidal symptoms or EPS; tardive dyskinesia or TD) and no increase in prolactin levels (Herrling, 1991). They may improve "negative" aspects of schizophrenia in addition to the conventional antipsychotic reduction of positive aspects. Positive and negative aspects of schizophrenia are shown in Table 22.3. Indeed, conventional antipsychotics may themselves induce secondary symptoms (side effects) similar to (and often confused with) as-

Table 22.3 *Positive and Negative Aspects of Schizophrenia*

Positive Aspects
- Delusions
- Conceptual disorganization
- Bizarre thought content
- Hallucinations
- Excitement, agitation
- Hostility, suspiciousness, aggression
- Grandiosity
- Poor impulse control
- Tension, fear

Negative Aspects
- Blunted affect
- Emotional and social withdrawal
- Passive, apathetic attitude
- Lack of spontaneity and flow of conversation
- Rigidity
- Stereotyped thinking
- Depressive mood
- Motor retardation, catatonic posturing
- Poor attention
- Guilt feelings
- Somatic preoccupations
- Negative (failure to do what is situationally suggested; characterized by stupor or stereotyped repetitive movement

Data from Lindenmayer, 1994, and clinical experience.

pects of schizophrenia (Gerlach & Peacock, 1994). Mental and motor side effects of conventional antipsychotics are listed in Table 22.4. Gerlach and Peacock (1994) note that patients complain more of the mental side effects, while physicians focus mainly on objective movement/motor side effects. Unfortunately, there is no pharmacologic cure for schizophrenia, only control of its symptoms, which is usually lost when antipsychotics are discontinued (Kane & Freeman, 1994). Given the predominant need for continued treatment, relative reduction of side effects and normalization of thought and mood through use of atypical antipsychotics are important advances in psychotherapy.

Table 22.4 *Side Effects of Conventional Antipsychotic Drugs*

Mental Side Effects

- Emotional indifference
- Blunted affect
- Anhedonia, lack of pleasure
- Reduced initiative, apathy
- Reduced energy, weakness, asthenia
- Depression
- Slow or retarded thinking
- Lack of social drive or interest
- Anxiety
- Subjective restlessness

Movement/Motor Side Effects

Extrapyramidal Symptoms (EPS)

1. **Dystonia**: Exaggerated, stretched posturing of head, neck, jaw, trunk, back, arms, legs, and other movable body parts; fixed aberrant gaze; hyperextension; distorted, twisted, repetitive postures with prolonged muscle contractions; sustained spasms.
2. **Akathisia**: Inability to sit still; intolerance of inactivity; pacing, restless movement, rocking, tapping, and shifting of weight while standing or sitting.
3. **Akinesia**: Rigidity, stiffness, and slowness of voluntary movements; mask-like facial immobility; stooped posture, shuffling gait; slow, monotonous, hesitant speech.
4. **Tremor**: Regular rhythmic oscillations of hands and fingers.
5. **Tardive Dyskinesia**: Orofacial protruding and idling of tongue; lip-sucking, rabbit syndrome (repetitive mouth movement resembling a rabbit's munching); twitching of orofacial, masticatory, and tongue muscles, sometimes spreading to limbs. Typically develops after prolonged treatment, but may also appear at start or even at withdrawal of antipsychotic. Responds poorly to treatment and sometimes becomes permanent in older patients.

Data from Gerlach and Peacock, 1994; Rupniak, Jenner, and Marsden, 1986; and clinical experience.

Clozapine (Clozaril) was first synthesized in 1958 as one of over 1,900 tricyclic drugs modeled after the recently introduced antidepressant imipramine (McKenna & Bailey, 1993). Similar to chlorpromazine, it was anticholinergic and anti-adrenergic. Tested from 1961 to 1971 as an antipsychotic, it was approved for clinical use in 1971 and removed from general use in 1975 due to agranulocytosis (McKenna & Bailey, 1993). Restricted use continued in some European countries, and even in the United States on a humanitarian named-patient basis, due to the fact that it sometimes was quite efficacious for otherwise treatment-refractory patients and even improved neurocognitive function in some patients (Meltzer, Lee, & Ranjan, 1994). Indeed, clozapine has been shown in six of 13 research studies to be more effective than chlorpromazine, in contrast to the failure to find even a single study showing increased efficacy to chlorpromazine in 58 comparative research trials of other recognized conventional antipsychotics (McKenna & Bailey, 1993).

Prominent side effects of clozapine are weight gain, sedation, fatigue, hypertension, dizziness, tachycardia, constipation, sialorrhea (drooling, excess saliva), hyperthermia, seizures, and agranulocytosis (Meltzer, Alphs, Bastani, Ramirez, & Kwon, 1991). Evidently, despite its advantages in comparison to conventional antipsychotic drugs, it is far from a safe and tolerable pharmacological treatment for schizophrenia. Sedation and weight gain due to blockade of histamine H_2 receptors and weight gain due to serotonin blockade are particular problems with both currently available atypical antipsychotics, clozapine and risperidone (both have a far stronger antihistamine action than the conventional over-the-counter antihistamine diphenhydramine; Richelson, 1994). Seizure rate has been reported as 0.6–2% for doses below 300 mg, 1.8–4% for doses of 300–599 mg, and 5–14% for doses of 600–900 mg (Garcia, Crismon, & Dorson, 1994; Toth & Frankenburg, 1994). The typical clinical dose for clozapine is 200–700 mg/day (Fleischhacker et al., 1994).

Clinically significant weight gain occurs during the first six to 12 months of clozapine treatment and continues yearly at a lower rate, so that the cumulative incidence of patients reaching 20% or more overweight (a definite health risk) may be over 50%, and 75% of treated patients may gain at least 10 to 20 pounds (Lamberti, Bellnier, & Schwarzkopf, 1992; Umbricht, Pollack, & Kane, 1994). This degree of weight gain is considerably more than occurs with most conventional neuroleptics (weight gain is also a particularly severe problem with thioridazine, which can be considered a somewhat atypical antipsychotic). It is startling to note that prior extensive reviews (generally from limited inpatient studies) of clozapine clinical experience and "guidelines for clinical management" have reported weight gain in less than 1% of treated patients (Lamberti et al., 1992).

The degree of sexual dysfunction in patients treated with clozapine has not yet been studied. However, given its side-effect profile, clozapine can hardly be considered a useful enhancer of sexual well-being, despite its frequent success in reducing negative aspects of schizophrenia. Given the efficacy of serotonin potentiators (SSRIs) for treating obsessive-compulsive disorder, it is interesting to note that clozapine has a peculiar effect of inducing or exacerbating obsessive-compulsive symptoms, possibly as a result of its strong antiserotonergic (anti 5-HT_2 action) (Baker et al., 1992).

Risperidone (Risperdal) is a potent antagonist of both 5-HT_2 and DA_2 receptors (Cohen, 1994). Given its strong antidopaminergic action, risperidone can have notable motor extrapyramidal side effects at doses over 10 mg/day, but it is typically efficacious at doses of 4–10 mg/day, at which levels these motor symptoms are only minimally greater than on placebo (Cohen, 1994). Other prominent side effects at therapeutic doses at or below 10 mg/day are insomnia, headaches, anxiety, tension, dizziness, constipation, weight gain, nausea, gastric upset, rhinitis, coughing, hyperthermia, tachycardia, and significant sexual dysfunction (Cohen, 1994; Marder & Meibach, 1994). Side effects more frequent on risperidone 6 mg/day (the optimum dose) compared to haloperidol 20 mg/day are anxiety, nervousness, headaches, dizziness, nausea, gastric upset, weight gain, rhinitis, sinusitis, coughing, fever, and tachycardia (Marder & Meibach, 1994). Strongly dose-dependent side effects include diminished sexual desire and erectile deficiency, fatigue, sedation, weight gain, and tachycardia (Lindenmayer, 1994; Marder & Meibach, 1994). Distinct advantages of risperidone over other antipsychotics are decreased negative symptoms of schizophrenia such as emotional withdrawal, depression, blunted affect, thought and speech, as well as improvement of attention, cognition, and brain information processing toward normal (Wagner & Clayton, 1995). Given risperidone's relatively strong antagonism of DA_2 receptors compared to clozapine, occasional elevation of prolactin and development of tardive dyskinesia is more likely with prolonged use than on clozapine.

Risperidone's sexual side effects are significantly greater than on placebo and include decreased desire and erectile dysfunction, orgasm/ejaculation problems, menstrual disturbance, and menorrhagia (Lindenmayer, 1994; Marder & Meibach, 1994; Meltzer et al., 1994). Long-term complaints directly affecting compliance are weight gain and the above sexual problems (Lindenmayer, 1994). Some instances of priapism have already been noted during risperidone treatment (Lindenmayer, 1994). It is interesting that weight gain and sexual dysfunction are also prominent on thioridazine, which may be considered an atypical antipsychotic due to its relatively low level of movement/motor side effects. The weight gain that occurs on risperidone is not as great as on clozapine, and there is no special danger of agranulocytosis, less risk of seizure, and greater cognitive improvement on risperidone compared to clozapine.

23

Stimulants/Anorectics: Mazindol, Fenfluramine, Diethylpropion, Methylphenidate, Phenylpropanolamine

OBJECTIVES

- To compare and evaluate the sexual side effects of commonly prescribed and over-the-counter anorectic stimulants
- To examine the sexual side effects of the non-anorectic stimulant methylphenidate (Ritalin)

Stimulants are predominantly used (and often abused) by women for appetite control. The number of women using stimulants nonmedically to control weight rose during the 1980s (Clayton, Voss, Robbins, & Skinner, 1986). Use and overuse of diet pills have reached epidemic levels. Nonprescription stimulants for weight loss are used largely outside the context of medical supervision, making it impossible to assess the scope of abuse. Phenylpropanolamine (PPA) and caffeine pills are available over the counter and are only loosely regulated by health authorities or the Federal Drug Administration. Furthermore, phenylpropanolamine is in a remarkable number of other drugs such as decongestant "cold" remedies.

The diet stimulants currently available are the same ones that were available 20 to 30 years ago. Because research on the side effects of these stimulants has been largely limited to their abuse, surprisingly little is known about the general or sexual side effects of anorectics at "therapeutic" non-abuse dosages. Partly in response to pressure groups, the Federal Drug Administration tightly controls all prescription stimulants and has discouraged the development of new drugs. Ironically, while pressure groups appropriately point out the dangers of abuse, there are few unbiased replicated studies showing serious dangers associated with these diet pills for women or men at "therapeutic" doses. This chapter reviews prescription stimulant anorectics and phenylpropanolamine, which is the main ingredient in most nonprescription stimulants. (Caffeine, a common nonprescription xanthene stimulant, was covered in Chapter 11.) Methylphenidate (Ritalin), which is not used as an anorectic, is also discussed.

OVERVIEW OF STIMULANTS/ ANORECTICS

Amphetamine/PEA derivative anorectics:

- *amphetamine* (Dexedrine, etc.) schedule II control
- *diethylpropion* (Tenuate) schedule IV control

- *fenfluramine* (Pondimin, etc.) schedule IV control
- *mazindol* (Sanorex, Mazanor) schedule IV control
- *phentermine* (Fastin, etc.) schedule IV control
- *phenylpropanolamine* (generic nonprescription)
- *methylphenidate* (Ritalin) (not an anorectic) schedule IV control

Amphetamine anorectics work chiefly through adrenergic stimulation and, to a lesser extent, through dopaminergic stimulation. An exception is fenfluramine (Pondimin), which stimulates serotonin and has more specific anorectic properties rather than stimulant properties (it can even cause sedation). Stimulants generally activate catecholamines – dopamine and norepinephrine – as well as other excitatory chemicals in the brain. Their actions on serotonin are somewhat mysterious and the mix of excitatory and inhibitory serotonergic actions has not been explored. All of the stimulant anorectics except for mazindol (Sanorex, Mazanor) are phenylethylamine (PEA) derivatives. Due to their amphetamine nature, they are controlled, scheduled drugs. However, they vary widely in abuse and dependence potential. Diethylpropion (Tenuate) and mazindol have low abuse potential. Although fenfluramine (Pondimin) also has low abuse potential and a particularly effective weight-reducing effect, it has the potential for brain damage exceeding even that of amphetamine. Apparently, brain damage occurs through excess serotonin release, which occurs with both fenfluramine and amphetamine. Mazindol inhibits serotonin 5-HT-uptake, but does not cause excess serotonin release; it also inhibits dopamine uptake, which may prevent the excess chemical release and synaptic activity that leads to toxic neuronal exhaustion.

The stimulant action of diethylpropion is far less than that of amphetamine. It has a stronger effect when taken orally than when injected, suggesting that it works through an unidentified hepatic-derived metabolite. Hepatic metabolism of diethylpropion may change as the dosage is raised, limiting incremental stimulant response when dose is increased in an abusive fashion. There is very little abuse reported for diethylpropion and practically none for mazindol.

Sexual Dysfunction

Researchers and physicians are commonly unaware of the direct sexual manifestations of stimulant drugs. The adrenergic activation of stimulants can affect sexual function in both directions. It can either heighten or interfere with sexual desire and/or response, depending upon the situation, the emotional state of the individual, and the dose of the stimulant.

While the adrenergic arousal level necessary for appetite control may not excessively affect overall behavior, it may impact more subtle levels of sexual responsibility and "genital tone" (i.e., erection turgidity, rigidity, flaccidity). The vascular responses of the male genitals are under tonic adrenergic inhibitory control.* Adrenergic activation by anorectic/amphetamine-like medications may increase the inhibitory action on vascular sensitivity. As a result, the penis may be abnormally limp and an increased amount of sexual stimulation may be necessary for erection to occur. It is unknown if there is an analogous effect within female genitals.

Stimulants may also restrict the "dynamic range" of sexual response. Excitatory orgasmic response is normally preceded by decreased local genital adrenergic arousal, which occurs during the vasodilation stage of the sexual response (lubrication or erection). Orgasm is then experienced as a rebound reaction (release from local inhibition of adrenergic tone). There is evidence that orgasm is triggered when heat increases to a certain "flashpoint"; orgasmic release then may function as a cooling mechanism (Blumberg & Moltz, 1988). With the use of stimulants, orgasm can be reached more readily, but it may not have the explosive, satisfying quality generated by the buildup of sexual tension.

Speculation on stimulant restriction of the

*Tonicity is defined as the normal state of slight contraction or readiness to contract of healthy muscle fibers.

sexual response cannot be furthered by any evidence presently available in the literature. In our clinical experience, we have found that even the mild effects of legal, non-abused stimulants can and do restrict the range of sexual response and reduce the resting "tone" of the penis (the penis is more contracted than in its usual resting state). We have also observed this resting "limpness" and "shrunkenness" in the penis with the use of stimulating antidepressants such as amineptine (Survector, available in Europe) and nomifensine (Merital, now withdrawn from the market).

A reverse of the contracted resting tone seems to be the case with bupropion (Wellbutrin), a stimulant antidepressant that does not have the potent adrenergic action common to most amphetamines. However, even with bupropion there may be an adrenergic facilitation in occasional patients that leaves the penis unusually limp in the resting state. This "limp penis," suggesting a tonic "epinephrine response," occurred for a few weeks in two of our male research patients on bupropion, but resolved with a lowering of the drug dose. The drug affected only the size of the nonerect penis. Erections were not noticeably affected.

Excess weight often decreases sexual attractiveness and undermines a positive body-image. As weight is lost, sexuality may improve in response to a better body image and increased self-esteem. However, obesity may be a protective camouflage for an aversion to sex. A man or woman who does not want to be touched may consciously or unconsciously resort to making themselves sexually unappealing. When the weight is lost, the previously masked sexual aversion becomes evident, causing problems in the relationship.

Male/Female Differences

In a 1986 National Institute of Drug Abuse (NIDA) publication, it was stated that "the clearest gender difference in medical use of psychotherapeutics is for stimulants. . . . The Federal research agenda . . . require(s) attention [to] the use of stimulants by women, particularly younger women, to lose weight, and the relationship of such use to anorexia and bulimia" (Clayton et al., 1986). The potency of catecholaminergic anorectic stimulants in women is increased by a decrease in serotonin that occurs naturally with dieting. Cowen and his colleagues (Anderson, Parry-Billings, Newsholme, Fairburn, & Cowen, 1990; Goodwin, Fairburn, & Cowen, 1987) have found serotonergic deficits due to dieting only in women and have suggested that this reduction of serotonin makes women especially susceptible to eating disorders. Dieting reduces the serotonin precursor tryptophan in both women and men, but the reduction is greater in women and produces exaggerated prolactin responses to intravenous-injected tryptophan only in women. Anderson et al. (1990) hypothesized that, due to reduced serotonin function associated with reduced tryptophan in dieting women, there is impaired satiety, a tendency to binge-eat, poor impulse control, and depressive symptoms, all of which can generate eating disorders. Given the greater levels of brain serotonin (McBride, Tierney, DeMeo, Chen, & Mann, 1990) and greater rate of serotonin turnover (Young, Gauthier, Anderson, & Purdy, 1980) in women than men, women are particularly sensitive to changes in tryptophan availability. Estrogen and progesterone appear to work synergistically with serotonin, partially explaining why sensitivity to serotonergic changes is greater in women (DiPaolo, Masson, Daigle, & Belanger, 1987).

Reduced levels of serotonin in mildly overweight, dieting women could result in increased susceptibility to sexual stimulation. Hypothetically, decreased serotonin generated by weight loss and increased dopamine generated by anorectic stimulants, together with preexisting female sensitivity to the stimulant effects of dopamine, would lead not only to increased sexual desire and sensation, but also to a shift toward more active, masculine sexual behavior. As part of this shift, however, the perverse aspects of male sexual desire may be experienced by women, leading to sexual perversion dysfunctions usually found chiefly in men. Ellinwood (Ellinwood & Rockwell, 1975) has noted that "female chronic amphetamine abusers reported increased pleasure and sexual behavior, as well as increased promiscuity, compulsive masturbation, prostitution, and intensification of sadomasochistic fantasies." Milder forms of this type of sexual behavior may occur due to chronic use of anorectic stimulants. In light of the possibility of serotonin depletion with dieting in mildly overweight women, use of anorectic drugs with distinct serotonergic actions (e.g., mazindol, fenfluramine) may be advisable for those already susceptible to alcohol and drug abuse or those who have sexual obsessive-compulsive disorders. When eating is reduced and sexual activity unavailable, other strong positive environmental or relationship reinforcers are often necessary to avoid attraction to drug abuse.

In animal research, response to amphetamines has been found to be greater in female rats than in male rats (Robinson & Becker, 1986). There is also greater sensitization with continued use. Apparently, sensitization is decreased by testosterone in males, since castrated male rats also show increased sensitization to the level found in females. The greater sensitivity to amphetamines in female rats is paralleled by a greater sensitivity to a variety of stressors (e.g., immobilization, forced running). Whereas the male response to stressors is more phasic, as shown by acute secretion of epinephrine (adrenaline), the female response is more tonic, as shown by extended cortisol elevation.

Sexual Benefits

In *Chemistry of Love* (1983) Liebowitz suggested that phenylethylamines (PEA) were endogenous amphetamines that generated high levels of sexual desire and activity. He proposed that the chemistry of romantic love involves endogenous chemicals that are both sexually stimulating and appetite suppressing. Phenylethylamines are stimulants with both adrenergic and dopaminergic activation.

While stimulants may relieve sexual sluggishness, it should also be noted that the hyperarousal generated by amphetamine-like substances has rarely been shown to facilitate sexual behavior in normal, sexually active animals. In humans, the agitation of hyperarousal (the "speed" effect) induced by stimulants often isolates the individual, preventing the relaxation necessary for intimacy and sexual comfort.

Alternatives

The stimulant antidepressant bupropion, which has been shown to treat both bulimia (Horne et al., 1988) and inhibited sex drive (Crenshaw, Goldberg, & Stern, 1987), is contraindicated for use in bulimic women due to a possible increased risk of seizure. The alternative antidepressant treatment of bulimia is fluoxetine (Prozac), which itself reduces sexual desire and response. Fluoxetine is currently under FDA review for treatment of obesity (it was approved for the treatment of bulimia in 1994). If fluoxetine is shown to cause weight loss equivalent to amphetamine-like stimulants, the Federal Drug Administration would be faced with sanctioning the widespread use of a psychologically powerful prescription drug. Consequently, FDA approval of fluoxetine for treatment of obesity is unlikely, even if it proves to be relatively effective. Even for bulimia, higher fluoxetine doses than those used for depression are usually required (40–80 mg/day), which increase the risk of sexual side effects. The present anorectic stimulants are like to remain the chief alternatives for weight control for some time to come.

MAZINDOL (SANOREX, TERONAC, MAZANOR)

On the basis of its sexual side effects, mazindol (Sanorex, Teronac, Mazanor) use is more appropriate for women than men. Though recognized as a stimulant on the basis of its dopaminergic and noradrenergic uptake inhibiting properties (Hauger et al., 1986), it also has serotonergic action involving 5-HT uptake inhibition (Carruba, Zambotti, Vicentini, Picotti, & Mantegazza, 1978). Furthermore, mazindol has an indole structure characteristic of serotonin. Men may be bothered by this as yet undefined serotonergic effect. Exogenous serotonergic activity may be more comfortable for women than men because higher levels of such activity are present at birth in females and are potentiated by estrogen. For weight reduction, this serotonergic action can supplement the catecholamine stimulant anorectic property of mazindol. Mazindol apparently has no effect on pituitary hormones or testosterone (Dolecek, 1980).

Mazindol is perhaps the safest anorectic stimulant in terms of abuse potential. When given to drug abusers (six male, six female) in normal clinical doses (.5–2 mg), it had only dysphoric subjective effects and was given a negative rating on a drug-liking scale (Chait, Uhlenhuth, & Johanson, 1987). Compared to placebo in this study, mazindol was actually considered to be aversive. Side-effect profiles of mazindol are generally similar to those of other anorectic stimulants. Mazindol has been in use with little evidence of toxicity since 1974. However, some discomfort has been reported. In an incontinence study, Woodhouse and Tiptaft (1983) noted unpleasant feelings of dizziness, light-headedness, insomnia, and dry mouth at high doses (3–4 mg/day) and cautioned that treatment should be initiated at low doses. Table 23.1 summarizes the properties and side effects of mazindol.

Sexual Dysfunction

Australian surveillance monitoring has reported that 19% of the adverse drug reaction reports for mazindol up to 1985 were for sexual dysfunction, including decreased sex drive, impotence, and testicular pain (Mashford, 1985). This relatively high figure was not paralleled in the United States labeling, however, in which impotence and changes in sex drive are indicated to occur only rarely. Apparently, most or all of these sexual side effects occurred in men.

Symptoms of genital pain have been reported by male patients treated with mazindol in our clinical practice, but no similar discomfort seems to occur in women on mazindol. The chief reference for testicular pain due to mazindol was a report of eight spontaneous adverse drug reactions to the Australian and Netherlands Adverse Drug Reaction monitors (McEwen & Meyboom, 1983). In many of these cases, the testicular effect quickly disappeared after mazindol was discontinued and reappeared upon successive rechallenge. The symptom initially was diagnosed as prostatitis, but was later differentiated due to its contiguous relation to mazindol use. Symptoms manifested within hours of the first dose in some cases and in others took up to two months to develop. (Dosage was either 0.5 mg or 1 mg daily; therapeutic dose is 1–2 mg.)

The range of symptoms reported to monitors was fascinating and, in a few cases, reminiscent of spontaneous emission/ejaculation, which has occasionally been found with serotonergic antidepressants (clomipramine, imipramine, fluoxetine). A summary of the cases reported by McEwen and Meyboom (1983) follows.

Case 1: Within 48 hours, testes became painful, retracted, and hard. Dysuria with interrupted erratic urination also occurred. Symptoms recurred on four subsequent occasions within 24 hours of ingesting the drug.

Case 2: Within one month, painful testes became sore to touch and dysuria developed. Symptoms resolved within 24 hours of discontinuing the drug and reappeared three times within 12 hours upon rechallenge.

Case 3: For about one month, testicular pain, swelling during urination, and seminal discharge with each bowel movement were noted. These symptoms were treated unsuccessfully as prostatitis, but resolved when mazindol was discontinued. Symptoms began four hours after first dose.

Case 4: Within two hours of first dose, severe pain in testes and groin appeared, recurring three more times when rechallenged. The patient complained of "penile shrinkage" and transient impotence.

Case 5: After eight weeks of treatment, the patient developed impotence, sore testes, and non-orgasmic spontaneous ejaculation. Withdrawal of mazindol resolved these symptoms.

Case 6: On three separate occasions of mazindol treatment, prostatitis-like reaction occurred with painful urination, painful testes, and lower abdominal pain.

Case 7: "Tender" testes developed within an hour and lasted two hours after taking each dose.

Table 23.1 *Profile of Mazindol*

	Daily Dose
Sanorex	1 mg TID
Teronac	or
Mazanor	2 mg QD

COMMON INDICATIONS
Obesity

MECHANISMS OF ACTION (GENERAL)
Increases catecholamine activity
Inhibits dopamine and norepinephrine uptake
Inhibits 5-HT uptake

MECHANISMS OF ACTION (SEXUAL)

Positive	*Negative*
Increased adrenergic ($alpha_1$) activity	Increased adrenergic ($alpha_2$) activity
Increased adrenergic ($beta_2$) activity	Increased cortisol
Increased dopamine	Increased serotonin (5-HT)

DIRECT SEXUAL SIDE EFFECTS

Desire disorders	Erection difficulties	Orgasm/ejaculation irregularities
• Inhibited sexual desire (male) • Hypersexuality (female)	• Inability/difficulty obtaining/maintaining erection • Decreased quality of erection • Ejaculation through flaccid or semi-erect penis	• Difficulty or inability to be orgasmic • Ejaculatory inhibition • Ejaculation without orgasm • Dyspareunia

INDIRECT SEXUAL SIDE EFFECTS
Discomfort caused by dryness of skin, mouth, mucous membranes, weight loss, nausea, rash/itching, urinary problems (retention)
Mood disorders resulting in anhedonia, nervousness, anxiety, detachment
Neurological disturbances resulting in dizziness, headache, pain, sedation, sleep disturbances

SEXUAL CONTRAINDICATIONS/BENEFITS

Avoid with prior condition of	*May be useful for*
Desire disorders	Sex drive disorders
Genital pain	Hypersexuality
Pain with ejaculation	Desire disorders
Urinary tract symptoms	Urinary incontinence
Prostatitis	
Erectile dysfunction	
Orgasmic dysfunction	

ALTERNATIVES
Fenfluramine (Pondimin)
Fluoxetine (Prozac)
Bupropion (Wellbutrin)

Case 8: Prostatitis-like pain in perineal region and urge to urinate within one hour of each dose were reported. These symptoms occurred again upon rechallenge.

Male/Female Differences

Since there are many isolated reports of sexual stimulation of women treated with serotonergic agents (e.g., fenfluramine, fluoxetine, clomipramine, trazodone, tryptophan), sexual stimulation can be expected to occur occasionally in women on mazindol. This same serotonergic action can be expected to interfere with male orgasm/ejaculation and sex drive. While instances of spontaneous genital pain with mazindol have not as yet been noted in women, Zahorska-Markiewicz and Kucio (1984) have shown that pain sensitivity is increased by mazindol in both obese and lean women given electrical shocks to their hands.

Sexual Benefits

Since obesity and urinary incontinence are major causes of sexual dysfunction in women (Vereecken, 1989), mazindol use could be helpful in restoring sexual function by treating these problems. In a placebo-controlled study, Woodhouse and Tiptaft (1983) found a 68% positive response in both women and men on mazindol (2–3 mg/day for three weeks) for the treatment of incontinence. The authors also noted "startlingly good control of voiding" in patients with incontinence due to sphincter and detrusor causes. Other sympathomimetic anorectic stimulants such as ephedrine and norephedrine have been used to treat incontinence by raising urethral pressure, thereby increasing outlet resistance (Wein, 1991). Mazindol is not as commonly recognized as these drugs in the treatment of incontinence.

A case report by Friesen (1976) suggested aphrodisiacal properties of mazindol in some women. A 40-year-old patient treated with mazindol developed such a sexual "hunger" that she coerced her husband into changing jobs so that he would be more available for sex. Friesen reported more moderate increases in sexual desire in 5% of his women patients. His finding has not been supported by other reports in the literature. Positive sexual effects in women may occur as a result of the drug's combination of dopaminergic and serotonergic actions, which facilitates weight-reduction action. However, this same combination of serotonin with dopamine can also induce mania with hypersexuality as a symptom.

FENFLURAMINE

Fenfluramine (Pondimin, Ponderal, Ponderox) is an anorectic amphetamine derivative. Due to modification of the amphetamine structure, it primarily releases serotonin rather than dopamine. Consequently, it has sedative effects characteristic of serotonin rather than the activation characteristic of dopamine. Fenfluramine's anorectic effect is supplemented by a thermogenic action that aids in weight loss. Fenfluramine is a mixture of d- and l-isomers. Subsequently, the d-isomer dexfenfluramine (Isomeride) has been shown to have a more potent anorectic effect than l-isomer, with fewer side effects due to its specificity for serotonin transmission. Due to its greater potency and specificity, dexfenfluramine at the suggested therapeutic dose of 30 mg/day has the same therapeutic effect as 60 mg/day of dl-fenfluramine. The l-isomer has been shown to block dopaminergic activity in the rat striatum and nucleus accumbens, causing a compensatory increase in dopaminergic activity and an increase in the HVA dopamine metabolite (Invernizzi, Bertorelli, Consolo, Garattini, & Samanin, 1989). Dexfenfluramine is now available in Europe and should be marketed in the United States late in 1995.

The inhibitory effect of fenfluramine on dopamine is characteristic of neuroleptics. Dopamine inhibition by l-fenfluramine has also been shown to make male rats less competitive, less assertive, more submissive, and less active (File & Guardiola-Lemaitre, 1988). This altered dopamine activity may have a toxic effect on brain dopamine receptors similar to that of amphetamine. With d-fenfluramine, toxicity should occur only at brain serotonin receptors and should be less than with dl-fenfluramine because of the lower dose used. However, a neurotoxicity study by Kleven and Seiden (1989) showed equal or greater neurotoxicity with d-fenfluramine than with l-fenfluramine or dl-fenfluramine.

Metabolic effects of fenfluramine can be positive for antihypertensive and diabetic patients whose health is further compromised by excess weight. Brun et al. (1988) found decreased LDL cholesterol and triglycerides and increased HDL cholesterol. Fenfluramine and dexfenfluramine have both been shown to reduce blood pressure and plasma norepinephrine levels, and to reduce blood glucose while increasing glucose tolerance (Andersson et al., 1991). These actions appear to occur independent of weight loss in some cases.

Stunkard (1984) has suggested that fenfluramine lowers the set-point for weight, but does not achieve the lasting results of behavior therapy. He found that an average of 15 kg was lost during six months of fenfluramine alone or fenfluramine combined with behavior therapy; 11 kg was lost on behavior therapy alone. However, at one-year follow-up, behavior-therapy patients had regained only 1.9 kg, whereas the fenfluramine and fenfluramine/behavior therapy groups had regained 8.2 kg and 10.7 kg, respectively. Behavior therapy alone was effective, but the behavior therapy given with fenfluramine was not sufficient to prevent rebound weight gain that presumedly occurred due to an upward adjustment of the weight set-point when the drug was discontinued. Since weight set-point is modulated in the same hypothalamic area of the brain that governs sexual activity, regulation of sexual desire in the brain may be disturbed either during or after fenfluramine treatment.

In common with other serotonergic drugs, including fluoxetine (Prozac) and buspirone (BuSpar), fenfluramine increases cortisol levels in animals and humans (Lewis & Sherman, 1984; McElroy, Miller, & Meyer, 1984). The serotonin-induced release of corticotrophin-releasing factor (CRF) may be partly responsible for fenfluramine's anorectic action, because CRF is a potent anorectic (Le Feuvre, Aisenthal, & Rothwell, 1991). A decrease in this CRF response with daily fenfluramine (Serri & Rasio, 1989) may be partly responsible for the tolerance that develops to the anorectic action of fenfluramine. It is also possible that, with long-term use of fenfluramine, serotonin levels are decreased, resulting in lowered levels of CRF and cortisol (Serri & Rasio, 1989).

Raleigh et al. (1986) found that 70 days of chronic fenfluramine treatment of male vervet monkeys produced decreased levels and metabolism of serotonin, which was reversed when fenfluramine was discontinued. Parallel to this decrease in serotonin, there was an increase in active, antagonistic, aggressive behavior. When injected into the brain of female rats, CRF potently inhibited receptive lordosis sexual behavior and generated aggressive rejection of males' attempts to mount (Sirinathsinghji, Rees, Rivier, & Vale, 1983). CRF was also shown to inhibit LHRH secretion and decreased testosterone (Miskowiak, Janecki, Jakubowiak, & Limanowski, 1986; Reichlin, 1987), which are needed to activate and sustain sexual stimulation. However, fenfluramine has not been shown to decrease these sexual hormones in normal clinical use. CRF activity induced by fenfluramine also increased hypothalamic beta-endorphin (Sirinathsinghji et al., 1983) and met-enkephalin (Harsing & Yang, 1984), endogenous opiates that reduce sexual behavior (Almeida, Nikolarakis, Sirinathsinghji, & Herz, 1989). Serotonin, CRF, and opiates/endorphins all have powerful inhibiting actions on sexual behavior. However, other cortical factors such as ACTH (adrenocorticotrophic hormone) can stimulate sexual behavior (Bertolini, Vergoni, Gessa, & Ferrari, 1969), and it is unclear how ACTH interacts with CRF, opiates, and serotonin.

Both fenfluramine and CRF acutely increase the release of epinephrine and norepinephrine, thereby stimulating the sympathetic nervous system. Even low doses of CRF can induce neural excitation in the amygdala, which can increase fear and aversive reactions (Valentino & Foote, 1986). Inability to start and stop epinephrine activity efficiently and purposefully characterizes states of fear, aversion, and free-floating anxiety. By stimulating epinephrine when it is not needed, fenfluramine may undermine appropriate triggering and cessation of the epinephrine pump; with chronic activation, the epinephrine pump may become exhausted and unreliable.

The serotonergic activation by fenfluramine causes a clear, dose-dependent increase of prolactin in animals and humans. For example, the prolactin responses of male and female volunteer subjects to 60 mg fenfluramine was blocked by the serotonin receptor antagonist metergoline (Quattrone et al., 1983). Furthermore the acute prolactin response to fenfluramine is often used as a test of serotonergic responsiveness in physical and mental disorders (Maes, Jacobs, Suy, Minner, & Raus, 1989). When given to rats, both fenfluramine and fluoxetine increased corticosteroids, but only fenfluramine increased prolactin (Fuller, Snoddy, & Robertson, 1988). Therefore, the increase in prolactin was probably due to the serotonin-releasing action of fenfluramine rather than to its serotonin uptake inhibiting action. This abrupt elevation of serotonin in the neural synapse due to fenfluramine-induced release appears to cause both prolactin secretion and receptor deterioration. In contrast, because serotonin uptake inhibitors do not release serotonin, excessive actions are less likely to occur and the serotonin receptors do not "burn out."

Rats given fenfluramine show increased levels of oxytocin (Saydoff, Rittenhouse, Van de Kar, & Brownfield, 1991). Oxytocin can generate migraine in humans, increase prolactin, decrease eating, stimulate erections, and increase female receptive lordosis (Elands, van Doremalen, Spruyt, & de Kloet, 1991). It increases rather than decreases male copulatory behavior (Arletti, Bazzani, Castelli, & Bertolini, 1985). Differences between the behavioral effects of oxytocin and fenfluramine are partly due to the fact that oxytocin works synergistically with dopamine, whereas fenfluramine works synergistically with serotonin and therefore antagonistically (at least in the case of l-fenfluramine) to dopamine.

Of all the anorectic/weight-loss drugs, fenfluramine appears to be the most effective. However, because of its amphetamine-like action of exhaustive serotonin release, it can be toxic to the brain. Although destruction of serotonin neurons has not been shown in humans, in animals fenfluramine's brain toxicity potential is greater than amphetamine, occurring at doses only two times the therapeutic dose for obesity. Comparable or greater neurotoxicity has been shown for fenfluramine than for the amphetamine psychedelic derivative MDMA (Grob, Bravo, & Walsh, 1990; Wagner & Peroutka, 1988). The fenfluramine doses shown to be toxic in animals are from 1.25 to 5 times greater than those used therapeutically (Schuster & Johanson, 1985; Schuster, Lewis, & Seiden, 1986). (Neurotoxic doses for fenfluramine are closer to the therapeutic dose than neurotoxic doses of d-amphetamine are to its therapeutic dose.) However, the risk of reaching these toxic levels with fenfluramine is unlikely. Due to its dysphoric effect (sedation, lethargy, and nausea), abuse is discouraged.

Serotonin cell degeneration (dark neurons) in fenfluramine-treated rats was found by investigators in 1975 and subsequently replicated (Harvey & McMaster, 1977). Reduced levels of serotonin were also shown. A Federal Drug Administration committee review of possible neurotoxicity in 1978 considered the toxicity evidence from animal studies, deciding that pathological changes due to fenfluramine were not significant. Further toxicity studies were not funded.

Subsequently, Schuster, Ricaurte, Seiden, and their colleagues at the University of Chicago conducted a series of studies investigating neural damage from a variety of amphetamine-related substances including fenfluramine (Kleven, Schuster, & Seiden, 1988; Seiden & Ricaurte, 1987). The neural damage shown in dopamine and serotonin neurons was widely publicized as evidence of brain damage caused by abusing stimulants. The equal or greater damage caused by fenfluramine was clearly stated by Schuster (Schuster et al., 1986) but was disregarded by the Federal Drug Administration, due to lack of evidence of toxic brain damage in humans over many years of use. (However, such damage in humans due to amphetamine or MDMA (Ecstasy) use was also not verified for many years.) The position of Charles Schuster, who subsequently became head of the National Institute of Drug Abuse, was stated in 1986 and still seems relevant today (Schuster, Lewis, & Seiden, 1986):

> What are the implications of the pre-clinical laboratory evidence regarding long-term changes in 5-HT neurons for clinicians? When fenfluramine is used in the treatment of obesity, one must ask whether the therapeutic benefits gained warrant even the slightest risk that long-term changes in 5-HT neurons are being produced. At the very least, clinicians should be aware of this possibility in order to make a decision as to whether the drug should be prescribed. . . . At the present time, however, the findings from animal studies strongly suggest that the therapeutic benefits produced by fenfluramine must be sizable and durable in order to outweigh the potential risk of long-term irreversible changes in 5-HT neurons in the brain.

Few studies of amphetamines taken orally at therapeutic doses have been conducted. In a review of therapeutic use of fenfluramine in autistic and other mentally retarded children, Aman and Kern (1989) provided a well-balanced history of the debate regarding fenfluramine toxicity. Since autism and other emotional disorders in children may be related in part to excess serotonin activity, destruction of some serotonin neurons may even be useful (Schuster et al., 1986).

In spite of contradictory animal studies, the pharmacological differences between d- and l-fenfluramine strongly suggest greater safety with d-fenfluramine. Continued use of dl-fenfluramine in the United States is unfortunate, particularly since this drug is used predominantly by women, who are especially sensitive to stimulant brain neurotoxicity. Reduced neuronal serotonin due to fenfluramine appears to persist longest in the hippocampus and cortex (Contrera, Battaglia, Zaczek, & DeSouza, 1988), where such loss has been shown to cause subtle learning and performance deficits (Segal & Richter, 1988) in rhesus monkeys as well as in rats. Table 23.2 summarizes the properties and side effects of fenfluramine.

Sexual Dysfunction

The sexual side effects of fenfluramine are similar to other serotonergic potentiators, such as SSRIs, monoamine oxidase inhibitors, and tricyclic antidepressants. The powerful serotonergic action of fenfluramine stimulates cortisol and prolactin, which have adverse effects on sexual function (Altomonte et al., 1987; Lewis & Sherman, 1984; McElroy et al., 1984; Quattrone et al., 1983). Due to its serotonergic potency, fenfluramine can be expected to decrease sexual desire and genital sensitivity and possibly to inhibit orgasm. Animal studies have found that fenfluramine and similar anorectic drugs can elicit erection but inhibit copulation, indicating that erection alone does not eliminate the possible presence of sexual dysfunction.

Theoretically, stimulation of norepinephrine sympathetic activity during early fenfluramine treatment could cause vascular constriction in the penis, resulting in reduced erection. However, with continued use, fenfluramine appears to block norepinephrine. Since norepinephrine stimulates eating (especially "stress eating"), chronic adrenergic stimulation by amphetamines can backfire, activating rather than inhibiting appetite.

Fenfluramine may also have a specific stimulatory action on 5-HT_{1B} and 5-HT_{1C} receptors, which would significantly reduce both eating and sexuality. Such specific 5-HT_{1B} and 5-HT_{1C} receptor activity has been shown for d-fenfluramine but not for l-fenfluramine (Garattini, Borrini, Mennini, & Samanin, 1978). In rats, fenfluramine seems to have effects opposite to 5-HT_{1A} agonists (i.e., 8-OH-DPAT and buspirone). 5-HT_{1A} agonists increase male sexual activity and feeding in rats, while decreasing body temperature, aggressive behavior, and female receptive lordosis. In contrast, when fenfluramine is given to rats, male sexual activity and feeding are decreased and body temperature, aggressive behavior, and (possibly) female receptive lordosis behavior are increased.

Fenfluramine side effects have not been systematically evaluated. Inadequate monitoring of these side effects in published weight reduction and eating-disorder studies suggests an inattention to fenfluramine toxicity in general clinical practice, even though it is a scheduled drug. The purported absence of sexual side effects becomes meaningless when monitoring is superficial and unsystematic. Even fluoxetine (Pro-

Table 23.2 *Profile of Fenfluramine*

	Daily Dose
Pondimin	20–40 mg TID
Ponderal	
Ponderax	

COMMON INDICATIONS
obesity, autism

MECHANISMS OF ACTION (GENERAL)
Increases amphetamine-induced release and stimulation of serotonin reduces dopamine activity
Increases thermogenesis

MECHANISMS OF ACTION (SEXUAL)

Positive	*Negative*
Increased adrenergic ($alpha_1$) activity	Increased adrenergic ($alpha_2$) activity
Increased growth hormone	Increased cortisol
Increased oxytocin	Increased prolactin
	Increased serotonin

DIRECT SEXUAL SIDE EFFECTS

Desire disorders	Erection difficulties	Orgasm/ejaculation
• Hyposexuality (males)	• Inability/difficulty obtaining erection	• Anorgasmia
• Hypersexuality (females)		• Orgasmic inhibition
		• Retarded ejaculation

INDIRECT SEXUAL SIDE EFFECTS
Discomfort caused by diarrhea, urinary problems (nocturia, polyuria), weight loss
Mood disorders resulting in anxiety, nervousness, depression
Neurological disturbances resulting in dizziness, fatigue, headache, sedation, weakness
Vascular disturbances resulting in orthostatic hypotension

SEXUAL CONTRAINDICATIONS/BENEFITS

Avoid with prior condition of	*May be useful for*
Desire disorders	Premature ejaculation
Impotence	
Ejaculatory dysfunction	

ALTERNATIVES
Mazindol (Sanorex, Teronac, Mazanor)
Fluoxetine (Prozac)
Bupropion (Wellbutrin)

zac) has shown few or no sexual side effects in eating-disorder controlled clinical trials (Fluoxetine Bulimia Nervosa Collaborative Study Group, 1992; Marcus et al., 1990). Side effects that have been associated with fenfluramine treatment include drowsiness, tiredness, lethargy, sedation, dizziness, headache, loss of energy, and nervous disturbances which sometimes occur due to anorexia-generated weight loss. Transient but serious depression has also been noted upon withdrawal from fenfluramine (Oswald, 1974). All of these side effects may adversely affect sexual function.

Male/Female Differences

Fenfluramine is the only amphetamine available that decreases eating through activation of serotonin rather than dopamine. Women usually react better to serotonergic agents than to dopaminergic agents, possibly because the serotonin system is especially well-developed in women. Also, serotonin works synergistically with estrogen and antagonistically to testosterone, suggesting more compatibility with female patterns. Carlsson, Svensson, Eriksson, and Carlsson (1985) have shown that the early development of the serotonin nervous system in female rats is distinctly more complete than in males.

Fenfluramine was previously reported to reduce both lordosis and male copulation (Everitt, Fuxe, & Hokfelt, 1974; Meyerson & Malmnas, 1978), but more recent studies have shown facilitation of lordosis. In addition, even though it decreased male copulatory behavior, fenfluramine (dose-dependent) increased spontaneous erection in rats (Berendsen & Broekkamp, 1987; Szele, Murphy, & Garrick, 1988). Anorectic serotonin agonists active at 5-HT_{1B} and 5-HT_{1C} receptors also stimulate erection and female receptive lordosis in rats (Berendsen & Broekkamp, 1987).

An unusual "aphrodisiac effect" occurred in two bulimic women on fenfluramine (Stevenson & Solyom, 1990), perhaps due to breakthrough oxytocin stimulation. A 37-year-old woman treated for bulimia with 80 mg fluoxetine complained of fatigue, lifelessness, suicidal thoughts, lack of libido, and no pleasure from sexual activity. When switched to fenfluramine (60 mg/day), she began to feel frequent sexual arousal. At 120 mg, she felt incessant "embarrassing" sexual urges:

> She started to proposition old friends. She had many erotic dreams. She was continuously preoccupied with sex and had about six partners in a two-week period. She had multiple orgasms, which she had not experienced previously . . . for the next 10 days . . . she had intercourse 11 times, masturbated once, had seven sexual partners, had 28 orgasms with intercourse, experienced intense pleasure sensations with most intercourse, and had reduced time to orgasm. . . . She said, "Everything I do makes me think of it [sex]; I get involuntary vaginal contractions; I feel the desire for intercourse—not foreplay—just intercourse; masturbation doesn't help; I'm orgasmic within a few seconds—but within a half-hour I want more; even when I'm too tired, I still have a mental need. . . . I'm constantly aware of increased vaginal lubrication; even the nature of my thoughts have changed—I'm no longer concerned about a steady relationship—I'd sleep with 17 men if I could . . . it's driving me crazy; it's a living hell."

Sexual arousal returned to normal within days of stopping fenfluramine. A second woman treated for bulimia with 120 mg fenfluramine also complained of increased sexual arousal for two weeks, which disappeared when fenfluramine was withdrawn.

Sexual Benefits

A decrease in genital sensitivity due to fenfluramine may delay ejaculation and therefore could be useful in the treatment of premature ejaculation. The serotonin antagonist cyproheptadine (Periactin) acts in an opposite way to fenfluramine on serotonin receptors and facilitates genital excitement and orgasm. Cyproheptadine can reverse the anorgasmia caused by therapeutic serotonergic drugs such as fluoxetine and clomipramine. This opposing pattern suggests that fenfluramine might delay or block orgasm, but such an effect has not been noted in the research.

Alternatives

When prescribing fenfluramine for weight control, several strategies may be considered in an effort to limit or avoid its side effects and brain toxicity.

Prescribe fenfluramine for weight reduction for a limited time (one to two months), during which tolerance to its anorectic action occurs, thus decreasing its efficacy. Then switch to a dopaminergic anorectic stimulant such as mazindol (preferable for women), diethylpropion (preferable for men), or phentermine for a few months so that the anorectic effect continues but tolerance in the serotonin system is allowed to dissipate. Although dopaminergic anorectics may not have the thermogenic activity of fenfluramine, they can help prevent weight lost on fenfluramine from being regained. A study of obese patients has shown that fenfluramine followed by phentermine facilitated more weight loss than continuous fenfluramine treatment over the same period or treatment with phentermine followed by fenfluramine (Carruba, Garosi, et al., 1986).

Fenfluramine damage to serotonin neurons apparently occurs due to excessive release of serotonin so that these neurons become exhausted. Fenfluramine prescribed in combination with a SSRI such as fluoxetine, sertraline, or paroxetine can prevent excessive release and synaptic influx of serotonin. It seems that the 5-HT uptake inhibiting action of fenfluramine itself is not sufficient to restrain excess serotonin activity. The combination of fenfluramine and SSRI antidepressants may be as effective as and safer (in terms of brain toxicity) than fenfluramine alone. Unfortunately, side effects with such combinations have not been studied; these possible side effects include severe anxiety, lethargy, mania, or even hallucinatory/psychotic episodes. Nevertheless, this approach may be worth consideration on a case by case basis.

A number of thermogenic substances are currently being developed for weight reduction and treatment of obesity, but these drugs may have more side effects and be more toxic than fenfluramine. The obvious available serotonergic alternative to fenfluramine is fluoxetine (Prozac). Its manufacturer is seeking Federal Drug Administration approval for its use in treatment of obesity. However, for this use fluoxetine must be used at higher doses (60–80 mg/day), which increases the risk for side effects; moreover, it is too expensive for most patients (in 1991, four to six dollars per day). The other SSRIs soon to be marketed do not seem to have the weight-reducing potency of fluoxetine.

DIETHYLPROPION (TENUATE)

Diethylpropion (Tenuate) has amphetamine-like pharmacological properties, but was introduced in 1957 as a safer alternative to amphetamines for appetite control. As a stimulant, it is only about 20% as potent as d-amphetamine (Hoekenga, Dillon, & Leyland, 1978). Prescriptions reached a peak in the 1960s and 1970s but precipitously declined in the 1980s as concern about dependence increased (Carney, 1988).

Diethylpropion is a phenethylamine (PEA) molecule modified by the inclusion of a ketone (carbonyl) structure. Chemically it is somewhat similar to bupropion, but bupropion is further designed to avoid amphetamine effects, which are the basis for therapeutic action of diethylpropion. The side effects of diethylpropion are similar to those with other stimulants: insomnia, nervousness, restlessness, dry mouth, and constipation. Norepinephrine and dopamine levels in the brain are increased by diethylpropion, much as with d-amphetamine at comparable anorectic doses. In contrast to amphetamines, fenfluramine, and mazindol, there is practically no effect of diethylpropion on serotonin activity. As with dopamine uptake inhibitors (e.g., cocaine, methylphenidate), the catecholamine-induced locomotor stimulation on diethylpropion is blocked by reserpine rather than the toxin alpha-methyltyrosine, which blocks amphetamine-induced catecholamine stimulation. Consequently, diethylpropion should not have the toxic catecholamine-depleting toxic action associated with amphetamines. There is little possibility of toxic actions on serotonin neurons due to the absence of serotonergic chemical effects.

Abuse and dependence are far less likely on diethylpropion than on amphetamines and, perhaps, only a little more likely than with over-the-counter stimulants and diet pills. Diethylpropion has been shown to function as a reinforcer in monkeys (an indication of abuse potential), but has far less potency than amphetamines, cocaine, and even methylphenidate (Johanson & Schuster, 1975). Nevertheless, psychoses and abuse are occasionally reported on diethylpropion. The few reported cases (less than 20) of psychoses have mostly occurred in middle-aged female patients with a history of stimulant abuse and/or with the use of abnormally high doses of diethylpropion (Carney, 1988; Khan, Spiegel, & Jobe, 1987; Martin & Iwamoto, 1984). Presenting symptoms in these cases have included paranoid, manic, and depressive states, which were resolved upon withdrawal from diethylpropion and/or short-term treatment with neuroleptics. The use of diethylpropion was often discovered only with questioning and urine drug screens, even though the drug was taken legally as treatment for obesity.

It is probable that abuse and psychoses occur much more frequently than reported. However, reports to Drug Abuse Warning Network in the United States from 1973 to 1975 (when diethylpropion use was near peak levels) showed minimal abuse—even less than with fenfluramine, which is not a reinforcer in animals (Hoekenga et al., 1978). In a review of epidemiological surveys of drug abuse and the medical literature, Cohen (1977) found almost no abuse or dependence. Nevertheless, diethylpropion is a moderately strong amphetamine and can be expected to increase the risk of psychoses and depression, particularly when there is a predisposition to affective disorders or a history of substance abuse. Table 23.3 summarizes the properties and side effects of diethylpropion.

Sexual Dysfunction

Diethylpropion can be expected to affect sexual function in a manner similar to other stimulants. Its stimulation of noradrenergic sympathomimetic activity can cause constriction of the penis and possibly premature ejaculation. Nervousness or anxiety generated both by dieting and diethylpropion treatment may make relaxation for sexual activity difficult, and the stimulation received from diethylpropion may compete with sexual drive, so that patients are functional but personally withdrawn. Facilitation of orgasm in hyperactive women by diethylpropion has never been reported. The lack of serotonergic properties may allow gradual sensitization to masculine sexual obsessions and perversions in men or women, which had previously been repressed.

Alternatives

There has been no evidence that phentermine (Fastin), the chief alternative to diethylpropion, has pharmacological or psychological effects that are any different from those of diethylpropion. There is a possibility that phentermine's properties and side effects are closer to those with amphetamines and that diethylpropion's are closer to those with cocaine or methylphenidate. At this time, however, such a difference is purely speculative. Neither of these mild amphetamine-like stimulants reliably maintains weight loss with extended use, and the probability of stimulant sensitization causing tension and dependence is great. Therefore, although it has only a weak weight-loss effect, bupropion (Wellbutrin) is a far better alternative as a mild stimulant for long-term use. Prescribing bupropion is less complicated because it is not a scheduled drug, but it must be more closely monitored for side effects. For those who are already on diethylpropion or phentermine and feel the need to continue, bupropion may serve as a substitute for maintenance treatment.

METHYLPHENIDATE (RITALIN)

Methylphenidate (Ritalin) was introduced over 30 years ago as a safer but less potent anorectic alternative to amphetamine. Although it releases both dopamine and norepinephrine, the stimulant potency of methylphenidate is chiefly due to inhibiting the uptake of these catecholamines. Furthermore, like cocaine, it releases dopamine only from stored reserves (reserpine-sensitive) rather than from newly synthesized pools, as with amphetamines. Limitation of dopamine release to these stored reserves avoids the neurotoxicity found with amphetamines. Also unlike amphetamines, methylphenidate does not prominently affect serotonin and generally does not increase cortisol levels. Because of its relative safety, this drug is used widely with prepubertal children who have attention deficit disorder with hyperactivity; more recently, it has also been used with adults who have attention deficit disorder. (Due to its stimulant potency, methylphenidate became a controlled Schedule II drug in 1971.)

In 1988 considerable controversy was generated concerning the side effects (including violent behavior and psychotic manifestations) of methylphenidate when used in children (Cowart, 1988a, 1988b). Ingrid Rimland, an educational psychologist in the California public

Table 23.3 *Profile of Diethylproprion (Tenuate)*

Daily Dose
25 mg TID

COMMON INDICATIONS
Weight gain, obesity

MECHANISMS OF ACTION (GENERAL)
Amphetamine-like derivative catecholamine stimulant
Increases dopamine and norepinephrine activation

MECHANISMS OF ACTIONS (SEXUAL)
Positive
Increased adrenergic ($alpha_1$) activity
Increased dopamine

DIRECT SEXUAL SIDE EFFECTS

Desire disorders (in both sexes)	Erection difficulties	Ejaculation disorders
• Hypersexuality	• Inability/difficulty obtaining/maintaining erection	• Retarded ejaculation facilitated
	Orgasm facilitated (in both sexes)	• Ejaculation without orgasm facilitated
		• Premature ejaculation aggravated

Menstrual disorders	Breast disorders
• Amenorrhea	• Gynecomastia

INDIRECT SEXUAL SIDE EFFECTS
Discomfort caused by: dryness of skin, mouth, mucous membranes, constipation, nausea, rash/itching, urinary problems (incontinence), weight loss

Mood disorders resulting in anxiety, nervousness, detachment, irritability, mania, psychoses

Neurological disturbances resulting in dizziness, sleep disturbances, tremor

Vascular disturbances resulting in arrhythmias, headache, peripheral vasoconstriction

SEXUAL CONTRAINDICATIONS/BENEFITS

Avoid with prior condition of	*May be useful for*
Sex drive disorders	Ejaculatory inhibition
Premature ejaculation	Anorgasmia
Menstrual disorders	

ALTERNATIVES
Phentermine (Fastin)
Fluoxetine (Prozac)
Mazindol (Sanorex)
Fenfluramine (Pondimin)

school system, who has worked in 40 schools encompassing five districts, has noted stunted growth in children receiving daily treatment with Ritalin in up to 70% of cases (personal communication, 1994). She and many of her colleagues have expressed concern that Ritalin is being prescribed too liberally and without full appreciation of the development consequences.

Reservations about the use of stimulants in general has prevented further evaluation of methylphenidate's potential benefits in treating depression, fatigue, and neurasthenia in the elderly or medically ill. In the past, stimulants have been advertised for the treatment of mild depression, fatigue, and neurasthenia. Early reports in the 1930s, which had originally recommended amphetamines (Benzedrine) for psychotropic treatment, emphasized their use for fatigue and nervous exhaustion (Myerson, 1936). Subsequently, amphetamines were liberally provided to soldiers during World War II and the Korean War, and their use rose: eight billion were legally prescribed in 1968 (equal to 35 to 50 pills a year for every American). Given this history of stimulant overuse and abuse, treatment of mild depression and fatigue with methylphenidate has not been studied. Nevertheless, many doctors, discouraged by the severe side effects of tricyclics, do prescribe methylphenidate. Dosage used for mild depression, geriatric, or illness-related depression is 10–60 mg/day. Table 23.4 summarizes the properties and side effects of methylphenidate.

Few alternative medications have been available. Nomifensine (Merital), an antidepressant with methylphenidate-like chemical actions, was used for many years in Europe. It was approved for use in the United States in 1985, but in 1986 it was withdrawn worldwide due to serious hemolytic anemia and periodic fatal reactions from a "flu-like" syndrome. Presently, the only available antidepressant with stimulant properties is bupropion (Wellbutrin). Methylphenidate and the other dopaminergic drugs available (bupropion, deprenyl, bromocriptine) offer an alternative to tricyclics and SSRI antidepressants, which have frequent adverse sexual effects. Unfortunately, as a Schedule II stimulant drug, methylphenidate is unlikely to be generally available to treat mild depression. Several prominent psychiatrists have suggested wider use of stimulants such as methylphenidate for depression (Ayd, 1985; Chiarello & Cole, 1987; Pitts, 1982a, 1982b; Warneke, 1990). Although the few controlled studies on the overall efficacy of methylphenidate as an antidepressant have shown inconsistent, marginal results (Satel & Nelson, 1989), uncontrolled, non-placebo studies have indicated that methylphenidate may be effective, with few side effects and little abuse, when used in depressed medically ill (e.g., cancer, post-stroke) patients (Fernandez, Adams, Holmes, Levy, & Neidhart, 1987; Lingam, Lazarus, Groves, & Oh, 1988) or depressed, apathetic, or withdrawn geriatric patients (Branconnier & Cole, 1980; Kaplitz, 1975).

Sexual Dysfunction

Since methylphenidate treatment is generally kept confidential due to its Schedule II status, it is difficult to determine the incidence and prevalence of such side effects. Published case reports of its use have not indicated sexual effects. Beneficial sexual effects could be attributed to recovery from depression and fatigue or to a general stimulating action. Negative sexual effects would only be indicated in cases of abuse and addiction as evidence of toxicity. Nevertheless, the dopaminergic action of methylphenidate could be expected to cause sexual reactions of a stimulatory nature that either benefit or otherwise alter sexual desire and responsivity.

Often patients on stimulants do not notice any sexual changes, but their partners report becoming aware of a gradual withdrawal from sexual activity—a common behavioral tendency with both stimulant and benzodiazepine tranquilizer drugs. Physicians should consider consulting privately with the spouses of patients treated with methylphenidate and other stimulants to be sure that negative psychological and sexual changes are not occurring. Possible negative sexual changes include disinterest, aversion, compulsive sexuality, lack of concentration during sex, premature ejaculation, and failure to maintain a firm erection.

Male/Female Differences

Of particular interest is a report by Askinazi, Weintraub, and Karamouz (1986) which showed a much better response for female than for male depressed elderly and ill patients (6 of 8 = 75% females versus 1 of 5 = 20% males). Such a differential response may be due to women's greater sensitivity to stimulants. However, women may also be expected to experience more

Table 23.4 *Profile of Methylphenidate (Ritalin)*

Daily Dose 10–60 mg/daily	
COMMON INDICATIONS	
Attention deficit disorder	
Hyperactivity disorder	
MECHANISMS OF ACTION (GENERAL)	
Central nervous system stimulation through dopamine and norepinephrine uptake inhibition	
MECHANISMS OF ACTION (SEXUAL)	
Positive	*Negative*
Increased adrenergic ($alpha_1$) activity	Increased cortisol
Increased dopamine	
DIRECT SEXUAL SIDE EFFECTS	
Desire disorders (in both sexes)	Ejaculation disorders
• Hypersexuality	• Premature ejaculation aggravated
• Sexual aversion	• Impotence aggravated
Orgasm facilitated	Menstrual disorders
	• Amenorrhea
INDIRECT SEXUAL SIDE EFFECTS	
Discomfort caused by constipation, nausea, rash/itching, weight loss	
Mood disorders resulting in anxiety, nervousness, irritability, psychoses	
Neurological disturbances resulting in dizziness, sleep disturbances, tremor	
Vascular disturbances resulting in arrhythmias, headache	
SEXUAL CONTRAINDICATIONS/BENEFITS	
Avoid with prior condition of	*May be useful for*
Aversion	Anorgasmia
Hypersexuality	Inhibited ejaculation
Impotence	
Premature ejaculation	
ALTERNATIVES	
Mazindol (Sanorex)	
Fenfluramine (Pondimin)	
Diethylpropion (Tenuate)	

bothersome side effects, especially insomnia, anorexia, and anxiety.

Sexual Benefits

Children taking methylphenidate as treatment for attention deficit disorder with hyperactivity (ADDH) are usually taken off the drug prior to puberty. However, within the past few years, methylphenidate treatment has been extended successfully to postpubertal adolescents (Wender, Wood, & Reimherr, 1985); but there has been no discussion of how the drug may affect the increased sexuality accompanying the hormonal changes of puberty. It has now been recognized that attention deficit disorder (ADD) often does not necessarily disappear with childhood and adolescence, but continues to cause problems in adults. Currently, adult (residual) attention deficit disorder (AADD) is included in the *DSM-IV* as a diagnosis. Symptoms include impulsivity, distractibility, restlessness, anxiety, and demanding, short-tempered, and socially unstable behavior. Paul Wender (Wender, Reimherr, Wood, & Ward, 1985) has conducted a number of studies showing psychostimulant efficacy without abuse or tolerance for treatment of a limited group of adult patients with clear-cut residual AADD continuing from childhood. In a preliminary trial with 15 patients (Wood, Reimherr, Wender, & Johnson, 1976) 8 of 13 (53%) adults improved on methylphenidate, 5 of 15 (33%) on pemoline, and only 1 of 13 (8%) on tricyclic antidepressants. Methylphenidate dose ranged from 20 to 60 mg/day.

Of note sexually, two women in Wood et al.'s study who had never experienced orgasm during intercourse became orgasmic and five patients with unhappy marriages reported improved relationships with their spouses. Facilitation of orgasm could be expected because methylphenidate's chief mechanism of action appears to be dopamine uptake inhibition. We have found evidence of facilitation of orgasm in women on bupropion, another dopamine uptake inhibitor. The MAO-B inhibitor l-deprenyl (selegiline/Eldepryl), currently used solely to treat Parkinson's disease, is also a weak dopamine uptake inhibitor. There is evidence that both bupropion and l-deprenyl have therapeutic actions on low sex drive in animals and humans. Methylphenidate may have similar sexual benefits hitherto unrecognized.

Alternatives

Alternatives to methylphenidate include pemoline (Cylert), which is much less effective, and bupropion (Wellbutin), which is closer in chemical action to methylphenidate and is free of prominent adrenergic amphetamine-like effects.

PHENYLPROPANOLAMINE (PPA)

Phenylpropanolamine (PPA) was first synthesized in 1910 as an ephedrine derivative. Ephedrine is a natural stimulant used for centuries as an orally effective epinephrine-like substance. It is the chief ingredient in the popular Oriental herb ma huang. The American ephedra plant is sometimes referred to as "Mormon tea" because the Mormons used it as a tea to treat cold and kidney disorders and as a "blood purifier" and "spring tonic." It was also used by natives in Mexico to treat syphilis. Ephedrine and phenylpropanolamine were promoted for use in Western medicine by the pharmacologist K.K. Chen in the 1920s (Silverman, 1985). They were first used as digitalis or epinephrine-like cardiovascular stimulants and to treat allergies such as hay fever, asthma, rhinitis, urticaria, edema, and bronchospasm. Medical use of phenylpropanolamine as a nasal decongestant became popular in 1936 (Morgan, 1985). In 1939, Hirsch reported that PPA reduced appetite in obese patients.

The Federal Drug Administration has been concerned, not with the intrinsic safety of this drug, but with its applications: indiscriminate use and excessive advertising claims for weight-reduction effects have caused alarm. Phenylpropanolamine (PPA) is the main ingredient in over-the-counter anorectic stimulants currently in use. In addition, it is widely used in other over-the-counter drugs (nasal decongestants, cough, cold, and anti-allergy preparations, to name a few) in which a stimulant is needed to counteract sedative effects. From the 1950s to the 1970s, prescription amphetamine stimulants were used extensively for weight reduction, but during the 1970s availability of these prescription anorectics declined. Phenylpropanolamine, freely marketed over-the-counter, filled the void, often used in combination with caffeine and herbal stimulants. By the 1980s, the overuse of phenylpropanolamine was recognized and debated, but little action was taken. Recently, its use has been somewhat curtailed, and in 1983, the Federal Drug Administration banned combination phenylpropanolamine-caffeine diet pills, due to potentially dangerous interactions between these two stimulants.

The most well-known over-the-counter PPA anorectic products are probably Dexatrim, Acutrim, and Ayds candy, but the list of other phenylpropanolamine drugs is nearly endless. The form of phenylpropanolamine sold in the United States is mainly the mixed (±) isomer dl-norephedrine (recommended diet dose, 75 mg/day). The single isomer d-norephedrine and d-norpseudoephedrine, which are much more stimulating, are chiefly used as anorexiants in Europe.

Despite its adrenergic sympathomimetic properties, phenylpropanolamine is not classified as an amphetamine-like anorectic stimulant (Morgan, 1985). It is considered to have minimal CNS action, but has been shown at high doses to have dopaminergic effects in rats (Lee, Stafford, & Hoebel, 1989). While at therapeutic anorectic doses phenylpropanolamine lacks the euphoric and energizing properties of amphetamines or dopamine stimulants, its sympathomimetic actions may cause vasoconstriction, tension, and dizziness. In persons susceptible to or actively experiencing panic attacks, phenylpropanolamine is a major hazard because it triggers or facilitates many of the somatic signs of panic.

Recent drug discrimination studies have shown that phenylpropanolamine is unlikely to be abused except by entrenched stimulant abusers, who may use excessive doses of phenylpropanolamine drugs on occasion to satisfy their drug craving. Normal volunteers or patients being treated for obesity have not shown a preference for phenylpropanolamine over placebo (Lamb, Sannerud, & Griffiths, 1987). Normal volunteers may identify phenylpropanolamine (75 mg) as an amphetamine (Chait, Uhlenhuth, & Johanson, 1986), indicating that it does have significant CNS effects; but it is not reinforcing enough to maintain either human or monkey behavior (Chait, Uhulenhuth, & Johanson, 1988; Lamb et al., 1987). Combination caffeine-ephedrine-phenylpropanolamine look-alike stimulants are subject to abuse, but the reinforcement in these combinations is apparently due to ephedrine and caffeine rather than to phenylpropanolamine.

Phenylpropanolamine has a small but consistent weight-reduction effect consisting of reduced appetite and a slight adrenergic thermogenic action. It is too weak to have a major effect on obesity, but may complement other behavioral means of weight reduction. The average user of phenylpropanolamine as an anorexiant is a woman under 45 years old who is less than 10 pounds (4.5 kg) above her ideal weight (Bray, 1985). In various surveys, 20–50% of women have used PPA anorexiants at some time as compared to less than 10% of men (Vener & Krupka, 1985). PPA is generally used as a stimulant by men (Vener & Krupka, 1985); the majority of emergency-room "speed" amphetamine reports have been for men, whereas nonprescription diet pills are widely abused by bulimic women. In one study of 158 bulimic women patients, 65.8% had used diet pills periodically and 18.4% had used them regularly for at least a year (Mitchell, Pyle, & Eckert, 1991). In another sample of 275 bulimic patients, 52% had used diet pills for weight control and 25.1% had used them on a daily basis (Mitchell, Hatsukami, Eckert, & Pyle, 1985). Women using diet pills also frequently report diuretic, laxative, and enema abuse to reduce weight. Among 57 bulimic cocaine abusers, 32 (56%) had also abused diet pills, 11% had abused laxatives, and 18%, diuretics (Jonas, Gold, Sweeney, & Pottash, 1987). Diet-pill use is therefore only one aspect of general substance abuse in bulimics. It is tempting to speculate that use of more effective prescription anorectic drugs would decrease abuse of these other substances. (Table 23.5 summarizes the properties of phenylpropanolamine.)

Sexual Dysfunction

It is not known to what extent oral therapeutic doses (75 mg) of phenylpropanolamine cause changes in penile vascular adrenergic tone. Sympathomimetic activation may cause vasoconstriction that prevents maintenance of erection sufficient for climax and ejaculation. However, increased sympathetic muscle tone may lead only to irregular spasms that interfere with the erection-ejaculatory-emission sequence.

Though there is no evidence in the literature, it may be assumed that phenylpropanolamine can cause or worsen premature ejaculation. Anxiety and adrenergic stimulation can both cause spontaneous ejaculation. The delay of ejaculation that may initially occur with cocaine or amphetamines is due to powerful neurotransmitter interactions not present with phenylpropanolamine. Free-floating anxiety generated in some

Table 23.5 *Profile of Phenylpropanolamine*

Daily Dose
75 mg

COMMON INDICATIONS
Weight gain, obesity

MECHANISMS OF ACTION (GENERAL)
Increases of catecholamine activity (norepinephrine and dopamine)

MECHANISMS OF ACTION (SEXUAL)

Positive	*Negative*
Increased adrenergic ($alpha_1$) activity	Increased adrenergic ($alpha_2$) activity
Increased adrenergic ($beta_2$) activity	Increased cortisol

DIRECT SEXUAL SIDE EFFECTS

Erection difficulties	Orgasm/ejaculation irregularities
• Inability/difficulty obtaining/maintaining erection	• Premature ejaculation
• Decreased quality of erection	

INDIRECT SEXUAL SIDE EFFECTS
Discomfort caused by constipation, nausea, weight loss
Mood disorders resulting in anxiety, nervousness, tension
Neurological disturbances resulting in sleep disturbances, tremor, dizziness
Vascular disturbances resulting in headache, peripheral vasoconstriction

SEXUAL CONTRAINDICATIONS/BENEFITS

Avoid with prior condition of	*May be useful for*
Decreased sex drive	Ejaculatory incompetence
Impotence	
Premature ejaculation	

ALTERNATIVES
Prescription anorectics: chiefly diethyproprion (Tenuate)
bupropion (Wellbutrin)
fluoxetine (Prozac)

individuals by chronic phenylpropanolamine use and weight loss can also disrupt normal body function, including the buildup to orgasmic climax. For a few individuals, actual panic and subsequent phobia may cause either severe premature ejaculation or ejaculatory incompetence. Also, excessive use of phenylpropanolamine along with caffeine, nicotine, excessive exercise, and poor diet may deplete and exhaust the body, resulting in difficulty with orgasm and ejaculation.

It is unknown whether $alpha_1$ adrenergic sympathetic drugs like phenylpropanolamine can facilitate orgasm in women. While it may be helpful for some individuals, we would expect that most women would be more likely to become tense, which would further inhibit orgasm. Relaxation and concentration on erotic cues and sensations could also be undermined.

Zorgniotti et al. (1987) identified impotence induced by chronic use of phenylpropanolamine nasal decongestants in 16 patients. Few of these patients had risk factors for impotence (e.g., diabetes, hypertension, smoking). The authors suggested the possibility of some kind of connection between nasal and penile vasodilation and observed that some men experience nasal congestion during sexual excitation. However, additional research has indicated that the reverse may also be true: Men with rhinitis experienced alleviation of nasal congestion during sexual excitement and a return to congestion following ejaculation (Blumberg & Moltz, 1988).

Sympathetic arousal is normally phasic (rises and falls in relation to the external situation), but the arousal generated by phenylpropanolamine and other stimulants is tonic. To the extent that one is too active to eat due to an anorectic stimulant, one may also be too active to make love. While it is clear that nervousness can prevent erection by not allowing smooth muscle in the cavernosum to relax, its effect on swelling, lubrication, and clitoral sensitivity is unknown. The increase in adrenergic stimulation that results from stimulants such as phenylpropanolamine could have either positive or negative effects on coital reflex circuitry. Unfortunately, no research has been conducted to investigate the effect of phenylpropanolamine and other anorectic stimulants on adrenergically mediated muscle tone.

Sexual Benefits

Phenylpropanolamine apparently has no direct, sexually stimulating effect in normal, sexually active persons. However, sexual enjoyment may be facilitated indirectly by phenylpropanolamine due to weight loss and the consequent physical and psychological changes that occur in body comfort, self-esteem, and sense of attractiveness. However, phenylpropanolamine and other sympathomimetic drugs containing adrenergic $alpha_1$ stimulants such as phenylephrine (e.g., synephrine) and pseudoephedrine (e.g., Sudafed) are used medically to correct retrograde ejaculation or "ejaculatory incompetence" (Stewart & Bergant, 1974; Thiagarajah, Vaughn, & Kitchin, 1978; Thomas, 1983). However, Stockamp, Schreiter, and Altwein (1974) found that alpha-adrenergic stimulants could not correct primary emission dysfunction associated with certain surgeries or neuropathies. With diabetic neuropathy or surgical damage (i.e., retroperitoneal lymphadenectomy), there may not be sufficient alpha-adrenergic receptors remaining to adequately respond to sympathomimetic drugs (Sandler, 1979). Improvement is more often found with idiopathic retrograde ejaculation that occurs intermittently. While normal ejaculation may be facilitated by these drugs, speed of ejaculation and semen volume, not sperm content, are affected.

Published case reports (Stewart & Bergant, 1974; Thiagarajah et al., 1978) have cited the use of phenylpropanolamine in Ornade preparations (75 mg phenylpropanolamine and 12 mg chlorpheniramine) once or twice a day, or one or two hours prior to intercourse, to facilitate ejaculation. Any preparation with 75 mg phenylpropanolamine, including over-the-counter diet pills, may work equally well. Nasal sprays with phenylephrine may be used alone after erection occurs or in combination with previously ingested phenylpropanolamine drugs. It should be noted that excessive use of these sympathomimetic drugs will eventually interfere with erection.

Alternatives

The chief new alternative to anorectic stimulants and phenylpropanolamine is fluoxetine (Prozac). Particularly when a serious affective disorder is also present, fluoxetine can have a therapeutic benefit not available from phenylpropanolamine. Although many women show remarkable benefits from fluoxetine, it has far more serious side effects and abuse potential than phenylpropanolamine. Widespread use of fluoxetine for weight reduction, even under medical supervision, could cause sexual problems far beyond the effects of phenylpropanolamine. Bupropion (Wellbutrin) is an obvious alternative, but probably has even less anorectic action than phenylpropanolamine.

Part VI

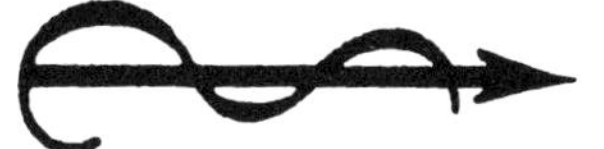

DRUGS FOR INTERNAL MEDICINE

24

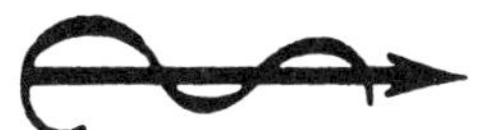

Antiulcer Drugs

OBJECTIVES

- To clarify the differences in sexual impact among histamine-2 antagonists
- To review the extensive literature on cimetidine and ranitidine
- To discuss interaction of cimetidine with other drugs

There are 60 million ulcer patients in the United States alone, many taking ulcer drugs. In fact, ranitidine (Zantac), an ulcer drug, is the most widely prescribed drug in the world. Histamine-2 antagonists are the most common medications used to treat ulcer disease. Within this group, cimetidine (Tagamet) has numerous adverse sexual properties while the other three—ranitidine, famotidine (Pepcid), and nizatidine (Axid)—are relatively benign sexually.

In the early 1980s, cimetidine was the most widely prescribed drug in the United States. During the course of its clinical use, adverse sexual side effects associated with it became increasingly apparent. A shift in prescription habits was reflected in its fall from first place as the drug of choice. In the early 1990s ranitidine was the most commonly prescribed ulcer medication (American Medical News, 1991); the newer ulcer drugs, famotidine and nizatidine, are becoming more widely prescribed with time. In 1995, famotidine (Pepcid) was the first of the antiulcer drugs to be sold over-the-counter (OTC) in the United States, and now cimetidine (Tagamet) and ranitidine (Zanac) have also been approved as OTC drugs to be used at low doses for treatment of "heartburn."

Cimetidine and ranitidine are the best known and most extensively studied of the histamine-2 receptor antagonists. Consequently, most of the data presented will concentrate on these two drugs. In spite of their many similarities, the drugs are more different than alike in regard to their sexual properties; as noted, cimetidine is associated with more significant sexual problems than ranitidine and the other histamine-2 antagonists. Prospective studies comparing histamine-2 receptor antagonists are dismally lacking; the Federal Drug Administration has not required anything beyond a general side-effect inquiry in the course of approving histamine-2 antagonists, even the newer ones. A six-month prospective study of all of these drugs, comparable to the 1986 captopril antihypertensive quality-of-life studies (Croog et al., 1986), would be helpful. Indeed, such a study is particularly important given the impending approval of over-the-counter status for cimetidine and ranitidine.

In the absence of ideal data, it is still possible to draw some conclusions regarding sexual effects of histamine-2 antagonists from the existing literature. The mechanisms of action for cimetidine's sexual effects are well-defined and the consequences have been well researched in other settings. Ranitidine and the other histamine-2 antagonists have occasional adverse sexual consequences associated with their use, but such reports are far less frequent than with cimetidine. In fact, there are several documented examples of disappearance of negative sexual side effects when cimetidine is replaced by ranitidine, and none (to our knowledge) when ranitidine is replaced by cimetidine.

The following sections describe the similarities and differences between histamine-2 antagonists from the point of view of sexual function. Prescribing considerations should include sensitivity to patients' sexual health when suitable alternatives exist that are less sexually toxic. Additional stress due to sexual dysfunction is clearly undesirable with ulcer disease. In the context of a comprehensive treatment plan, the probabilities are that medication, when required, can be provided at the lowest optimum dose, minimizing adverse side effects of all kinds, including sex. Table 24.1 summarizes the properties and side effects of histamine-2 antagonists.

MALE SEXUAL DYSFUNCTION ON CIMETIDINE

Unlike other histamine-2 antagonists, cimetidine is known to be antiandrogenic in humans. Its sexual effects (including gynecomastia, impotence, and decreased sperm count) have been attributed to this antiandrogenic activity.

The first clinical reports of negative sexual effects in humans were not published until 1979, more than a year after cimetidine had been approved for use in the United States (August, 1977). Comments that associate cimetidine with adverse sexual effects have routinely appeared in American Medical Association (AMA) peer review journals and Continuing Medical Education presentations. For example, the first sentence of an article that appeared in the AMA's *Archives of Internal Medicine* (Lardinois & Mazzaferri, 1985) stated: "Hyperprolactinemia, gynecomastia, decreased sperm count, loss of libido, and impotence may occur in patients treated with cimetidine hydrochloride" (p. 920). Similarly, the January 1990 report of research supported by the General Clinical Research Centers Program of the National Institute of Health Division and the National Cancer Institute of Environmental Health Sciences (Collins, 1990) stated that:

> Scientists at Rockefeller University Hospital in New York City report that cimetidine, a widely prescribed ulcer medication, interferes with the catabolism or metabolic degradation of the female sex hormone estradiol in men. The increased hormone levels produce abnormally enlarged breasts—gynecomastia—and sexual impotence in some men. (p. 1)

Further, the *Physicians Desk Reference* (1991a) compared cimetidine unfavorably with ranitidine with respect to sexual side effects: "Controlled studies in animals and man have shown no stimulation of any pituitary hormone by Zantac [ranitidine] and no antiandrogenic activity, and cimetidine-induced gynecomastia and impotence in hypersecretory patients have resolved when Zantac [ranitidine] has been substituted" (p. 1066).

Impotence

Although cimetidine's manufacturer (SmithKline Beecham) maintains that impotence is only a concern in patients treated with very high doses for hypersecretory states, the literature contradicts their position with numerous cases demonstrating the relationship between cimetidine and impotence at normal therapeutic dosages.

- Galeone et al. (1978) reported loss of erection in one of 15 men treated with 1200 mg/day cimetidine. Erection became normal two months after discontinuing cimetidine.
- Biron (1979) reported a 51-year-old man treated for ulcer with 800 mg/day cimetidine over six weeks, whose wife complained that intercourse had decreased from twice a week to once in two weeks.
- Peden, Cargill, Browning, Saunders, and Wormsley (1979) reported three cases of sexual dysfunction during cimetidine ulcer treatment. A 33-year-old man treated for four weeks (1,000 mg/day) spontaneously complained that he lost his sexual desire during the first week and thereafter could not get an erection. His desire and erectile function returned to normal four days af-

Table 24.1 *Profile of Histamine-2 Antagonists*

	Daily Dose
Cimetidine (Tagamet)	400–1600 mg HS
Famotidine (Pepcid)	20–40 mg HS
Nizatidine (Axid)	150–300 mg HS
Ranitidine (Zantac)	150–300 mg HS

COMMON INDICATIONS
Ulcer, reflux esophagitis
Gastric hypersecretory states

MECHANISMS OF ACTION (GENERAL)
Reduce gastric acid secretion through histamine-2 receptor antagonism

MECHANISMS OF ACTION (SEXUAL)

Negative	CIM	FAM	NIZ	RAN
Decreased adrenal androgen (DHEAS)	+ + + +			
Increased prolactin	+ +			+
Decreased testosterone activity	+ + +			+
Increased estrogens	+ +			
Decreased zinc	+ +	+ +	+ +	+ +
Increased serotonin	+			
Decreased serotonin				+ +

DIRECT SEXUAL SIDE EFFECTS
Desire disorders (in both sexes) (cimetidine only)
Erection difficulties
- Inability/difficulty obtaining/ maintaining erection
- Decreased or absent noctur-nal/morning erection

Infertility (cimetidine only)
- Decreased sperm

Breast disorders
- Gynecomastia
- Galactorrhea
- Pain, tenderness

INDIRECT SEXUAL SIDE EFFECTS
Neurological disturbances resulting in dizziness, headache

SEXUAL CONTRAINDICATIONS/BENEFITS
Avoid with prior condition of (cimetidine only)
Desire disorders
Impotence
Anorgasmia
Ejaculatory disorders

ALTERNATIVES
Helicobacter pylori antibiotic treatment
Antacids (Di-Gel, Maalox, Tums, etc.)
Sucralfate (Carafate)
Omeprazole (Prilosec)
Cisapride (Propulsid)

ter discontinuing cimetidine. Long-term use of cimetidine may have permanent consequences, however. A 50-year-old man treated with 1,000 mg/day experienced loss of sexual desire followed by gradual loss of erectile function within three weeks. He did not complain to his doctor for seven months and his desire did not return to normal when he discontinued cimetidine after nine months. He subsequently required ulcer surgery. Lastly, a 51-year-old man experienced decreased sexual desire and erection on 1,000 mg/day treatment for 11 months, yet did not complain until he was specifically questioned by his doctor. He reported that he had lost his sexual desire soon after starting on cimetidine and subsequently became impotent. No improvement was noted when the drug was discontinued.

- Peden et al. (1979) also noted that in three years of market availability, 23 cases of impotence due to cimetidine had been reported to the government monitor in men 37 years of age or older within one to seven months after starting treatment.
- In the initial cimetidine postmarketing surveillance report, Gifford, Aeugle, Myerson, and Tannenbaum (1980) noted "sex inhibition" in a man and a woman, loss of sexual desire in one man, and "poor" erection in another man.
- Peden and Wormsley (1982) reported impotence and gynecomastia in a 50-year-old man treated over 18 months for ulcer with 1,000 mg/day cimetidine. All hormone measurements were normal. When switched to ranitidine, the gynecomastia regressed and the patient regained normal erection.
- Jensen et al. (1983) treated 22 patients with gastric hypersecretion (20 had Zollinger-Ellison syndrome) with high dose cimetidine (mean = 5300 mg/day). Within two to five months on the highest dose, nine patients showed erectile dysfunction for at least two months, and five of the nine experienced complete inability to become erect for those two months. Seven of the nine men also developed gynecomastia. Impotent cimetidine patients were switched to ranitidine. All recovered normal erectile function within four weeks on ranitidine, which continued to treat effectively the gastric hypersecretion. In three of the cimetidine patients who became totally impotent during cimetidine treatment, objective NPT monitoring showed that nocturnal erections nearly disappeared while on cimetidine but returned to normal on ranitidine.
- Gough et al. (1984) conducted a double-blind trial of maintenance ulcer therapy with 400 mg/day cimetidine or 150 mg/day ranitidine, each taken before sleep. Two of 186 male patients on cimetidine experienced sexual dysfunction versus none on ranitidine. One patient noted difficulty maintaining erection one month after starting on cimetidine; another patient on cimetidine was withdrawn after eight months due to partial impotence. His erection improved within a month of discontinuing cimetidine.

Lowered Sperm Count

Van Thiel, Gavaler, Smith, and Paul (1979) reported in the *New England Journal of Medicine* that seven sexually normal male patients who were treated for gastritis or ulcers with a normal therapeutic dose of 1200 mg/day for nine weeks showed on average 43% reduction in sperm count compared to untreated controls. The sperm counts of cimetidine patients returned to baseline levels two to three months after cimetidine was discontinued (noted in Bleumink, 1983). Although testosterone levels actually increased in these men, action due to such increased production would be blocked at the receptor sites. Several years later, Van Thiel, Gavaler, Heyl, and Susen (1987) conducted a comparative study of patients treated with cimetidine, nizatidine, or placebo. Once again, they found a reduced sperm count in men treated with cimetidine (1,600 mg/day for six weeks). Cimetidine was tested double-blind against placebo and 300 mg/day nizatidine. In the cimetidine patients, no significant changes were found in LH reactions, testosterone, or prolactin. Placebo and nizatidine caused no change in sperm count or hormones.

In all studies of the effects of cimetidine on sperm count, it should be noted that even significant reductions in sperm count left men with adequate concentrations for fertility. Therefore, it appears that men with normal sperm counts have no cause for concern. However, no sperm count studies have been performed to evaluate the effect of cimetidine on men with low or borderline sperm counts. It is conceivable that men whose fertility is borderline could be adversely affected. Until studies clarify this issue, cimetidine probably should be avoided in men who have concerns about fertility.

Surprisingly, the current *Physicians Desk Reference* labeling (1994) for cimetidine states that it does not decrease sperm count. Inquiry to cimetidine's manufacturer revealed that the basis for this assertion was a study by Paulsen, Enzmann, Bremner, Perrin, and Rogers (1983), which showed a dose-dependent though nonsignificant reduction of sperm count with the normal therapeutic dose of 1,200 mg/day cimetidine over six months. (Apparently the other studies were disregarded.) However, several problems with this study should have prevented it from serving as evidence for the lack of an effect on sperm count by cimetidine. For example, a decrease in sperm count from 92.7 to 70.4 mill/ml did occur on the normal 1,200 mg/day dose. No reduction occurred with a smaller, nontherapeutic dose of 400 mg/day (96.2 to 97.4) and a much smaller reduction occurred on placebo (82.8 to 68.8). Thus, Van Thiel's and Paulsen's studies *both* showed reduction in sperm count on therapeutic dose cimetidine. Furthermore, Paulsen's article was not peer reviewed. It appeared in a 1983 supplement of *Drug Therapy* from a symposium of the Royal Society of Medicine. In contrast, Van Thiel's 1979 study was published in the *New England Journal of Medicine* after strict peer review, which would have included approval of the statistical analysis, adding considerate credibility.

Yet another weakness in Paulsen's study: It is not clear whether the subjects in the study were volunteers or ulcer patients, making results difficult to interpret. If they were ulcer patients, leaving them on either placebo or subtherapeutic doses for six months would be unethical. Additionally, the data from these men would be confounded by their continued illness when compared to the men given the therapeutic dose. If the subjects were not ulcer patients, then the drug was being tested in a population other than that indicated for the drug, which would disqualify the study as definitive evidence for *Physicians Desk Reference* labeling.

Van Thiel's 1979 study was done with older patients on cimetidine for therapeutically indicated gastrointestinal problems. Paulsen's men were aged 20 to 39, whereas Van Thiel's 1979 subjects (mean, 40 years old) were closer to the mean age of ulcer patients. Older man are generally more vulnerable to sperm deficiencies, which are a normal consequence of aging.

The high percentage of patients with symptoms of gynecomastia in all groups of Paulsen's study is particularly baffling. The baseline profiles *prior* to cimetidine treatment showed more than 50% of the men *already* had gynecomastia (17 of 30). During treatment, gynecomastia increased in *both groups* (22 of 30 men, placebo and cimetidine). The authors stated that physicians did not note any occurrence of cimetidine-related gynecomastia, but accurately identifying cimetidine effects in this area would have been rendered unlikely due to the pre-existing condition.

Lastly, the group on the therapeutic dose, which showed substantial yet "nonsignificant" reduction in sperm count also showed a significant increase in prolactin (16.3 to 21.0 ng/ml). An increase in prolactin, which could be associated with gynecomastia, was not shown with placebo or the lower 400 mg/day dose. The authors stated that this difference was "significant only at the $p = .05$, but not at $p < .05$." Significance usually is defined as equal or lower than the chosen criteria (i.e., .05 level). Minimizing the difference by calling it "only significant at $p = .05$" suggests a bias toward finding nonsignificant effects and the possibility of post hoc statistical manipulation.

FEMALE SEXUAL DYSFUNCTION ON CIMETIDINE

Since androgens enhance sex drive in women as well as men, cimetidine's antiandrogen action should cause sexual deficits in women as well as men. Blockade of dihydrotestosterone (DHT) binding to peripheral receptors could directly reduce androgen-mediated sensitivity of the clitoris or vulva. Central and peripheral androgen inhibition in women could decrease sexual desire and orgasmic capacity. In fact, the adverse sexual effects of cimetidine due to androgen inhibition could occur more frequently in women than in men, because women have less androgen at baseline and often are more prone to decreased sexual desire and orgasmic difficulties (McConaghy, 1993). Additional deficits to already decreased sexual desire caused by cimetidine may be recognized even less often than in men. Nevertheless, reports of cimetidine-induced sexual dysfunction in women are unexpectedly rare. The fact that 94.7% of gastroenterologists are male (Elixhauser, McMenamin, & Witsberger, 1991) may have a bearing on reporting patterns. Women are reluctant to discuss sexual matters with the opposite sex and male physicians are more likely to perceive such problems in their same sex.

The only published case report of a cimetidine-induced sexual deficit in a woman appeared in 1983 (Pierce, 1983). A 40-year-old woman with duodenal ulcer was treated with 1200 mg/day cimetidine. Within three days she noted depression and loss of sexual desire, but continued on cimetidine for one month. Reduction of dosage to 600 mg/day did not resolve her loss of desire. Within 24 hours of discontinuing cimetidine, however, her libido "dramatically returned" and her depression lifted.

ANTIANDROGEN EFFECTS OF CIMETIDINE

Decreased sexual desire in a woman was also noted in the initial cimetidine postmarketing surveillance report (Gifford et al., 1980). The dearth of published reports is predictable for two reasons: First there is the erroneous notion among many clinicians and researchers that an antiandrogen would only affect men; second, when a woman complains of reduced desire, there is a tendency to automatically attribute it to the relationship or an emotional disorder.

Antiandrogens can cause impotence and gynecomastia. As an antiandrogen, cimetidine interferes with the sex hormone testosterone. Prescribing information for cimetidine has specific warnings/precautions about the possibility of impotence and gynecomastia, whereas no such warnings/precautions are required for ranitidine labeling, although it does note those possibilities under "other adverse reactions." There is a clear distinction, mandated by the Federal Drug Administration, between "warnings/precautions" and "adverse reactions." None of the other histamine-2 antagonists have been demonstrated to have antiandrogenic properties.

Antiandrogenic properties have been documented to affect sex drive in both men and women (Eskin, 1984; Sherwin, 1988a). Cimetidine has such pronounced antiandrogenic properties that it has even been studied as a possible treatment for hirsutism in women (Golditch & Price, 1990; Lissak et al., 1989; Vigersky, Mehlman, Glass, & Smith, 1980). Lissak et al. (1989) showed reduced DHEA adrenal androgen in 12 women treated for hirsutism with 1,500 mg cimetidine for three months. Their testosterone levels were unchanged. Despite the drop in DHEA, cimetidine did not treat hirsutism successfully. The decrease in DHEA may have been due to inhibition of P-450 enzymes rather than to a direct antiandrogen effect. DHEA is also reduced by ketoconazole (Nizoral) which, like cimetidine, is an imidazole drug with antiandrogen effects. A decline in DHEA is characteristic of aging past 30 or of disease. Thus, cimetidine affected this hormone in a way that is characteristic of aging, disease, and sexually negative drugs such as ketoconazole.

In addition to causing sexual problems, cimetidine's direct inhibition of peripheral androgen receptor binding could subtly alter secondary sex characteristics (genital size, hair growth, etc.). Androgen receptors are not blocked by ranitidine (Brittain et al., 1982; Pearce & Funder, 1980) and have not been reported to be blocked by other histamine-2 antagonists. In spite of these antiandrogenic effects, cimetidine has been recommended for use in women, based on its potential to prevent osteoporosis. Most women, if informed, would not willingly jeopardize their sex drive for this feature, especially when there are more effective ways of preventing osteoporosis readily available (Levin, 1991; Pogrund, Bloom, & Menczel, 1986).

Lardinois and Mazzaferri (1985) showed subnormal testosterone levels (170 ng/dl; normal = 300–1,000) in a 66-year-old man treated for ulcers over 12 months with 300–1200 mg/day cimetidine. Within a month of stopping cimetidine, his testosterone level returned to normal.

Teratologic Hypoandrogenization

Although the Physicians Desk Reference (1991a) does not attribute teratogenic (fetal malformations) effects to cimetidine, some research has indicated that this issue warrants further study before reassuring patients. A 1977 toxicological profile of cimetidine prepared by its manufacturer for FDA approval (Lesley & Walker, 1977) and a 1987 toxicological paper from company scientists (Walker, Bott, & Bond, 1987) failed to find any indications of demasculinization of male pups due to perinatal maternal exposure to cimetidine. Similarly, Shapiro, Hirst, Babalola, and Bitar (1988) and Shapiro and Bitar (1991) found that perinatal cimetidine exposure had no long-term effects on sexual development of male or female offspring and no effect on steroidal enzymes, including the P-450 enzyme group. However, Ryan and Levin (1990) found a decrease of estradiol 2-hydroxylation due to perinatal exposure to cimetidine, a P-450 catalyzed step that could result in elevated estradiol in offspring. Furthermore, a 1982 *Science* article by Anand and Van Thiel reported hypoandrogenization in male rats from prenatal and neonatal exposure to cimetidine. In both cases, gonadal tissue was reduced and the males' sexual behavior at maturity was diminished. Testicular prostate and seminal vesicle weights, as well as serum concentration of testosterone, were all significantly reduced in male offspring at 55 days of age. At 110 days of age, mount latency and frequency were greatly reduced. These findings suggested the possibility of an antiadrogen effect that may be neither mild nor irrelevant. The authors concluded that cimetidine has an unpredictable, undefined, and probably underdiagnosed antiandrogen effect. When experienced prenatally and neonatally, it may also be an irreversible effect.

A subsequent study by Van Thiel's group (Parker, Udani, Gavaler, & Van Thiel, 1984) replicated these negative antiandrogen effects of cimetidine in a controlled comparison to placebo and ranitidine. None of the toxic antiandrogen effects occurred with either placebo or ranitidine. The cimetidine and ranitidine doses used in this rat study were equivalent to the doses used clinically for treatment of ulcers. The authors concluded: "The present study . . . adds yet another concern to the widespread and, at times indiscriminate use of cimetidine. Specifically, it suggests that the use of cimetidine but not ranitidine by pregnant women might result in unwanted feminization of male fetus(es) and also have long-term adverse effects on adult male sexual behavior of male progeny of such women" (p. 317).

Gynecomastia and Prolactin Increases

Spence and Celestin (1979) reported gynecomastia in five of 25 male patients after four months of ulcer treatment with 1,600 mg/day cimetidine. Patients complained of breast swelling and soreness in their nipples. Due to satisfaction with cimetidine's therapeutic effect on their ulcers, all patients completed 12 months of treatment. Nipple soreness disappeared a few days after discontinuing cimetidine and gynecomastia soon regressed. The authors pointed out that the gynecomastia reported by their patients took months to develop, indicating that the condition may not appear within a short four- to six-week treatment period. Finding no circulating hormonal changes in the gynecomastia patients, they attributed the effect to antiandrogenic receptor blockade in the local breast tissue.

In the first postmarketing surveillance trials of cimetidine, Gifford et al. (1980) noted 18 cases of gynecomastia that were "considered related to cimetidine therapy" among 4,404 men monitored. Jensen, Collen, McArthur, et al. (1984) and Jensen, Collen, Pandol, et al. (1983) found breast changes (11 instances) including gynecomastia (five instances) in 22 patients treated for gastric hypersecretion. Patients with impotence in this study have been discussed above. All breast problems resolved when patients were switched to ranitidine. Breast tenderness resolved within eight weeks, but gynecomastia required two months or more to disappear.

A 1984 cimetidine postmarketing survey (Humphries et al., 1984) reported a .2% gynecomastia rate for treatment under six months, but a .8% (fourfold increase) for treatment over six months.

A 12-month English postmarketing surveillance of cimetidine reported gynecomastia as a discharge diagnosis in 20 of 6,240 male patients (.32%); it was the principal diagnosis in 11 (Colin-Jones, Langman, Lawson, & Vessey, 1985). In 13 of these patients, gynecomastia was attributed to cimetidine. In comparison, only a single control patient developed gynecomastia during the year (attributed to spironolactone treatment for heart failure). The authors stated that "gynecomastia is a well-described adverse effect of cimetidine which . . . usually reverses on stopping therapy." Apparently, the possibility of gynecomastia increases with continued use of cimetidine. Formal test trials of histamine-2 antagonists very rarely extend beyond three months. Because of the high relapse rate for ulcers, patients may be treated intermittently with cimetidine, so that total exposure is frequently greater than three months. Sexually adverse effects are rarely observed on the 400 mg continuous maintenance dose of cimetidine.

Gynecomastia has been noted only rarely with ranitidine or nizatidine. Indeed, there were no case reports of ranitidine-induced gynecomastia until 1982, when Tosi and Cagnoli reported a case of painful gynecomastia after eight days treatment with 150 mg/day of ranitidine. A 1994 cohort study (Rodriguez & Jicks, 1994) of 81,535 men treated with cimetidine, misoprostol, omeprazol, or ranitidine for ulcer showed a significantly increased risk of gynecomastia only in cimetidine-treated patients (37,202 men). The risk compared to nonusers (55,763 men) ranged from a 3.4-fold increase at low doses (under 600 mg) to a 43.5-fold increase at higher doses (over 1000 mg). Cimetidine-induced gynecomastia has been eliminated occasionally by substituting ranitidine (Jensen, Collen, McArthur, et al., 1984; Jensen, Collen, Pandol, et al., 1983).

Gynecomastia is listed as a rare side effect in the Physicians Desk Reference for both ranitidine and nizatidine, but not for famotidine. In a summary report of nizatidine side effects in 3,800 patients, the frequency of gynecomastia, impotence, or reduced libido was less than 0.8% and no different from placebo (Cloud, 1987). Only one case of gynecomastia was noted among 6,346 famotidine-treated patients in a 1987 postmarketing survey (R.N. Shackelford, personal communication, August 3, 1991).

Although histamine stimulates prolactin secretion through histamine-1 receptors, it inhibits prolactin through histamine-2 receptors (Knigge, Thuesen, & Christiansen, 1986). Consequently, any histamine-2 antagonist can theoretically increase prolactin by blocking inhibition of prolactin secretion at histamine-2 receptors. In clinical practice only cimetidine seems to have this capability. While cimetidine-induced prolactin increases at normal doses are rarely reported in the literature, there is, nevertheless, some evidence that this may occur. Although 800–1,200 mg/day cimetidine is currently recommended for ulcer treatment, 1,600 mg/day is the recommended therapeutic dose for gastroesophageal reflux. The maintenance dose is typically 400 mg. At normal therapeutic doses, consistent prolactin increases usually do not occur (Barber & Hoare, 1979). Delle Fave et al. (1977) noted increased prolactin in seven ulcer patients treated with 1,600 mg/day cimetidine for eight weeks, but no prolactin increases in three patients who received 1,000 mg/day. A small but significant prolactin increase from 16.3 ng/ml to 21.0 ng/ml was noted by Paulsen et al. (1983) in 10 men given 1,200 mg/day cimetidine for six months. Finally, Leonard, Nickel, and Morales (1989) noted impotence in a hyperprolactinemic patient treated with cimetidine; erectile function and prolactin levels normalized when cimetidine was withdrawn.

In summary, cimetidine may have a prolactin-increasing effect at normal therapeutic oral doses, contrary to claims that it does not. Since increases in prolactin have been associated with erectile dysfunction, a rise in prolactin due to normal therapeutic doses of cimetidine could cause sexual difficulties.

Increases in prolactin have been shown with intravenous infusion of cimetidine in men (Bohnet et al., 1978; Carlson & Ippoliti, 1977; Knigge et al., 1986) or women (Belisle, Patry, & Tetreault, 1982; Carlson, 1981; Iodice, Lombardi, Tommaselli, Rossi, & Minozzi, 1981). Delitala, Devilla, Pende, and Canessa (1982) reported comparable increases in prolactin with intravenous injections of 300 mg ranitidine or 200 mg cimetidine. A dose of 300 mg ranitidine *is from 5 to 10 times as potent* for acid inhibition as a 200 mg dose of cimetidine (McGuigan, 1983). Consequently, cimetidine is much more likely to cause increased prolactin than ranitidine. Famotidine and nizatidine do not appear to affect prolactin.

Knigge et al. (1986) attributed some of cimetidine's effect on prolactin to its antiandrogen properties and a possible central action on brain neurotransmitters (such as increasing serotonin). Kertesz, Somoza, D'Eramo, and Libertun (1987) reported that large increases in prolactin due to cimetidine injections in male rats could be blocked by the nonselective serotonin blockers, methysergide or metergoline (Iodice et al., 1981) or by the specific 5-HT_2 blocker ketanserin. Shi, Patterson, and Sherins (1986) hypothesized that the serotonergic, estrogenic, and antitestosterone effects of cimetidine could synergize to increase prolactin.

A few animal studies have suggested a GABA link in cimetidine's prolactinergic effect, which would identify another mechanism whereby sexual potential could be adversely affected (Lakoski, Aghajanian, & Gallager, 1983; Sibilia, Netti, Guidobono, Pagani, & Pecile, 1985). However, there is no evidence for this effect in humans.

Ranitidine has shown inhibitory effects in humans on serotonin (Lai, Cho, Ogle, & Wang, 1986; Noppen, Jacobs, Van Belle, Herregodts, & Somers, 1988) and estrogen (Berta et al., 1988), and it does not have antiandrogen effects. Without these mechanisms facilitating prolactin secretion, ranitidine appears much less likely than cimetidine to increase prolactin.

Breast Changes in Women

Breast changes in women during cimetidine treatment have been noted only rarely, but that may be due to the fact that any subtle enlargement would be masked by the woman's preexisting breast size. Galactorrhea has been noted in association with hyperprolactinemia in a woman treated with oral cimetidine (1,600 mg) for two months (Delle Fave et al., 1977). Three instances of breast pain or tenderness occurred among 436 patients (sex unspecified) on long-term, low-dose ranitidine maintenance therapy (Penston, 1990).

CIMETIDINE-INDUCED ESTROGEN INCREASES IN BOTH SEXES

Cimetidine has hyperestrogenic side effects in both men and women, secondary to inhibition of estradiol 2-hydroxylation. Increased estrogen levels may diminish sex drive and response in men (Segraves, 1988) and are contraindicated for women with estrogen-dependent breast cancers (Raymond, 1987).

Galbraith and Michnovicz (1989), working at Rockefeller University on grants independent of drug company support, have reported that therapeutic doses of cimetidine increased estrogen in both animals and humans. Levels of exogenous estrogens contained in oral contraceptives are also increased by cimetidine treatment, so it was thought that endogenous estradiol would be similarly increased by cimetidine. However, Galbraith and Jellinck (1989a) found in male rats that cimetidine inhibited the 2-hydroxylation step in estradiol breakdown, as well as other enzymes involved in metabolism of endogenous estradiol. Estradiol metabolism was not changed in female rats, despite a generalized decrease in P-450 enzyme content and activity. Increased estradiol has a negative sexual effect in men and a potentially positive effect in women. The lack of an effect in *female* rats is predictable and does not indicate that the drug is sexually benign.

Galbraith and Jellinck (1989b) also reported that cimetidine reduced the metabolism of both estradiol and testosterone in male rats. No effect on estradiol metabolism or P-450 enzyme content was found with either ranitidine or famotidine. Galbraith and Jellinck (1989a) summarized the complexity of cimetidine's enzyme actions:

> We interpret these results to suggest that cimetidine may exhibit multiple differential inhibitory actions on the metabolism of various endogenous and exogenous substrates in the rat. The resulting inhibitions are dependent on dosage, method of administration, and the sex of the animal, and likely reflect differing susceptibilities of different isoenzymes of cytochrome P-450 to the action of cimetidine. (p. 317)

Recent research articles (Lissak et al., 1989; Michnovicz & Galbraith, 1991) have reported that cimetidine increases estrogen levels through metabolic inhibition and reduces DHEAS adrenal androgen levels apparently through inhibition of P-450 and other enzymes (e.g., 17–20 lyase). Reduced DHEAS may be related to reduced sexual desire and activity in males, as well as to reduced health in many other areas of essential body functions (for example, the immune system; see Chapter 9). Experts on male aging have reported renewed nocturnal erections in multiple sclerosis patients treated for neuropathy with DHEAS supplementation (Eugene Roberts, 1987, personal communication). Raised estrogen levels are also associated with impotence and other male degenerative diseases; in fact, estrogen administration can cause impotence (Ellis & Grayhack, 1963). The effects of cimetidine on estrogen and DHEAS levels have been found at therapeutic doses. The antitestosterone effect of cimetidine, while relatively small, can still cause serious adverse sexual side effects in both men and women through P-450 enzyme alterations, even at the low doses used to treat the common ulcer.

In women, the cimetidine effect differed in premenopausal and postmenopausal women. Michnovicz and Galbraith (1991) found that 1,600 mg/day cimetidine treatment of postmenopausal women for one month increased estradiol and decreased the 2-hydroxylation step. A decrease in 2-hydroxylation was also found with only two weeks of treatment on 800 mg/day. No effect was found in premenopausal women. A previous study (Moller, Lindvig, Klefter, Mosbech, & Jensen, 1989) reported no increased risk of breast or uterine cancer in women on long-term cimetidine. However, the possibility of increased cancer risk in particular subpopulations still remains to be determined through further surveillance.

Cimetidine can cause increased estrogen levels through a second mechanism: inhibiting the metabolism of alcohol, which may increase estradiol levels (Caballeria, Baraona, Rodamilans, & Lieber, 1989b; Van Thiel, 1980). Chronic alcohol consumption has been shown to increase estrogen and decrease testosterone (Gordon et al., 1979; Van Thiel et al., 1985). Increased levels of alcohol due to decreased metabolism can also be expected to decrease testosterone levels, given alcohol's toxic effect on testosterone production (de Moraes & Capaz, 1983). Ranitidine can also inhibit alcohol metabolism, though to a lesser degree than cimetidine. Furthermore, ranitidine does not have a documented estrogenic effect similar to cimetidine. It should be noted that many studies on cimetidine-treated patients have not found altered estrogen levels. For example, Barber (1979) reported no change in estrogens, testosterone, or prolactin in 10 men after 12 weeks of 1,600 mg/day cimetidine ulcer treatment.

Famotidine and ranitidine have not been found to elevate estrogen levels. Berta et al. (1988) showed that on 300 mg/day ranitidine, which is the therapeutic dose for ulcers equivalent to 1,200 mg/day cimetidine, 24 male patients treated for ulcers for one month showed *decreased* estradiol (33.26 pg.ml to 15.81), unchanged testosterone, and increased prolactin (9.03 ng/ml to 21.5 ng/ml). These patients had not received prior histamine-2 antagonist treatment; therefore, their hormonal responses were uninfluenced by prior treatment. Ten men treated with 40 mg famotidine showed no changes in estradiol, testosterone, or prolactin.

In summary, cimetidine appears to increase estrogens, ranitidine to decrease estrogens, and famotidine and nizatidine to cause no change.

CIMETIDINE INHIBITION OF P-450 ENZYMES

Soon after the introduction of cimetidine, reports began to appear on cimetidine's interference with the metabolism of other drugs such as theophylline, beta-blockers, anticonvulsants, and oral contraceptives. Cimetidine increases blood levels of these drugs by inhibiting their metabolic breakdown by P-450 liver enzymes and other enzymes dependent on P-450 activity. The P-450 enzyme system is particularly important for steroid metabolism. As mentioned, cimetidine appears to inhibit P-450 enzymes necessary for the formation of the adrenal androgen DHEAS. Cimetidine's inhibition of P-450 enzymes is due to its imidazole ring structure (though there may be a contributory effect from its cyano side chain). Other histamine-2 antagonists do not have this imidazole ring, so they either do not inhibit P-450 or do so only indirectly through unexplained chemical mechanisms. Drugs with possible adverse sexual effects that have been shown to interact with cimetidine include (Sorkin & Darvey, 1983):

- alcohol
- alprazolam (Xanax)
- carbamazepine (Tegretol)
- chlordiazepoxide (Librium)
- clorazepate (Tranxene)
- desipramine (Norpramin, Pertofrane)
- diazepam (Valium)
- digitoxin (Crystodigin, Furodigin)
- flurazepam (Dalmane)
- furosemide (Lasix)
- imipramine (Tofranil)
- ketoconazole (Nizoral)
- labetalol (Trandate, Normodyne)
- metoprolol (Lopressor)
- metronidazole (Flagyl)
- morphine
- oral contraceptives
- penicillins and various antibiotics
- phenobarbital (Luminal)
- phenytoin (Dilantin)
- proprandolol (Inderal)
- quinidine (Duraquin, Quinidine)
- theophylline (Theo-Dur)
- warfarin (Coumadin)

Cimetidine slows hepatic metabolism and clearance of these drugs, most of which have their own dose-dependent effects on sexual function. The potential for adverse sexual side effects from these drugs is increased when they are taken concomitantly with cimetidine. Therefore, these drugs may have to be used at lower doses or be discontinued altogether when cimetidine is added.

Ranitidine has been shown to bind to cytochrome P-450 only in vitro. In laboratory tests, the affinity of ranitidine was five-fold less than that of cimetidine (Hoensch, Hutzel, Kirch, & Ohnhaus, 1985). However, many drugs have not been tested for cimetidine interactions, so that doctors must closely monitor patients on cimetidine when other medications are taken concomitantly. Impaired drug metabolism due to cimetidine occurs quickly (often within 24 hours or sooner) and usually does not exhibit tolerance with prolonged use. This effect is rapidly reversible, so that there may be a sudden drop in blood levels of concomitant drugs when cimetidine is discontinued. To prevent this effect, in some cases cimetidine should be tapered gradually rather than discontinued abruptly.

INHIBITION OF ALCOHOL METABOLISM

Perhaps the most controversial drug interaction of histamine-2 antagonists is the inhibition of alcohol metabolism, which in turn increases blood alcohol levels. Cimetidine, ranitidine, and nizatidine (but not famotidine) all increase blood alcohol concentrations, presumably by interfering with gastric alcohol dehydrogenase (ADH), which breaks down alcohol in the gastrointestinal tract (Caballeria, Baraona, Rodamilans, & Lieber, 1989a; Holt, 1991; Palmer, 1989). According to Holt (1991), blood alcohol concentrations can be raised by cimetidine or nizatidine from "legal to illegal levels." Caballeria, Baraona, Rodamilans, and Lieber (1987) measured blood alcohol concentrations in male volunteers after one week of treatment with 800 mg/day cimetidine; blood alcohol concentration almost doubled. Both the magnitude and duration of alcohol concentration were increased.

Since cimetidine and ranitidine will now be sold over-the-counter, albeit at lower than prescription doses, they could become a contributing factor to the toxic effects of alcohol use and abuse. Alcohol consumption can itself cause digestive problems requiring histamine-2 antagonist treatment (Holt, 1990). Conversely, alcoholism occurs more frequently in gastrointestinal/ulcer patients than in the general population (Holt, Skinner, & Israel, 1981).

Holt (1991) has shown that cimetidine may have more consistent effects on alcohol metabolism than other histamine-2 antagonists. It is not clear whether cimetidine's inhibition of liver P-450 enzymes is involved in this impact. Toxic alcohol effects such as hyperestrogenic states and interactions with other drugs may be worsened if alcohol and cimetidine are regularly used concomitantly. Furthermore, dangerous combinations such as alcohol and Valium could be potentiated by cimetidine.

Apparently, all histamine-2 antagonists can slow drug metabolism in the gastrointestinal tract through decreased blood flow and inhibition of gastric acid secretion. Sturniolo et al. (1991) found that zinc absorption in men and women was reduced by either cimetidine or ranitidine treatment. Although no studies have indicated zinc deficiency with any histamine-2 antagonists, such a deficiency could have a serious negative effect on gonadal function (Apgar, 1985; Mahajan et al., 1982).

CONCLUSIONS

Most of the histamine-2 antagonists have been associated with some adverse sexual consequences. However, there is a large disparity between the adverse sexual effects of cimetidine and the other three drugs:

- Cimetidine has measurable antiandrogenic properties that interfere with testosterone metabolism and receptor binding.
- Used at normal therapeutic doses, cimetidine reduces DHEAS, which could adversely affect sexual function in both men and women.
- Cimetidine increases estrogen metabolism, which can cause impotence in men.
- Cimetidine intensifies the toxic effects of other drugs by interfering with their metabolism; many of these drugs are themselves sexually toxic.
- Cimetidine appears to decrease sperm count.
- Cimetidine inhibits P-450 enzyme activity.

ALTERNATIVES

Patients who are sexually dysfunctional should not be treated with cimetidine unless there are overriding concerns. Most patients without sexual problems would prefer to receive a drug that does not have the potential to compromise sexual function. Men concerned about fertility should probably avoid cimetidine; women for whom estrogens are contraindicated should take one of the other histamine-2 antagonists. All the histamine-2 antagonists, except famotidine, can potentiate alcohol. Therefore, famotidine seems the best alternative for alcohol drinkers, especially chronic alcoholics. Ranitidine has few adverse sexual side effects and may even improve sex drive in some cases. Because famotidine and nizatidine are newer histamine-2 antagonists, less is known about their impact on sexual function. Based on their mechanisms of action and chemical structures, it is quite possible that they are less sexually toxic than their predecessors.

In addition to diet programs, aggressive treatment with combination antibiotic therapies may reduce or eliminate the need for histamine-2 antagonists.

Helicobacter Pylori Infection

A recent remarkable discovery has established that possibly the majority of cases of gastritis and ulcer are due to infection with the bacteria *Helicobacter pylori (H. pylori)* (Hopkins & Morris, 1994). Indeed, H. pylori may be one of the most common human infections and was long ignored because it was so widespread among asymptomatic individuals. In developed countries, infection occurs in more than 50% of adults, while infection rates may reach 90% in developing countries (Hopkins & Morris, 1994).

Only a minority of infected individuals will develop H. pyloric-induced gastrointestinal pathology in their lifetimes, despite frequent infection during childhood (Hopkins & Morris, 1994). Why some individuals are more vulnerable or susceptible to infection and pathological progression than others is currently unknown. Low socioeconomic status is associated with unhygienic conditions that increase the probability of H. pylori infection (Hopkins & Morris, 1994). In the United States, infection with H. pylori in African-Americans and Hispanics is twice that seen in Caucasians, even after adjustment is made for socioeconomic factors (Graham, Malaty, & Go, 1994). Relatively higher rates of infection have been shown in individuals with low socioeconomic status during childhood, regardless of their current socioeconomic status (Graham et al., 1994).

Ulcers and ulcer complications or gastric cancer occur in 15–40% of H. pylori-infected individuals (Graham et al., 1994). Ulcer disease usually runs in families, and twin studies show a genetic predisposition to H. pylori infection (Graham et al., 1994). Morbidity may be related to high intrinsic gastric-acid secretion, which may be limited by H_2 antagonist gastric-acid inhibition, but cured only by appropriate antibiotic treatment supplemented by an acute pharmacological reduction in gastric-acid secretion (Hopkins & Morris, 1994; Tytgat, 1994). Consequently, though individuals may have been infected with H. pylori since early childhood, they may be bothered by symptoms such as dyspepsia, gastritis, and ulcers only after periods of stress that increase chronic gastric-acid secretion. In such cases, the typical medical treatment is OTC antacids or prescription of H_2 antagonists; however, the problem may be cured within a few weeks by antibiotic eradication of the H. pylori infection.

Gastric inflammation and ulcer may also be caused by oversensitivity or overuse of nonsteroidal anti-inflammatory pain relievers (NSAIDs), in which case, bacteria infection may be irrelevant and treatment consists of control of further damage by gastric-acid inhibition with the synthetic prostaglandin E-analog misoprostol (Cytotec) and discontinuance of NSAIDs (misoprostol can cause chronic diarrhea but should not have adverse sexual side effects).

Eradication of H. pylori may cure duodenal and gastric ulcer disease, and this cure may last as long as there is no reinfection, regardless of stress levels (Tytgat, 1994). However, pharmacological treatment of H. pylori infection is successful only 50–90% of the time, and various treatment regimes may be necessary to achieve eradication (Rune, 1994). Simple and accurate diagnostic tests for post-treatment confirmation of H. pylori eradication are not yet available (Rune, 1994).

The ideal treatment for H. pylori-induced gastric pathology has not been agreed upon. Currently, triple therapy with bismuth subcitrate, metronidazole, and tetracycline is considered the initial treatment of choice (Hopkins & Morris, 1994). Omeprazole (Prilosec) may be added for short-term profound inhibition of gastric secretion. Side effects of this triple therapy may be unpleasant (nausea 31%, diarrhea 7%, dizziness 4%, drowsiness 4%, and burning in the mouth 4%) (Hopkins & Morris, 1994). The conventional length of treatment is 14 days with this or alternative treatments. The most promising alternative therapy with less side effects is the combination of omeprazole (40 mg) with amoxicillin (2000 mg) or clarithromycin (1000 mg) for 14 days, which typically achieves eradication in over 80% of cases (Axon, 1994; Labenz, Leverkus, & Börsch, 1994; Rune, 1994).

Alternative Drugs for Gastric Symptoms

Drugs used for heartburn and gastroesophageal reflux include antacids (Di-Gel, Maalox, Mylanta, Tums, etc.) and H_2 antagonists. Metoclopromide (Reglan) and domperidone (Motilium in Canada, not yet available in the United States) are antidopaminergic prokinetic drugs used for these symptoms, which may cause tardive dyskinesia and hyperprolactinemia—serious side effects that are aversive to sexual drive and function and to general well-being (Medical Letter, 1994).

Cisapride (Propulsid) is a prokinetic drug recently approved for gastroesophageal reflux, which acts through serotonin stimulation to release acetycholine, thereby increasing gastrointestinal motility and accelerating gastric emptying (Medical Letter, 1994). Cisapride has also been shown to reduce dyspepsia and gastroparesis (Medical Letter, 1994). Omeprazole (Prilosec) may be used over short periods for resolution of acute inflammation (healing) and is a more potent blocker of acid secretion than H_2 antagonists (Medical Letter, 1994). It will be interesting to see if cisapride proves effective in treating constipation associated with irritable bowel syndrome. Sexual side effects of cisapride have not yet been studied.

Sucralfate (Carafate) is an aluminum salt that adheres to gastrointestinal tissue and protects against gastric acid inflammation with a viscous mucosal barrier. It may be used along with antacids for gastritis or ulcerative conditions. Its most common side effect is constipation.

25

Miscellaneous Drugs

OBJECTIVES

- To highlight several categories of drugs that fit into no previous category
- To demonstrate that little information exists regarding sexual side effects
- To encourage further research and investigation of the sexual side effects of little-researched drugs not in these categories

Most drugs not described in *Sexual Pharmacology* have either not been studied in respect to their impact on sexual function, or there is such a paucity of information available that no meaningful conclusions could be drawn.

The drugs discussed in the preceding chapters were included in this volume because they were verified in the research (both animal and human) as sex offender drugs, or because anecdotal information volunteered by patients has suggested the possibility of their adverse effects. Much less is known about the sexual effects of the drugs discussed in this chapter. Nonetheless, their inclusion is important. The following drug groups are discussed:

- cold/allergy medications
- asthma medications
- anticonvulsants
- anticancer drugs
- cardiac drugs
- hypolipidemics (cholesterol reducers)

COLD/ALLERGY MEDICATIONS

- chlorpheniramine (Chlor-Trimeton)
- cough medicine (guaifenesin-expectorant, dextromethorphan-synthetic morphine, antitussive)
- diphenhydramine hydrochloride (Benadryl)
- diphenhydramine citrate (Bufferin AF, Excedrin PM)
- phenylephrine hydrochloride (Neo-synephrine)
- pseudoephedrine (Sudafed)
- triprolidine/pseudoephedrine (Actifed)

Cold treatments include antihistamines such as diphenhydramine, which are discussed in Chapter 19; decongestants such as pseudoephedrine or PPA products are discussed in Chapter 23. Since cholinergic and histaminergic activity appears to be involved in sexual function, these drugs with anticholinergic and/or antihistaminergic effects may adversely affect sexual function. Sympathetic stimulation from decongestant medications may cause constriction of blood flow so that erection may be compromised; on occasion, some of these sympathomimetics are used to treat ejaculatory inhibition (whether drug induced or spontaneous). Nevertheless, the sexual impact of cold and allergy medications only becomes noticeable with chronic use.

ASTHMA MEDICATIONS

Sexual dysfunction is frequent in patients with pulmonary diseases of all kinds. In cases of chronic obstructive pulmonary disease, impotence rates of 19–35% have been shown; in addition, a decrease or cessation of intercourse may occur in over 50% of patients (McSweeny & Labuhn, 1990). Patients with breathing difficulties are often anxious and irritable, so that sexual and marital difficulties may exist prior to initiation of drug treatment. Dyspnea occurring during sexual activity can cause further anxiety, irritability, and weakness.

Beta$_2$ Agonists and Sympathomimetics

- albuterol (Proventil, Ventolin)
- metaproterenol (Alupent, Metaprel)
- terbutaline (Brethine)
- epinephrine (Adrenalin Bronkaid Mist, Primatene Mist)
- isoproterenol (Isuprel, Medihaler-ISO)

The prominent adverse reactions of beta-agonists include nervousness, tremor, tachycardia, arrhythmias, palpitations, nausea, and headache (Lulich, Goldie, Ryan, & Paterson, 1986). The therapeutic aspect of the sympathomimetic action appears to be the formation of cyclic adenosine monophosphate (cAMP), the natural mediator of respiratory smooth muscle tone. Additionally, there are increases in mucociliary transport and airway surface water and decreases in mast cell sensitivity. Advantages of medications utilizing beta$_2$ agonists over general sympathomimetics include longer duration of action (4–6 versus 1–2 hours) and beta$_2$ selectivity. However, these agents have a slower onset of action. Beta$_2$ stimulation is chiefly responsible for bronchial relaxation and muscle tremor. Tachycardia, palpitations, anxiety, nausea, and hyperglycemia are chiefly alpha and beta$_1$ adrenergic reactions. Through stimulation of adrenergic activity and tissue relaxation, beta$_2$ agonists may have positive effects on psychogenic impotence, but nervousness and tremor counteract these gains.

Beta$_2$ agonists treat only asthmatic symptoms, not the disease itself. Asthmatic wheezing, coughing, and difficulty breathing are apparently generated by exaggerated responsiveness to bronchoconstrictor stimuli, due to an inflammatory process that is not reduced by beta$_2$ agonists (Frew & Holgate, 1993). Indeed, prolonged and continuous treatment with beta$_2$ agonists may lead to a decreased response (tachyphylaxis) and may cause rebound effects (e.g., severe acute bronchoconstriction, increased hypersensitivity) when these agonists are withdrawn, resulting in a deterioration in asthma control and airway/lung function (Cheung et al., 1992). Consequently, there may be increased asthma-related morbidity and mortality (Tattersfield, 1994).

Xanthines

Xanthines such as theophylline have long been used as medium potency bronchodilators. While they increase cAMP by phosphodiesterase inhibition, their chief mechanism of action is still not known. It is very likely that they stimulate by blocking inhibitory adenosine receptors (E. Richelson, personal communication, 1993). Toxicity increases noticeably slightly above therapeutic levels and includes seizures, nervousness, nausea, diarrhea, headache, insomnia, cardiac arrhythmias, and hyperglycemia. We have noted unpredictable psychiatric side effects (including anxiety, panic, hostility, and hypersensitivity) when theophylline is used concurrently with antidepressants. Irritability and restlessness occur frequently during regular use and may cause interpersonal overreactivity leading to argument, and hostility. This nervousness and irritability generated from xanthines are negative to sexual desire and function. While these negative effects have been noted in our clinical practice, such effects have yet to be documented in the literature.

Trental, which is discussed later in this chapter, is an atypical xanthine; it doesn't block adenosine, has little in common with theophylline or caffeine, and is not used to treat asthma.

Corticosteroids

Corticosteroid use is based on the recognition that asthma and bronchospasm often involve inflammation of bronchial and throat tissue. This inflammation can lead to epithelial damage and leucocyte infiltration through an increase in eosinophils, T-cells, platelets, macrophages, and cytokine mediators (Frew & Holgate, 1993). Corticosteroids such as beclomethasone (Beclovent, Beconase Inhaler) and triamcinolone (Azmacort) are particularly effective in reducing allergic and hypersensitive reactions, but can cause reduced tissue sensitivity and inconsistent mental attention. Fungal infections such as oral candidiasis are frequent. Rash, hoarseness, dry mouth, and suppressed hypothalamic-pituitary-adrenal function are additional disturbing physical reactions, not to mention osteoporosis, which may occur with long-term treatment. Psychiatric reactions such as delirium and steroid-like psychoses (including paranoia, euphoria-dysphoria, depression, and aggression) should be carefully monitored and avoided. Sodium and fluid retention, easy bruising, and weight gain due to increased appetite can decrease personal attractiveness. In addition, since corticosteroids decrease tissue sensitivity and oppose testosterone and DHEAS production, they may be expected to have adverse sexual effects which increase with dose and extended use. These negative consequences of corticosteroids should be weighed against the probability that they directly treat the underlying inflammatory disease. They may be used on an acute intermittent basis more effectively than $beta_2$ agonists.

Anticholinergics

Anticholinergic agents have been used to treat bronchial obstruction and spasm since antiquity. The anticholinergic side effects on the bladder, gut, heart, eyes, mouth, and secretory glands have always been a limiting factor in their use. Given these side effects, anticholinergics can potentially interfere with kissing and intercourse by causing dry mouth and dry vagina. They also have the potential to interfere with erection and orgasm. The commonly prescribed anticholinergic is ipratropium (Atrovent), a methylated analogue of atropine, with a greater selectivity for bronchial tissue. It only minimally crosses the blood-brain barrier, does not affect mucus secretion, does not have significant cardiovascular effects, and is poorly absorbed by oral or gastric mucosa. It is administered by aerosol inhalation, like most bronchodilators. Compared to $beta_2$ agonists, it causes more nausea and cough but less tremor and worsening of asthmatic symptoms (Tashkin et al., 1986). However, it is less potent than other bronchodilators and is considered a second-line treatment.

Alternatives

Of the available bronchodilators, the $beta_2$ agonists appear to be the least sexually toxic. Tolerance to their hyperstimulating influence often occurs, and their cAMP molecular effect should not interfere with sexual function. However, very little research has been conducted on the sexual effects of $beta_2$ agonists. Benelli, Zanoli, and Bertolini (1990) have shown that clenbuterol improved copulatory behavior in sexually sluggish rats, but disturbed the behavior of sexually vigorous rats. However, after seven days the decrement in sexually vigorous rats was no longer present, while the beneficial effect on sexually sluggish rats persisted.

ANTICONVULSANTS

Seizure disorders have been associated with both hypersexuality and hyposexuality. Hypersexuality and sexual deviancy, including fetishism, exhibitionism, orgasmic dyscontrol, and transvestism, have all been reported (Toone, 1986). However, hyposexuality is far more characteristic of epileptics, especially those on medication. In a study by Morrell (1991) using retrospective self-report of sexual drive and behavior, the incidence of sexual dysfunction ranged from 14% to 66%. In another study comparing 50 women (mean age = 36.6 years) treated with anticonvulsants for epilepsy to a community control, Bergen, Daugherty, and Eckenfels (1992) noted that the epileptic women were less likely to report sexual desire and activity at the highest level and more likely to report severely decreased sexual desire and frequency of intercourse. Toone (1986) found that only 36% of epileptic patients showed sexual activity leading to orgasm within a year time period; 44% had never experienced sexual activity leading to orgasm. Toone (1985, 1986) has described hyposexuality among epileptic patients in a series of reviews during the 1980s.

Though typically attributed to temporal lobe epilepsy (Gastaut & Collomb, 1954; Sorensen & Bolwig, 1987), hyposexuality can occur in patients with all forms of epilepsy (Toone, 1986). (It seems to be more frequent when the epileptic condition is associated with intellectual, neurological, or psychiatric degeneration.) In fact, patients with epilepsy show hyposexuality as well as reduced fertility more than the normal population, regardless of whether they are treated with anticonvulsant medication (Toone, 1985).

The incidence of decreased sexual desire and responsiveness among men and women with temporal lobe epilepsy ranges from 31-67% in different studies (Herzog, Seibel, Schomer, Vaitukaitas, & Geschwind, 1986a, 1986b). This statistic is not surprising, given that the temporal lobe includes limbic structures (such as the amygdala) that prominently affect sexual desire. Despite the obvious prevalence of sexual abnormalities associated with this condition, there has been little investigation of sexual side effects of the anticonvulsant drugs. One exception is the work of Herzog et al. (1986b), who studied sexual dysfunction in women with temporal lobe epilepsy. A variety of physical conditions were noted: amenorrhea (14–20%), menorrhagia (43%), overall menstrual dysfunction (56%), polycystic ovarian syndrome (20%), and infertility (46%). Decreased sexual desire appeared to be associated with EEG abnormalities lateralized to the right temporal lobe (which is assumed to be more sensitive to emotional content than the more language-oriented left hemisphere). Seven of 13 women with right-sided seizure focus were found to have decreased sexual desire, compared to zero of nine with a left-sided focus. Herzog reported that menstrual disorders in women with temporal lobe epilepsy were as frequent in patients not treated with anticonvulsants (60%) as in those treated (53%).

Herzog et al. (1986a) found decreased sexual desire or potency in 55% (11/20) of male patients with temporal lobe epilepsy. The average age of these patients was 35 and the average duration of their seizure disorder was 13 years. Thus, they suffered from sexual and reproductive dysfunction during their peak reproductive years. No relation between sexual dysfunction and side of epileptic focus was found. Abnormalities of sperm morphology and motility that may occur in epileptic men may be due to LHRH-LH dysfunction or various hormonal and chemical deficiencies that occur during long-term anticonvulsant therapy.

Valproate, Valproic Acid (Depakote, Depakene)

Valproate (available as divalproex sodium, Depakote, an enteric-coated combination of sodium valproate and valproic acid) and valproic acid (Depakene) have long been available as treatments for epilepsy, but their use has increased during the last five years. They have broad-spectrum efficacy for all seizure types and also have been used to treat bipolar disorders (findings on valproate are the same for valproic acid). The use of valproate has been restricted as a result of associated hepatic dysfunction and damage as well as thrombocytopenia. In addition, teratogenicity renders this drug contraindicated for pregnant women (Cotariu & Zaidman, 1991). Alopecia, weight gain, and tremor may also discourage its use. Dizziness, motor complaints, sedation, and gastrointestinal distress are similar to the symptoms found with other anticonvulsants. Skin rash occurs less frequently on valproate than phenytoin, but weight gain may be greater (Mattson, 1990).

Isojarvi, Parkarinen, Ylipalosarri, and Myllyla (1990) have shown desirable hormonal effects with valproate treatment compared to treatment with other anticonvulsants. The chief feature that distinguishes valproate is its lack of an inhibitory action on the adrenal androgens DHEA/DHEAS. Levesque et al. (1986) have shown that lowered DHEAS in treated temporal lobe epileptics was due to anticonvulsant treatment, not to the seizure disorder itself. Since optimum levels of DHEA/DHEAS are essential to sexuality, health, and longevity, preservation of normal DHEA/DHEAs levels with valproate is an excellent reason to select it over other anticonvulsants. Also in contrast to other anticonvulsants, thyroxine and free thyroxine are not lowered by valproate, and sex hormone-binding globulin (SHBG) is not increased. Furthermore, the overall free testosterone index may increase with valproate. Franceschi et al. (1984) found that all anticonvulsants except valproate increased basal and stimulated prolactin levels. The benign nature of valproate/valproic acid is apparently due to the fact that it is not an inducer of liver enzymes (Mattson, Cramer, Williamson, & Novelly, 1978). Due to its overall hormonal profile, we would anticipate that less impotence, fatigue, and skin toxicity would occur with valproate. Its lack of androgen inhibition suggests that decreased sex drive would be minimal. MacPhee et al. (1988) recommended valproate for epileptic patients reporting sexual dysfunction. Renri et al. (1990) have also shown that anticonvulsants can cause bone atrophy, which would appear to be avoided by the use of valproate.

Valproate has also been shown to be an effective treatment for acute manic states (Gelenberg, 1991; Gerner & Stanton, 1992) and bipolar disorder (Jacobsen, 1993; McElroy, Keck, Pope, & Hudson, 1992; Post, Weiss, & Chuang, 1992). It may be used in addition to lithium in difficult-to-treat manic or bipolar patients (McFarland et al. 1990).

Carbamazepine (Tegretol)

Carbamazepine (Tegretol) use has also increased over the last decade. It is reputed to be less teratogenic than other anticonvulsants (*Lancet* editorial, 1991), but hormonal abnormalities are common: DHEAS, free testosterone, and thyroxine are decreased; prolactin and SHBG are increased (Connell et al., 1984; MacPhee et al., 1988). Overall, the free testosterone index decreases with both phenytoin and carbamazepine. Dizziness and incoordination are similarly frequent on carbamazepine and phenytoin (Mattson, 1990). Bone marrow suppression and agranulocytosis or aplastic anemia occur only rarely, but are cause for great concern (Neppe, Tucker, & Wilensky, 1988). This hematologic toxicity limits carbamazepine use more than its hormonal alterations, which are not as well-known. Considerable weight gain may occur on carbamazepine, but not as frequently as on valproate (Lampl, Eshel, Rappaport, & Sarova-Pinchas, 1991). Carbamazepine also has a reputation for minimal but adverse cognitive and behavioral effects (Mattson, 1990; Wildin, Pleuvry, & Mawer, 1993). It has been investigated for other indications, including treatment of bipolar disorders, aggression and rage syndromes, and pain syndromes such as trigeminal neuralgia (Ballenger, 1988; Keck, McElroy & Friedman, 1992; Malcolmb, Ballenger, Sturgis, & Anton, 1989; Monroe, 1989; Patterson, 1988; Yatham & Mehale, 1988).

Phenytoin (Dilantin)

Despite its widespread use, phenytoin (Dilantin) is a fairly toxic medication. Neuropathy and cerebellar degeneration, indicated by side-to-side eyeball movements (nystagmus), as well as ataxia and incoordination are relatively frequent with chronic use (Mattson, 1990). Peripheral blood disorders such as leukopenia are frequent but rarely serious. Hypertrophic side effects are common, including thickened gums (gingival hyperplasia), excessive hair growth, and lymphoproliferative disorders. Dermatological effects occur more frequently than on other anticonvulsants, particularly androgenic alterations such as coarsened features, acne, and hirsutism.

Increases in SHBG with anticonvulsants, which decrease testosterone availability, may be due to liver enzyme induction (Dana-Haeri, Oxley, & Richens, 1982) (interactions with other drugs are also likely due to this enzyme induction). Although testosterone levels increase with phenytoin, SHBG, which binds testosterone, also increases, so that free testosterone does not increase during phenytoin treatment. Teratogenic effects, termed the "fetal hydantoin syndrome" (Hanson & Smith, 1975), include mental deficiency, coarse facial features, and small head circumference (Kaneko et al., 1984). Sexual effects of phenytoin are dose-related and are associated primarily with sedation and neurological disturbances. Since it increases prolactin and decreases DHEAS, phenytoin may be expected to have negative sexual effects with the extended use required for its therapeutic effect.

Primidone (Mysoline) and Phenobarbital

Primidone (Mysoline) and phenobarbital are barbiturates used to treat epilepsy and are more frequently associated with decreased sexual desire and potency than other anticonvulsants (Mattson & Cramer, 1985). Mattson (1990) suggested switching to carbamazepine or phenytoin when sexual dysfunction occurs during barbiturate treatment, but failed to note the frequent sexual dysfunction and hormonal abnormalities prevalent with these alternative anticonvulsants. On phenobarbital and primidone there is a high frequency of connective tissue pathology, including Peyronie's disease, Dupuytren's contractures (thickening of fibrous tissue of the palm, causing contraction of fingers), and generalized aches and pains (Mattson, 1990); sedation is also more noticeable than on other anticonvulsants (Beghi et al., 1986). While other barbiturate side effects often decrease over the first six months, sexual dysfunction may continue to increase with chronic treatment. In an extensive VA hospital study, complete seizure control with primidone and phenobarbital was less dependable than with carbamazepine (Mattson, 1990). However, the cost of generic phenobarbital is far less than other anticonvulsant drugs, which encourages its continued widespread use.

New Anticonvulsant Drugs

Many years have passed since any novel antiepileptic drugs have been marketed. A glycine-receptor antagonist (Upton, 1994), felbamate (Felbatol), was marketed in 1993, but removed from the market due to potential severe toxicity in 1994. Regulation of seizure activity through direct modulation of the glutamate/excitatory amino acid, NDMA receptor system, as with felbamate, remains a promising mechanism of action for the development of highly effective anticonvulsants with lowered levels of hormonal abnormalities and sexual side effects.

Other new anticonvulsants that work chiefly through enhancement of inhibitory GABA-mediated activity (gabapentin and vigabatrin) have shown efficacy in clinical testing (Upton, 1994). Gabapentin (Neurontin) was approved by the Federal Drug Administration in 1994 as an anticonvulsant. Another newly marketed anticonvulsant, lamotrigine (Lamictal), apparently acts through stabilizing membrane cation conductance, preventing the pathological release of excess glutamate and other excitatory neurotransmitters (Upton, 1994). Lamotrigine is currently approved for use in addition to other anticonvulsants in adults with partial seizures (*Medical Letter*, 1995).

One way or another, these new anticonvulsants inhibit or regulate glutamate/excitatory amino acid activity in limbic areas of the brain that effect cognition and sexual desire (Graves & Leppik, 1991). It remains to be seen whether they can effectively control epilepsy without significantly impairing cognition and sexual motivation.

Hopefully, some of these novel anticonvulsants will be relatively free of teratogenic fetal death and abnormalities. Of existing anticonvulsants, phenobarbital has been associated with the highest rate of major abnormalities (23.8%), phenytoin the next highest (10.7%), and carbamazepine the least (3%) (Waters, Belai, Gott, Shen, & De Georgio, 1994). Fetal deaths and neural tube defects, including spina bifida, have been noted in women treated with any available antiepileptic medication, including carbamazepine and valproic acid, but phenytoin and barbiturates (phenobarbital and primidone) seem most likely to cause pregnancy, infant deaths, and birth defects (Hiilesmaa, 1992; Waters et al., 1994).

ANTICANCER DRUGS

- alkylators (decarbazine, hexamethylamine, busulphan, chlorambucil, cyclophosphamide)

- vinblastine (Velban, procarbazine, methotrexate—4-amino-10-methylfolic acid)
- 5-fluorouracil (Efudex)
- alkeran melphalan—L-phenylalanine mustard
- l-asparaginase (Elspar)

Medical attention to cancer treatment has not generally concerned sexual side effects. Understandably, the focus has been on preservation of life, retarding cancer growth, and prevention of pain and organ degeneration. The pharmacological treatment of cancer remains largely limited to toxic drugs that have acute and system-wide suppressive effects that could be expected to extend to the area of sexual function. Usually, the adverse sexual effects disappear after treatment is discontinued, but not always. In one study, half of the men treated with chemotherapy for Hodgkin's disease reported decreased sexual desire at the time of diagnosis, 85% reported decreased desire during chemotherapy, and 40% reported decreased desire long after treatment had ended (Chapman, Sutcliffe, & Malpas, 1981). Even when sexual desire is maintained, orgasmic intensity is often decreased and dry orgasm may occur. Sexual dysfunction that develops during chemotherapy may be accompanied by irritability and sometimes physical violence.

Of the few anticancer substances that have been evaluated from a sexual perspective, procarbazine, busulfan, chlorambucil, and cyclophosphamide have been shown to cause azoospermia, testicular damage, and amenorrhea (Averette, Boike, & Jarrell, 1990; Chapman, 1984). While women treated for cancer often claim that their sexual desire does not change, examination of sexual activity indicates a decrease (Chapman, Sutcliffe, & Malpas, 1979). Sexual desire frequently shifts to a desire for intimate closeness, distinct from actual sexual activity. Within three years of chemotherapy, Chapman (1984) reported that 70% of the women in his study acknowledged decreased or totally absent sexual desire. Sexual deficits increased with ovarian failure/premature menopause due to cancer treatment and were worsened by increased insomnia, irritability, and hot flashes. Women under 30 may be especially disturbed by their loss of reproductive function, associated with a concomitant loss of self-confidence and self-esteem. Campos (1972) found that continued chemotherapy and radiation treatment caused a "continuous positive aging" pattern.

Certain cancers and the associated surgeries can cause sexual dysfunction without other adjunctive treatments. Colon and rectal cancer cause physiological sexual disruption as well as shame associated with colostomy. Forty percent of male colostomy patients have been found to suffer impaired erection due to organic lesions from surgery, and sexual intercourse decreased in 75% of patients (Burnish, Meyerowitz, Carey, & Morrow, 1987).

Depressed mood has been proposed to promote cancer by causing a decline of the immune system (Linkins & Comstock, 1990; Noyes & Kathol, 1986). Depressive illness has been shown to occur more frequently in a two-year period in cancer patients treated with combination cyclophosphamide, methotrexate, and 5-fluorouracil than in those treated with melphalan or not given chemotherapy (Noyes & Kathol, 1986). Depression seems to occur most often with vinblastine, l-asparaginase, and the alkylating drugs decarbazine and hexamethylamine (Noyes & Kathol, 1986).

In Israel a new approach to chemotherapy is being used with some success. Instead of taking treatment intravenously or orally, the site of the cancer is isolated surgically and chemotherapy is applied locally. Using this method, the concentration given can be considerably higher and there are no general side effects. Patients do not experience the nausea and hair loss for which chemotherapy is so infamous. Temporary and long-term sexual effects are probably eliminated as well.

Tamoxifen (Nolvadex) Treatment for Breast Cancer

Over the last ten years tamoxifen (Nolvadex) has been shown to reduce the incidence of relapse in women treated for breast cancer and to reduce the incidence of breast cancer when used prophylactically (Plowman, 1993). Given the controversy involved in treating healthy women with a hormonally-active drug prior to actual disease, a $68 million-dollar nationwide clinical trial was initiated in the United States in 1992 to test definitively whether tamoxifen is safe and effective for prophylactic use in healthy women at risk (Marshall, 1994). Despite scandal and suspicion created by the revelation of fraudulent data by a trial investigator, and the evidence of an increase in endometrial cancer in tamoxifen-treated women, as well as possible liver damage and increased thrombosis (Marshall, 1994), the trial is continuing. Tamoxifen is expected to be very effective for prevention of breast cancer and, serendipitously, has been found to have estrogen-like effects in reducing cardiovascular morbidity and mortality as well as preserving bone mass and thus reducing the risk of osteoporosis (Plowman, 1993). Apparently, tamoxifen works as an anti-estrogen agonist in other parts of the body.

It should be noted that endometrial cancer is relatively infrequent and often curable, whereas metastatic breast cancer is frequent and often fatal (Jordan, 1992). Other toxic effects of tamoxifen, such as liver damage, have not been proved, and would be so rare as to be irrelevant, given tamoxifen's health benefits. Tamoxifen itself is used as chemotherapy for the treatment of liver cancer (hepatocellular carcinoma) (Jordan, 1992). More than a million women around the world are currently being treated with tamoxifen (Jordan, 1992). Reduction of cardiovascular disease with tamoxifen treatment is apparently due to an estrogen-like lowering of total cholesterol and low-density lipoprotein (LDL) cholesterol levels (Dewar et al., 1992; Love et al., 1991). A remarkably comprehensive survey, published in *Lancet* by the Early Breast Cancer Trialists' Collaborative Group (1992) of 133 randomized trials involving 31,000 recurrences and 24,000 deaths among 75,000 women treated for breast disease, showed a 25% reduction in annual rates of recurrence, a 17% reduction in annual rates of mortality, and a 39% reduced risk of development of contralateral breast cancer. Prominent side effects of normal doses (10–40 mg) of tamoxifen treatment include hot flushes, tachycardia, cessation of menstruation in premenopausal women, nausea, edema, leukopenia, vaginitis, vaginal discharge, even loss of top octaves in singers' voices (Goodare, 1992; Plowman, 1993; Rostom & Gershuny, 1992).

Despite noting that tamoxifen therapy has far less impact on female sexuality than other kinds of chemotherapy (Kaplan, 1992b), Helen Singer Kaplan (1992a) reports that some women on adjuvant tamoxifen therapy complain of drying and constriction of the vagina, though in most patients vaginal lubrication is "totally unaffected." Some women on tamoxifen report increased vaginal lubrication. One postmenopausal female carried a towel with her on which to sit, because her lubrication became so copious in response to the drug. However, some women treated by Kaplan also complained of decreased libido and orgastic response—symptoms that resemble those of androgen deficiency (Kaplan, 1992a).

Many perimenopausal and postmenopausal women treated for breast cancer with tamoxifen experience vaginal dryness and decreased libido and sensation that is a long-term result of estrogen deprivation rather than an effect of androgen deficiency (which commonly occurs in women who are aging or have disease states). Bird, Masters, Sterns, and Clark (1985) found no reduction in testosterone, free testosterone, or DHEAS in a careful endocrine study of six postmenopausal women treated with tamoxifen for breast cancer. In female rates treated with tamoxifen (Whalen, 1984), there was an increase in the display of male-typical mounting responses, indicating an androgen-like effect. Similarly in male chickens (cockerels), tamoxifen enhanced male secondary sex characteristics, testes growth, sperm, volume, and sexual activity (Rozenboim, Dgany, Robinzon, Arnon, & Snapir, 1989). Tamoxifen treatment of infertile men leads to a decrease in prolactin and no change or an increase in sperm, testosterone, sexual activity, libido, and orgasm (Comhaire, 1976; Gooren, 1985; Lewis-Jones, Lynch, Machin, & Desmond, 1987; Noci, Chelo, Saltarelli, Donaticori, & Scarselli, 1985).

It is interesting that tamoxifen was originally formulated in 1966 as an oral contraceptive, but was found to stimulate rather than inhibit ovulation (Fentiman & Powles, 1987). However, recent findings from premenopausal women have shown that menstruation may cease in up to 50% of those treated with tamoxifen (Goodare, 1992). Tamoxifen (20 mg/day over three months) has been shown in placebo-controlled trials to reduce premenstrual pain (mastalgia); and in clinical practice, tamoxifen can be effective at even 10 mg/day for the treatment of mastalgia (Fentiman, 1986; Fentiman, Caleffi, Rodin, Murphy, & Fogelman, 1989; Fentiman & Powles, 1987).

Herbs, Vitamins, and Minerals for Cancer Treatment

Paclitaxel (Taxol) is an extract from the bark of the Pacific yew tree recently approved by the Federal Drug Administration for treatment of ovarian cancer (Sifton, 1994). Investigational trials are being conducted to evaluate Taxol use in breast, lung, and other cancers. It is second-line therapy for use where primary chemotherapy has not been effective, and it must be given intravenously at a hospital or clinic (Sifton, 1994). There is no information on whether its sexual side effects are any more or less than other conventional anticancer drugs. To avoid allergic reactions, treatment with corticosteroids is often necessary (Sifton, 1994), which has an inhibitory effect on sexuality.

Selenium, a natural trace element mineral, is heavily promoted by alternative therapy/heath store organizations for cancer chemoprevention (Hocman, 1988). Evidence for its questionable efficacy was detailed by Birt (1989). Toxicity commonly occurs at doses somewhat higher than those used to treat cancer; symptoms include bad breath (garlic or sour mild odor) as well as nausea, diarrhea, and toxic degenerative changes in the hair and nails (Fan & Kizer, 1990).

Vitamins A, C, and E have limited but accepted anticarcinogenic actions (Birt, 1989; Jensen & Madsen, 1988). As with many lethal illnesses, increased intake of vegetables and fruits may contribute to successful immune function, and loss of excess weight is always recommended (Jensen & Madsen, 1988).*

CARDIAC DRUGS

- digitalis glycosides (Digitalis purpura/foxglove, digitoxin, digoxin)

In men, long-term digitalis treatment causes increased estrogen and decreased testosterone and luteinizing hormone (Stoffer, Hynes, Jiany, & Ryan, 1973; Tappler & Katz, 1979). Fourteen men (mean age = 34) with rheumatic heart disease on digoxin for two or more years were compared to 12 men with untreated rheumatic heart disease (Neri et al., 1980). Estradiol levels were twice as high in digoxin men compared to controls (62.07 pg/ml versus 31.83); testosterone (223 ng/ml versus 532) and luteinizing hormone (1.16 mIU/ml versus 2.49) were decreased by more than half. Average testosterone was lowered to a subnormal level (223 ng/ml). Sexual desire, erectile function, and frequency of sexual activity were reduced in five of 14 men on digoxin but in none of the 12 controls. Sexual reductions occurred in the men with the most severe hormonal changes who had been on digoxin for five to 10 years. Anderson (noted in LeWinn, 1984) reported a 53-year-old man who was impotent during three-to-five month periods on digitalis leaf (100 mg per day), but not when the drug was periodically discontinued.

Gynecomastia was first observed in the 1950s to occur during long-term use (months or years) of digitalis (LeWinn, 1984). Subsequently, estrogenic effects such as hyperplasia and hypertrophy of the breast and vaginal epithelial cell proliferation were noticed in postmenopausal women on digoxin or digitoxin (LeWinn, 1984). However, Stenkvist, Bengtsson, and Dahlquist (1982) found that breast tumors were less frequent, smaller, and more uniform in postmenopausal women treated with digoxin than those

*For further information on non-traditional approaches to cancer therapy, contact Lorraine Day, M.D., who produced a video entitled *Cancer Doesn't Scare Me Anymore*, and has extensive literature and references available.

not treated. This finding suggested that digitalis may compete with estradiol for estradiol receptors and thereby antagonize some estradiol toxic effects. In any event, the estrogenic effects of digitalis have usually been evaluated as benign. Digitalis has also been shown to increase performance in stressed animals and prevent adrenal hypertrophy induced by stress (LeWinn, 1984). Such a tonic effect may be similar to that found with ginseng, which also has estrogenic properties.

Antiarrhythmic Drugs

- amiodarone (Cordarone)
- disopyramide (Norpace)
- encainade (Enkaid) (removed from United States market)
- flecainide (Tambocor) (removed from United States market)
- mexiletine (Mexitil)
- procainamide (Procan, Pronestyl)
- propafenone (Rythmol)
- quinidine (Cardioquin, Quinidex, Duraquin)

Antiarrhythmic drugs were spotlighted when a large study with flecainide (Tambocor) and encainide (Enkaid) had to be terminated due to a 200% increase in mortality/sudden death compared to placebo (Graedon & Graedon, 1991). A meta-analysis of controlled quinidine (Cardioquin, Quinidex, Duraquin) trials showed reduction of atrial fibrillation, but a threefold increase in mortality compared to controls (Coplen, Antman, Berlin, Hewitt, & Chalmers, 1990). In light of these dire findings, patients may decide to limit therapy to potassium/magnesium supplements and avoidance of caffeine, if these measures alone can be effective.

There is little information on sexual side effects due to antiarrhythmic agents. Disopyramide (Norpace) has been shown to cause impotence in two case study reports. McHaffie, Guz, and Johnston (1977) described a 47-year-old man treated with disopyramide for maintenance of sinus rhythm who reported inability to maintain erection for intercourse after 10 months of treatment. The plasma concentration on his 300–400 mg dose was found to be an abnormally high 14 microgram/ml. When the dose was lowered, the impotence was resolved. Ahmad (1980) reported a 35-year-old man treated with 300 mg per day disopyramide who could not sustain an erection after three weeks of treatment. When the drug was discontinued, the impotence resolved in six days. When he was later restarted on disopyramide, impotence recurred; again it resolved one week after the drug was discontinued.

Most antiarrhythmic drugs cause fatigue. Amiodarone (Cardarone) has been associated with movement disorders including ataxia and tremor, pulmonary toxicity, neuropathy, photosensitivity and thyroid disorder (due to its high iodine content). However, it is a very effective antiarrhythmic. Given the lack of definite sexual side-effect information, quinidine still seems to be the antiarrhythmic drug of choice. Propafenone (Rythmol) is newly available and may have a beneficial stimulating action; however, it has yet to be sufficiently investigated.

PENTOXIFYLLINE (TRENTAL)

Pentoxifylline (Trental) is used to treat peripheral vascular disease—in particular, intermittent claudication, which affects blood flow to the legs—by decreasing the viscosity of blood. The exact mechanism by which this occurs has not been identified; it appears to improve erythrocyte flexibility, which enables blood cells to get through tight spaces, so to speak.

Many years ago it came to our attention that patients consulting us for symptoms of impotence who also had intermittent claudication could get a double benefit from treatment with Trental: improvement of erections along with treatment of claudication. Clinical effect, however, can take two to three months to manifest.

Trental is not without adverse side effects. Nausea, bloating, nervousness, dizziness, and flushing have been reported (*Physicians Desk Reference,* 1991a). Interestingly, so has anorexia, which adds to the list of sexually active drugs that are associated with weight loss.

A neurally active form of pentoxifylline called propentofylline, which exerts a stronger action on adenosine, is currently in clinical trials for treatment of Alzheimer's disease and dementia.

HYPOLIPIDEMICS (CHOLESTEROL REDUCERS)

- cholestyramine (Questran)
- clofibrate (Atromid)
- gemfibrozil (Lopid)
- lovastatin (Mevacor)
- pravastatin (Pravachol)
- probucol (Lorelco)

For most patients, high cholesterol and lipids are an invisible problem when not accompanied by obesity, but the cardiovascular risks have now been clearly identified and drug treatment is common. These drugs do not appear to have chemical actions that would lead to sexual dysfunction, and specific sexual side effects have rarely been noted. Lovastatin and pravastatin are members of a new class of drugs called *3-hydroxy-3-methylglutaryl-coenzyme A (HMG-CA) reductase inhibitors*, which enhance plasma LDL removal and thereby lower cholesterol (Bradford et al., 1991). Our impression is that older cholesterol reducers such as probucol (Lorelco) and gemfibrozil (Lopid) may cause fatigue in some patients. Lovastatin (Mevacor) and pravastatin (Pravachol) appear to be both effective and sexually safe, but they have only been available for a few years. To the extent that they can reduce arterial plaque, they may even be able to improve those aspects of sexual function that depend on blood flow. It should be noted that weight is not reduced by either lovastatin or pravastin (Bradford et al., 1991), so that neither drug will have the mental or physical benefits of reducing overweight to normal.

A continuing subject of controversy is whether excessively lowering cholesterol levels (below 160 mg/dl) leads to increased mortality from suicide, accidents, and other violent causes (Glueck et al., 1994; Horrobin, 1989; Modai, Valevski, Dror, & Weizman, 1994; Pekkanen, Nissinen, Punsar, & Karvonen, 1989; Vartiainen et al., 1994). While reduction in cholesterol reduces cardiovascular disease and death from heart disease, total overall mortality has not been found to be reduced, partly due to an excess of deaths related to violent causes in patients with very low cholesterol concentrations (Horrobin, 1989; Modai et al., 1994; Pekkanen et al., 1989). Additionally, an association between very low serum cholesterol values and impulsive or aggressive behavior has been suggested (Pekkanen et al., 1989). As far as we know, no direct association has been shown between the use of lovastatin or pravastatin to reduce cholesterol and increased suicide, violence, or aggression. Glueck et al. (1994) found that the incidence of very low cholesterol (below 160 mg/dl) was much greater in a sample of 203 patients hospitalized for affective disorder (20%) than in a self-referred community screening sample of 11,864 subjects (4%). However, they attributed the greater incidence of very low cholesterol in these affective disorder patients to subnutrition, malnutrition, and weight loss as components of the disorder morbidity (or alternatively, by implication, as a result of a steady diet of hospital food).

CONCLUSIONS

The most significant aspect of this chapter is what is absent—the drugs that cannot be mentioned because the research has not yet been performed. Where is the research investigating the effects of antibiotics on sexual function? Are there differences among the antibiotics we now use interchangeably? What about antimalarials? Patients living in endemic areas sometimes take these drugs for years; travelers, often for months. Especially important are medications like acyclovir, which are typically prescribed for long-term treatment.

Common drugs like aspirin, ibuprofen and other anti-inflammatories raise more questions than answers, although for most people—scientists and patients alike—the thought that aspirin could affect sex might never occur. We suspect that aspirin may actually enhance sexual functioning in a manner analogous to its newly discovered protective effect against stroke. After all, cerebrovascular accidents of the brain operate by the same mechanism that can obstruct genital vessels. While a strong beginning has been made, we expect to see an acceleration of interest in the area of sexual pharmacology. Relatively soon, investigation of the sexual effects of *all* medications will become routine practice.

Part VII

SEXUALLY EFFECTIVE DRUGS

26

Dopaminergic Drugs: Deprenyl, Phenylethylamine, Quinelorane, Lisuride, Bromocriptine, L-dopa, Minaprine, Amineptine

OBJECTIVES

- To compare and contrast the mechanisms of action, benefits, and contraindications of several drugs known to have potent sexual side effects

Since the beginning of time, humankind has searched for potions with "magical" sexual properties. The most unlikely substances have been tried, and the most outrageous claims have been made. The "menu" has included oysters, raw meat, rhinoceros horn, tiger penis brandy, snake soup, deer antler marrow, ginseng, vanilla bean, ginger, and many other questionable delicacies. Some are even dangerous poisons, like Spanish Fly (Cantharides)—a urinary tract irritant that can kill. Others are harmless to everything but the pocketbook and endangered species (i.e., tiger, rhinoceros). Understandably, the whole concept of aphrodisiacs has been suspect; purveyors of these products are usually disreputable characters—snake oil salesmen, hustlers, charlatans. Magic potions have not materialized. Instead, chemicals from alcohol to antihistamines have been sabotaging sex for centuries. By default, traditional medicine has not played a meaningful role until quite recently.

Chemicals that favorably affect sex do exist. In most cases, they were developed for other medical purposes and the sexual findings were incidental. The mechanism of action by which these chemicals affect sexual function is clear in some cases but not in others. Often the response is paradoxical: The same substance that improves sexual function at one dose interferes with it at another. The gradual accumulation of evidence that medications can help sexual function has attracted scientific interest and research. Consequently, our understanding of sexually relevant substances is increasing more rapidly than ever before. Like other medications, drugs that improve sexual function are not effective for all patients at all times. Some are consistent in their effect, some are paradoxical, but all have potential as valuable adjuncts to traditional sexual therapy.

The development of sexually useful drugs has the potential to transform sex therapy in the same way that psychotropics have contributed to psychiatry. Sexually effective drugs will not replace sex therapy, nor should anyone attempt to use them for this purpose. However, in some cases they will make the difference between success and failure in therapy; in many cases, they will be able to shorten therapy and contribute to its effectiveness.

While no drugs have been approved by the Federal Drug Administration for the specific purpose of treating sexual problems, there are a few drugs available by prescription for other purposes – antidepressants, some hormones, blood pressure medications – that have demonstrated positive sexual properties. Physicians can legally prescribe these medications for nonindicated purposes, but the Federal Drug Administration strictly forbids advertising based on unproven claims. In order for these medications to become clinically useful and available for the treatment of sexual dysfunction, more research is needed; in order for sexual indications to be approved, controlled trials must be conducted to the satisfaction of the Federal Drug Administration.

In addition to existing prescription medications, there are a number of drugs with promising sexual patterns in research and development and a handful of medications available outside the United States with potentially useful sexual attributes. Eventually, specific "sexual medications" will be developed, as pharmaceutical companies come to appreciate the potential of this new medical dimension. Eli Lilly, in fact, has already taken this step with one of their new substances, quinelorane. This is the first pharmaceutical company to initiate studies of a new drug specifically for its sexual properties.

We have included drugs in this section as "sexually effective" based on the strength of mechanism of action analysis, animal studies, human research, clinical experience, and anecdotal reports. When the human research is sparse, but the mechanism of action of a particular medication is clearly understood and conforms to mechanisms of action known to influence sexual function, the drug has been included as a potentially effective sexual medication based on an understanding of its known pharmacological properties. Certain drugs that have not been studied for their sexual properties in animals or humans will be discussed in theoretical and/or speculative terms, when their potential applications to sexual dysfunction are persuasive.

There is no such thing as an "aphrodisiac" – a single substance that makes sexual problems disappear. There is, instead, a variety of substances that affect sex in different ways, depending upon which mechanism or mechanisms they influence. Many of these medications affect men and women differently. Some drugs that have positive sexual effects on males have negative sexual effects on the females, and vice versa. For instance, a drug that makes orgasm easier for a woman may cause dysfunctional premature ejaculation in a man. Similarly, a drug may have positive effects on some sexual behaviors but negative effects on others. For example, erection or ejaculation may be increased, while sex drive is decreased. When possible, the paradoxical effects of the drugs will be delineated.

Sexual pharmacology is still in its infancy; there is considerably more to be learned. Because the study of sexually effective drugs is so new to traditional Western medicine, the data are sparse and often flawed. With the exception of Eli Lilly's efforts, most of the information pertaining to sexually effective drugs has emerged as an unexpected finding in the course of other research.

In the course of preparing this material, we have made an unanticipated discovery. There seems to be a connection between drugs that improve sexual function and drugs that promote longevity. At first, we merely noted with interest that many of the drugs that warranted inclusion in this chapter happened to be the same drugs chosen for study by those in the forefront of longevity research. However, it does not appear that this relationship is merely coincidental, since the association appears so frequently. We have included sections on longevity and quality-of-life when appropriate.

DOPAMINE—A COMMON DENOMINATOR

The common mechanism of action of several sexually active drugs – dopa, deprenyl, bupropion, amphetamine, and cocaine – is the stimulation of the neurotransmitter dopamine and/or dopamine receptors. Dopamine's clear influence on sex drive and sexual behavior has been demonstrated in experiments in both animals and humans. Dopamine has both direct and indirect sexual properties: It directly increases sex drive through its chemical action, and it indirectly affects sexual behavior through its activation of drive and motivation, especially in the pursuit of pleasure. Dopamine sometimes stimulates sex drive independently of sexual opportunity or available partners. The effect can be intense and undesirable, leading to hypersexuality and aberrant sexual behavior; or moderate, with a distinct and valuable impact on sexual function.

Mentally and physically activating, a central feature of dopamine's mental activation is to motivate the pursuit of pleasure; it is the chemical responsible for drive and motivation in general. Dopamine is also the primary neurotransmitter that controls movement—particularly, movement toward things that give pleasure. When movement occurs for its own pleasure, it is called *exercise*; when movement is used to achieve a goal that gives pleasure, it is called *reward* or *reinforcement*. Sexual behavior is both exercise and reinforcement. It is both inspired and stimulated by, dependent upon, and reinforced by, dopamine.

Dopamine activity can be increased by several mechanisms:

- increasing the amount of dopamine by providing precursors (e.g., L-dopa)
- prolonging action by inhibiting uptake of dopamine (e.g., bupropion, cocaine)
- prolonging its action by interfering with destruction of dopamine (e.g., l-deprenyl)
- increasing its release (e.g., amphetamine)
- directly stimulating dopamine receptors as substitute neurotransmitters (e.g., bromocriptine, lisuride, LY1635/quinelorane)
- imitating dopamine with synthetic agents

According to the "dopamine-positive/serotonin-negative sexual hypothesis" (Gessa & Tagliamonte, 1975), drugs that stimulate dopamine increase sexual drive and/or behavior, while drugs that stimulate serotonin decrease sexual drive and/or behavior. Serotonin generally complements, balances, or opposes dopamine. Drugs such as lisuride increase sexual activities through a dual mechanism that involves both dopamine and serotonin. By studying these complex interactions, it has become clear that while the dopamine-positive/serotonin-negative sexual hypothesis generally holds true, there is more involved than this simple formula. Indeed, there are exceptions to the rule that current research has been unable to explain, suggesting a more complex dynamic yet to be identified. The paradoxical reports of hypersexuality (for example, spontaneous orgasms) with drug stimulation of serotonin could either be extreme manifestations of a normal stimulatory process or manifestations of pathological sexual chemistry. Animal sex research with serotonergic drugs has progressed from categorizing various so-called paradoxical findings to the identification of specific receptor subtypes that have different and even opposite effects on sexual function (see Chapters 16 and 19 on serotonergic drugs). By its nature, the scientific method is often guided by where it is found to be wrong—a reasonable hypothesis that can no longer be followed due to contradictions discovered in experimental testing is replaced by a new, more encompassing hypothesis. Such is the case with the serotonin-dopamine hypothesis: While it remains fundamentally correct, new findings have refined, added to, and occasionally contradicted the original premise.

Sexually effective drugs are not panaceas. If they are improperly prescribed for patients who have been inadequately screened or have preexisting psychotic tendencies or aggressive disorders, the consequences can be severe and unpredictable. Since inhibition of DA-2 receptor activity is assumed to be the action of neuroleptic antipsychotic drugs, stimulation of these receptors by agonists like quinelorane can be expected occasionally to trigger psychotic behavior in predisposed individuals.

L-DEPRENYL (ELDEPRYL)

Distinct sexual effects in animals have demonstrated with l-deprenyl (selegiline). Although human research has been limited and anecdotal reports infrequent, the animal work has been so compelling that deprenyl's potential for affecting human sexual function is biochemically predictable: What we know about its dopaminergic effect—deprenyl increases catecholamines by inhibiting MAO-B enzymatic breakdown and dopamine uptake—allows us to predict certain sexual properties for humans.

L-deprenyl was patented in 1962 as a psychic energizer (Dow, 1993). In Germany during the 1970s, l-deprenyl was used to supplement L-dopa in the treatment of Parkinson's disease, helping to control the symptoms as well as the progression (Birkmayer, Riederer, Ambrozi, & Youdim, 1977). Little was done with deprenyl in the United States until 1985, when a group of researchers began investigations to determine if deprenyl could be used in combination with L-dopa to delay brain degeneration in Parkinson's patients. By 1988, l-deprenyl was proven to prevent a toxic syndrome resembling Parkinson's in animals and to delay the progression of Parkinson's disease in humans (Tetrud & Langston, 1989). In the movie *Awakenings*, Robert de Niro's character is revived with L-dopa; his relapse might have been delayed had l-deprenyl been available in the 1960s. Unfortunately, the actual delay in Parkinson's disease progression lasts for only a short period of time, perhaps less than a year, though relief of some mood and cognitive symptoms may continue over a longer period of time (Ward, 1994).

As a monoamine oxidase inhibitor, deprenyl was considered a safer alternative to other MAOI antidepressants used in the 1980s. However, without a major Western drug company to develop it, little research was conducted with deprenyl. Early work in Germany indicated that it was an effective antidepressant, but a few small trials in the United States showed only borderline effects at high doses.

Deprenyl remained relatively unknown to the general public until popularized in the 1990 December issue of the health magazine, *Longevity*. The author of this well-researched article termed deprenyl an "anti-aging aphrodisiac," based on Josef Knoll's research on "sexually sluggish old male rats" conducted in Hungary.

Although deprenyl is said to act through a metabolic process called MAO-B inhibition, which decreases enzymatic breakdown of dopamine, its positive effect on sexual function and movement is apparently due to stimulation of dopamine. L-deprenyl is selective for MAO-B enzymes at a dose of 10 mg/day (Liebowitz et al., 1985). Other currently available MAOI antidepressants inhibit MAO-A enzymes, increase serotonin and norepinephrine, and often have a negative effect on sexual function. At higher doses, l-deprenyl also inhibits MAO-A; however, at low doses l-deprenyl does not cause MAO-A inhibition and thus avoids adverse side effects, perhaps even potentiating sexual function. A single small dose of l-deprenyl causes extended inhibition of the MAO-B enzyme that destroys dopamine, resulting in elevated levels of dopamine. In other words, the sexual effects of l-deprenyl are probably due to elevated dopamine levels caused by interference with dopamine's normal enzymatic destruction. Inhibition of MAO-B usually decreases after one week but can last up to four to five weeks. In Knoll's 1981 study (Knoll, 1981), sexual activity of rats rose after 0.25 mg/kg l-deprenyl injection, but gradually decreased over the following four weeks, as MAO-B levels returned to normal. Tolerance developed over 30 weeks, so that l-deprenyl injections were required three times a week to maintain the positive sexual effect. The relationship of this tolerance to changes in MAO-B activity has not been determined.

In another related study on sexually "sluggish" male rats, Yen, Dallo, and Knoll (1982) compared the effects of l-deprenyl with other selective MAO-B inhibitor drugs. Only l-deprenyl caused an increase in frequency of ejaculation, despite the fact that one of the alternative MAO-B inhibitors was 20 times stronger than l-deprenyl. These researchers concluded that l-deprenyl's effect on sexual function was due mainly to its action as a dopamine uptake inhibitor, not to its inhibition of MAO-B.

Knoll's animal studies during the 1980s (Knoll, Yen, & Dallo, 1983; Yen et al., 1982) well demonstrated l-deprenyl's positive sexual effects. Sexually sluggish male rats were rejuvenated, often copulating successfully and ejaculating more frequently than untreated younger rats. They also lived longer than those on placebo, and for much of this extended life span remained sexually vigorous. Knoll also compared clorgyline (a selective MAO-A inhibitor) with l-deprenyl and placebo and found that, while a small sexual improvement occurred with clorgyline, it did not compare in intensity or duration with l-deprenyl.

In a 1986 study (Dallo et al., 1986), l-deprenyl's effect on sexual activity was compared to that of other dopamine stimulants (amphetamine, apomorphine, and bromocriptine), to evaluate the speculation that l-deprenyl's positive sexual effects were due to the fact that it is metabolized into a weak form of amphetamine in the body. A single injection of any of these dopaminergic drugs stimulated ejaculation in sexually sluggish rats, but the sexual effect occurred in less than 50% of the rats over the next three weeks (Dallo, Yen, Farago, & Knoll, 1988). A single injection of l-deprenyl had only a small effect in sexually inactive noncopulating rats, but injections three times a week over 17 weeks caused full sexual activity by the tenth week, which continued through week 17. Amphetamine-treated rats ejaculated more quickly than l-deprenyl-treated rats but became exhausted sooner and took longer to recover. This difference showed that the sexual effect of l-deprenyl is not due simply to its metabolism in the body to amphetamine.

Experiments with l-deprenyl use in monkeys have shown less encouraging results. Chambers and Phoenix (1989) found that two weeks of l-deprenyl treatment did not improve sexual behavior of old, sexually inactive male monkeys (20 to 26 years) or sexually sluggish younger monkeys (6 to 17 years). There was only a slight, nonsignificant increase in ejaculation. The authors speculated that long-term treatment of six months or more may be required for any effects to occur. Treatment with apomorphine or yohimbine also failed to increase sexual behavior in the sluggish male monkeys, despite consistently positive sexual effects of these drugs when tested in sluggish male rats.

Sexual Benefits

Given its few side effects at low doses (10 mg/day), l-deprenyl for three to four months could be helpful in the treatment of low sexual desire and is unlikely to be harmful. Women with low sex drive and orgasmic difficulties might benefit from low-dose l-deprenyl as an adjunct to sexual therapy; however, until further research is performed, no definitive conclusions can be drawn.

Further research will ultimately determine whether l-deprenyl has benefits for the treatment of sexual dysfunction. For now, the use of l-deprenyl for sexual dysfunction should be performed in research centers only, in conjunction with sex therapy guidance and monitoring. If l-deprenyl does show sexual benefits without the complications of abuse or other serious side effects, it could be a valuable adjunct to treatment of sexual dysfunction.

Paradoxical Effects

An interesting finding in Dallo et al.'s 1988 study was that a smaller sexual effect occurred when the dose of l-deprenyl was increased from 0.25 mg/kg to 1 mg/kg. At 5 mg/kg l-deprenyl, the sexual effect was small and nonsignificant. The researchers reasoned that at doses higher than 0.25 mg/kg, l-deprenyl was less selective for MAO-B. As more MAO-A was inhibited with increases in dose, serotonin was increased instead of dopamine. Serotonin reversed the positive sexual effect either by inhibiting sexual activity directly or by inhibiting dopamine's positive action.

The sexual effects associated with l-deprenyl in animals, and perhaps in humans, are difficult to interpret because of the complex and paradoxical properties of this drug. While some sexual effects have been clearly associated with dopaminergic properties and l-deprenyl-induced increases in phenylethylamine (PEA), other effects could be due to l-deprenyl's amphetamine or methamphetamine metabolites. Experience with initial sexual benefits due to amphetamine or cocaine use has shown that such sexual stimulation tends to disappear with time or leads to pathological and antisocial behavior.

As a drug that metabolizes in the body to even weak forms of amphetamine (l-amphetamine and l-methamphetamine), l-deprenyl use for mild depression, longevity, and sexual benefits may be controversial. A new form of deprenyl, called para-fluoro-deprenyl, which does not metabolize to amphetamines, is now available in Europe, but has not yet been studied in clinical trials. It shows benefits for longevity and sexual performance in male rats similar to those seen with l-deprenyl (Dallo & Knoll, 1992). Testing of l-deprenyl for stimulant abuse potential in rats and monkeys has shown little or no abuse liability (Nickel, Szelenyi, & Schulze, 1994; Winger, Yasar, Negus, & Goldberg, 1994; Yasar & Bergman, 1994). In humans, neither abuse nor dependence has been shown during l-deprenyl treatment of various disorders (Schneider, Tariot, & Goldstein, 1994).

During electroencephalogram studies in rats, l-deprenyl has been shown to significantly increase theta rhythm, which has been associated with sexual orgasm (see Chapter 9), while d-amphetamine has been shown to significantly decrease theta rhythm (Nickel et al., 1994). L-deprenyl also profoundly increases endogenous phenylethyamine levels (suggested by Liebowitz, 1983, to be the "chemical of love") and directly (through dopamine uptake inhibition) and indirectly (through increased phenylethylamine and metabolism to amphetamines) increases dopaminergic activity that facilitates sexual desire and response (Berry, Juorio, & Paterson, 1994; Youdim & Finberg, 1994).

Longevity

Knoll et al. (1983) demonstrated that rats treated with l-deprenyl lived much longer than those on placebo. On the basis of this research they hypothesized that:

> The significant increase of the incidence of depression in the elderly, the age-dependent decline in male sexual vigor, and the frequent appearance of Parkinsonian symptoms in the latter decades of life might be attributed to a decrease of dopamine and "trace amines" in the brain. . . . The possibility to counter-act these biochemical lesions of aging by chronic administration of (-)-l-deprenyl, a selective inhibitor of MAO-B, which facilitates dopaminergic and "trace-aminergic" activity in the brain and is a safe drug in man, was analyzed in detail. The restitution and long maintenance of full-scale sexual activity in aged male rats continuously treated with (-)-l-deprenyl was demonstrated as an experimental model in support of the view that the long-term administration of small doses of (-)-l-deprenyl may improve the quality of life in senescence. (p. 135)

Knoll et al.'s association of sex, longevity, and antidepressant effects conforms with the central theme of this book: that many drugs of most interest to the field of sexual pharmacology should be the focus of longevity research and are often characterized by weight loss, antidepressant effects, activating properties, and sexual improvements.

The company distributing l-deprenyl in the United States, Somerset Pharmaceuticals, apparently has no plans at this time to test l-deprenyl as an antidepressant or as a sexual stimulant. In fact, l-deprenyl was not tested in the United States for treatment of Parkinson's disease, until a group of prominent doctors ran a trial themselves. We may not have the answer to l-deprenyl's sexual properties until researchers take the initiative to explore these questions independently. Now that l-deprenyl has been approved by the Federal Drug Administration for use in the treatment of Parkinson's disease (approved in 1989), our most valuable information about the sexual effects of l-deprenyl in humans may emerge from the observations of astute geriatricians.

PHENYLETHYLAMINE (PEA)

A group of psychiatrists at Columbia University found that a form of depression called "hysteroid dysphoria" responded better to monoamine oxidase inhibitors (MAOIs) than to conventional tricyclic antidepressants (Liebowitz, 1983). Since MAOIs control the metabolism of phenylethylamine (PEA), the psychiatrists hypothesized that these patients were ill due to dysregulation of PEA, giving rise to the PEA theory of depression. This particular form of depression is characterized by manic states of romance that abruptly dovetail into severe depression when the romance ends. The usual depressive symptoms of loss of appetite and sleep and decreased mood reactivity are not present; rather, patients with this type of depression overeat, sleep too much, and are emotionally overreactive. Liebowitz speculated that PEA rose to exaggerated levels during romantic periods, as if the person were inebriated or addicted to romance. When the romance ended, PEA levels dropped precipitously and the person experienced a reaction similar to amphetamine withdrawal. MAOI antidepressants returned the PEA to normal levels, allowing patients to function normally again, with appropriate emotion and mood.

This subgroup of depressed patients with abnormally low PEA could also benefit from cotreatment with l-deprenyl. Birkmayer, Riederer, Linauer, & Knoll (1984) successfully treated depressed patients with a combination of 10 mg l-deprenyl supplemented by 250 mg l-phenylalanine. L-phenylalanine (which is sold in health food stores as a diet pill) provides amino acid for conversion into PEA. Sabelli and Giardino (1973) noted rapid mood elevation in nine of 10 depressives treated with a combination of 5 mg l-deprenyl, 1,000–6,000 mg l-phenylalanine, and 100 mg vitamin B_6. Three days later, six of the 10 patients felt they were no longer depressed. Improvement continued for six weeks. There was no mention of any sexual effects in this short report.

The association of romance with PEA was popularized in a book by Dr. Michael Liebowitz, who described in lay terms hysteroid dysphoric atypical depression and its treatment with MAOIs (Liebowitz, 1983). The defining characteristic of this disorder is that patients remain emotionally reactive to their environment and eat and sleep too much rather than too little. Liebowitz also mentioned that chocolate, which contains significant amounts of PEA, could be used as an antidote to the loss of a love. In the media, PEA was then cited as a "scientific" explanation for infatuation and lovesickness (with little or no scientific evidence), and chocolate craving was misleadingly given qualified therapeutic validation. In actuality, the small amount of PEA in chocolates is metabolized rapidly once ingested. Diet soda pop contains the artificial sweetener Nutrasweet, which contains a form of phenylalanine that is converted into PEA. Drinking diet soda pop should provide a PEA "high" more readily than eating chocolates. (However, any PEA "high" is more likely to feel like anxiety or migraine than romance.) A single dose (10 mg) of l-deprenyl would lead to a far higher level of PEA for a far longer time than a box of chocolates, yet no cases of sudden infatuation or "crazy love" have yet been noted during even prolonged l-deprenyl treatment, which maintains PEA levels far above normal.

Until the 1970s, the prevailing hypothesis explained depression as the result of catecholamine deficiency. At that time, research differentiating the action of dopamine from norepinephrine as an excitatory neurotransmitter was meager; both were categorized as catecholamines. The PEA theory suggested another explanation. In a series of papers, Sabelli and Giardina (1973) and Sabelli and Moshaim (1974) proposed that depression could be due to PEA deficiency and that mania or schizophrenia resulted from an excess of PEA. For Sabelli, the availability of l-deprenyl presented an opportunity to put this theory to the test. L-deprenyl is a reliable, safe way to achieve sustained, elevated levels of PEA. Normally, PEA is immediately metabolized by MAO-B enzymes, remaining in the body for a very brief time. Monoamine oxidase inhibitors that inhibit MAO-A can raise PEA somewhat, but they also increase serotonin and norepinephrine considerably more. Any positive sexual effects of PEA would be overwhelmed by the negative effects of serotonin.

L-deprenyl appears to increase PEA effectively by decreasing its metabolic breakdown by MAO-B enzymes (Berry et al., 1994; Youdim & Finberg, 1994). Even a few 10-mg doses of l-deprenyl per week produce maximal MAO-B inhibition and a tremendous increase in the body's PEA level (1,000–2,000% increase) (Knoll, 1985). While Knoll attributed l-deprenyl's sexual benefits to increased dopamine activity, PEA may also play a significant role.

Male/Female Differences

There is a strong suggestion in the literature that abnormally high PEA levels are primarily found in women rather than men (DeLisi et al., 1984). The elevated levels typically occur at ovulation (perhaps contributing to the peak sexual arousal that can characterize this time period) or later in the menstrual cycle. High levels are also associated with depression, mania, schizophrenia. Isolated findings of excessive PEA in patients with paranoid schizophrenia and other psychotic disorders suggest the possibility of a causative, or at least contributory, role (DeLisi, Dauphinais, & Hauser, 1989). The genetically identical Genain quadruplets, who were all schizophrenic, also had extremely high levels of PEA (DeLisi et al., 1984). Any sexually effective drug that involves increased levels of PEA may potentially trigger or aggravate psychotic behavior. Because women are more likely to have excess levels of PEA (DeLisi et al., 1984), they may be more at risk for such disturbances and should be closely monitored.

There is a danger that patients treated with stimulant drugs for sexual dysfunction may become susceptible to disruptive behavior requiring therapeutic intervention. Any patient showing indications of psychoses should not be treated with l-deprenyl or any other dopaminergic or PEA stimulant.

Sexual Benefits

As noted, one of the most fascinating aspects of PEA is the possibility that it somehow mediates the feelings of romance and love. While this theory involves far more speculation than proof, it also represents the first time that traditional researchers have ventured to explore the molecular underpinnings of love. Many would resist the concept that love, romance, and affection could be chemically motivated. Yet, in light of the evidence that sex drive in animals and humans is heavily dependent on hormones and peptides, it is not unreasonable to consider the possibility that the main reason we have so little information on the "molecules of love" is that few have looked and the relationship of sex to love or infatuation is obscure.

QUINELORANE (LY 1635)

Quinelorane (LY 1635) is the first therapeutic drug developed and tested by a pharmaceutical company (Eli Lilly) expressly for the treatment of sexual dysfunction.* Quinelorane was synthesized in the course of developing bromocriptine-like drugs for the treatment of Parkinson's disease. These drugs were intended to be specific for dopamine DA-2 receptors. Quinelorane has been shown to be more selective and potent than Lilly's prior DA-2 agonist drugs, pergolide (Cimax) and quinpirole (LY1715) (Foreman & Hall, 1987a). Quinelorane was tested in the late 1980s for use in treatment of sexual dysfunction. In a multi-site double-blind placebo-controlled protocol trial, 500 men and women were treated for desire, erection, and arousal dysfunctions. Results of this study are still confidential and unpublished. The initial FDA review of the study was inconclusive, citing side effects such as nausea and hypotension in more than 50% of patients as a complicating factor, and suggesting that indirect sexual side effects may compete with or cancel any positive direct sexual effects.

Quinelorane's chemical action as a DA-2 agonist is simple, well-identified, and specific. Quinelorane research is grounded in prior dopamine sex research and reinforces the concept that dopamine enhances sexual desire and responsitivity. While our review of the experimental work on animals is limited to the area of sexuality, there is a vast literature describing the effects of similar DA-2 agonists on all aspects of animal behavior and physiology.

Quinelorane stimulated full sexual responses, including mounting, intromission, and ejaculation, in both sexually inactive and sexually slug-

*Eli Lilly has made another laudable move: It has hired a scientific investigator with experience and knowledge of animal sexual behavior and drug effects to complement the human trials.

gish rats (Foreman & Hall, 1987a). This finding differed notably from Knoll's l-deprenyl studies, in which l-deprenyl's effect on sexually sluggish rats was strong but its impact on sexually inactive rats was often weak (unless injections were given several times a week for an extended period) (Dallo et al., 1988).

When quinelorane was given to sexually active rats who were already ejaculating, copulation speed increased and ejaculation occurred more quickly; the refractory period also shortened. However, at the lowest and highest doses many of the rats failed to ejaculate. At the lowest dose some appeared sedated, while at the highest dose many were too hyperactive, often engaging in stereotyped behaviors characteristic of excess dopamine or amphetamine, such as sniffing and chewing. Results were similar with oral intake or injection. Positive sexual stimulation continued to occur with repeated daily injections of quinelorane for 15 days. No tolerance occurred, despite the fact that tolerance is typical for many amphetamine-type dopamine stimulants. With direct dopamine agonists, animals may become more sensitive to the effects of the drug with repeated use, instead of developing tolerance. All stimulatory effects were eliminated by prior treatment with dopamine antagonists, showing that the sexual effects were due to quinelorane's stimulation of the dopamine receptor. The finding that high doses interfered with sexual behavior suggested that abuse of quinelorane would probably eliminate any sexual benefits.

Eaton et al. (1991) studied the effects of a range of quinelorane doses injected into the male rat limbic brain paraventricular nucleus, an area involved in the penile erection/stretching and yawning syndrome. They found that a low dose (1 μg) increased erections and caused the rats to start copulating sooner; a higher dose (10 μg) decreased erection and slowed initiation and rate of copulation; both dose levels quickened ejaculation once copulation had started. Hull et al. (1989) found similar effects when quinelorane was injected into the MPO sex center of male rats. Ejaculation occurred after fewer penetrations, but overall copulation rate (time between penetrations) was slower and rats were somewhat slower to begin copulation. Thus, studies of quinelorane injected directly into brain sex centers have indicated that while ejaculation is facilitated, overall sexual vigor (copulation rate) and drive (initiation) may be decreased. In effect, the drug could cause premature ejaculation, lower sex drive, and decrease frequency. In women it may conceivably increase orgasmic responsiveness but decrease desire.

Studies of quinelorane's effects on monkey sex drive indicated enhancement in both males and females (Davis, Goy, Baum, & Johnson, 1988). The animals were exposed to an opposite-sex monkey in a nearby cage, but were unable to make physical contact. Males showed increased erection and females showed increased solicitation/presentation behavior. Erection even increased in castrated monkeys. Increases in sexual behavior occurred only when the opposite-sex monkey was present, even if unavailable. In the same experimental situation, Pomerantz (1991, 1992) noted increased erection and masturbation in monkeys with a range of quinelorane doses. Yawning occurred at the lower doses, but yawning and sexual behavior both decreased at the highest dose. Spontaneous erection, masturbation, and ejaculation did not occur unless the female was present in the neighboring cage.

Sexual stimulation by quinelorane should be similar to that which occurs with apomorphine, since both drugs are DA-2 receptor agonists. Chambers and Phoenix (1989) failed to find copulatory improvement in sluggish male monkeys with apomorphine. Given quinelorane's similarity to apomorphine, it is possible that improvement in frequency of copulation may not occur despite these promising findings in separated monkeys.

Sexual Benefits

One quinelorane test protocol was limited to women who have had low sexual desire (*DSM-III-R* hypoactive sexual desire: HSD) for no longer than 10 years. A crossover six-month trial was run with placebo and low, medium, and high quinelorane doses. A focus on women with low desire may have resulted from observations consistent with our bupropion study: that dopaminergic drugs predominantly treat sex drive dysfunction, and that the treatment is most effective in women. A test protocol for treatment of erectile dysfunction was also conducted. Results of these trials remain confidential and unpublished.

Paradoxical Effects

Within a wide range of doses, quinelorane increases sexual response. However, as noted, response decreases at the highest and lowest doses. At very low doses (below 25 mg/kg), quinelorane has a negative effect on sexual function; only negative "autoreceptor" dopamine neurons are thought to be stimulated, which *decrease* dopamine activity. Dopamine *auto*receptors respond to lower doses of dopamine than do dopamine receptors in such a way that their firing decreases normal receptor activity. At these low doses, paradoxical effects such as sedation occur instead of the usual hyperactivity. Clinically lowering the dose (to avoid excess excitement or psychoses) might make a patient's sexual and emotional condition worse than no drug at all.

In a study with female rats (Foreman & Hall 1987b), complex and paradoxical effects were noted. In nonreceptive females, lordosis was increased, thus promoting sexual activity. However, in receptive females, lordosis was decreased. Reduction in lordosis was small at intermediate doses but greater at both lower and higher doses. At the highest dose, females were rendered almost totally unreceptive and actively resisted male attempts to mount. Paradoxical sexual effects also have occurred in male rats given brain injections of quinelorane (Eaton et al., 1991). Ejaculation was quicker once copulation started, but rats were slower to mount and copulated less frequently.

It is not clear whether quinelorane will have any of the general stimulating and energizing benefits found with bupropion and l-deprenyl. While it is dopaminergic, quinelorane does not appear to have the sympathomimetic PEA-like effects shared by bupropion and l-deprenyl. Direct DA-2 agonists such as bromocriptine or pergolide have primarily been used to treat patients with Parkinson's disease who are grossly dopamine deficient; as many as 15% of these patients develop psychotic symptoms such as hallucinations, confusion, paranoid delusions, and sexual deviation. The effect of DA-2 agonists in patients with normal levels of dopamine is not known. The chief concern is that drug-generated psychotic behavior would be misdiagnosed or mismanaged in sexually dysfunctional patients. Perhaps what must be said is that drugs with possible beneficial sexual effects (such as bupropion, l-deprenyl, yohimbine, and vasopressin) have a long history of safe clinical use not yet shared by quinelorane. Unfortunately, the human clinical studies testing quinelorane as a treatment for sexual dysfunction remain unpublished in 1994, and the fate of quinelorane remains on its manufacturer's shelf.

LISURIDE (LYSENYL)

Lisuride (Lysenyl) is a direct DA-2 agonist ergot available in Europe for treatment of headache and Parkinson's disease. Due to adverse side effects, lisuride is not currently available in the United States, nor is it likely to be (it was approved recently for use in Mexico and is available in Tijuana). Animal research has shown it to be one of the strongest sexual stimulants (it can stimulate sexual activity even in castrated rats), due to a combination of chemical actions on key neurotransmitter receptors (Keller, Bonetti, Pieri, & DaPrada, 1983). Like quinelorane, lisuride stimulates dopamine as a direct agonist at the DA-2 receptor; it inhibits serotonin through a complex mechanism including stimulation of the 5-HT_{1A} receptor (like 8-OHDPAT and buspirone) and mixed agonist/antagonist actions on the 5-HT_2 receptor; and it stimulates norepinephrine and epinephrine by blocking the adrenergic $alpha_2$ receptor (like yohimbine). When it is used to treat Parkinson's disease, instances of hypersexuality exceeding those found with L-dopa have been reported (Ruggieri, Stocchi, & Agnoli, 1986).

Animal Studies

Lisuride has been observed to stimulate male rat sexual behavior but inhibit the female receptive lordosis response (Dorner et al., 1987). When lisuride was given to male rats who were castrated at birth and given testosterone as adults, it caused nearly complete inhibition of lordosis (which is sometimes prominent among castrated male rats), but a remarkable increase in ejaculation compared to testosterone treatment alone. Similarly, in prepubertal ovariectomized female rats treated with testosterone, lisuride potently increased inhibition of lordosis and stimulated them to mount other sexually receptive females. Dorner stated that lisuride's masculinization effect on females was even stronger than surgical removal of the "female mating center," the ventromedial hypothalamus, and suggested that it might be useful clinically for correction of "female sexual orientation" in men, possibly as an adjunct to testosterone therapy.

Male-to-male and female-to-female mounting behavior was greater with lisuride than with the putative animal aphrodisiac PCPA (Keller et al., 1983). Lisuride stimulated mating behavior in prepubertal females even more than in adult females and males, and also affected 18-day-old weanling rats. If other rats were not available to mount, treated females mounted other species such as guinea pigs—and even dead animals or dummies. Induced mounting occurred within 30 minutes of injection and as many as 60 mounts occurred within a two-hour interval (mounting continued even when intromission was impossible). These extreme masculine sexual effects of lisuride have not been noted in other animal species.

Hlinak (1987) studied the effect of lisuride on lordosis and female proceptive soliciting behavior (darting, hopping). Female rats were ovariectomized and maintained on estradiol for maximum receptivity. Inhibitory sexual effects were induced by lisuride within 15 to 30 minutes of injection. Proceptive hopping and darting initially disappeared, followed by a decrease in presentation postures and a smaller decrease in lordosis. Behavior returned to normal within two to six hours. Apparently, lisuride not only blocks passive behaviors such as lordosis, but also blocks active female sexual approach behaviors, indicating a decrease in the female's sex drive and stimulation and a simultaneous increase in inappropriate masculine sexual behavior such as indiscriminate mounting.

Lisuride's potent stimulation of masculine sexual behavior strongly resembles testosterone effects. The more generalized effects of testosterone, such as aggression and dominance behavior, are not noted with lisuride. Lisuride-induced mounting behavior can be eliminated by serotonin (5-HTP) pretreatment. It is also decreased by dopamine antagonists (pimozide) and serotonergic antidepressants (trazodone, clomipramine, fluoxetine), which blunt lisuride's inhibition of serotonin transmission. Therefore, these intense sexual reactions are most probably due to a combination of forces: increased dopamine and reduced serotonin (DaPrada, Bonetti, Scherschlicht, & Bordiolotti, 1985).

Human Studies

Frajese (1989) conducted a placebo-controlled crossover study of lisuride effectiveness for treatment of psychogenic erectile dysfunction in 44 men carefully screened for organic/hormonal defects. With the exception of some measurable increase in nocturnal/morning erections, lisuride caused no significant sexual improvement. Nearly all the patients noted increased speed of ejaculation and some complained of premature ejaculation. A small increase in ejaculatory intensity and sexual desire was reported. There have also been indications of elevated sexual desire in Parkinson's patients treated with lisuride, sometimes accompanied by mild euphoria and manic mood (Ruggieri et al., 1986).

Lisuride has been shown to function as an antidepressant in otherwise refractory patients. All studies have been done in Europe. It is unlikely that lisuride will ever be available in the United States because of its adverse side effects such as nausea, vomiting, and sedation, which occur in the majority of patients treated for Parkinson's disease (Ruggieri et al., 1986). Orthostatic hypotension and weight gain (five to

15 pounds) are particularly bothersome. As many as 30% of patients show evidence of psychoses, including hallucinations, delusions, and hypersexuality (Critchley et al., 1986; Ruggieri et al., 1986).

It is possible that lisuride could improve woman's sexual assertiveness and orgasm at relatively low doses. Evidently, lisuride can be used to treat headache in women with tolerably few side effects, since it is marketed as a headache treatment in Italy. Given lisuride's quick and potent effect, it could possibly be taken shortly before intercourse for sexual effect. However, dysphoric reactions such as dizziness and fatigue are likely to occur as well.

Due to its promotion of sexual initiative and assertiveness, lisuride's greatest therapeutic potential may be as a treatment for female sexual dysfunction. However, its potent undesirable side effects and the potential for aberrant sexual reactions discourage further experimentation in humans. Nonetheless, experience with lisuride's powerful sexual effects better prepares us for identifying less toxic drugs with similar sexual properties in the future.

BROMOCRIPTINE (PARLODEL)

The ergot drug bromocriptine (Parlodel) has been available in Europe since 1970 and in the United States since 1978. It is used primarily to treat prolactin-secreting brain tumors. Elevated prolactin levels have a severe depressive effect on sexuality, particularly in men: Hyperprolactemia can cause decreased sex drive, impotence, ejaculatory dysfunction, amenorrhea, gynecomastia, and galactorrhea. The most clinically useful effect of ergots such as bromocriptine is suppression of elevated prolactin levels, which have been identified as an organic cause of sexual dysfunction (Spark, Wills, O'Reilly, Ransil, & Bergland, 1982). Bromocriptine also inhibits postpartum lactation, may be an effective antidepressant, and can be used to induce metabolic weight loss.

When bromocriptine was first used in Europe as a treatment for Parkinson's disease in the 1970s, it acquired a reputation as an aphrodisiac, similar to L-dopa. Since it had fewer side effects, it was considered more useful as a sexual stimulant than L-dopa. With the recognition of elevated prolactin levels as an organic cause of impotence (Spark, 1983), bromocriptine seemed a promising treatment; it was most effective in treating sexual dysfunction secondary to hyperprolactemia. However, when it was first used for other sexual problems, the results were not as encouraging.

Sexual Mechanisms of Action

Chemically, bromocriptine is an ergot similar to lisuride but is much less potent as a direct DA-2 agonist than either lisuride or quinelorane and only mildly antagonizes the DA-1 receptor. While it has actions on serotonergic receptors similar to other ergot drugs, again it is less potent than lisuride and does not have lisuride's atypical antiserotonergic actions. Despite its similarity to lisuride, bromocriptine shows less selectivity and potency for serotonin, dopamine, and norepinephrine receptor sites (Beart, McDonald, Cincotta, de Vries, & Gundlach, 1986). In rats trained to discriminate lisuride from saline, bromocriptine was not sufficiently similar to function as a substitute for lisuride (Schechter, 1984), indicating that sexual effects similar to those of lisuride, if they occurred at all, would be of lesser intensity. Apparently, lisuride's potent sexual effects and possible weight-gain action are due to antiserotonergic mechanisms not possessed by bromocriptine (which may cause weight loss).

Bromocriptine inhibits growth hormone as well as prolactin and is used to treat gigantism (acromegaly) (Spark & Dickstein, 1979). However, ergot effects on growth hormone, which promotes fat metabolism, lean body muscle mass, and can have pleasant psychological effects that might facilitate sex, have been inadequately studied and specific sexual effects due to these hormonal changes have not been demonstrated.

Bromocriptine corrects testosterone and luteinizing hormone deficits that occur in hyperprolactemia by reducing prolactin. It is commonly used to treat infertility by stimulating luteinizing hormone and normal pituitary function. However, at the genital level it can inhibit the testosterone production of Leydig cells and decrease sperm volume (Chambon, Grizard, & Boucher, 1985). There is an unproven hypothesis that bromocriptine can decrease genital blood flow due to the same ergot vasoconstriction property that is useful in the treatment of migraine. (Dihydroergotamine/PHE and lisuride are approved migraine treatments.) The interplay between bromocriptine's dopaminergic vasodilating effects and its serotonergic vasoconstricting effects has not been sufficiently studied or compared to other direct DA-2 agonists. The vasodilation effect of bromocriptine's DA-2 activity can cause dizziness, headache, nausea, and flushing.

Chemically, bromocriptine is closely related to lisergic acid diethylamide (LSD) and can metabolize into LSD. As LSD use became popular in the 1960s development of ergot drugs was discouraged, but research continued on their remarkable blend of dopaminergic and serotonergic actions. Bromocriptine was synthesized as a nonhallucinogenic ergot that could be used safely to treat prolactin/endocrine disorders. However, psychotic episodes replete with hypersexuality and sexual compulsions still occur unpredictably in both men and women with bromocriptine use. Indeed, hypersexuality is a reliable sign of toxic ergot overdosage; moderate increases in sexuality may occur with non-toxic doses of bromocriptine. Paradoxically, bromocriptine can also cause erectile dysfunction. Cleeves and Findley (1987) reported four Parkinson patients who complained of impotence, which was reversed when bromocriptine was withdrawn.

If bromocriptine is discontinued due to side effects or any other reason, a prolactin rebound increase can cause depression and even suicidal ideation. Sexual dysfunction associated with withdrawal is probably due to high prolactin along with exhaustion of the dopamine system (Dackis & Gold, 1985). Tapered dose withdrawal and close medical supervision can protect against these consequences. A realistic and comprehensive description of bromocriptine's sexual effects is not yet available in the literature.

There is considerable clinical evidence that bromocriptine can be used to treat depression, including double-blind trials showing efficiency equal to imipramine and amitriptyline (Sitland-Marken, Wells, Froemming, Chu, & Brown, 1990). However, the average dose of 40 mg/day used in these clinical trials is over fourfold greater than that used for treatment of hyperprolactemia disorders (5–10 mg/day) and more than twice that used for Parkinson's disease (10–20 mg/day). Side effects mentioned in these studies have included increased sexual desire, but much more often nausea, vomiting, headache, dizziness, fatigue, and agitation (Nordin, Siwers, & Bertilsson, 1981; Theohar et al., 1981; Waehrens & Gerlach, 1981).

When abused, bromocriptine can lead to the psychotic or manic behavior characteristic of cocaine abuse. In spite of its abuse potential—perhaps because of certain similarities—bromocriptine has been suggested for treatment of cocaine and alcohol withdrawal and the subsequent depression that may occur (Giannini, Folts, Feather, & Sullivan, 1989; Herridge & Gold, 1988).

Sexual Effects in Men

Bromocriptine has not been shown to be effective for the treatment of erectile dysfunction in men with normal prolactin levels. Ambrosi et al. (1977) treated 30 men with psychogenic impotence with bromocriptine or placebo for up to six weeks. There was no significant difference in improvement between patients on bromocriptine (50%) or those on placebo (44%). Cooper (1977) found no psychological or physical changes in 15 middle-aged men with organic erectile dysfunction.

A small positive response to bromocriptine was noted in diabetic men with impotence. Legros, Chiodera, Mormont, and Servais (1980) treated 30 diabetic impotent patients for four weeks with bromocriptine or placebo. Nine of 16 on bromocriptine improved, compared to six of 14 on placebo. Pierine and Nusimovich (1981) treated impotent diabetics with 5 mg/day for 12 weeks. Only three of 15 (20%) showed any benefit, compared to 30 of 60 (50%) on L-dopa. (Five mg/day may be too small a dose for a noticeable effect.)

Male hyperprolactemia is associated with decreased erection and delayed or absent ejaculation (Grafeille, Joutard, & Ruffle, 1984). Usually, sexual dysfunction due to hyperprolactemia can be eliminated with bromocriptine treatment (5–10 mg/day for one to three months), which normalizes prolactin levels and reverses testosterone deficits (Carter et al., 1978; March, 1979). Spark, White, and Connolly (1980) treated eight impotent hyperprolactemic men with bromocriptine (5–10 mg/day). Six recovered normal sexual function, while two failed to respond. The two failures had discontinued bromocriptine due to gastrointestinal upset or continued inadequate testosterone below 300 ng/dl. One of the six men responding to bromocriptine recovered normal erection despite continued low testosterone (120 ng/dl), but still required supplemental testosterone injections. Tordjman (1982) treated six men with hyperprolactemia (over 60 ng/dl) who complained of decreased sex drive (all six), decreased erection (three), and lack of ejaculation (two). Treatment with 5–10 mg/day bromocriptine (for one to six or more months), supplemented by testosterone injections, improved or normalized sexual desire and response.

Weizman et al. (1983) treated four impotent hyperprolactemic patients undergoing chronic hemodialysis uremic treatment who reported decreased sex drive, decreased sexual activity, decreased orgasmic sensation, as well as decreased erection. Beneficial effects on erectile function occurred after three weeks of treatment with 3.75 to 5.0 mg/day bromocriptine. All aspects of sexual desire, activity, and response returned to normal in all patients. Muir et al. (1983) treated 23 impotent men with end-stage renal failure on maintenance hemodialysis in a placebo-controlled bromocriptine crossover double-blind study. Eight patients withdrew from the trial due to intolerable side effects such as nausea, vomiting, or hypotension. Of the 14 who completed the crossover trial, three showed no improvement, six showed some improvement, and five returned to normal desire and function. Improvements in desire were not differentiated from improvements in erection.

Grafeille et al. (1984) found that impotent men with mild hyperprolactemia (20–30 ng/ml) responded to one to three months of bromocriptine treatment (5 mg/day) in four of six cases (67%). In two impotent men with moderate or high prolactemia (31–224 ng/ml), bromocriptine (5 mg/day) restored normal erection within three weeks. Zini et al. (1986) treated 16 hyperprolactemic men with decreased sexual desire and response with bromocriptine 5–15 mg/day over three to eight months. Sexual function was normalized and prolactin was decreased (from 345 to 40 mean ng/dl). Free and total testosterone levels were increased to normal (free testosterone from 4.5 to 9.8 ng/dl; total testosterone from 206 to 482 ng/dl). However, there was still about 33% less testosterone in bromocriptine patients than in control subjects and lingering mild-to-moderate hyperprolactemia in some men.

Testosterone can be used to enhance bromocriptine in providing more effective treatment of impotence. Testosterone potentiates dopamine sexual effects (Dallo & Lekka, 1986), inhibits prolactin (Sinha et al., 1984), and has a synergistic effect with dopamine in brain sex centers such as the MPO. Even in the treatment of hyperprolactemia, testosterone might improve the often borderline effect of bromocriptine. However, testosterone supplementation increases the chance of psychotic reactions to bromocriptine, making concurrent sexual therapy advisable both for recovery and safety. A final note: Although bromocriptine has been effective in reversing impotence that is secondary to hyperprolactemia, men may also require sexual therapy for continuing problems, even after prolactin levels are normalized by the drug treatment (Buvat, Lemaire, Buvat-Herbaut, Fourlinnie, et al., 1985).

Sexual Effects in Hyperprolactemic Women

Hyperprolactemia in women is characterized by depression and hostility, which can generate sexual aversion. Sexual aversion often continues even after prolactin is reduced by bromocriptine. Given the possible presence of aversive responses interfering with renewed sexual drive and sensations due to bromocriptine treatment, women should receive concurrent counseling or sexual therapy in order to achieve the full benefit of treatment.

Fioretti et al. (1978) followed 11 women treated for hyperprolactemia amenorrhea over six months. Depression decreased and sexual desire increased significantly by three months and even more in six months. All women regained menstrual cycles.

Weizman et al. (1983) studied 21 women with elevated prolactin due to hemodialysis and found higher prolactin levels in patients with decreased sexual desire than in patients with normal sexual activity (prolactin levels: 140 ng/dl with decreased sex; 54 ng/dl with normal sex). Only one woman treated with bromocriptine reported return of normal sexual activity.

Tordjman (1982) found decreased sexual interest in four of six hyperprolactemic women, secondary sexual aversion in two, and secondary anorgasmia in three. When bromocriptine (5–7.5 mg/day) was supplemented with biweekly testosterone treatment over several months, sexual desire increased, aversion decreased, and anorgasmia was reversed in two of three women.

Grafeille et al. (1984) found hyperprolactemia (26–224 ng/dl) in 20 of 108 women complaining of decreased sexual desire. Nine of those women were treated with bromocriptine (5 mg/day) for at least two months and some for more than six months. All the women showed increased sexual desire.

Koppelman, Parry, Hamilton, Alagna, and Loriaux (1987) have suggested that hyperprolactemic women are less sexually active and reactive than non-symptomatic women. In a 10-week double-blind crossover placebo-controlled study, six hyperprolactemic women were compared to six unmedicated female controls. Despite reduction of prolactin, there was no significant change in any sexual behavior with bromocriptine compared to placebo. However, the five-week period of treatment was probably too short for adequate evaluation of sexual improvement and the population size too small to expect meaningful results.

Bromocriptine is also used to treat a naturally occurring form of hyperprolactemia in postpartum lactation. However, the side effects can be severe. Orthostatic hypotension, vomiting, hypertension, seizure, stroke, vasospasm, and heart attack have occurred (Ruch & Duhring, 1989; Watson, Bhatia, Norman, Brindley, & Sokol, 1989). Furthermore, bromocriptine can cause postpartum psychotic or manic reactions (Canterbury, Haskins, Kahn, Saathoff, & Yazel, 1987; Lake, Reid, Martin, & Chernow, 1987). Postpartum depression may be delayed until bromocriptine is discontinued and then occur unpredictably.

A 28-year-old woman given bromocriptine postpartum experienced several daily instances of painful clitoral tumescence lasting a few minutes (Blin, Schwertschlag, & Serratrice, 1991). She also reported increased sex drive, which she did not associate with the clitoral response. The tumescence disappeared when bromocriptine was discontinued, but quickly returned when it was again taken. Clitoral changes with bromocriptine use in women are rarely considered or monitored. The incidence and significance are therefore unknown.

Vaginal bromocriptine suppositories have been used successfully to treat hyperprolactemia (Katz, Schran, & Adashi, 1989; Vermesh, Fossum, & Kletzky, 1988). Vaginal administration seems to circumvent the side effects of nausea and vomiting, the main causes of bromocriptine intolerance. Although psychological side effects were not been observed with this treatment, further reports of vaginal administration are needed to assess whether these side effects are also lower than with oral bromocriptine.

Bromocriptine is used by about 700,000 women a year for suppression of lactation. The National Women's Health Network and the Public Citizen Health Research Group have pressured the Federal Drug Administration to ban this application of bromocriptine to inhibit lactation. An FDA panel concluded that bromocriptine benefited only 10% of lactation patients, leaving the other 90% with all the risks and none of the benefits (Waldholz, 1989). Considering its widespread use among physicians, this conclusion was puzzling. If further studies confirm that the therapeutic benefits of bromocriptine are so low in relation to lactation, such use will become less widespread. On the other hand, research may reveal more benefits than are currently validated, considering how routinely physicians prescribe it. Additional prospective controlled clinical trials are required to assess benefits and risks and to test other ergot drugs such as pergolide (Permax) for safe inhibition of postpartum lactation.

In summary, bromocriptine resembles both lisuride and quinelorane, but its effects are less intense. It is related to LSD and can metabolize into this hallucinogen. As with other dopaminergic stimulants, psychotic symptoms and hypersexuality can sometimes occur. Bromocriptine does not appear to improve sexual function in normal men and women. However, it does correct hyperprolactemia in both sexes, usually correcting the associated sexual symptoms. As with other sexually effective drugs, bromocriptine has antidepressant properties, some weight-loss potential, and the possibility of favorable effects on longevity.

Conventional ergot drugs such as bromocriptine and lisuride will soon be replaced by more refined derivatives that selectively stimulate either dopamine or serotonin, hopefully avoiding the unpredictable interaction between these two neurotransmitters responsible for the high level of poorly tolerated side effects.

L-DOPA

"L-dopa" is the abbreviated name for L-dihydrophenylalanine, a naturally occurring amino acid related to the amino acid l-phenylalanine. Because dopamine cannot cross the blood-brain barrier, L-dopa is used as a "raw material" precursor that can enter the brain where it is metabolized into dopamine. Usually, L-dopa is combined with the decarboxylase inhibitor, carbidopa (Sinemet), which prevents L-dopa from metabolizing to dopamine outside the brain.

L-dopa treatment of Parkinson's disease began in 1967. The notion of "love drugs" was popular during this time. A few years earlier, LSD had come into vogue. In 1969 a study was published in *Science* (Tagliamonte, Tagliamonte, Gessa, & Brodie, 1969) showing that PCPA (p-chlorophenylalanine) acted as an aphrodisiac in male rats ("induces long-lasting sexual excitement"). By 1970, L-dopa was established as an aphrodisiac (Taberner, 1985) in the public arena, and even appeared in an ad for an X-rated movie, *L-Dopa* ("an exclusive report on the new stimulant that will keep man and wife active through the problem years"). However, because L-dopa use was restricted to Parkinson's patients, the general public did not have access to it.

Although associated with other dopaminergic stimulants, L-dopa had been used only infrequently in animal research, until studies on its sexual impact in rats were initiated in response to its purported aphrodisiac effect in humans. Although the dopamine-increase/serotonin-decrease sex hypothesis was already well established early during its clinical use, published studies on L-dopa did not indicate strong sexual effects. The sexual effect of L-dopa in normal, sexually active rats was unremarkable (DaPrada, Carruba, Saner, O'Brien, & Pletscher, 1973; Gessa & Tagliamonte, 1974a, 1974b; Gray, Davis, & Dewsbury, 1974; Hyyppa, Lehtinen, & Rinne, 1971; Malmas, 1976). However, a significant positive sexual effect was found in sexually sluggish male rats (Gessa & Tagliamonte, 1974a, 1974b). Malmas (1976) showed that L-dopa inhibited lordosis in female rats and that lower L-dopa doses, which caused hyperactivity, were more sexually effective than higher doses.

Sexual Dysfunction

The use of L-dopa for the treatment of Parkinsonism became prevalent in the late 1960s and 1970s. It was rumored to cause hypersexuality in certain patients. However, published reports of L-dopa-induced hypersexuality were few and the sexual effects described were often merely a return to normal sexual function or only one aspect of manic and psychotic aberrations.

In 1970, Hyyppa, Rinne, and Sonninen reported increased sex drive in 10 of 41 Parkinson's patients treated with L-dopa. In a second study, 8% of their sample reported an increase in sexual activity or sex drive, but this was attributed to improved health. Next, Hyyppa, Falck, and Rinne (1975) conducted a comprehensive investigation of 11 Parkinson's patients (mean age = 60) before L-dopa treatment, during three months on L-dopa, and during the next three months off L-dopa. No sustained sexual effects of L-dopa were found.

The results may have been different in younger subjects. The authors attributed L-dopa-induced hypersexuality to transient mania or psychoses and other transient sexual effects to general improvement in health. Similarly, Duvoisin and Yahr (1972) had discounted any aphrodisiac effect in a large sample of patients, in which hypersexuality was observed only as an aspect of mania, psychoses, dementia, or past history of unusual sexual behavior.

Other reports have identified instances of hypersexuality attributed directly to L-dopa, without associated mania. Bowers, Van Woert, and Davis (1971) reported increases in sexual activity or desire in seven of 19 L-dopa patients. Quinn, Toone, Lang, Marsden, and Parkes (1983) reported two case studies in which L-dopa reactivated prior sexual deviances such as masochism or bondage, which became part of a pattern of compulsive hypersexuality. Tanner, Goetz, and Klawans (1986) reported nearly continuous sexual urge and incessant requests for sex in five male Parkinson's patients. The authors commented that such hypersexuality rarely appears in women patients. In a later article (Uitti et al., 1989), the same authors described two cases of hypersexuality in women, but one was apparently caused by bromocriptine.

The sexual properties of L-dopa are difficult to interpret from the rare instances of hypersexuality reported. Uitti et al. (1989) described hypersexuality during L-dopa treatment in 13 Parkinson's patients (11 male, two female). L-dopa was often taken with other dopamine agonists like bromocriptine or pergolide. Varied psychiatric disturbances such as mania and agitation accompanied hypersexuality. The authors suggested that, regardless of the relation to mania or other disturbances, hypersexuality in many of these patients was due solely to L-dopa treatment. Hypersexuality resolved in all patients when drug was withdrawn. Hypersexuality in these patients was characterized as perverse and a threat to the their relationships.

Abusive use of L-dopa has also been reported (Vogel & Schiffter, 1983). A patient showing protracted hypersexuality manipulated his prescriptions to obtain additional pills and then took large doses, which triggered extreme psychotic episodes. The authors pointed out that patients may abuse L-dopa to increase sexual feelings and recommended that doctors explicitly inquire about sex drive to alert them to this potential. Quinn et al. (1983) described a man on L-dopa who reverted to bondage compulsions experienced earlier in his life. As his sexual compulsion worsened, he hoarded his pills and then took many at once "to give himself a boost."

Sexual Benefits

Unfortunately, L-dopa's beneficial sexual effects are difficult to determine. Other than anecdotal reports and clinical monitoring, few studies (and none of any size) have been conducted to study L-dopa's possible therapeutic use as a treatment for sexual dysfunction. Benkert (1972; Benkert, Crombach, & Kockott, 1972) used L-dopa to treat impotence in eight patients, but found only transient increases in nocturnal and daytime erections that were not sufficient for intercourse. Pierini and Nusimovich (1981) reported that 30 of 60 (50%) impotent diabetic men experienced improved erectile function during 12 weeks of L-dopa treatment. Leyson (1987), in a urology convention presentation, reported that 60% of patients with spinal cord injury and multiple sclerosis achieved usable erections during L-dopa treatment.

Patients treated for Parkinsonism are generally over 50 years of age and experiencing the progression of their debilitating disease. Despite use of L-dopa and various dopaminergic adjunctive medications, a majority of Parkinson patients remain sexually dysfunctional. For example, five of the hypersexual patients in Uitti et al.'s (1989) study demanded daily sex but remained impotent. In another study (Koller et al., 1990) reduced desire was found in 44% of the male and 71% of the female Parkinson's patients medicated with L-dopa. Only 14% of the men could maintain erection and nearly 50%

were unable to ejaculate. Among women, 67% reported lowered arousal and 38% were anorgasmic.

Despite dopaminergic medications, sexual desire and activity remained impaired among the majority of elderly patients with Parkinsonism. No studies on L-dopa have been done in younger (below 50) healthy or sexually dysfunctional subjects. Until then, it is not possible to evaluate fully L-dopa's potential for therapeutic effect on sexual function.

MINAPRINE (CANTOR)

Minaprine (Cantor) is a unique antidepressant that has been used for many years in Europe, but has only recently been tested for use as an antidepressant in the United States (by Wyeth). Trials for the treatment of sexual dysfunction are ongoing outside the United States, sponsored by its French manufacturer. Due to its cholinergic properties, minaprine is also being tested for treatment of dementia and as a nootropic drug for aging. Minaprine has been shown to prevent neural degeneration (Araki, Nojiri, Kimura, & Aihara, 1987; Chaki, Usuki-Ito, Muramatsu, & Otomo, 1990) typical of senile dementia and is used in Europe to treat many of the problems associated with aging. Because of its unique structure, identification of minaprine's chemical effects is still not complete, despite its many years on the European market.

Minaprine's strong action on the hippocampus in the limbic system suggests that it may modulate cognitive aspects of sexual functioning and could be used to facilitate a cognitive approach to sexual therapy. Minaprine's effects on the septal and entorhinal inputs to the hippocampus theoretically would allow better integration of the sensory and cognitive aspects of sexual behavior appropriate to the higher level functioning of the human brain (Biziere, Kan, Souilhac, Muyard, & Roncucci, 1982). Tricyclic antidepressants, in contrast, have strong anticholinergic properties that can block integration of sexual and cognitive processing. With promising antidepressants such as minaprine, we can finally move beyond the outmoded view that emphasizes an opposition between pharmacological and cognitive therapeutic treatments for sexual dysfunction.

The French equivalent of the *Physicians Desk Reference* cites many indications for minaprine: inhibitory states characterized by withdrawal and psychomotor retardation, neurasthenia, lowered libido, decreased activity, lack of initiative, and memory and attention deficits. Although minaprine is categorized in Europe as a psychostimulant, it does not cause the intense hyperactivity and stereotypical movements characteristic of amphetamines. It has a positive dopaminergic effect and decreases prolactin levels, but the source of its dopaminergic action is still uncertain.

Some studies have shown minaprine to be a dopamine uptake inhibitor. Chemically, it resembles the reversible MAO-A inhibitor moclobemide. Moclobemide apparently has typical MAO antidepressant efficiency with far fewer side effects than currently available MAOIs and is now available in Europe. MAOI action could explain minaprine's ability to increase serotonin levels, but does not explain its strong cholinergic property. Ferretti et al. (1984) proposed that minaprine increases dopamine through an effect on MAO activity. If this is correct, then it may have sexual and aging benefits similar to l-deprenyl (selegiline/Eldepryl). Minaprine has serotonergic affinity at the 5-HT_2 receptor which may be involved in ejaculatory control. Muramatsu, Tamaki-Ohashi, Usuki, Araki, and Aihara (1988) suggested that it facilitates cholinergic activity by blocking 5-HT_2 or 5-HT_{1B} activity. In this respect, minaprine is similar to 8-OHPAT, which also seems to block 5-HT_2 and 5-HT_{1B} activity. Since 8-OHDPAT potently stimulates sexual behavior in animals, minaprine may also have some stimulatory properties; however, no studies on minaprine's sexual effects on animals have been published.

Maffla and de Garcia (1979) tested minaprine for treatment of mild to moderate depression mainly related to sexual function. Forty patients (27 male and 13 female) were treated for 30 days. Sexual dysfunction was defined as impotence or frigidity. (The choice of terms may be misleading, since in many parts of the world impotence refers to any male sex deficiency, including low libido, and frigidity refers to absence of desire, arousal, and/or orgasm.) None of the patients had organic sexual problems. Two of the female patients, who presented with sexual arousal deficits due to prior tricyclic antidepressant treatment, reported significant improvement on minaprine. Sixty percent of the patients improved sexually but the nature of the improvement was not described. Thus, while this study indicated some benefits in the treatment of depression associated with sexual dysfunction, the precise effects are not clear.

Therapeutic sexual benefits of minaprine were reported in a 1972 clinical study published in a French journal (Muyard, 1972). Twenty-four patients were treated for various affective disorders, including neurasthenia, anxiety, fatigue, and nervousness. A 31-year-old impotent inpatient experienced renewed nocturnal erections and a spontaneous ejaculation two days after starting on minaprine. The nocturnal erections disappeared when minaprine treatment was interrupted. Increased nocturnal erections were noted in some other patients and impotence was ameliorated in six. However, it is not clear whether the sexual improvement was part of the antidepressant response. Improvements in sexual drive and activity were also noted. The authors noted disinhibition and elevated sex drive in some patients early in minaprine treatment.

Minaprine's side-effect profile reflects its activating action: The most common side effects are insomnia, nervousness, gastrointestinal upset, dizziness, and anxiety (Amsterdam et al., 1989). Its positive action on excitatory amino acid transmission appears due to a partial agonist action and blockage of glycine inhibition. Consequently, minaprine has convulsant potential similar to bupropion, a drug that also has positive though undefined actions on dopamine and excitatory amino acid transmission. Comparison of these two unusual drugs with somewhat similar effects, including beneficial sexual arousal, could help clarify the mechanism(s) of action of drugs that affect sexual function. However, because minaprine is not available in the United States, it is not possible to compare these two antidepressants. The neural activating effect of both minaprine and bupropion can aid alertness even when taken with alcohol, whereas tricyclic sedative effect is worsened by alcohol. Each has been used in children to treat hyperactive attention deficit disorder. Despite an apparent central analgesic action, minaprine caused some headache during its antidepressant clinical trial in the United States (Amsterdam et al., 1989).

In conclusion, the suggested psychostimulant and cholinergic properties of minaprine indicate that it could be used to treat sexual inhibition, depression, and fatigue. However, its dopaminergic and serotonergic chemical actions are unclear and must be further explored. Until controlled trials are conducted with minaprine in the United States, its proper dose levels and side-effect profile cannot be determined. Once again, an antidepressant drug exhibiting sexual properties is associated with longevity. The recurring association of these three variables, often accompanied by mild weight loss, is unlikely to be coincidental.

AMINEPTINE (SURVECTOR)

In Europe, amineptine (Survector) is considered to have a specific therapeutic effect on sexual dysfunction, independent of its antidepressant action (Tatarelli, Giraldi, & Vella, 1984). It is a preferred antidepressant (or "psychotonic") for treatment of retarded depression, neurasthenia, hypochondria, and chronic fatigue. When the stimulating antidepressant nomifensine (Merital) was withdrawn from use in Europe in 1986, many patients were switched to amineptine due to its similar stimulant properties and lack of side effects. Use in Italy has steadily increased until it has become the most prescribed antidepressant among general practice doctors during the early 1990s (Balestrieri, Bragagnoli, & Bellantuong, 1991). Apparently due to reports of liver toxicity (Geneve, Larrey, Amouyal, Belghiti, & Pessayre, 1987), it has not been tested for use in the United States.

As with minaprine, its sexual and activating properties are attributed to dopamine stimulation (De Leo, Dalla Barba, & Dalla Barba, 1986). Although it has a tricyclic structure, amineptine has an unusual chemical action that includes dopamine release and uptake inhibition (Bonnet, Chagraoui, Protais, & Costentin, 1987; Ceci, Garattini, Gobbi, & Mennini, 1986) coupled with norepinephrine uptake inhibition. It is free of tricyclic side effects such as anticholinergic symptoms, cardiotoxicity, sedation, and weight gain.

Due to its stimulant action, amineptine is subject to abuse. Between 1978 and 1988, 186 cases of abuse were noted in surveillance monitoring (Castot, Benzaken, Wagniart, & Efthymiou, 1990). Eighty percent of these cases were women and the majority occurred in patients between 20 and 40 years old. Associated with this abuse was benzodiazepine use (40%), insomnia, agitation, psychoses, and anxiety. Marked weight loss occurred in 22 cases and acne in 17. Ginestet, Cazas, & Branciard (1984) described two cases of abuse/dependence in women successfully treated for depression with asthenia. Insomnia, weight loss greater than 20 pounds, irritability, and heightened physical sensations (hyperaesthesia) were conspicuous in these cases.

In a small double-blind comparison of amineptine or amitriptyline antidepressant treatment in women, sex drive improved on amineptine and worsened on amitriptyline, but the difference between the drugs was not significant (De Leo et al., 1986). A similar double-blind trial with depressed men and women also showed a decrease in depression-related sexual dysfunction on amineptine but not on amitriptyline (Van Amerongen, 1979).

A study of amineptine using normal volunteers showed increased REM sleep and improved attention and concentration in the morning (Bramanti et al., 1985). Given the association of EEG theta rhythm with REM sleep and orgasm (Cohen, Rosen, & Goldstein, 1985), amineptine's sleep effects indicate a potential for sexual stimulation. Amineptine and other known dopaminergic sexual stimulants, including bupropion, apomorphine, and lisuride, all induce EEG theta in rabbits (Bo et al., 1984) and l-deprenyl induces theta in rats (Nickel et al., 1994). Theta rhythm, which is associated with cholinergic and dopamine DA-1 receptor activation, is driven from the limbic hippocampus and septum, where cognitive and emotional stimuli are integrated. The connections of amineptine to these sleep and theta phenomena and its apparent special stimulant properties for women suggest that it could facilitate female orgasm (see Chapter 27).

27

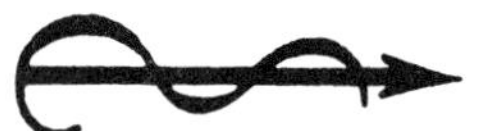

Bupropion

OBJECTIVES

- To analyze the pharmacological properties of and clinical indications for bupropion
- To describe the first large placebo-controlled trial (the Crenshaw Clinic research protocol) to investigate the positive sexual properties of a drug
- To report the results and analyze the strengths and weaknesses of the study

Bupropion (Wellbutrin) is a novel antidepressant that works through an unknown chemical mechanism, producing relief of depression comparable to other antidepressants, but without their unpleasant side effects (patients often report no side effects whatsoever; side effects that do occur are usually activating, similar to other mild stimulants). The drug was developed in the United States and approved for marketing in 1985. However, seizures in four female patients treated for bulimia caused its manufacturer to withdraw it from the market early in 1986 for further tests. Its seizure rate was subsequently found to be tolerably low (0.4%) and it was re-released in 1989. The popularity of bupropion is gradually increasing due to its relative absence of adverse side effects and its potential to improve sex.

Bupropion is comparable to fluoxetine (Prozac) in its relatively low level of side effects: Even though the side effects of each are different, both are sufficiently low-grade that a majority of patients can take medication without feeling a chemical "knockout." Fluoxetine is a better drug for anxiety or panic because of its serotonergic properties; bupropion is better suited for depression without significant anxiety components because of its dopaminergic activating properties. When depression occurs without anxiety, bupropion is preferable because it has so few adverse sexual effects. In addition to being an antidepressant and a sexual stimulant, bupropion causes weight loss rather than the weight gain associated with the majority of other antidepressants (except fluoxetine and newer SSRIs). It also has properties that make it a promising drug for longevity research. Table 27.1 summarizes the properties and side effects of bupropion.

BUPROPION-INDUCED LIMBIC ACTIVATION

Bupropion's sexual action appears to involve activation of the limbic system, including the amygdala, septum, hippocampus, and entorhinal cortex. These areas govern cognitive and emotional evaluation of the sensory and social stimuli that either generate or repress sexual desire and response.

The amygdala is a limbic structure which activates learning, memory, and evaluation of emotional reactions that occur during positive as well as stressful social interactions (including sex). As part of its general alerting effect on the brain, bupropion probably stimulates the amygdala as well as other limbic structures that mediate the interplay of thought and emotion. Bo et al. (1984) have shown that bupropion generates specific EEG stimulation in the hippocampus. The occasional propensity of bupropion to induce seizure activity could be explained by this potentiation of limbic activity. Its failure to alleviate panic

Table 27.1 *Profile of Bupropion (Wellbutrin)*

Daily Dose
200–450 mg/day

COMMON INDICATIONS
- Depression
- Manic-depressive disorder

MECHANISMS OF ACTION (GENERAL)
- Dopamine uptake inhibition
- Weak norepinephrine uptake inhibition action

MECHANISMS OF ACTION (SEXUAL)
- *Positive*
  - Increased adrenal androgen (DHEAS)
  - Increased adrenergic (alpha-1) activity
  - Increased dopamine
  - Decreased prolactin

DIRECT SEXUAL SIDE EFFECTS
- Desire disorders
  - Hyposexuality (improves)
  - Inhibited sexual desire (improves)
  - Sexual aversion (improves)
  - Hypersexuality (aggravates)
- Erection difficulties (improves)
- Lubrication (improves)
- Orgasm/ejaculation
  - Orgasmic inhibition (improves)
  - Anorgasmia (improves)
  - Diminished number of orgasms (improves)
  - Anesthetic ejaculation (improves)
  - Painful ejaculation (aggravates)
- Menstrual disorders
  - Amenorrhea (aggravates)

INDIRECT SEXUAL SIDE EFFECTS
- *Appearance/body-image* such as dryness of skin, mouth, mucous membranes, weight loss
- *Discomfort* caused by dryness of skin, mouth, mucous membranes, constipation, nausea, rash/itching
- *Mood disorders* resulting in aggression, anxiety, irritability, nervousness, psychoses
- *Neurological disturbances* resulting in dizziness, headache, sleep disturbances, tremor

SEXUAL CONTRAINDICATIONS/BENEFITS
- *Avoid with prior condition of*
  - Hypersexuality
  - Menstrual disorders
- *May be useful for*
  - Desire disorders
  - Inhibited ejaculations

ALTERNATIVES
- Fluoxetine (Prozac)
- Trazodone (Deseryl)
- Nefazodone (Serzone)

disorder, in contrast to most other antidepressants (Sheehan, Davidson, Manschreck, & Van Wyck Fleet, 1983), may also involve a special limbic activating feature. Though limbic activation is associated with cholinergic stimulation, activation by bupropion could be due to its uninvestigated actions on excitatory amino acids through the brain sigma receptor (Ferris, Russell, & Topham, 1987).

The positive aspect of limbic activation would be facilitation of attention and cognitive processing of sensory input. The same type of overexcitation that is involved in seizure may also be involved in orgasm which, to a large extent, is a response from the limbic septal area (Heath, 1972). The appearance of EEG theta activation in the right hemisphere during orgasm (Cohen et al., 1976) indicates limbic activation. Theta and limbic activation is also characteristic of REM "dream" sleep; theta rhythm has also been shown to be selectively increased in rats given l-deprenyl (Nickel et al., 1990; Nickel et al., 1994). The positive sexual effects of bupropion and l-deprenyl may be due in part to such theta activation or to stimulation of limbic structures such as the septum that generate theta.

As a dopaminergic stimulant, bupropion has an excitatory effect on the nucleus accumbens (NACC), a small area at the base of the limbic system adjacent to the basal ganglia and in front of the hypothalamus. Positioned in a reinforcement pathway from the ventral tegmentum and the median forebrain bundle connected to the mesolimbic dopamine regions (governing thought and emotional reactions) and to the nigrostriatal area (governing movement), the nucleus accumbens appears to function as a nodal interface between dopaminergic motivation drives and the behavior necessary to satisfy these drives. If there are areas in the brain that get a "charge" during vigorous and pleasurable activities, the nucleus accumbens is certainly one of them. NACC activity is increased prior to and during sexual activity, feeding, exercise, and other pleasurable activities.

The nucleus accumbens receives direct neural projections from the limbic structures that govern emotional and sexual reactions: amygdala, septum, hippocampus, entorhinal cortex, cingulate gyrus, and prefrontal cortex. Technically, the nucleus accumbens and the hypothalamus are transitional structures between the lower (reptilian) brain and the middle brain limbic structures (MacLean, 1990). In lower animals, chemical sexual stimuli like pheromones pass directly to the reptilian brain, sometimes called the smell brain. As the brain evolved, sexual stimuli were increasingly routed for evaluation to cognitive areas in the cortex and limbic area. Parallel to this evolution, critical sexual stimuli shifted from the sensory domains of smell and touch, which are direct and reflexive, to sight, which allows decisions of desire to be made at a distance. The desires and attractions are recorded as higher-order perceptions, so that they can be remembered and acted on in the future. Appropriately, the nucleus accumbens, which is fired when these attractions actually occur, is located next to the olfactory nucleus at the forward base of the brain. The nigrostriatal brain structures governing initiation, direction, and modulation of physical movement operate in tandem with the nucleus accumbens, allowing intentions, thoughts, habitual and stereotyped actions, and emotional reflexes to be translated into purposeful and routine activity. Thus, limbic and cortical learning and memory may be expressed through appropriate action. The nucleus accumbens may work to some extent as a transformer, resonator, or charger within this circuit.

In humans, smell and touch stimuli are remembered in the context of their cognitive associations. We remember that someone has a pleasing or displeasing odor and/or touch from our memory of that person. The additional brain area in the prefrontal cortex allows us to anticipate smelling and touching a particular person, even when he or she is not physically present. When the person is present or immediately expected, the nucleus accumbens receives an alerting charge from memory structures to move toward the desired person. Thus, evolution of the brain has facilitated a cognitive-emotional interface far more complex than simple hormone-driven sexuality. If these reinforcement areas of the brain do not charge when appropriate, then behavior is unresponsive, even listless. Sexual overtures and initiatives from the partner will not evoke arousal behavior, and pleasurable activities in general, such as eating and playing, will also fail to evoke response. Such a lack of anticipatory responsiveness to pleasurable stimuli may underlie bulimic and addictive behaviors, in which one is satisfied only while directly involved in the addicting activity.

The evidence that the nucleus accumbens functions as a pleasure resonator is very strong. However, few researchers appreciate that pleasure and reinforcement are central to the whole nervous system. The prevailing view concentrates on the role of pleasure and reinforcement in abuse and indulgence that corrodes or stops the system from performing normally.

Various studies have shown different aspects of NACC involvement in active pleasurable and resourceful behavior. Dopamine appears to be the chief stimulant of NACC activation. Unfortunately, most of the experimental work in this area has been done on rats. In higher animals, NACC involvement may be more intricate or may be obscured by less direct expression of desire. Nonetheless, this research constitutes a starting point:

- Bos & Cools, 1989
- Costall, Naylor, Mardsden, & Pycock, 1976
- Hernandez & Hoebel, 1988
- Jones, Neill, & Justice, 1990
- Maj, Wedzony, & Klimek, 1987
- Nurse, Russell, & Taljaard, 1985
- Phillips, Blaha, & Fibiger, 1988
- West & Michael, 1990
- Wise, Fotuhi, & Colle, 1989
- Yu & Han, 1990

Specific activation of the NACC by sexual stimuli and sexual activity also has been shown by:

- Ahlenius, Carlsson, Hillegaart, Hjorth, & Larsson, 1987
- Alderson & Baum, 1981
- Deminiere, Piazza, Le Moal, & Simon, 1989
- Di Chiara & Imperato, 1986
- Everitt, Cador, & Robbins, 1989
- Everitt & Hansen, 1983
- Heath, 1972
- Koene, Prinssen, & Cools, 1990
- Mas, Gonzalez-Mora, Louilot, Sole, & Guadalupe, 1990
- Mitchell & Gratton, 1990
- Morgenstern, Fink, Ott, & Parvez, 1988
- Pfaus et al., 1990
- Pfaus & Phillips, 1991
- Pleim, Matochik, Barfield, & Auerbach, 1990
- Rivas & Mir, 1990

There are strong indications that bupropion positively affects the nucleus accumbens, indicating a possible central mechanism for bupropion's sexual stimulation and antidepressant efficacy. Remember, most of this research has been done with rats, which are considerably less sensitive to bupropion than mice, monkeys, and probably humans. Rats also do not show breakdown of bupropion to active metabolites, which accumulate to high levels in monkeys and humans.

Infused directly into the rat nucleus accumbens, bupropion had the same effect as cocaine or the dopamine releaser pipradol (Rosenzweig-Lipson, Chu, Delfs, & Kelley, 1990). All three drugs increased spontaneous activity, rearing, and responding for conditioned reinforcers. Bupropion also elevated dopamine activity stimulation in the nucleus accumbens by inhibiting NACC dopamine uptake (Stamford, Kruk, & Millar, 1988). Systemic injection of bupropion into rats raised NACC dopamine levels in a dose-dependent manner (Nomikos, Damsma, Wenkstern, & Fibiger, 1989). While 1 mg/kg bupropion had no effect, dopamine levels in the nucleus accumbens were clearly increased (170%) by 10 mg/kg, which is close to the antidepressant dose in rats (8–9 mg/kg). The increase appeared to be due to inhibition of dopamine uptake, not to dopamine release characteristic of amphetamines. In other research, bupropion prevented the chemical destruction of dopamine by the depletors 6-OHDA and alpha-MPT (Ferris, Cooper, & Maxwell, 1983). Such protection of neuronal dopamine is due to bupropion's dopamine uptake inhibiting action, which reduces entry of toxins into dopamine neurons. However, toxicity to noradrenergic neurons is not affected. This protective action could block toxic degeneration of neuronal dopamine in the nucleus accumbens and other parts of the dopamine pleasure-incentive sex-movement circuit.

With the evidence that bupropion stimulates and possibly alleviates depressed firing of the nucleus accumbens, we can begin to speculate on its positive effect on deficient sexual desire. The nucleus accumbens appears to act as a pleasure "power booster" in a circuit from the medial preoptic hypothalamus (sex center) and limbic structures (sensory-thought-memory centers) to the nigrostriatal area (movement/action center) (Mogenson, Jones, & Yim, 1980). The chief neurotransmitters in this circuit are dopamine and excitatory amino acids (glutamate transmission). Most antidepressants, including the tricyclics, indirectly sensitize (recharge) dopaminergic reactivation of this region over the course of three to six weeks of chronic administration, paralleling the recovery from overall depression. However, these antidepressants also have various neurotransmitter actions (serotonergic, noradrenergic) that inhibit the normal activation of the nucleus accumbens and limbic centers. Bupropion's general antidepressant action may be less potent than tricyclic or serotonergic antidepressants, but its dopaminergic stimulant action (and possible glutamate activation through sigma receptors) is directly targeted to this NACC/nigrostriatal/limbic pleasure circuit. Consequently, sexual stimulation from limbic areas and the MPO sex center is reinforced by bupropion, so that sensory and motivational stimuli can be translated into sexual action.

In this schema, bupropion does not directly *generate* sexual stimuli; rather, it *reinforces* sexual stimuli that are already occurring. Furthermore, bupropion does not have the directive action of testosterone and estrogen (though in women it may have such an action through stimulation of the adrenal androgen DHEAS). If sexual stimuli are not present through lack of exposure or are blocked by emotional conditioning, then there is no opportunity for the bupropion "boost" to manifest in increased sexual activity.

DHEAS STIMULATION

Bupropion treatment has been associated through our research with a significant increase of DHEAS in women patients, which was reversed when the women were switched to placebo (Crenshaw et al., 1987). No other therapeutic drug was known to increase DHEAS at the time of our research finding. However, recently calcium channel blockers and the diabetic drug metformin have been shown to increase DHEAS during the course of their normal therapeutic use. As discussed in Chapter 9, increased DHEAS may be beneficial to sex and health.

There is evidence that a large decrease in DHEAS can cause loss of sexual desire and that DHEA supplementation can have positive sexual effects. In a landmark study in the 1950s, Waxenberg found that sexual drive remained relatively unaltered after hysterectomy and ovariectomy, but decreased precipitously after the adrenal glands, the source of DHEAS, were removed (Waxenberg et al., 1959). Roberts (1986) reported the return of nocturnal erections in some patients treated with DHEA for neuropathy.

As noted previously, there is no known vital function for DHEA or DHEAS. Experimentation in animals may not be very meaningful because substantial adrenal secretion of DHEAS occurs only in humans, although primates show much greater activity than rats. Roberts (1986) and Regelson et al. (1988) have linked decline in DHEAS to aging and disease pathology. Roberts' work indicated a connection between DHEAS, cholinergic, GABA, and limbic activity, which may be relevant to bupropion's apparent stimulatory effects on limbic transmission and its seizuregenic propensity. DHEAS levels are lower in various disease states, including diabetes; conversely, DHEAS has been shown in animals to reduce obesity, autoimmune toxicity, and cancerous tumors (Schwartz, 1985). Barrett-Connor et al. (1986) have related lower DHEAS in men to heart disease and shorter life expectancy. However, this relationship was not shown for women.

Since declining levels of dopamine and DHEAS are two major toxic effects of aging, bupropion could have considerable benefit for longevity due to its stimulating action on both substances. However, DHEAS has been shown to antagonize GABA actions, which prevent seizures, so that its increase with bupropion, even if transient, could increase seizure susceptibility. However, the apparent excitatory influence of DHEAS could simultaneously benefit cognitive activity of the limbic system, which declines with age. Furthermore, DHEA supplementation in women at physiological doses has been shown to increase insulin growth factor (IGF-1), which could have beneficial effects on physical health during aging (Morales, Nolan, et al., 1994).

STIMULANT PROPERTIES OF BUPROPION

Bupropion satisfies both the reinforcer and discrimination criteria for abuse and dependence potential similar to cocaine, but has far less potency and risk; it resembles stimulants in general and cocaine in particular in its ability to serve as a reinforcer in animals.* Bupropion has been shown to be self-administered by monkeys (Johanson, 1986; Lamb & Griffiths, 1990; Melia & Spealman, 1991; James H. Woods, personal communication, 1983) and to cause rats to prefer a compartment associated with it (Ortmann, 1985).

Most of the evidence for bupropion's similarity to cocaine comes from research with monkeys and has been performed by key researchers in behavioral pharmacology who specialize in evaluation of drugs as reinforcers and drug dependence. While drug reinforcement and discrimination procedures tested on animals have identified many drugs as reinforcers (including the antidepressant nomifensine), such drugs may not cause abuse or dependency during human clinical use. However, doctors should be alerted to the possibility that abuse *may* occur in order to properly monitor patients and screen those with a history of prior stimulant abuse.

In a landmark article in *Science*, Ritz, Lamb, Goldberg, and Kuhar (1987) identified dopamine uptake inhibition as the chief aspect of cocaine's reinforcement action. It was shown that self-administration (reinforcement) of cocaine and its derivatives and other cocaine-like drugs (but not amphetamines) was directly related to their potency at the dopamine uptake inhibitor site. They then proposed that cocaine substance abuse was due to this uptake inhibitor property. A later study by Ritz (Ritz & Kuhar, 1989) indicated that self-administration of amphetamine-type drugs was related to dopamine and norepinephrine *release* rather than to dopamine *uptake inhibition*. Furthermore, self-administration of amphetamine (but not cocaine) was decreased by serotonergic drugs such as fluoxetine (Porrino et al., 1989). The toxic destruction of serotonin brain receptors that is caused by amphetamines does not occur with cocaine. In fact, amphetamine-induced brain toxicity can be blocked by dopamine uptake inhibitors such as cocaine and bupropion (Marek, Vosmer, & Seiden, 1990; Snyder, Stricker, & Zigmond, 1985). Consequently, although bupropion and cocaine share a common stimulant reinforcing property (that of dopamine uptake inhibition), possession of this property does not mean that bupropion will have amphetamine-like toxic effects or be abused. However, its chronic use could sensitize prior stimulant addicts to cocaine and other stimulant craving.

A researcher at the National Institute of Mental Health has suggested that "benign" dopamine uptake inhibitors like bupropion and nomifensine could even be used as safe substitutes for cocaine (Rothman, 1990). Bupropion is currently being tested by psychiatrists at Yale to see if it will reduce cocaine abuse in their patients (Margolin, Kosten, Petrakis, Avants, & Kosten, 1991). However, bupropion may be expected to be too weak in stimulant potency to satisfy craving in cocaine abusers. While it may be safe for some former cocaine abusers to use bupropion as a substitute, the dangers of bupropion use in

*Lever-responding in animal research identifies a drug as a reinforcer. The National Institute of Drug Abuse criterion for drug abuse potential is whether a drug acts as a reinforcer, reasoning that "liking" a drug indicates a risk for drug abuse and dependency (Johanson, 1990). An additional indication of abuse potential is identification with abused drugs in the drug discrimination paradigm.

patients with addictive personalities have already been shown in bulimics (Mitchell et al., 1991).

The negative degenerative effects that occur with cocaine abuse have not been shown with bupropion during its short history of clinical use. However, as noted, seizures can be generated by both cocaine and bupropion. With adequate monitoring, bupropion is remarkably safe; with inadequate monitoring and prescription to patients with drug abuse and psychotic tendencies, bupropion can be dangerous. Unfortunately, if bupropion is shown to be dangerous to a few patients prone to stimulant abuse, it may again be removed from the market.

Given that bupropion is a unique dopaminergic therapeutic drug, findings in regard to its benefits and toxicity will advance our knowledge of dopaminergic stimulation free of the risks that characterize amphetamine-derivative stimulants. While dopamine and its body metabolites also inhibit norepinephrine uptake, bupropion's effects in research and clinical practice indicate that its chief action is through dopamine, PEA, and sigma actions, rather than through conventional norepinephrine actions.

ABSENCE OF SEXUAL DYSFUNCTION

Due to its apparent lack of sexually negative mechanisms of action, bupropion should have no negative sexual side effects except those due to nervousness generated from its stimulant action. Indeed, the dopamine potentiation that occurs on bupropion should have generally positive effects on sexual desire and response. However, since dopamine quickens ejaculation, premature ejaculation may sometimes occur. It would be difficult to discriminate a direct dopaminergic facilitation of orgasm/ejaculation from ejaculation precipitated by bupropion-induced anxiety. We assume that nervousness from stimulants is due to their norepinephrine action; dopamine-induced quickening of ejaculation may be due to increased release of dopamine or to a direct agonist action on the dopamine DA-2 receptor. However, bupropion appears to have only a relatively mild effect on norepinephrine receptors and does not release dopamine or have a DA-2 agonist action. These properties make premature ejaculation less likely.

In practice, we have not found that bupropion causes premature ejaculation or the general limp (contracted/vasoconstricted) tone in the penis often induced by stimulants (diethylpropion, pseudoephedrine) and stimulating antidepressants (nomifensine, amineptine). In fact, some patients noticed the opposite effect—that the resting penis was larger than usual. Conceivably, nervousness or tenseness due to bupropion could interfere with erection. This effect would occur within two to four weeks of beginning the treatment. In such cases, dosage can be lowered and the patient reassured that his agitation is most probably due to a transient stimulant effect. This nervousness may be the most frequent side effect of bupropion occurring in male patients.

A recent convention report by Fossey and Hamner (1994) on the treatment of 30 depressive males with a sustained-release formulation of bupropion (not yet marketed) noted erectile dysfunction in eight of the patients (26.7%) and decreased sexual interest in five (16.7%). Such a finding should remind doctors that bupropion may be excessively stimulating, resulting in sexual dysfunction due to nervousness and hypersensitivity, which could be avoided by careful dose adjustments downward. At the same time, positive sexual effects may not occur in males unless the dose is kept near the upper limit (450 mg/day), which is well-tolerated by most male patients (in contrast, 300 mg/day is more appropriate for female patients).

A side-effect table in bupropion's *Physicians Desk Reference* labeling includes decreased libido in 3.1% of patients versus 1.6% with placebo and 3.4% impotence versus 3.1% on placebo. Increased libido and decreased sexual function are indicated as prominent "neuropsychiatric" side effects. In contrast, fluoxetine (Prozac) is listed in the *Physicians Desk Reference* as having only 1.6% decreased libido versus 0% on placebo and 1.9% sexual dysfunction versus 0% on placebo. According to the *Physicians Desk Reference,* bupropion has more frequent negative sexual side effects than fluoxetine: 3.1% decreased libido and 3.4% impotence on bupropion versus 1.6% decreased libido and 1.9% sexual dysfunction on fluoxetine. In this case, the *Physicians Desk Reference* is not only unhelpful but misleading. Our findings and the cumulative findings in the literature do not support the statistics in the *Physicians Desk Reference*, either on bupropion or fluoxetine. Bupropion rarely decreases libido, and often *increases* it. Fluoxetine so potently reduces desire and inhibits orgasm that it is being used to treat premature ejaculation. Curiously, the Federal Drug Administration allows bupropion's manufacturer to advertise bupropion (Wellbutrin) as free of sexual side effects in contradiction to *Physicians Desk Reference* labeling; in contrast, the prominent, adverse sexual side effects for fluoxetine are required in the labeling. A 1991 trial comparison of bupropion versus fluoxetine (Feighner et al., 1991) sponsored by bupropion's manufacturer showed no sexual side effects on bupropion, but also very few on fluoxetine (only single cases of impotence, anorgasmia, and decreased libido).

Gardner (1983) demonstrated that bupropion could relieve sexual symptoms caused by tricyclics. He selected a group of 40 patients intolerant of tricyclic side effects: While taking tricyclics, seven of 11 (64%) of the men in this group complained of sexual dysfunction, including erectile failure and decreased libido. However, no adverse sexual side effects were noted in 29 females, so that overall only 17% of tricyclic intolerant patients complained of sexual dysfunction. When switched to bupropion, only two of the seven men continued to complain of sexual dysfunction. In a later study, Gardner and Johnston (1985) reported that sexual dysfunction ("drive or performance") was resolved in 24 of 28 male patients switched from various antidepressants (mostly tricyclics) to bupropion. It was unclear whether this sample included the men studied in the initial 1983 report. The authors noted that "due to the complexity of the female sexual response and the in-depth interviewing required, only data from male patients were used." Gardner (1983) either failed to note sexual dysfunction in women patients or chose to exclude women (Gardner & Johnston, 1985). The 1983 report was published in a supplement sponsored by bupropion's manufacturer. The absence of sexual side-effect information for women reflected the prevailing attitude of the drug industry—that women need not be investigated for antidepressant "sexual pathophysiological action."

A recent study funded by bupropion's manufacturer included both women and men (22 females, 17 males) who had side effects of anorgasmia or delayed orgasm on fluoxetine (Walker, Cole, Gardner, et al., 1993). These patients were switched to bupropion treatment, and 31 of the 39 completed four weeks of treatment. Of these 31 patients, 29 (94%) reported partial or complete resolution of their drug-induced orgasm problems and 25 (81%) reported improvement of libido from the level experienced while treated with fluoxetine. Unfortunately, a comparison group of patients switched from fluoxetine to a more conventional antidepressants (e.g., desipramine) was not included.

MALE/FEMALE DIFFERENCES

Bupropion has a side-effect profile and sexual benefits particularly attractive to women. However, women may also be at greater risk for adverse effects (seizure, psychoses) from the stimulant properties of bupropion. The total number of seizures reported by patients on bupropion is small: 12 seizures in 3,000 patients (0.4%) (Davidson, 1990). The generally accepted estimate of seizures with most available antidepressants at recommended doses is three to six seizures per 3,000 patients (Davidson, 1989). A few available antidepressants (maprotiline and clomipramine) have seizure rates of 1% or over. There is no information on the comparable seizure risk in women and men on other antidepressants. Apparently, seizures that do occur on bupropion are benign, with quick and uncomplicated recovery. In contrast, seizures due to accidental or intentional overdose of tricyclic antidepressants occur with other toxic reactions that can be fatal. Overdose with bupropion alone is seldom, if ever, fatal. (Three fatal drug overdoses involving bupropion were recently reported, but the toxic drugs carbamazepine and thioridazine were also detected in one case, and toxic levels of diphenhydramine were detected in a second case [Friel, Logan, & Fligner, 1993].)

Seizure risk due to bupropion is greater for women than for men (Goldberg, 1990). Prior to the post-approval surveillance trial investigating seizure prevalence, few seizures had been noted at recommended therapeutic doses of 450 mg/day. Those that did occur in patients not predisposed to seizures were almost always in women (12 seizures in women versus one in men). Considering all factors, the risk for seizures at recommended doses was three to eight times greater for women than for men. In the surveillance trial of 3,277 patients, which excluded patients with risk factors for seizures and eating disorders, the difference between women and men still occurred but was small: 0.46% for women versus 0.30% for men (Davidson, 1990).

The general seizure threshold of women is much lower than in men. As measured during electroconvulsive shock therapy in depressed patients, men must be given a larger shock dose (158%) than women to elicit seizures (Sackeim, Decina, Prohownik, & Malitz, 1987). The lower charge required for women was partly attributed by the authors to higher cortical blood flow, neurometabolism, and neural excitability in women. The higher cerebral blood flow in women is most noticeable in frontal regions that influence emotion and activity (Daniel, Mathew, & Wilson, 1988). Figiel and Jarvis (1990) also reported that bupropion substantially increased and prolonged induced seizures during electroconvulsive shock therapy in a 60-year-old depressed woman. In animal research, females show greater sensitization (increased response with repeated doses) to dopaminergic stimulants than males (Robinson & Becker, 1986). In standard tests of neural dopamine sensitivity (e.g., rotational behavior, stereotyped behavior, locomotion), female rats showed more initial reaction to a given amphetamine dose than males, and a greater increase in sensitivity with chronic administration. Apparently, testosterone lessens sensitization reactions in males. Removal of the ovaries causes no change in sensitization, but castration of males results in increased sensitization comparable to that shown by females. Female rats were also more reactive to cocaine and reacted to lower doses of cocaine than male rats (Glick, Hinds, & Shapiro, 1983). The authors speculated that female rat brain asymmetries are particularly sensitive to the dopamine uptake inhibitory property of cocaine.

WEIGHT REDUCTION

One of the appealing features of bupropion is its tendency to facilitate weight loss. Weight loss can promote sexual desire and response by increasing sexual attractiveness and energy. Patients who had gained weight on various antidepressants lost this excess weight when switched to bupropion (Gardner, 1984). Harto-Truax, Miller, Cato, Stern, and Sato (1983) showed that bupropion consistently caused an average weight loss of 1–3 kilograms (2–7 pounds). (The incidence of this slight weight loss is consistent and usually statistically different from placebo [0–1 kg weight gain] and tricyclic antidepressants [2–4 kg/3–9 lb gain].) From 26% to 39% of overweight patients treated with bupropion showed a weight loss of five pounds or more. Case studies have also shown that bupropion can eliminate chocolate craving (Michell, Mebane, & Billings, 1989).

Shown to reduce or eliminate bulimia (Horne et al., 1988), bupropion is now contraindicated in this population due to seizure side effects. However, bupropion may be efficacious in disorders characterized by concern with weight gain due to hyperphagia (atypical depression) or lack of energy and exercise (fatigue syndromes). Goodnick and Extein (1989) reported positive results using bupropion as treatment for atypical depression characterized by hyperphagia and/or hypersomnia; in the same study fluoxetine (Prozac) showed little benefit. Case studies have also shown that bupropion can reverse the symptoms of chronic fatigue syndrome (Goodnick, 1990). Duffy and Campbell (1994) reported cases of a 40-year-old woman and a 38-year-old man successfully treated with bupropion for fatigue and irritability associated with multiple sclerosis. Energy increased and irritability decreased with no adverse side effects in both patients over an extended period. As more reports are published on these weight control and fatigue reduction features of bupropion, its unique blend of stimulant and antidepressant actions will be better understood.

While serotonergic antidepressants (SSRIs) such as fluoxetine can cause weight loss and treat obesity, they can also cause fatigue and possibly reduce body metabolism (e.g., Hoehn-Saric, Lipsey, & McLeod, 1990; Lewis, Braganza & Williams, 1993), so that weight gain occurs with long-term use. In contrast, bupropion may initially cause only slight weight loss compared to fluoxetine, but with long-term use its energizing properties can facilitate further weight loss. However, since it lacks fluoxetine's appetite reduction impact and the anorectic actions of amphetamine-like stimulants, bupropion is unlikely to be useful for the treatment of obesity except as an adjunctive medication.

Bupropion may be suitable for preventing the seemingly inevitable weight gain that occurs when a person quits smoking, while also treating the depression that may occur with cessation of this habit. The usual weight gain upon quitting smoking (2–7 lbs) is matched by the typical weight loss (2–7 lbs) experienced on bupropion. In addition, stimulating, reinforcing, and antidepressant features of bupropion may facilitate withdrawal from smoking and prevent relapse. The same benefits may occur in alcohol withdrawal, with the further advantage that bupropion can reduce the sedating and intoxicating effects of alcohol. J.M. Jonas (among others) has proposed that "binge eating and psychoactive substance abuse are both expressions of the same underlying biological vulnerability" (1990). Bupropion was being tested for the treatment of alcohol withdrawal when its use was suspended in 1986. Apparently, this protocol has been abandoned. However, it is intriguing to speculate that one medication might possess these multiple clinical features: weight loss, addiction management potential, and antidepressant properties.

Reduction of weight and fatigue with bupropion use may encourage sexually "sluggish" or dysfunctional patients to become more active in this area. The dopaminergic action of bupropion should further activate sexual initiative when physical inhibitions such as overweight and fatigue are removed. Any bupropion-facilitated withdrawal from smoking and alcohol will help eliminate related impediments to physical sexual function.

INSOMNIA

Delay of sleep onset and abnormal waking is a characteristic feature of bupropion. However, this side effect is often masked by preexisting sleep difficulties (insomnia is a baseline symptom of depression). When the need for benzodiazepines to treat insomnia begins after initiation of bupropion treatment, the sleep disruption can be seen as an effect of bupropion distinct from depressive symptomatology. (Despite its concern with seizures, which are often preceded by or generated during insomnia, the Federal Drug Administration has never required a study of bupropion's sleep effects.) The Crenshaw Clinic study of bupropion described in the last section of this chapter was not complicated by preexisting insomnia, due to the fact that depressed patients were excluded from the study. However, insomnia was a major dose-limiting side effect of bupropion, occurring chiefly among female patients. Overall, 57% of bupropion subjects experienced insomnia versus 30% in the placebo group, a significant difference. Sixty-three percent of bupropion-treated women had moderate to severe, dose-related insomnia versus 21% of placebo-treated women. Serious insomnia was infrequent in male subjects, whether on bupropion or placebo. Bupropion-induced insomnia can be minimized by limiting dose increases until they are tolerated without sleep upset.

PSYCHOSES

A definite risk of psychoses is associated with the use of bupropion, primarily due to its dopaminergic and activating properties. At usual therapeutic doses (200–450 mg/day), the stimulation of dopamine activity is probably low and unlikely to induce psychoses, except in patients already predisposed. However, bupropion's influence on excitatory amino acids (EAA) through the sigma receptor (Ferris et al., 1987) has not been investigated. Considering the fact that phencyclidine (PCP—"angel dust") seems to induce psychoses through an effect on excitatory amino acids, and that there is an investigatory antipsychotic drug (rimcazole) that appears to block psychoses by antagonizing sigma receptor activity (Ferris et al., 1987), there is a possibility that bupropion can worsen psychotic and schizophrenic tendencies through its undefined actions at the sigma receptor. (The affinity of bupropion to the sigma receptor is equivalent to that of the neuroleptic sigma antagonist rimcazole [Ferris et al., 1987].)

The effect of bupropion on glutamate transmission through the sigma receptor is unknown. However, it can be assumed to be a sigma agonist because its stimulant effects are similar to those of excitatory amino acid-glutamate transmission. Bupropion induces movement, generates seizures, aggravates psychoses, and in general, causes limbic activation typical of EAA/glutamate stimulation. Such EAA stimulation would reinforce the possibly marginal dopamine action of bupropion on the nucleus accumbens at therapeutic dose levels. There is considerable evidence (Cheramy et al., 1990; Imperato, Honore, & Jensen, 1990) that EEA/glutamate stimulates dopamine activation of the nucleus accumbens, inducing locomotor behavior. EEA/glutamate antagonists injected into the nucleus accumbens reduce amphetamine and cocaine hyperactivity (Pulvirenti & Koob, 1990). Because the nucleus accumbens is critically involved in pleasure-seeking behaviors, including sex, bupropion may exert a stimulant action on it through dopamine and EEA/glutamate potentiation. Since antagonists of dopamine and EEA/sigma antagonists (such as rimcazole) are used as antipsychotics, bupropion may also aggravate psychotic behavior through dopamine and EEA stimulation. Many commonly used antipsychotic drugs (including haloperidol) have strong affinity to both dopamine and sigma receptors.

It is likely that PEA and EAA sigma activity are the "hidden ingredients" that interact with bupropion's dopaminergic action to induce therapeutic increases in sexual drive and function. When bupropion generates an overload of EAA-dopamine activity or increases PEA activation, it may cause hypersexuality or compulsive sexual thoughts and activity (sex addiction?).

Becker and Dufresne (1982) reported psychotic/schizophrenic reactions in bupropion-treated patients consisting of perceptual alterations, increased sensory intensity, increased activity, decreased inhibitions, vivid dreaming, increased emotionality, and distractions from competing stimuli. Patients generally found these states to be "pleasurable and helpful" because they included increased awareness of others and emotional involvement which helped resolve "issues that had been depressing to the patient." These reactions occurred in 40–70% of 12 hospitalized depressed patients. They started within 3–12 days of bupropion treatment (mean dose = 561 mg/day). Clearly psychotic or schizophrenic episodes occurred in only three patients who had been previously diagnosed with schizophrenia. There was no indication of how many of these patients were women. Bupropion doses above 450 mg are no longer recommended.

The most complete investigation of bupropion-induced psychoses was reported by Golden and his colleagues at the National Institute of Mental Health (Golden et al., 1985). All four cases were women being treated for depression, who had no prior history of schizophrenia or schizo-affective disorder. However, three of the four patients had had brief psychotic episodes years earlier. Only one was prescribed bupropion at a dose (500 mg/day) higher than the currently recommended limit of 450 mg/day. Visual or auditory hallucinations were present in all four cases, agitation in two, and paranoia in one. Other adverse effects, including nausea, headache, and restlessness, occurred prior to or coincidental with the psychoses.

Later papers by Golden and his colleagues (Golden, Rudorfer, Shere, Linnoila, & Potter, 1988; Golden et al., 1988) reported lack of therapeutic response or aberrant chemical reactions in bupropion-treated patients with psychoses (some of these patients discussed were in their 1985 article). The dopamine metabolite homovanillic acid (HVA) and bupropion chemical metabolites showed excess levels in these patients as compared to patients with therapeutic response. It appeared from this study that female patients are more at risk than males for such high HVA levels. Since bupropion-induced seizures occurred more frequently in women patients and were dose-dependent (Goldberg, 1990), there should be a clear warning that women are at risk for excess reactions to bupropion compared to males and side effects should be closely monitored to avoid toxic doses even within the 450 mg/day limit. There may be a relationship between seizures and psychoses, such that either may occur in response to stimulation by high levels of bupropion or its metabolites.

It has been established that bupropion can exacerbate psychotic symptoms in schizo-affective or psychotically depressed patients (Goode & Manning, 1983). However, these reports apparently occurred during earlier clinical investigation, when doses higher than the currently recommended 450 mg were used. Some reports have noted that combining the dopamine DA-2 receptor antagonist haloperidol (Haldol) with bupropion was sufficient to block psychotic symptoms, yet allowed optimum treatment of schizoaffective and psychotically depressed patients (Goode & Manning, 1983; Manberg & Carter, 1984; Wright et al., 1985). However, Dufresne, Kass, and Becker (1988) found that the addition of bupropion to neuroleptic (thiothixene) treatment of schizophrenic depressed patients disrupted therapeutic effects of the neuroleptic alone. Since neuroleptics and bupropion each have some seizuregenic potential, their combination may increase the risk of seizure.

BIPOLAR DISORDERS

Bupropion seems especially useful in treating bipolar and schizo-affective disorders (Shopsin, 1983; Wright et al., 1985). Tricyclic antidepressants are often contraindicated in such patients because they can trigger mania and may increase the swings between depression and mania (Wehr & Goodwin, 1987). Often the only pharmaceutical alternative to treat manic-depressive patients is lithium. However, lithium can cause intolerable weight gain, mild depression, as well as some sexual dysfunction. Haykal and Akiskal (1990) successfully treated rapid cycling manic-depressives with combinations of bupropion and lithium.

It is expected that bupropion will be increasingly used to treat manic-depression (bipolar disorder) and schizo-affective disorders. As such use increases, it may be expected that more cases of mania (Bittman & Young, 1991; Masand & Stern, 1993) and delirium (Liberzon, Dequardo, & Silk, 1990; Dager & Heritch, 1990) during bupropion treatment will be reported. Stoll et al. (1994) have observed that mania induced by bupropion may be milder than typically seen with either tricyclic antidepressants or fluoxetine. Use of bupropion with lithium can increase seizure risk because both drugs can induce seizures.

Perhaps the safest combination for treating bipolar and schizo-affective disorders is bupropion and valproate (Depakote). Each of these drugs has been effective in treating manic-depression and valproate, as an anticonvulsant, can protect against the possibility of seizure with bupropion use alone. John Feighner (personal communication, 1990) has found that the use of bupropion with valproate is safe and effective for his patients, but this combination has not been subject to controlled testing.

THE CRENSHAW CLINIC STUDY

Due to its apparent dopaminergic action and occasional findings of improved sex drive during antidepressant trials, bupropion has been investigated in controlled trials for treatment of sexual dysfunction (Crenshaw et al., 1987; Goldberg & Crenshaw, 1992; Klein, Mendels, Lief, & Phillips, 1987). We had the opportunity to perform a series of research studies with bupropion to evaluate the sexual side effects that had been reported during depression trials and determine whether they were the predictable consequence of the successful treatment of depression or the independent positive sexual actions of bupropion. Use of a new drug in a field in which there is no previous experience with established testing instruments is problematic. Criteria for sexual dysfunction remain ambiguous, with no consistent research standard. Reversal of sexual dysfunction by any drug has yet to be established. Consequently, research design must be original, using testing instruments either "borrowed" from other settings or newly developed. The drawbacks of new questionnaires are obvious: They have not been standardized or verified. Results may be borderline, uncertain, or not reproducible. In addition, testing a small (less than 100) number of patients at a single site risks failure to show benefit (false negative), which discourages further testing. These were some of our concerns as we approached this research project. We were fortunate that, in spite of the numerous obstacles characteristic of novel projects of this sort, we were able to demonstrate statistically significant results and have our study report accepted by a major medical journal with stringent peer review.

In order to address the question, we selected patients with sex drive disorders and other *DSM-III-R* sexual dysfunctions excluding premature ejaculation. None of these patients was clinically depressed, so relief from depression could not be the significant factor in sexual improvement and normalization. We structured this research so that the results could be statistically significant and trustworthy, to the extent that any single study can. We took the opportunity to address and correct many of the inadequate study aspects and parameters we had identified in previous research. We had a relatively large population of 60; and there was an equal number of women and men in the study. We used standardized questionnaires and included the sexual partners in our interviews.

All subjects were in excellent health and generally not on other drugs except for contraceptives or estrogen replacement. They showed no evidence of organic cause for sexual dysfunction and all were in steady sexual relationships of at least six months' duration. Most subjects experienced some form of desire disorder: low sexual desire, inhibited sexual desire, or sexual aversion. Some subjects had associated erectile dysfunction or anorgasmia. The intention was to focus on low sexual desire, but subjects were accepted for the study if they had any *DSM-III-R* sexual drive or function disorders. The purpose of including other disorders was to obtain some indication of which sexual disorders might be affected to guide future research directions. Consequently, subjects represented a cross-section of sexual disorders normally treated by sex therapy, rather than a special group with only one dysfunction. An eight-week single-blind placebo lead-in period enabled us to establish baselines without medication, thus neutralizing the placebo effect that so strongly influences most sexual side-effect research. We also double-blinded the study with a crossover extension so that, in addition to having a placebo group that was separate, patients also served as their own controls.

From an analysis of the sexual mechanisms of this drug, bupropion appeared to be relatively benign. We also had identified it as a drug with the potential to have independent sexual effects of its own, but we were not optimistic about confirming this hypothesis because no such study had been done previously and the dopaminergic properties appeared to be relatively weak. More important was the potential to define the sexual side effects of this antidepressant drug in hopes of finally identifying one that had no adverse sexual consequences. We were richly rewarded initially in that bupropion demonstrated so few adverse sexual properties. As the study progressed, we became fascinated and surprised when we began to identify sexual improvements that we suspected were drug-related.

Approximately three weeks into the double-blind drug treatment phase of this study (weeks 10–12 overall), patients began to report sexual effects that led us to suspect bupropion over placebo. Research subjects described sexual responses, genital sensations, and physical experiences that we not only had never seen reported on placebo but had not been able to achieve through the sex therapy. One of our positive responders, who reported regaining his sex drive and erectile function, had gone through our treatment program without success, was referred elsewhere, and had undergone two additional therapies without success. Several of the women described experiencing throbbing vaginal sensations during the day, unrelated to sexual activity or thoughts which were, however, of a distracting sexual nature and which they felt compelled to act on when they next had the opportunity. For these reasons, we began to form opinions about who was on medication and who was not.

Critics might contend that our suspicions regarding these patients somehow distorted our results. Perhaps they did, but we do not believe this to be the case, since the study was carefully double-blinded and evident drug side effects were relatively few and benign. Also of note was the fact that, as patients achieved therapeutic levels in the 450 mg range (which was the upper limit recommended at that time), activating side effects such as insomnia became apparent in women, rendering the study less blinded at higher levels of medication.

The therapeutic sexual effect of bupropion required two to four weeks to manifest, the typical latency for its antidepressant effects. While improvement increased with further treatment, sexual desire and response reached maintenance levels and were sustained, sometimes even beyond drug discontinuation. Sexual drive and behavior did not seem to increase beyond normal except in a few patients, and any noted abnormal intensity diminished within three to 10 days. Bupropion has not been investigated in normal, sexually active persons to determine whether or not it can precipitate hypersexuality.

Our study suggested that bupropion could increase genital and orgasmic sensitivity in women, but this premise has yet to be investigated and confirmed. Its stimulant actions may also increase assertiveness and energy, which may become excessive and disruptive. Consequently, improved sexual desire and function could occur within the context of a general activation which, for some couples, could be counterproductive. Nevertheless, bupropion appears to be an excellent adjunctive drug treatment in the context of sex therapy—and vice versa: Sex therapy can help couples integrate the new assertive behaviors into their relationships.

The sexual and activating effects of bupropion appear to be due to dopamine uptake inhibiting action, which increases dopaminergic tone. While dopaminergic drugs are often abused for their stimulating effects, bupropion's gradual onset of action, characteristic of its antidepressant nature, suggests that it would not be subject to abuse, dependency, or tolerance typical of cocaine or amphetamines.

Placebo Condition (Single-Blind)

Historically, the chief problem with sexual dysfunction treatment trials has been a large placebo response rate (30–40%), which makes it difficult to differentiate a true drug effect (Benkert, 1975). This large placebo response has engendered skepticism and exasperation regarding study outcomes, especially claims regarding drug-induced improvement of sexual function. While this excessive placebo response has occurred mainly with impotence treatment, the assumption is that it would occur with treatment for any sexual dysfunction. Indeed, since the placebo response is assumedly psychological, it should be greater for disorders of sexual desire than for impotence, which often has organic aspects limiting a therapeutic response. In contrast, sexual desire is particularly sensitive to the psychological and social environment.

An unusually long placebo lead-in period of eight weeks was used in our study to maximally control for placebo responses while providing educational group therapy to subjects and their partners. The group sessions consisted of sex education and discussion of relationship problems related to sexual activity. Group sessions were lead by highly experienced clinical sex therapists independent of research visit reviews.

Patients appeared to be quite discerning in separating benefits of the sex education groups from possible drug-induced improvements, often noting improvement in sexual awareness and their relationships due to the groups but no noticeable change in their own sexual state. Consequently, patients entering the double-blind phase at week 9 had already shown proper study compliance and lack of placebo response. The few patients who did show a placebo response were continued in the study but not counted as subjects.

Evaluation Forms

Due to the lack of standard instruments for evaluating sexual dysfunction with drugs, we had to work with untested forms. The content of the forms was designed by the Crenshaw Clinic and modified by sponsor decisions in relation to FDA evaluation of drug efficacy. Weekly information and rating forms were answered by patients and brought to evaluation reviews. Clinical global dysfunction severity and improvement evaluations (CGI) were completed separately by the investigator and patient during the reviews. Weekly evaluation forms were also included, but not required, for rating by the patients' partners, but these forms were not always completed and returned. Initial patient evaluation included Hamilton Depression Scale ratings by independent psychiatrists, physical exams by independent physicians, and the remarkably comprehensive structured sexual interview, the Kinsey Questionnaire, conducted by highly trained and experienced sex therapists during a two-hour visit.

The essential ratings for change in sexual dysfunction were the CGI ratings. To rate improvement or deterioration, investigator and patient used a seven-point scale (1 = *very much improved*; 2 = *much improved*; 3 = *minimally improved*; 4 = *no change*; 5 = *minimally worse*; 6 = *much worse*; 7 = *very much worse*). In accord with standard clinical and FDA practice, a rating of 2 or 1 (*much* or *very much improved*) represented a positive response to treatment. (Improved evaluation forms and a new baseline sex evaluation instrument equivalent to a "sexual MMPI"—the Crenshaw-Goldberg Sexual Desire Inventory (CGSDI)—was subsequently developed from our experience with bupropion and used in our yohimbine treatment protocol described in Chapter 30.)

Double-Blind Phase

According to the scale 2 or "much improved" CGI criteria, 63% of bupropion-treated patients were positive responders compared to only 3% of those on placebo (though many placebo-treated patients noted minimal improvement). Table 27.2 shows the progressive improvement during the initial 20-week protocol at the four evaluation points for all patients and for men and women separately. These scores for treatment of sexual dysfunction are equal to or better than those found with bupropion treatment of depression. As is typical, investigator ratings show improvement before patient ratings. (Many antidepressant trials do not include patient ratings, which are less often significant than those of the investigator.) Although men showed greater improvement than women in the first double-blind phase, women patients showed greater improvement during the crossover phase. Improvement began during treatment weeks 2 through 4, as is also typical of antidepressant effects. Improvement became clearer by week 4, became consistently significant statistically by week 8, and continued through week 12. Since improvement and differentiation from placebo were still occurring at week 12, additional weeks of treatment may have resulted in more impressive changes in sexual behavior. Global dysfunction severity scores decreased as improvement increased. Based on these standard global efficacy measures, bupropion was shown to be effective in the treatment of sexual dysfunction in a prospective placebo-controlled double-blind study. Improvement on bupropion but generally not on placebo was shown between patient groups (first 12 weeks) and within the crossover group (from placebo in the first 12-week double-blind to bupropion in the crossover).

Statistical analysis showed that improvement score differences between bupropion and placebo were significant at all review points for investigator ratings and at the week 8 and week 12 ratings for patient ratings. As can be seen from the week 8 placebo baseline ratings, patients generally rated themselves as unchanged or minimally improved during the placebo lead-in phase. Placebo responding occurred in three male patients with erectile dysfunction, who did not have sexual desire deficiencies.

The CGI severity of illness rating decreased as improvement increased. As with the improvement scores, the differences between bupropion and placebo were significant from week 2 for-

Table 27.2 *CGI Improvement Scores from Placebo Month 2 Baseline Through 12-Week Double-blind Phase: Investigator and Patient Rated*

	Investigator-Rated		*Patient-Rated*	
Double-Blind Study Week	*Bupropion*	*Placebo*	*Bupropion*	*Placebo*
All Patients (n = 60)				
Placebo Baseline (Week 8)	3.90	3.77	3.57	3.57
2	3.00	3.63	3.03	3.43
4	2.43	3.33	2.93	3.27
8	2.17	3.53	2.83	3.33
12	2.13	3.70	2.43	3.70
Female Patients (n = 30)				
Placebo Baseline (Week 8)	3.81	3.86	3.63	3.71
2	3.31	3.86	3.19	3.57
4	2.62	3.29	3.00	3.21
8	2.25	3.93	2.69	3.64
12	2.38	4.14	2.56	4.14
Male Patients (n = 30)				
Placebo Baseline (Week 8)	4.00	3.69	3.50	3.44
2	2.64	2.44	2.86	3.31
4	2.21	3.38	2.86	3.31
8	2.07	3.19	3.00	3.06
12	1.86	3.31	2.29	3.31

5 = minimally worse; 4 = no change; 3 = minimally improved; 2 = much improved; 1 = very much improved

ward in the investigator ratings but only after week 4 in the patient ratings. Thus, moderate to marked dysfunction decreased nonsignificantly to moderate by placebo week 8. In the double-blind phase, dysfunction was reduced significantly to borderline or mild in bupropion patients, but remained moderate on placebo. The severity ratings by the investigator and patients showed that half of the patients (15) on bupropion still had mild to moderate sexual dysfunction after 12 weeks of bupropion treatment. The difference between bupropion and placebo in these week-20 improvement ratings was statistically significant by a wide margin ($p < 0.001$). On average, for both women and men, moderate to marked dysfunction in the bupropion group was reduced to mild to borderline.

Crossover Phase

During the double-blind crossover phase, 17 of 23 (74%) patients who were switched from placebo to bupropion showed positive responses, despite failure to show response during 20 weeks of placebo treatment (8 weeks single-blind, plus 12 weeks double-blind). Ten of 17 (59%) patients who improved initially on bupropion maintained their positive response through 12 weeks on placebo, while 7 of 17 (41%) reverted to minimal or no improvement.

Maintenance of response beyond drug treatment indicated that once sexual drive and function are improved toward normal, this improvement can continue without the drug. Return to prior levels of sexual dysfunction was more frequent for women than for men. Provision of group therapy, close monitoring of improvement, the 12-week extended period on drug, and lack of knowing that drug had been discontinued—all these factors may have facilitated later maintenance of response. In any event, response to drug during crossover can only be compared to the patients' own baseline. Bupropion-treated patients showed a definite, long-lasting carry-over effect to placebo treatment, which suggested that crossover studies of drug treatment for sexual dysfunction could be confounded by carry-over effects that do not disappear even after two or three months.

Of the 12 female patients who showed no response over the initial 20 weeks on placebo and were crossed over to bupropion during the extension, 10 (83%) showed positive responses. Of the 10 bupropion-treated women crossed over to placebo, four who had failed to improve on bupropion continued unchanged during placebo. Of the six who had shown positive responses on bupropion, three (50%) continued to show improvement on placebo, but in two of these three, CGI decreased from 1 (*very much improved*) to 2 (*much improved*). The remaining three women lost their positive response during placebo. Two of these three women further complained of the return of weight that had been lost while on bupropion.

Of the 12 male placebo-treated patients who were crossed over to bupropion, seven showed a positive response to the drug, four did not improve, and one maintained improvement experienced on placebo (placebo responder). Thus, seven of 11 (64%) men with minimal or no improvement during 20 weeks on placebo showed a positive response when switched double-blind to bupropion. Of the four who failed to show improvement, one complained of erectile dysfunction despite normal sex drive, two experienced both drive and erection dysfunctions, and one reported sex drive and erection dysfunction possibly related to post-traumatic stress syndrome from combat experience in Vietnam.

Bupropion-treated men were better able to maintain improvement (or claimed to be so) than women when switched from bupropion to 12 weeks of placebo treatment. The difference between men and women in actual CGI scores during the crossover was especially impressive. Despite an initial decline at crossover week 2, possibly indicating withdrawal, CGI scores for men did not significantly change (investigator CGI score: 1.75 at baseline week 20; 2.17 at crossover week 12). In contrast, CGI scores declined by more than a whole step, from *much improved to minimally improved*, in women switched from bupropion to placebo (investigator CGI score: 2.20 at baseline week 20; 3.40 at crossover week 12).

Summary of CGI Results

Statistically significant improvement occurred for both men and women treated with bupropion for mild to severe psychogenic sexual dysfunction. Many patients were convinced that they had become relatively normal, despite continuing or even new problems in their sexual relationships. These patients considered the improvement as a beginning and saw a need for couples sexual therapy. Hardly any patients focused on the drug as the source of improvement or as necessary to maintain improvement. It was only through the double-blind masked differentiation of improvement that it became evident that real improvement usually occurred with bupropion, not with placebo. From the CGI scores, it was clear that patients were able to discriminate between improved attitudes, knowledge, interest, and communication generated by the group sexual education sessions and a real change in their sexual energy and appetite.

Changes in desire and activity were dependent upon and confounded by differences in relationships, dysfunctional diagnoses, male and female sexual attitudes, and various limitations on sexual opportunities and stimulation. Improvements shown in sexual desire and activity measurements were less definite than those shown in the CGI integrated assessments. Given the diversity of diagnoses and relationships, this was to be expected.*

Bupropion did not appear to have a reliable effect for many patients. The small, overall changes shown here in desire and activity suggested that it was certainly no substitute for sex therapy for many of our patients. Its chief effect appeared to be in the area of sexual desire, despite some remarkable improvements in physical genital responses. Consequently, its efficacy in treating

*More clarity could be achieved by an increased number of subjects so that subgroups could be differentiated by more specific diagnostic criteria for the type of sexual dysfunction treated.

impotence is questionable. Perhaps its most notable effect, which is probably mediated by its dopaminergic property, is the stimulation of genital sensations and orgasmic response in women. How frequent or reliable this effect is cannot be answered without more specific research and clinical investigation.

Average strength of sex drive in bupropion-treated patients increased compared to placebo during the first four weeks (month 1) of double-blind treatment. It remained at the normal level through the remaining eight weeks (months 2–3). Sex drive in the placebo group decreased during the second and third months to a level below that shown at screening and at the end of placebo baseline. The differences in sex drive between bupropion and placebo were statistically significant for each of the three months. During the crossover phase, sex drive in placebo patients switched to bupropion gradually increased to normal from the low levels shown at the end of placebo treatment. Overall sex drive in bupropion patients switched to placebo remained at normal during the crossover phase, despite the loss of positive response in some patients. Bupropion alleviated self-rated low sex-drive problems, and these gains were maintained at "acceptable, normal levels."

Female sex drive ratings remained below male ratings throughout the study. Even when male patients who did not complain of sex-drive deficits (those with erection and ejaculation problems) were eliminated from the ratings, female drive ratings remained lower. Such a lower overall sex drive rating is typical of normal population surveys. (It is not clear whether this discrepancy represents a true difference between male and female sex drive in general, or whether men have a tendency to rate their drive as higher in accord with stereotyped notions of their preconceived role as initiators of sexual activity.) With bupropion, many women appeared to become more aware of sexual sensations localized in the vagina and clitoris. As they became aware of their improved physical reactivity, their sex drive also improved—even when orgasmic difficulties remained and their partners were uncooperative or unattractive. However, since most of the women patients in our study identified their sexual problem as one of low desire, the study sample was inadequate to test bupropion's explicit effects on physical sexual sensations and responses per se. Psychological specifics of bupropion-induced improvement in sex drive were also inadequately examined.

Pharmacological resolution of sexual desire dysfunction should not be attributed to aphrodisiacal effects, which may be more measurable because they express changes beyond normal. The change in sex drive in our bupropion study occurred in a subtle region of normalcy where quantitative measurement becomes infeasible. Sexuality is not a consistently present drive, need, or activity like hunger/eating or rest/sleep. It may occur irregularly and does not necessarily have immediate physical consequences if an opportunity for expression is not available.

During the first double-blind phase, sexual thoughts, feelings, and activity increased in all categories during bupropion treatment and decreased in all categories but one during placebo treatment. Decreases in the placebo group may have reflected the discontinuance of the educational groups or the fact that improvement failed to be noted. The increases in the bupropion group were sometimes small and nonsignificant, indicating either a rather weak drug effect or limitations due to relationships and circumstances.

Increases in strength of sex drive with bupropion compared to placebo were statistically significant for each of the three double-blind months. More specific sexual desire and activity ratings on the graduated Likert scales showed smaller and less consistently significant differences for bupropion compared to placebo. Crossover desire ratings showed that patients initially treated with placebo improved sexually when switched to bupropion even more than the initial bupropion group. In particular, intercourse frequency more than doubled, although masturbation frequency did not increase. Despite worsening of sexual drive during prior placebo treatment, these patients reached the "normal" point on the sex drive scale by the last month of the crossover to bupropion.

Although extensive data were gathered on orgasm, ejaculation, and erection, our sample was too small to draw any conclusions. Until studies are conducted of treatments for specific sexual dysfunctions, bupropion can only be said to treat lowered sexual desire. Individual patients on bupropion, but not on placebo, reported notable improvements in sexual response. Some of these response improvements could have been due to increases in sexual desire, but others (such as genital sensitization) were almost surely due to direct physical effects of bupropion.

Stimulation of DHEAS

In our study, bupropion treatment caused an impressive increase of adrenal androgen DHEAS levels in women patients, which was reversed when they were switched to placebo. Although DHEAS levels were also higher in men on bupropion compared to placebo, the difference was small and nonsignificant. Statistically significant increases occurred in women initially randomized to bupropion treatment and in women switched from placebo to bupropion during the crossover phase, so that this consistent effect was replicated within the study. No evidence of change in DHEAS levels occurred in the women randomized to placebo treatment, but these same women showed increased levels when switched to bupropion during the crossover phase. DHEAS levels declined significantly in women switched from bupropion to placebo during the crossover phase, so that it was shown to increase when women were switched from placebo to bupropion and subsequently to decrease when switched back to placebo. There were no changes in other hormones measured, even in cortisol, which is also secreted from the adrenal gland. No changes were found in levels of total testosterone, free testosterone, estradiol, estrone, progesterone, luteinizing hormone, follicle stimulating hormone, cortisol, or prolactin. Hormones were measured at screening and at the end of each double-blind phase as a safety measure.

Weight Loss

Our study showed consistent weight loss of from two to six pounds (1–3 kg), which was significantly different from placebo treatment in which minimal (0–1 kg) weight gain occurred. Patients lost weight on bupropion and regained weight when switched to placebo; conversely, patients who showed little weight change over 20 weeks on placebo showed only slight weight loss when switched to bupropion. Loss of appetite or nausea, which can induce weight loss on SSRIs such as fluoxetine (Prozac), was rare. Rather, energy and activity levels seemed to be increased by bupropion, along with a possible stimulation of metabolism. Weight loss and energy gain on bupropion could be partly responsible for the therapeutic increase in sex desire. Table 27.3 summarizes the results of our study.

Table 27.3 *Summary of Bupropion Study Results and Conclusion*

- Sexual desire deficiency usually corrected to normal; hypersexuality was rare.
- Normalized sexual desire often not accompanied by change in frequency of sexual behavior.
- Sexual dysfunction usually reduced to mild/minor but not fully eliminated.
- Sexual effects and improvement appeared after characteristic antidepressant latency (2–3 weeks).
- Specific acute genital sensations experienced by some female patients.
- Majority of patients with positive response to bupropion remained sexually restricted due to partner rejection/aversion.
- Significant efficacy of bupropion during crossover phase replicated efficacy in 20-week study.
- Positive sexual effect of bupropion often reversed during double-blind return to placebo.
- Placebo response rate low.
- No indication of physiological dependence on bupropion or of withdrawal when switched to placebo.
- Small and nonsignificant therapeutic effect on psychogenic impotence in subsequent study lacking clinical therapy groups (47% response on bupropion vs. 33% on placebo).
- Adjunct clinical sex therapy may be required for reliable therapeutic drug effect.

TREATMENT OF ERECTILE DYSFUNCTION: FOLLOW-UP STUDY

A later 12-week controlled trial comparing bupropion to placebo specifically for the treatment of psychogenic impotence failed to show improvement with bupropion. The study was executed by the sponsor at our clinic and at another site that had no experience with bupropion. Our site ran 30 patients, 15 on each, bupropion and placebo. Patients not responding at the end of 12 weeks were run in a 12-week bupropion open extension. (Placebo lead-in weeks were not used.)

Frequent improvement occurred during the 12-week open extension in placebo subjects switched to bupropion (they were told that they were now receiving bupropion, but were not told whether they had been on bupropion or placebo during the double-blind phase). Of 10 placebo patients continuing into the extension, eight (80%) improved. Of six bupropion-treated patients who continued into the extension due to lack of response, three (50%) became responders to bupropion during the extension. In sum, of 25 patients who completed both the initial double-blind and the open extension (24 weeks total), 72% showed a positive response.

CONCLUSIONS

The advances of our protocol to the field of sexual pharmacology were the inclusion of women in equal proportion to men; the basic structure of the study (long placebo lead-in period, double blind, crossover extension); and duration of treatment (three months) on drug. Weak points of our study were the questionnaires and testing instruments, which were not tested and standardized; and the lack of an explicit measure of sexual aversion.

At the time of the study, sexual aversion was not yet listed in the *DSM* manual (it has been included in the recent *DSM-IV* edition).

Subsequent to our studies, a bulimia study that was ongoing at the time bupropion (Wellbutrin) was first marketed, evidenced the seizure incidents that brought a halt to the release of bupropion (Horne et al., 1988). It also brought a halt to new funding for further research on the drug, since its future was so uncertain. Burroughs-Wellcome seriously considered abandoning the drug or selling it to another company. There were intense negotiations with the Federal Drug Administration to determine the scope of studies necessary to satisfy them regarding seizure incidents. In the interim, management was changed throughout the company. Continuity and concept were lost almost simultaneously.

Once we identified positive sexual effects in nondepressed sexually dysfunctional individuals, the natural question emerged: Since this drug is going to be prescribed to depressed but not necessarily sexually dysfunctional patients, what effect will bupropion have on patients who report normal sexual functioning? An intelligent use of time, money, and research would be to establish baselines in normal subjects to ensure that this medication does not stimulate any aberrant or hyperactive sexual patterns. Another natural course of research would be to evaluate bupropion in hypersexual individuals and among sex offenders to ensure that it does not aggravate these symptoms.

In the absence of these studies, we strongly recommend that baseline sexual histories be carefully evaluated prior to prescribing bupropion, and that patients with normal sex drive and function be monitored carefully during the first two to six weeks of treatment. Individuals with criminal sexual records or tendencies should not be given prescriptions for this medication.

28

Serotonin Antagonists: PCPA (P-Chlorophenylalanine)

OBJECTIVES

- To identify the toxic side effects of PCPA
- To explore implications of PCPA's effects on sexual function in animals and humans
- To explore the relationship among serotonin, testosterone, and dopamine in the context of PCPA effects
- To speculate regarding relevance of PCPA research to sexual orientation research

Serotonin uptake inhibitor antidepressants (SSRIs) have some of the most prominent sexual side effects of all drug categories. In general, these drugs have some value for male sexual dysfunction, but typically interfere with or complicate female sexual desire and responsiveness. Anorgasmia, inhibition of orgasm, and decreased desire are common. Orgasms triggered by yawning are rare. Erectile dysfunction and inhibited ejaculation in the male may occur as sexual side effects.

The serotonin depletor P-chlorophenylaline (PCPA) is a toxic drug that promotes aggression, insomnia, and aberrant sex. A report on the dramatic sexual properties of PCPA came from visiting Italian researchers, Tagliamonte and Gessa, at the United States National Heart Institute's Pharmacology Lab (Tagliamonte et al., 1969), where they described group sex in animals with male-to-male mounting. Sexual excitation lasted for several hours and was characterized by frenetic group behavior in which all the animals in one cage attempted to mount each other at the same time. Similar extreme hypersexual behavior was reported in cats treated with PCPA (Ferguson et al., 1970).

PCPA has such toxic side effects that, under ordinary circumstances, it is not advisable for use in humans. It is discussed here to demonstrate the sexual impact of serotonergic antagonists and to advise caution in the development of modified substances suitable for use in humans. This drug demonstrates beyond any doubt that manipulating certain neurotransmitters (in this case, serotonin) can dramatically alter the normal sexual behavior of animals. In the process of researching this effect, tremendous insight was gained into previously unappreciated sexual mechanisms of action.

The study of sexual pharmacology changed dramatically in 1969 with Tagliamonte's et al. report of PCPA's sexual effects. Prior to this research, the focus of "aphrodisiac" research was to identify sexual stimulants. With the discovery of PCPA's powerful sexual activity, interest shifted to removing the inhibitory action of serotonin on sex. PCPA selectively depletes brain serotonin by inhibiting the metabolism of tryptophan to serotonin. Norepinephrine and dopamine remain unchanged. Tryptophan is a naturally occurring amino acid that is converted into serotonin. Without new serotonin from tryptophan, brain reserves of serotonin radically decrease within one to three days. The result of decreased serotonin seems to be an intense form of compulsive, even bizarre sexual behavior. PCPA was first used to treat patients with carcinoid syndrome who had abnormally high levels of serotonin secreted by intestinal tumors. For such a serious use, considerable toxicity was tolerated. However, the adverse side effects of PCPA are sufficiently severe to contraindicate its use for most other conditions.

HYPERSEXUALITY

Michael Sheard (1969) at Yale published a study on male rats, using both placebo and PCPA, and noted behavior changes only with PCPA. Treated males increased mounting and pelvic thrusting with both males and females. PCPA-treated females mounted and thrusted on other females as well as on smaller males. Sheard found that aggressive behavior (including mouse-killing) increased "strikingly" on PCPA in both male and female rats. Though males who killed mice were not aggressive toward female rats, females who killed mice were openly aggressive toward male rats. Abnormally restless sleep and hypersensitive arousal were also observed.

The Italian pharmacological researchers Gessa and Tagliamonte (1974a) believed that sexual behavior was increased by dopamine and decreased by serotonin. They administered PCPA to male rats that were closely confined, expecting an increase in sexual behavior due to serotonin depletion. In a 12-hour test, 16 of 60 rats showed some mounting of other males. When dopamine was increased by adding the MAO-B inhibitor pargyline to the PCPA, the mounting increased dramatically to 58 of 80 rats—38 of them mounting more than 10 times in a single session. When the PCPA-pargyline combination was subsequently injected into male rabbits, compulsive sexual behavior continued for up to three days.

The researchers used special conditions to accentuate the possibility of hypersexual behavior. Animals were kept in isolation until released for testing into small cages with other males; isolation increases aggressive and reactive behavior. Testing was done at the start of the "dark phase" of the 24-hour day, when animals become most active. A rather small dose of PCPA was used to minimize side effects and to select for the serotonin effect. These conditions maximized activity and social response.

In addition to intensification of mounting behavior, there was excessive grooming, scratching, and a mutual smelling of each other's genitals. Rabbits frequently show male-to-male mounting even without PCPA; but when put together, untreated rabbits were usually mounted by treated rabbits. PCPA-treated rabbits also mounted male or female cats and small dogs. In both of these studies, hypersexual behavior disappeared when replacement serotonin was provided by 5-HTP injections. The rapid reversal of PCPA sexual effects by adding a serotonin precursor proved that hypersexuality, in these cases, was caused by serotonin depletion.

When 26 cats were given daily PCPA injections, intense sexual behavior, including male-to-male mounting, occurred within three to five days (Ferguson et al., 1970). Tests were not conducted on females or between males and females. Concurrent with PCPA-induced hypersexuality, there was a disturbing increase in aggressive behavior. Most of the cats became vicious, attacking and mauling their handlers and other cats. When rats were put in with the PCPA cats, many of the cats showed a dramatic increase in rat killing, which escalated into bizarre and savage behavior. The cats also became voracious in general, sometimes becoming obese due to overeating.

Bizarre perceptual behavior corresponding to progressive effects of PCPA also became noticeable. Cats were restless and unable to sleep, paced incessantly in their cages, became overreactive to the slightest stimulus changes, stared at imaginary objects, and struck out at unseen objects. By the tenth day the cats had quieted down, but would still mount other males and become violently irritable if pinched.

PCPA did not cause hypersexual male mounting in castrated rats (Gessa, Tagliamonte, & Brodie, 1970). Testosterone injections alone also did not cause such hypersexuality. However, when castrated rats were injected with both testosterone and PCPA, there was remarkable sexual stimulation, greater even than in normal rats treated with PCPA alone. Finally, when normal rats were given testosterone and PCPA together, even higher levels of mounting hypersexuality occurred.

A few months after the papers by Tagliamonte and Ferguson, two more papers appeared in *Science* contradicting the aphrodisiac findings. Whalen and Luttge (1970) tested sexually vigorous and experienced rats with receptive females. Either no change or reduction of sexual behavior was found with PCPA or PCPA combined with pargyline. Later, Luttge (1975) noted PCPA-induced sexual increases in castrated rats. Subsequent studies of PCPA effects showed that sexual behavior in normal or vigorous heterosexual male copulators often did not increase on PCPA, but rats did ejaculate more quickly (Larsson & Ahlenius, 1986). However, sexual activity increased in sexually sluggish or castrated male rats.

Zitrin, Beach, Barchas, and Dement (1970) refuted Ferguson's findings in male cats. These researchers could find no sexual change in male cats given PCPA. They noted that cats showed male-to-male mounting even prior to PCPA under normal conditions and sexual behavior did not increase with PCPA. Furthermore, none of the restless, vicious, or bizarre behavior noted by Ferguson et al. occurred in this study. However, that same year another study confirmed Ferguson's work, demonstrating a pronounced sexual effect in cats. A kinder, gentler PCPA study with cats was performed in England during 1970 by three researchers (Hoyland, Shillito, & Vogt, 1970). Four groups of young cats (three- to four-month-old male and female kittens and seven- to 15-month-old young adults) were studied in group observation rooms (not isolated in barren cages). PCPA was given orally in daily capsules.

After several days, sexual changes occurred that were similar to those reported by Ferguson et al. (1970). During the first two days, the cats were slow-moving, shaky, and scratched their backs excessively. Then they became somewhat restless, meowed a lot, and made loud purring "request or greeting" calls for contact. The cats who earlier had been most responsive to their human handlers now incessantly rubbed up against other cats, including untreated cage-mates. When touched, they made treading movements, lifting their tails and flattening their backs as if in estrus. Several of the male cats began mounting other males during the third day. Dominant males mounted submissive males and equals mounted equals, but the dominance hierarchy was not changed. Male mounting included much pinning behavior, frequent erections and thrusting movements. Untreated cats and some treated cats increasingly avoided the PCPA mounters, resisting mounting attempts with hisses, growls, and swatting with their paws. In females treated with PCPA, only increased scratching, rubbing, and treading occurred. When serotonin was restored by 5-HTP injections, the unusual sexual behavior of PCPA mounters and other PCPA-treated cats soon disappeared, with many quickly falling asleep. With the return to normal behavior, the untreated cage-mates became less tense and more playful, sitting near the treated cats rather than as "far away as possible."

SEROTONIN AND PCPA

Increased sexual activity, exaggerated responses to the environment and sensory stimuli, increased aggressiveness, irritability, abnormal sleep patterns, and bizarre social behavior are characteristic of serotonin-depleting brain lesions (Baumgarten & Schlossberger, 1984). Aggressive, overactive, hypervigilant, and irritable behaviors are also characteristic of PCPA-treated monkeys in social colonies (Raleigh, McGuire, & Brammer, 1988). Thus, the PCPA-induced behavior changes observed by researchers appear typical of serotonin depletion. Sexual stimulation and hyperactivity are also characteristic of REM sleep deprivation: sexual changes on PCPA could have been aggravated by sleep disruption secondary to the drug. Failure to note any increases in sexual, aggressive, and bizarre behaviors by some research groups is difficult to explain and should not diminish the significance of these remarkable findings.

TESTOSTERONE AND PCPA

Since PCPA's sexual effects are apparently due to decreased serotonin, and since testosterone strongly potentiates the sexual effect of this serotonin depletion, a second hypothesis, termed "serotonin down/testosterone up," explaining the increased sexuality was developed. There is substantial evidence that serotonin and testosterone are mutually inhibitory. Serova, Kudriavtseva, Popova, and Naumenko (1987) showed that a decrease in serotonin blood levels in male mice could be caused by either by an injection of testosterone or the presence of a receptive female. More directly, sexual arousal in a receptive female caused elevation of a male's testosterone, which could potentially trigger a decrease in serotonin. Conversely, castration or estrogen treatment can also increase serotonin blood levels. Biswas, Mazumder, Bhattacharya, and Das (1985) showed that an elevation of serotonin due to excess tryptophan could decrease testosterone, possibly by inhibiting LHRH activity.

DOPAMINE AND PCPA

Dopamine may also be involved in the reciprocal inhibition between testosterone and serotonin. Dopamine is increased by testosterone injection, by the presence of a sexually receptive female, or by sexual activity itself (Mitchell & Stewart, 1989). Castration reduces dopamine in contrast to the increase of serotonin. As evidence of this dynamic interaction of testosterone and dopamine, Benkert (1973) showed that L-dopa as well as testosterone potentiated PCPA-induced hypersexuality. In addition to the theory that sexual stimulation was controlled by testosterone, two additional methods of increasing sexuality have been identified: *increasing dopamine* and *decreasing serotonin.*

The interaction of all three of these substances (testosterone, dopamine, and serotonin) may be typical of natural sexual function. A deficiency in any can depress normal sexual drive and behavior.

THE EFFECTS OF PCPA ON FEMALES

The combination of lower testosterone and higher serotonin is a natural state in female animals and women. Apparently, this innate biological formula depresses sexuality and aggression in comparison with men. Drugs that increase testosterone and decrease serotonin could be expected to have the opposite effect. As noted, Sheard (1969) reported that female rats treated with PCPA not only mounted other females and smaller males, but also behaved more aggressively toward males. Some mounting females even showed thrusting body jerks similar to male ejaculatory behavior.

Nevertheless, PCPA effects on female rat sexual receptive behavior have been inconsistent. Several groups have found that PCPA stimulated lordosis in female animals (Everitt et al., 1975; Wilson, Bonney, Everard, Parrott, & Wise, 1982), while others found no effect or even reduction of lordosis (Gorzalka & Whalen, 1975; Sodersten, Larsson, Ahlenius, & Engel, 1976). There may be no effect on passive lordosis, but an increase in female active proceptive sexual behaviors, so that the nature of the PCPA sexual effect may depend upon what sexual behaviors or sexual situations are studied (Sodersten et al., 1976).

While the majority of studies in female animals identifies a serotonin effect, there are a few studies that fail to find it. Wilson et al. (1982) attributed the increased lordosis to an early depletion of norepinephrine by a PEA amphetamine-like metabolite of PCPA. Wilson et al. (1982) noted stimulation of lordosis four to six hours after PCPA injection, when serotonin levels were still normal (depletion requires 24 to 48 hours). The increase in lordosis was not prevented by adding 5-HTP serotonin supplementation, so it was not explained by a decrease in serotonin. There was no PCPA-induced sexual effect 24 hours later, when serotonin levels reached depletion.

Everitt et al. (1975) devised a female sex behavior model to compare the sexual effect of PCPA to testosterone. Removal of the adrenals from female monkeys impaired female proceptive sexual behavior. Proceptive behaviors can be restored by testosterone injections. When PCPA was substituted for testosterone, active sexual behavior was still restored. The PCPA effect disappeared when the females were given 5-HTP to bring their serotonin levels back to normal. Apparently, lowering serotonin with PCPA had a sexually stimulating effect similar to testosterone.

The inconsistent findings concerning the effects of PCPA on female sexual behavior may be due to other adverse side effects or to the fact that the drug's actions are not sufficiently selective for serotonin. However, even with a "clean," selective serotonin inhibitor, results could be paradoxical. Since estrogen and serotonin appear to work together, depletion of serotonin could deregulate estrogen and progesterone function.

HUMAN STUDIES

PCPA has not been tested for treatment of sex drive or orgasmic problems in men or women. Due to its side effects, it would not be approved for clinical use, even if its value were shown. However, other serotonin-inhibiting drugs currently available, such as cyproheptadine (Periactin) and methysergide (Sansert), may have sexual benefits. Interestingly, cyproheptadine is currently used to relieve anorgasmia and lack of ejaculation caused by drugs that increase serotonin activity (such as fluoxetine and other antidepressants) (Goldbloom & Kennedy, 1991).

Open studies by Benkert (1973) and Sicuteri (1974) used PCPA in combination with testosterone or other androgen supplements to treat erectile dysfunction, with minor sexual improvements. Despite encouraging results, dosage was limited by side effects such as irritability, fatigue, vertigo, and headaches. In a placebo-controlled double-blind study of 10 men on PCPA for four weeks (Benkert, 1975), no benefits were shown except in the case of one man who had much improved erections during intercourse. In a separate study Benkert showed that 12 days of PCPA treatment in healthy volunteers did not cause any changes in testosterone or luteinizing hormone. This double-blind trial of PCPA-testosterone treatment of impotence also failed to show any benefits greater than with placebo.

The lowering of sexual responsivity with serotonin potentiators may be accompanied by beneficial behavioral effects in animals, such as decreased defensiveness, increased relaxation, huddling, and grooming (Raleigh et al., 1983). Both excitement and relaxation can result in a positive change in sexual desire and/or behavior. The initial relaxation and decreased defensiveness with serotonergic drugs may improve sexual compliance, desire, and responsiveness in humans. However, it is likely that sexual benefits will decrease with long-term serotonin elevation, either due to tolerance or to negative feelings generated by a deprivation of genuine sexual excitement and pleasure. Treatment of negative sexual behaviors, such as paraphilias, sexual aggression, and various sexual compulsions, addictions and perversions, may be possible with serotonin potentiators.

Sexual Orientation

Clearly, current research has indicated that the serotonin hypothesis is far more complex than it appears on the surface. For example, we have already discussed numerous serotonin-enhancing drugs that can facilitate sex in certain individuals. Drugs such as fenfluramine, clomipramine, fluoxetine, and trazodone discussed in Part V all have paradoxical effects on sex—some negative, some positive.

What is particularly interesting is that, among serotonin-antagonist drugs and in regard to serotonin per se, male/female sexual differences become the most dramatically apparent. In animals, the serotonin depletor PCPA can make females behave sexually like males. It alters the sexual orientation of both sexes; although it appears to promote homosexual behavior, the impact is far more general: These animals not only mount the same sex but also become indiscriminate and mount different species. These drugs can also provoke deviant sexual behavior in animals, including attempted sex with dead animals. Are there currently unappreciated or unidentified biochemical determinants involved in these behaviors?

To date, there is little research pertaining to the biological determinants of sexual orientation. This subject is so clouded by ideologies, belief systems, and political stands that few scientists have dared to pursue the questions. Simon LeVay, an openly homosexual scientist, has proposed the existence of certain brain differences between homosexual and heterosexual men (LeVay, 1991), similar to brain differences found between female and male rats (Gorski, 1987). However, this study (LeVay's) has not been replicated. There are truly more questions than answers. With the insights generated by animal studies demonstrating the ease of altering sexual orientation with chemical manipulations, someday we may find parallels in humans.

CONCLUSIONS

An underlying characteristic theme of PCPA hypersexuality is an impulsivity suggestive of serotonin depletion. Bursts of activity, lack of self-control, and release from inhibitions are the result of a suppression of serotonin inhibitory action. Serotonin neurons fire at a slow and steady pace, which has a general restraining effect on activating transmitter neurons like dopamine receptors. In sexually sluggish animals, serotonin can prevent activity from occurring altogether; it can also suppress improper and oversensitive reactions in normal animals, allowing them to pace themselves. Excessive serotonin can delay orgasm and pleasurable sensory feedback indefinitely. With current serotonergic drugs like fluoxetine (Prozac), the crescendo of sexual excitement can be totally eliminated. This sexual dampening is not an occasional or bizarre effect of fluoxetine; rather, it is inherent in the drug's serotonergic mechanism.

PCPA's toxicity and the disturbing effects of extended serotonin depletion make any useful therapeutic sexual benefit unlikely for men or women. A serious problem in evaluating PCPA effects in the female sex is that females of various species are controlled by different hormones than the basic estrogen-progesterone combination in the rat. For the female cat and rabbit, sexual receptivity is more dependent upon estrogen, with progesterone, testosterone, and adrenal androgens playing limited roles. Also, monkey and human females are less bound by hormonal and behavioral constraints (sexual function is not limited to hormonally determined estrus cycles and the lordosis reflex). Consequently, even if PCPA's effects on female rat sex were consistent, the effects on female monkeys or humans probably would be significantly different.

PCPA research has shown that sexual reactivity is increased when serotonin is decreased. However, the unpleasant and sometimes perverse quality of PCPA-induced hypersexuality is also evident from this research. Reduction of serotonin has a positive sexual effect, but it cannot be isolated from the concomitant negative effects it provokes. Furthermore, the nature of the PCPA-induced reduction of serotonin activity and the precise effects on various serotonin receptors have not been adequately defined.

The PCPA animal studies, although not reliable as analogical indicators of human sexual response, nonetheless raise provocative questions. For example, if serotonin depletion in animals causes violent, perverse, aggressive, and homicidal sexual behavior, does this finding contain implications about the biochemical nature of violent sex offenders? Could there be a biologically determined neurotransmitter dysfunction governing their behavior? Is this dysfunction correctable? Could there be a chemical way to modulate their behavior toward normal? Psychopharmacology has successfully proceeded in this manner with regard to the treatment of depression: identifying neurochemical imbalances and correcting them. It can be seen that animal research with serotonin depleting drugs has profound implications, not just for the field of sexual pharmacology, but for the study of criminal pharmacology as well—a new field to consider.

29

Peptides: Oxytocin, Vasopressin, LHRH

OBJECTIVES

- To examine the endogenous dynamics of these multifaceted peptides
- To examine the effects of exogenous synthetics
- To encourage further research into the complex, interactive roles of these sexually significant substances

The analysis and interpretation of the sexual effects of the peptides oxytocin, vasopressin, and luteinizing hormone-releasing hormone (LHRH) are among the most fascinating areas of sexual pharmacology. Oxytocin, for example, has "multiple personalities" that reflect its essential role in a variety of sexual responses. It is associated with the birth process, breast-feeding, and orgasm. Masters and Johnson originally compared the uterine contractions associated with orgasm and those that occur during labor, finding them to be virtually identical. It may well be that oxytocin is the common denominator—although why one experience is so painful and the other so pleasurable remains a mystery. Oxytocin is also involved in one of the most curious of sexual phenomena: the penile erection and yawning reflex. As yet, we have no explanation for the connection between yawning and sexual arousal, although we have identified some of the chemicals that trigger the process. While oxytocin is associated with orgasm, uterine contractions, and other specific genital phenomena, it also has a much more global effect. It sensitizes the skin to touch, promotes affectionate behavior, and affects interpersonal relationships. One of the most fascinating attributes of this peptide is how it is influenced by the human environment.

Vasopressin has been of interest in the treatment of aging due to its apparent ability to improve cognitive behavior. Longevity researchers and popular writers have focused on its effect on learning, attention, and memory. However, clinical medicine in the United States has limited the focus on this drug to its antidiuretic properties. However, there are preliminary indications in the literature that vasopressin potentiates male sexuality, either directly or by potentiating other hormones and/or neurotransmitters. While much more research is necessary before we have a comprehensive profile of this multifaceted substance, its influence on sexuality and quality of life appears to be substantial. Animal studies on the female suggest that vasopressin may reduce receptive sex (lordosis) while not diminishing or potentiating proceptive sex drive. Its thermostatic effect on temperature regulation seems to extend to the heat that rises in the sexual response itself.

LHRH exerts much of its influence by regulating the relative levels of testosterone and estrogen. It is pulsatile in nature and challenging to study. When used therapeutically, it can have unpredictable and paradoxical effects on sex, depending upon dose, timing, and method of administration (i.e., pulsatile versus constant). It has been tested as a means of increasing sex drive and erection, of "chemically castrating" the male, and as a male contraceptive—all with varying degrees of success and failure. One fact, however, is clear: LHRH is integrally involved in sexuality, sexual response, fertility, and the lack thereof, and has even been implicated indirectly in sexual orientation.

OXYTOCIN

Because it is a pulsatile hormone, appearing in short bursts followed by a refractory period, oxytocin is difficult to measure. Excessive or prolonged doses of this peptide block these pulsatile effects, so that rhythmic contractions of labor become tetanic or the breast mammary nerve becomes insensitive to further stimulation. Given that oxytocin reaches saturation levels rapidly, refractory intervals are a natural part of the rhythmic flow of highly intense sexual stimulation. This same principle works for the pituitary regulation of sex through LHRH pulsatility. When this pulsatile action is overwhelmed by excessive concentrations, the system becomes refractory. Dopamine, which stimulates sex, fires in a relatively rapid, irregular burst pattern; in contrast, serotonin, which mutes sex, fires at a slow, regular beat that would not be responsive to the sudden changes in excitement characteristic of intense sexual activity. Oxytocin and dopamine may pace one another by mutual reinforcement.

Oxytocin is an *interpersonal* chemical, easily conditioned during intimate contact to outside stimuli, including smells, events, and other people. Similar to salivation in response to Pavlov's bell, we release oxytocin in response to conditioned circumstances near and dear to us. This diffusion of variables together with the intimacy of the circumstances renders oxytocin too "soft" for objective study. Newton (1978) noted that inattention to oxytocin in the research arena could be due to a "reluctance to study hormones involved in strongly emotional acts." Actions of oxytocin are also confounded by the influence of an "incestuous array" of other neurotransmitters, hormones, and peptides. A mutual interaction exists between oxytocin and other key sexual chemicals such as dopamine, LHRH, testosterone, estrogen, prostaglandin, vasopressin, and epinephrine. Oxytocin serves as an inconspicuous reactive hormone that underlies attachment and possibly orgasm (by mediating libido, affection, and nurturance). With such interdependencies and complications, predictable responses may be difficult to find. Oxytocin is often seen as secondary and less important to sexual drive and response, which may not be the case. In the realm of peptide and molecular psychopharmacology, oxytocin offers most interesting possibilities for sexual enhancement. Table 29.1 summarizes the properties and side effects of oxytocin.

Effect on Females

Oxytocin has a profound effect on women, influencing sexual behavior and, indeed, all aspects of reproduction (pregnancy, birth, and nursing). Vaginal and cervical distension both stimulate oxytocin release, which increases prior to the onset of female sexual receptivity (proestrus), during mating, prior to labor, and during delivery. Furthermore, tactile sensitivity and grooming during copulation, after copulation, during parental behavior (even for males), and during nursing/suckling are all potentiated by oxytocin.

Niles Newton studied oxytocin for over 30 years before the landmark 1978 article, "The Role of the Oxytocin Reflexes in Three Interpersonal Reproductive Acts: Coitus, Birth, and Breast-Feeding." Subsequently, Pedersen, Caldwell, and Jirikowski studied sexual bonding facilitated by oxytocin in a series of papers during the late 1980s (Caldwell, Jirikowski, Greer, & Pedersen, 1987; Caldwell, Jirikowski, Greer, Stumpf, & Pedersen, 1988; Jirikowski, Caldwell, Stumpf, & Pedersen, 1988; Jirikowski, Caldwell, Pilgrim, Stumpf, & Pedersen, 1989). While stimulation of the medial preoptic nucleus (MPO) and administration of dopaminergic stimulants have been shown to elicit and maintain active "masculine" sex behavior, they inhibit female receptive lordosis. In contrast, oxytocin stimulates copulation and lordosis even when injected

Table 29.1 *Profile of Oxytocin*

	Daily Dose
Oxytocin nasal spray (Syntocinon) (Pitocin injection)	1 spray
COMMON INDICATIONS	
Postpartum milk ejection during nursing	
Initiate or augment labor	
Postpartum contraction of uterus	
MECHANISMS OF ACTION (GENERAL)	
Peptide hormone secreted from posterior lobe of pituitary	
Stimulates tone and contractions of smooth musculature of uterus and of alveoli	
MECHANISMS OF ACTION (SEXUAL)	
Increased adrenergic ($alpha_1$) activity	
Increased cholinergic activity	
Increased dopamine	
Increased estrogen (female)	
Increased LHRH	
Increased prostaglandins	
Increased prolactin	
Increased serotonin	
Increased testosterone	
Increased VIP	
Increased vasopressin	
Decreased opiates	

into the medial preoptic nucleus. Its function appears to be to keep sexual partners and progeny literally "in touch."

The prescription oxytocin nasal spray Syntocinon has been used safely for many years, generally to facilitate breast-feeding, milk let-down, or to induce labor and control postpartum uterine bleeding. The spray conceivably could be used to stimulate touch and sensitivity as well as to facilitate orgasm. The suggested dosage for nursing is one spray into each nostril two to three minutes prior to breast contact. This dose may not be sufficient to have any sexual effect. However, it should not be too difficult to determine an effective dose in a research or clinical setting—if, indeed, one exists. If Syntocinon spray were used only prior to sexual activity, side effects probably would be tolerable and minor; however, daily use could cause cognitive side effects. Studies with acute use prior to sexual activity a few times a week have not been done. Any valid statement of efficacy and safety must await such research.

Effect on Human Males

Oxytocin potentiates human male erection, copulation, and orgasm/ejaculation. It is present throughout the male genital tract, including the tunica albuginea around the erectile cavernosum and in and around the skin and muscle of the penile spongiosum and glands. Contraction during orgasm/ejaculation may be dependent upon its pulsatile release; it peaks during and after ejaculation (Murphy, Checkley, Seckl, & Lightman, 1990; Murphy et al., 1987).

A Swedish study by Lidberg and Sternthal (1977) has shown beneficial effects of oxytocin on impotence in 48 subjects. In a double-blind placebo-controlled trial, nine men were given a 300 IU capsule of oxytocin, 10 were given 600 IU, and 10 were given placebo for an average duration of eight weeks. Sexual interest, fantasies, and desire for intercourse significantly improved with oxytocin. Sexual capability (including erection sufficient for penetration and partner satisfaction) was greater on oxytocin than on placebo but the difference was only marginal. The lower dose was more effective than the higher one.

Normally, oxytocin is not taken orally. We do not know where oral capsules were obtained for this research or how effectively they were absorbed. Ingested orally, oxytocin is degraded in the stomach and poorly absorbed, making control of dosage imprecise and unpredictable. Consequently, it is usually administered by injection or by a nasal spray (Synotocin).

Oxytocin appears to have less impact on males than females. Men may find the influence of oxytocin more difficult to integrate into affectionate relationships. Even the experience of oxytocin during and after orgasm/ejaculation may be undermined by men's notion of ejaculation as the "end of it" rather than part of an emotional and biological process. The locus of oxytocin in sensory ganglia makes the skin of the entire body complement the special intensity within the genitals and the breasts. In males, the tactile sensitivity may be less intense, perhaps because of lower estrogen levels.

Secretion During Sexual Activity

Oxytocin increases during sexual activity in both men and women, spiking during orgasm. Murphy et al. (1987) found a sharp rise in oxytocin at orgasm/ejaculation, which was still slightly elevated 10 minutes after ejaculation. Volunteers used their own fantasies or "sexually explicit material" to become aroused and then masturbated until ejaculation. A catheter for blood collection was inserted into one of their arms throughout the session. Oxytocin did not increase during the pre-masturbation arousal period, during which genital stimulation was not allowed. Carmichael et al. (1987) measured oxytocin in nine men and 13 women from six minutes before masturbation to five minutes after orgasm/ejaculation. Blood was collected from catheters and electromyographic activity was measured with an anal probe. No breast stimulation was used by the subjects. Four women subjects were multiorgasmic. Oxytocin levels rose gradually from the start of masturbation through orgasm/ejaculation, were higher in women than in men, and showed a steeper increase as orgasm approached. In the multiorgasmic women oxytocin continued to increase through the second orgasm. For both men and women, oxytocin levels remained elevated for five minutes following orgasm.

The presence of elevated oxytocin after orgasm has yet to be related to either decreased or increased arousal states. It is also difficult to relate oxytocin to differences in orgasmic potential or to explain the different postcoital patterns of men and women. Differences in oxytocin reactions between men and women may explain some of the sex-linked differences between sexual desire and orgasm. Oxytocin may be involved in the postcoital inertia that typically follows orgasm in men. Oxytocin generates a characteristic EEG theta afterreaction in rabbits (Kawakami & Sawyer, 1959) that resembles this refractory state consequent to male orgasm/ejaculation. This theta response occurs at orgasm in both men and women and is associated with activation of the right hemisphere (Cohen et al., 1976). Sedation during the postejaculatory period may be a refractory effect of the oxytocin orgasmic "flush."

Animal Research

Stimulation of Stretching-Yawning/Penile-Erection Syndrome Oxytocin plays a central role in the distinctive stretching-yawning/penile erection syndrome (SY/PE) of male rats (Argiolas, 1989, 1992) (see Chapter 3). Oxytocin injection can elicit this syndrome directly, or dopaminergic drugs can generate it through the stimulation of oxytocin activity. Drugs that block dopamine will not block oxytocin-induced SY/PE (Argiolas, 1989, 1992), but a drug that blocks oxytocin will prevent the syndrome from being triggered by oxytocin or dopaminergic drugs. Thus, dopaminergic drugs may have their stimulatory effect on sexual response through an oxytocinergic mechanism. This mechanism applies to both erection and orgasm/ejaculation.

Studies from 1985 to 1990 showed that yawning-erection in rats was induced by oxytocin and oxytocin/dopamine (e.g., Argiolas, Melis, & Gessa, 1988). When dopamine or oxytocin was injected into various brain regions, stretching-yawning/penile erection syndrome was elicited only with injections into the paraventricular nucleus, which secretes oxytocin and vasopressin throughout the brain (Melis et al., 1986). Conversely, paraventricular nucleus lesions prevent yawning and erection induced by both apomorphine (dopamine) and oxytocin (Argiolas, Melis, Mauri, & Gessa, 1987). (The paraventricular nucleus also contains magnocellular neurons that release oxytocin to the posterior pituitary, where it acts as a birth and lactation hormone in women.) The medial preoptic nucleus functions synergistically with the paraventricular nucleus to stimulate sexual and parental behavior. Additionally, progesterone and estrogen from the ventromedial nucleus (VMN) receptive sex lordosis center activate female sexual initiation behavior at least partly by stimulating neighboring oxytocinergic neurons of the paraventricular nucleus and the dorsomedial nucleus (Schumacher et al., 1990). The curious yawning-erection behavior reaction has enabled us to recognize these crucial chemico-anatomical bases for sexual and reproductive activity.

The recent availability of potent oxytocin antagonists has led to further understanding. Argiolas and his colleagues (Argiolas, Melis, Mauri & Gessa, 1987; Argiolas, Melis, Vargiu, & Gessa, 1987) showed that dopamine-induced yawning, erection, and male copulatory behavior in rats depended upon oxytocin; these behaviors were blocked by oxytocin antagonists. Furthermore, oxytocin antagonists eliminated ejaculation in normal male rats (Argiolas, 1992; Argiolas, Melis, Mauri & Gessa, 1987; Argiolas, Melis, Vargiu, & Gessa, 1987).

Oxytocin-induced yawning and erection can be blocked by the cholinergic antagonist atropine, indicating that oxytocin requires some cholinergic activity for its stimulation of this yawning and erection syndrome. However, cholinergic stimulation alone, such as with physostigmine, causes yawning but does not induce erections (Gower et al., 1984). Parvicellular oxytocin neurons of the paraventricular nucleus project to cholinergic areas of the limbic system (hippocampus, septum, and amygdala) and the spinal cord. Apomorphine dopaminergic injection elevates oxytocin levels in the hippocampus while inducing yawning and erection (Melis et al., 1990). Oxytocin can also elicit yawning and erection by direct injection into the hippocampus (Argiolas & Gessa, 1987). Oxytocin itself stimulates the release of LHRH (Johnston, et al., 1990). Potency studies of the stretching-yawning/penile-erection syndrome have shown that the oxytocin receptors that stimulate erection are similar in intensity to oxytocin receptors that stimulate uterine contraction and breast milk ejection (Melis et al., 1988).

In summary, research has indicated that oxytocin apparently activates erection by triggering a complex circuit involving the cholinergic limbic system through the dopaminergic hypothalamus to the pituitary and into the spinal cord. This effect is sensitized by testosterone, estrogen, vasopressin, and possibly ACTH and epinephrine, and can be blocked by the anticholinergic antagonist atropine and by morphine (Argiolas & Gessa, 1987).

When oxytocin is given to male rats, they become maternal when exposed to newborn pups (Insel, 1992; Insel & Shapiro, 1992). In animals, the sensitization to touch induced by oxytocin facilitates mating, grooming, and cuddling for both males and females; when given to female rats during ovulation, oxytocin heightens efforts to contact males and intensifies lordosis (Insel, 1992). Through its association with smell (through estrogen sensitization), it integrates bodily reactions to pheromones (Fahrback, Morrell, Pfaff, 1985).

Some researchers believe that activation of oxytocin during orgasm and ejaculation for both males and females facilitates sperm transport. Oxytocin and vasoactive intestinal polypeptide (VIP) are mutually stimulating in the hypothalamus (Bardrum, Ottesen, Fahrenkrug, & Fuchs, 1988); and VIP is stimulated by suckling, by electrical stimulation of the mammary nerve, or by oxytocin infusion (Eriksson & Uvnas-Moberg, 1990). Therefore, oxytocin may facilitate VIP secretion in the penis to promote erection, and VIP secretion may stimulate increased oxytocin, culminating in orgasm/ejaculation. Similarly, oxytocin can synergize with prostaglandins to heighten penile sensitivity and stimulate ejaculation (Manso, Sanchez, Hidalgo, & Andres-Trelles, 1986).

A key function of oxytocin may be to oppose the blunting action of opiates on the sexual response. Naloxone increases brain oxytocin release in rats 100–173% by blocking endogenous opioids that powerfully inhibit oxytocin release (Bicknell & Leng 1982; Bondy, Gainer, & Russell, 1988; Zhao, Chapman, & Bicknell, 1988). However, Honer, Thompson, Lightman, Williams, and Checkley (1986) found no effect of naloxone on normal oxytocin levels in humans, while Seckl, Haddock, Dunne, and Lightman (1988) showed that the oxytocin response to stimulation such as smoking can be released from opioid inhibition by naloxone injection. Alcohol can also inhibit oxytocin release, partly through opioid stimulation (Auerbach & Schreiber, 1987).

Oxytocin inhibits tolerance to opioids, suggesting that oxytocin itself may trigger an opioid-like feeling as a result of opioid disinhibition (Kovacs et al., 1987). Part of yohimbine's stimulating sexual effect is apparently related to oxytocin metabolism through reduction of dynorphin opioid tone. Combining yohimbine with naloxone and oxytocin could antagonize dynorphin-induced sexual inhibition. However, Murphy et al. (1990) showed that naloxone inhibited rather than facilitated men's oxytocin release at orgasm. This inhibition was accompanied by a decrease in arousal and pleasure during orgasm, indicating that endogenous opioids could add to pleasure experienced during orgasm.

Oxytocin increases both centrally and peripherally during and after coitus. Stoneham et al. (1985) have shown oxytocin release during coitus in male rabbits, usually occurring at ejaculation, but sometimes occurring during preliminary pelvic thrusting or in anticipation before entry of the female. The same group of researchers (Hughes, Everitt, Lightman, & Todd, 1987) found oxytocin increments in cerebrospinal fluid after ejaculation in male rats, but no change when males were positioned with sexually unreceptive females.

Increased oxytocin levels are promoted by repetitive positive sexual interchanges and may provide the basis for bonding, attachment, and reproduction. When sexually inexperienced rats were allowed their first night of copulation, oxytocin activity declined; however, after weeks of nightly experience, oxytocin increased considerably (Jirikowski, Caldwell, Stumpf, & Pedersen, 1988).

Satiation Mechanism

Oxytocin is also released when there is a sense of fullness in the genitals or the stomach. In the rat, feeding, stomach distension (by a balloon), and injection of the satiating peptide CCK all caused release of oxytocin (Uvnas-Moberg, 1990). Indeed, part of the appeal of heroin is that it generates such an oxytocin-like satiation response. Chessick (1960) has written a fascinating description of this "pharmacogenic orgasm," in which he refers to the psychoanalyst Rado, who compared the heroin rush to the primal satiation after feeding at the mother's breast. This thrill is experienced as an "alimentary orgasm" that is centered in the abdomen. Heroin addicts interviewed about the sensations associated with the state of euphoria described warm feelings in the stomach, the skin, and the genitals and a sense of fullness in the stomach "as if something had been put inside of me with a jolt or a bang" (Chessick, 1960). Despite the tingling felt in the genitals, all addicts reported reduced sexual drive and said that "it is beside the point to masturbate."

In fact, withdrawal from heroin causes hypersecretion of oxytocin (Bicknell, Leng, & Russell, 1987), sometimes coincident with erection and ejaculation in men and sexual craving in women (Sawyer, 1966). Kovacs et al. (1987) have shown that oxytocin reduces tolerance to morphine and heroin, which in turn allows lowering of the opiate dose (it also reduces tolerance to alcohol). It is as if oxytocin competes with the addictive process. Oxytocin might help an addicted woman stay off heroin once she begins breast-feeding. On the other hand, morphine potently inhibits oxytocin action, just as it inhibits orgasm.

Survival Value?

The inexplicable discrepancies frequently found in drug actions on sexual behavior (particularly opposite effects on active male behavior versus passive female lordosis) are not present with oxytocin, suggesting the possibility that oxytocin may be a trigger for transition from purely sexual behavior to reproductive behavior and attachment. While consideration of sexual behavior as a continuum extending from masturbation and copulation to nursing and grooming may seem too far-ranging, the nervous system, in fact, has evolved to accommodate these behaviors in a mutually facilitating manner. Oxytocin plays a central role in mediating behaviors along this continuum from the intense peak of orgasm to the restful "valley" of grooming.

Occasional attempts to use the nasal oxytocin spray (Syntocinon) for the treatment of schizophrenia, depression, and obsessive-compulsive disorder have shown little or no benefit and bothersome side effects (e.g., Ansseau et al., 1988). Mild psychotic reactions as well as memory, attention, and concentration losses occur. With so little human clinical work done with oxytocin, the seriousness, persistence, and prevalence of disturbing side effects have not been determined. In animal studies oxytocin has been shown to disrupt learning and memory, in contrast to the related peptide vasopressin, which enhances learning and memory (Fehm-Wolfsdorf, Born, Voigt, & Fehm, 1984). Perhaps this amnestic effect of oxytocin was useful as a survival mechanism: Oxytocin-induced forgetting could foster peaceable relations with others (and promote more pregnancies) by blocking sustained reactions of anger that would result in avoidance and rejection. Its release during coitus, orgasm, cuddling, and childbirth would allow all that is negative to be forgiven—or at least forgotten for the moment.

VASOPRESSIN

Vasopressin is another fascinating peptide secreted from the same areas of the brain as oxytocin. Popular as a treatment for problems of memory during aging, it is somehow involved with thermoregulation and sexual activity, as well as cognitive behavior. Diapid spray, derived from lysine-vasopressin, is a favorite drug promoted by authors of life-extension books as a nootropic that enhances learning, attention, and memory. Durk Pearson, author of *Life Extension,* contended that it gives him "great" erections and orgasms (Pearson & Shaw, 1982). However, it is not clear how he differentiates the effects of Diapid from the effects of the other vitamins, minerals, amino acids, and drugs that he uses. As with oxytocin nasal spray (Syntocinon), which is made by the same drug company as Diapid, vasopressin has few FDA-approved uses. It has been available for many years and is no longer promoted or investigated for additional uses. Oxytocin and vasopressin were once used together in a posterior pituitary extract to facilitate labor and birth. Vasopressin alone is an antidiuretic hormone that prevents water and salt depletion by stimulating thirst and inhibiting urination. The only current indication for Diapid in the *Physicians Desk Reference* is for the treatment of diabetes insipidus to control body water regulation (polydipsia, polyuria, and dehydration). The vasopressin derivative desmopressin has additional indications, such as facilitating alertness and cognition, because it lacks vasopressin's possible cardiac and peripheral complications.

Howard Moltz (1989) has conducted a series of studies in rats demonstrating that vasopressin modulates sexual behavior by keeping it from "overheating"—an aspect of the substance's fever-reduction action. In this role of temperature modulation, vasopressin has been seen as inhibitory to male copulatory activity. We believe, however, that this modulatory function can have positive effects on sexual behavior due to a mutual facilitating interaction with testosterone and cholinergic activity. (During winter hibernation of hamsters, a decrease in testosterone causes vasopressin inactivity in the septal region that regulates body temperature [Hermes et al., 1989].)

The logic of the body's sexual chemistry seems to assign vasopressin a supportive role in male sexual behavior, despite whatever specific negative effects it may have. All of the body's chemicals work in concert with one another. Within this dynamic balance, vasopressin interacts with other chemicals that generate sexual desire and behavior (see Table 29.2).

Testosterone Dependence

Vasopressin is dependent on the presence of testosterone for its sexual actions. During early development, testosterone differentiates vasopressin innervation into a male-specific pattern (De Vries, Buijs, & Sluiter, 1984). Castration in adult male rats can decrease vasopressin-binding in specific areas of the brain (De Vries, Buijs, Van Leeuwen, Caffe, & Swaab, 1985). Testosterone replacement can restore vasopressin activity in castrates (Ikeda et al., 1990). Thus, vasopressin shows a sexual dimorphism separate from anatomical sexual dimorphism in the brain, with increased activity dependent upon increased androgens.

Table 29.2 *Vasopressin Interactions*

CHEMICALS/DRUGS THAT INCREASE VASOPRESSIN

- *Positive Sexual Consequences*
  - Testosterone
  - Estrogen
  - Acetylcholine
  - Epinephrine (at $alpha_1$ receptor)
  - Dopamine (at DA_1 receptor)
  - Yohimbine
  - Naloxone
  - Picrotoxin
  - Substance P
- *Negative Sexual Consequences*
  - Angiotensin II
  - NPY
  - Dynorphin
  - Nicotine

CHEMICALS/DRUGS THAT DECREASE VASOPRESSIN

- *Negative Sexual Consequences*
  - Progesterone
  - Serotonin
  - Opiates
  - Endorphins
  - GABA
  - Epinephrine (at $alpha_2$ receptor)
  - Alcohol
  - Clonidine
  - Neuroleptics

If short- or long-term castrated rats are given a single injection of vasopressin into the sensitive medial amygdala, they will display offensive behavior typical of testosterone (Albeck et al., 1991). Similarly, Bohus and Koolhaas (1985) have shown that injection of vasopressin into castrated male rats can delay the decline in their sexual behavior. Testosterone supplementation may also treat declining vasopressin activity. Goudsmit, Feenstra, and Swaab (1990) pointed out that testosterone restores vasopressin innervation when given to old rats with declining levels in brain regions essential to movement, alertness, and pleasure (substantia nigra, locus coeruleus, and ventral tegmentum). Vasopressin stimulates social behavior characteristic of testosterone. In the hamster, flank marking and flank grooming are stereotyped actions that spread odors/pheromones to communicate an animal's social status. They serve to preserve dominant/subordinate relationships among hamsters. Injections of vasopressin into the anterior hypothalamus or the septum stimulated intense flank marking activity, while injection of a vasopressin antagonist inhibited flank marking (Ferris, Pollock, Albers, & Leeman, 1985). The relevance of this testosterone link is the suggestion that vasopressin may facilitate assertiveness and confidence.

Potentiation of Cholinergic Activity

Vasopressin has been shown to have positive attentional, memory, and other cognitive effects in humans, indicating its activating role in limbic system function (Beckwith, Petros, Couk, & Tinius, 1990). Vasopressin reinforces cholinergic (mental) processes of the limbic system (amygdala, septum, hippocampus, entorhinal cortex), which can control attention to and evaluation of sexual cues involved in active sexual behavior.

Neurotransmission by dopamine and serotonin involves less than one percent of human nervous system activity. The excitatory amino acid system and glutamine transmission, a separate neurotransmitter system, are currently the focus of advances in molecular pharmacology. Vasopressin action within the limbic areas may stabilize functional connections between cholinergic and glutamate nervous activity, which in humans represents the cognitive control of the "basic" drives associated with dopamine and serotonin.

Cholinergic mechanisms in the limbic area mediate reactions to sexual stimulation. It is important to remember that the limbic area around the septum was once the "smell brain," where pheromone cues were received in lower animals. During the evolutionary process, sexual stimuli were increasingly routed through the cortex for evaluation and learning and then sent back into the limbic system for action-based decisions. It appears that dopamine localizes in the lower brain (hypothalamus), where it influences sex drive, while the higher brain (limbic, cortex) controls sexual thoughts. In the transitional limbic structures, vasopressin appears to sensitize cholinergic and glutamate activity involved in thoughts and learning.

The theta rhythm generated from the limbic area is specifically associated with orgasm and REM sleep. When Heath (1972) stimulated the septum in humans with electrodes, ecstatic reactions resembling orgasm occurred. Vasopressin could strengthen the theta potential for these sexual reactions.

Sexual Benefits

Vasopressin helps keep sexual functioning within safe thermostatic limits, properly paced and avoiding the excessive exertion that leads to exhaustion. In physical terms, neurogenic fever can be produced by damage to the medial preoptic nucleus, which regulates both body temperature and sexual activity. Excess emotional activity can compete with stable regulation of body temperature because both are driven from the same area of the brain. During REM sleep characterized by nocturnal erection, the medial preoptic nucleus control of body temperature shuts down, as if to give the brain "full reign" to its cognitive capacities. Consequently, periods of REM sleep must be limited so that the brain itself does not overheat.

When there is excess emotion in a dream, the dreamer may wake up in a sweat. Normally, the REM sleep cycle severs dreaming before it overheats the body. During REM sleep, cholinergic activity is prominent, as indicated by the abundance of theta. Consolidation of learning and memory, including sexual memory, seems to occur during REM sleep. Appropriately, vasopressin activity is activated coincident with this cholinergic surge. A deficit of vasopressin causes a reduction of REM sleep, which can be reversed by vasopressin supplementation (Danguir, 1983).

Inhibitory chemical activities of serotonin are completely deactivated during REM sleep, allowing mental play that may include sexual fantasy or even sexual nonsense. Erection and lubrication that occur during REM sleep may be a physical indication of this release from inhibition. Nocturnal erection is coincident with dreaming, but the dreams are usually not sexual in nature. As an antidiuretic hormone, vasopressin secretion during REM sleep reduces the need to urinate, and the genitals can freely switch over to their sexual mode. Vasopressin also allows rapid onset and maintenance of higher temperature in the medial preoptic nucleus, while limiting temperature to a lower level in other parts of the brain (Naylor, Ruwe, & Veale, 1986).

Evelyn Satinoff (1982) has written elegantly on the parallels between thermoregulation and sexual behavior. Particularly important for her is the somewhat similar specialization of each system:

> One of the reasons it has taken so long to recognize that sexual behaviors are relatively independent (as is true for thermoregulation) is probably that (again, as in thermoregulation) one area of the brain is so overwhelmingly important in integrating the behaviors. After medial preoptic lesions, males of several species do not copulate. . . . Electrical stimulation of the preoptic area potentiates copulation in rats. . . . Finally, copulatory behavior of castrated rats can be restored by preoptic implants of testosterone. (p. 233)

Effect on Females

Evidence indicates that vasopressin decreases lordosis behavior (Sodersten, DeVries, Buijs, & Melin, 1985; Sodersten, Henning, Melin, & Ludin, 1983), but enhances cortical arousal (Fehm-Wolfsdorf, Bachholz, Born, Voigt, & Fehm, 1988). Such cortical enhancement can be favorable to male copulatory behavior but is inhibitory to lordosis. Surgical removal of the cortex in female rats increases the frequency and duration of lordosis.

Similarly, while limbic septal action is potentiated by vasopressin, removal of the septum facilitates lordosis and electrical stimulation of the septum inhibits lordosis. Thus, vasopressin and stimulation of higher cognitive areas of the brain inhibit lordosis; lordosis is not disturbed and may even be facilitated by removal of the higher areas of the brain involved in thought. However, until we get a better understanding of the expression of female sexual behavior, any effect of vasopressin is difficult to interpret. Certainly a behavior such as lordosis, which improves when thought areas of the brain such as the cortex and septum are removed, can represent only a partial, isolated reflex expression of female sexual motivation and activity.

LUTEINIZING HORMONE-RELEASING HORMONE (LHRH)

Luteinizing hormone-releasing hormone (LHRH) is a powerful hypothalamic chemical that regulates the relation between testosterone and estrogen. It was among the first of the sexual hormones to be appreciated for its pulsatile, rhythmic release nature. Research with this drug has been challenging for that reason alone and therapeutic administration of synthetic LHRH or LHRH analogues is complicated for the same reason. LHRH receptors are concentrated in the lower hypothalamus, close to the pituitary extension. Highest levels are found in the medial preoptic nucleus, the arcuate nuclei, and the median eminence. Hormonal disturbances that inhibit sex, such as hyperprolactemia or stress-related elevated cortisol, can suppress LHRH release. The peptide nature of LHRH allows it to be sensitive to and influenced by a multiple array of neurotransmitters and hormones. For this reason, simply injecting exogenous LHRH into an animal or person may not have any effect, because the endogenous system is so comprehensively controlled by the particular interaction of neurotransmitter and hormonal influences at any given moment.

LHRH has opposite effects, depending upon whether it is administered intermittently or continuously. Since LHRH operates in a functional manner with these chemicals (e.g., during ovulation), its interaction with other body chemicals cannot be said to be either positive or negative. For instance, at different times, it may have a positive or negative relation to dopamine. Consequently, manipulations of LHRH have unpredictable and often contradictory pharmaceutical actions, which have limited investigation of its apparently positive sexual influence. Since LHRH is the brain trigger for production of testosterone, LHRH users may assume that they are stimulating their sexual system by increasing testosterone. However, new potent LHRH analogues such as leuprolide (Luprin) and goserelin (Zoladex) inhibit the production of testosterone by overwhelming the feedback loop through constant stimulation. For men who are "chemically castrated" with these LHRH analogues, decreased libido and loss of erection may be inevitable (J.A. Smith et al., 1985). Continuous (pump) administration of LHRH has also been tested as a male contraceptive, but the subjects lost their sex drive concurrent with the reduction of testosterone and sperm (Andreyko et al., 1987).

Impressive animal research in the 1970s and early 1980s (discussed later) demonstrated that LHRH reliably increased mating and sexual behavior. The fact that it increased both male copulation and female lordosis suggested that it might be a general hormonal stimulus to improved sex drive in both men and women. LHRH has been shown to improve sex drive in men with hormonal deficiencies (hypogonadal), but has failed to show anything more than slight benefits for the treatment of impotence when tested in controlled trials against placebo (Benkert, Jordan, Dahlen, Schneider, & Gammel, 1975; Kastin, Ehrensing, Coy, Schally, & Kostrzewa, 1979; Moss & Dudley, 1979). Unfortunately, LHRH has not been tested in women as treatment for deficient desire or low arousal.

Pulsatile Rhythms

Only LHRH pulsatile activity at an appropriate physiologic frequency can correct hypogonadal hormone deficiencies (Knobil, 1980). LHRH works in a feedback loop to the pituitary in response to testicular testosterone in men and estrogen levels in women. For men, LHRH increases when testosterone is low; for women, LHRH production is triggered by changes in estrogen level. This neuromodulator activity within the brain appears to actively facilitate sex drive, but has not been adequately studied because of difficulties in delivering LHRH in appropriate pulsatile rhythms. Portable infusion pumps were devised to stimulate ovulation in women and potency in men (Filicori & Crowley, 1983; Hoffman & Crowley, 1983). For hypogonadal men, the effect of this pulsatile delivery of LHRH was an increase in testosterone, testes size, spontaneous erections, nocturnal emissions, and even acne typical of androgen stimulation (Hoffman & Crowley, 1983).

Animal research has shown that, when synthetic LHRH is given in abnormally large amounts, the LHRH system becomes desensitized and refractory. LHRH receptors no longer respond, preventing LHRH and follicle stimulating hormone (FSH) release from the pituitary and decreasing available testosterone. Essentially, the system is overwhelmed and shuts down. Given the availability of highly powerful and long-lasting LHRH analogues, the androgen system could be reliably suppressed. By contrast, the endogenous pulsatile rhythm of the LHRH receptor stimulates its own receptor. Firing one LHRH neuron triggers others, so that distinct bursts of activity accumulate quickly (similar to oxytocin's induction of its own activity). Coordination of sexual feedback in the body requires the sharp, clear signals generated from this pulsatile mode. Peak intensities are most effective in inducing the firing of neighboring receptors. The strong, distinct signals of pulses or bursts can also be integrated into coded rhythms which can control sequential patterns essential to the operation of a system.

This pulsatile pattern of momentum, rhythm, and crescendo typifies sexual function and is sensitive to stimulation from the environment. For example, the appearance of an attractive woman would trigger LHRH release in a man, while the sudden appearance of a threatening intruder would quickly shut down the release of the substance. The LHRH-testosterone production circuit in men is particularly dependent upon how they are coping with the outside world (Moss & Dudley, 1984). Likewise, women's menstrual cycles can become irregular due to emotional difficulties interfering with LHRH and other chemical rhythms. The complex modulation of LHRH activity in response to changes in the internal and external environments requires a complicated and precise regulation that these pulsatile rhythms provide.

Animal Research

Sexual effects of LHRH have been shown in frogs, lizards, pigeons, mice, rats, horses, and monkeys. LHRH injections facilitate male copulatory behavior (Moss, 1978), female lordosis (Pfaff, 1973), and female proceptive sexual behavior (Kendrick & Dixson, 1985). These positive effects, which have been demonstrated in various experimental situations, were quite sensitive to the animal's hormonal status. For example, Moss, Dudley, Foreman, and McCann (1975) found that copulation was facilitated by LHRH in normal male rats as well as in castrated rats given marginal low testosterone supplements, but no sexual effect occurred in castrated rats without testosterone. (LHRH is clearly not strong enough to have an effect separate from testosterone, as occurs with lisuride or sometimes with PCPA.) Similar to males, a minimal amount of another hormone (estradiol, in this case) is necessary for female monkeys to show LHRH-induced sexual activity (Kendrick & Dixson, 1985).

While sexual stimulation with LHRH has been demonstrated in routine tests of copulation, few studies have investigated the effect of LHRH on sex drive. McDonnell, Diehl, Garcia, and Kenney (1989) observed that sexually sluggish stallions stimulated by LHRH injection spent more time near mares, sniffing, licking, nuzzling, and nipping. Stallions injected with LHRH also showed frequent "flehmen responses," which constitute the characteristic male indication of sexual excitement (lip curls while sniffing urine, feces, or vaginal secretions, apparently allowing the passage of pheromones to the nostrils). Castrated horses (geldings) quickly began showing flehmen responses in the presence of estrus females when they were injected with testosterone and LHRH, but not with LHRH alone (McDonnell et al., 1989). However, the LHRH-testosterone combination elicited a more powerful response than testosterone alone, demonstrating that LHRH has a sexually stimulating effect independent of testosterone production.

Cooper, Seppala, and Linnoila (1984) have shown in female rats that synthetic LHRH agonists may not have the sexually stimulating effect of natural LHRH. Consequently, testing for sexual effects with these synthetic agonists may tell us nothing about the effect of natural LHRH and may discourage attention to this potentially useful peptide.

Sexual Effects in Humans

LaFerla, Anderson, and Schalch (1978) and LaFerla, Labrum, and Tang (1982) reported substantial increases in LHRH in men or women watching sexually arousing videotapes. LHRH treatment may have some pleasant effects on male libido, but it has not been significantly effective in treating erectile dysfunction. Evans and Distiller (1979) found marginal facilitation of erection and ejaculation in normal male volunteers injected with LHRH prior to masturbating. Davies et al. (1977) found no improvement in 10 men with psychogenic impotence injected with LHRH for four weeks. However, significant but small increases in sex drive and spontaneous erections occurred. When Ehrensing and Kastin (1976) gave three-day sequences in two weeks of LHRH injections to six men with decreased sexual desire, only one man showed any benefit different from placebo.

Kastin et al. (1979) conducted a comprehensive placebo-controlled trial with daily injections of LHRH for four weeks. Nine men with psychogenic impotence failed to show therapeutic effects beyond those on placebo. Moss, Riskind, and Dudley (1979) reported no effects for 10 to 14 days of LHRH injections on sexually inactive men with psychogenic impotence. However, there was more sexual activity in men who still masturbated than occurred with placebo. It was not clear whether there was any therapeutic effect on erection or just an increase in interest and activity.

In summary, LHRH has not been shown to be useful as a treatment for men with psychogenic impotence. Pleasant increases in sexual desire may sometimes occur, but these are relatively small and not much different from placebo when compared in controlled trials. LHRH has not been tested for sexual dysfunction in women, despite significant findings of LHRH-induced increases in sexual activity in female animals.

30

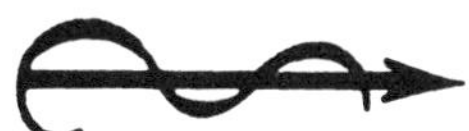

Yohimbine

OBJECTIVES

- To examine the mechanisms of action of yohimbine
- To distinguish among synthetic, herbal, and homeopathic formulations
- To evaluate the use of yohimbine combination drugs
- To evaluate the use of yohimbine as an adjunctive medication
- To examine anxiety-related side effects

Yohimbine, which comes from the bark of an African tree, is one of the oldest remedies for sex. It has been studied in herbal, homeopathic, and pharmaceutical forms and has been sold as a tonic for impotence rather than as a nonspecific "aphrodisiac." Although it is usually combined with other substances believed to potentiate erection (such as testosterone, strychnine [*nux vomica*], and thyroid supplements), there is no evidence that these adjunctive substances either increase or decrease yohimbine's efficacy. Yohimbine combinations have been cause for medical and Federal Drug Administration scrutiny and some combination drugs (like Afrodex) have been withdrawn from the market. The prescription drug yohimbine HCL is a synthetic salt and is only one of several forms of yohimbine found in the natural bark. It is not an herb and does not come from the "yohimbe" tree (yohimbine HCL is a white powder; natural yohimbine bark is rust-brown in color).

Most research studies of yohimbine have been small, interesting, but unreliable. More recently, however, well-controlled studies have been performed. From the perspective of these reports, it appears that yohimbine acts centrally on sex drive, affecting erection indirectly. Indeed, an analysis of yohimbine's sexual mechanisms of action (see Table 30.1) reveals that yohimbine positively influences so many sexual mechanisms, it would be surprising to find that this medication did *not* affect sexual function in humans. In general, yohimbine has been found to have more pronounced results for psychogenically impotent men than for organically impotent men, although its beneficial effects in the treatment of diabetic impotence have also been reported. The drug has also been helpful in treating peripheral neuropathy in these diabetics, which suggests that it may be affecting neural as well as vascular dimensions. In addition, because of its chemical mechanisms, yohimbine has shown significant potential as an enhancer of health and longevity, which has yet to be explored.

In 1989 the Federal Drug Administration stated that yohimbine was not effective or safe for the treatment of sexual dysfunction. This position means that the drug has not been *proven* to be effective, based on the fact that studies have not been submitted to the Federal Drug Administration for formal approval. Many positive studies exist, however. Therefore, while yohimbine may not be *labeled* as a treatment for impotence, doctors may *prescribe* it.

The folklore basis of yohimbine's reputation as an aphrodisiac is that it causes blood to rush to the penis, producing an erection. The standard text on pharmacognosy (the pharmacology

Table 30.1 *Profile of Yohimbine*

	Daily Dose
Yohimbine hydrochloric acid (HCL) (Yocon, Yohimex, generics)	15 mg/day
Yohimbine bark (YBRON, Yohimbe, herbal generics)	

COMMON INDICATIONS
Impotence, orthostatic hypotension, diabetic neuropathy

MECHANISMS OF ACTION (GENERAL)
Antagonizes $alpha_2$ inhibitory adrenergic receptor
Inhibits platelet aggregation and is a calcium channel blocker

MECHANISMS OF ACTION (SEXUAL)

Positive
Increased adrenergic $alpha_1$ activity
Decreased adrenergic $alpha_2$ activity
Decreased benzodiazepine (GABA)
Increased cholinergic activity
Decreased opioids
Increased oxytocin
Increased phenylethylamine
Decreased progesterone
Increased substance P
Increased vasoactive intestinal peptide
Increased vasopressin

Negative
Increased prolactin
Increased cortisol

DIRECT SEXUAL SIDE EFFECTS
Yohimbine has no adverse sexual effects

Desire enhanced	Erection	Orgasm/Ejaculation
• Inhibited sexual desire improves	• Obtaining erection enhanced • Maintaining erection enhanced • Quality of erection enhanced • Flaccid or semi-erect penis helped • Nocturnal, morning erections enhanced	• Retarded ejaculation helped

INDIRECT SEXUAL SIDE EFFECTS
Discomfort caused by indigestion, nausea
Mood disorders resulting anxiety, nervousness
Neurological disturbances resulting in dizziness, headache, paresthesia, tremor
Vascular disturbances resulting in arrhythmias, headache

SEXUAL CONTRAINDICATIONS/BENEFITS

Avoid with prior condition of	*May be useful for*
Panic/anxiety states	Sex drive disorders
Sexual obsessive-compulsion	Impotence (psychogenic and organic)
Sexual phobias	

ALTERNATIVES
Bupropion (Wellbutrin)
Penile Injection Therapy (PIE)

of natural plant drugs) by Tyler, Brady, and Robbers (1981) described the effect of the yohimbine herb: "The drug dilates the peripheral blood vessels and lowers blood pressure. Alleged aphrodisiacal effects are attributed to the enlargement of blood vessels in the sexual organs and increased reflex excitability in the sacral region of the spinal cord" (p. 501). However, more recently, it has been determined that yohimbine does not have a direct vasodilating effect. Due to its release of norepinephrine, yohimbine can even shrink the penis when injected into the corpus cavernosum (Lue, 1988). These findings point to other, non-local causes, such as stimulation of areas of the brain facilitating sexual activity (Clark, 1991).

Although many texts conclude that yohimbine has no effect on sexual desire, a positive effect on erection has been acknowledged (Tyler et al., 1981). According to one author, "although it has been promoted as an aphrodisiac for many years, in actuality it stimulates erectile tissue without increasing sexual desire and thus is not a true aphrodisiac" (Brysson, 1989, p. 90).

Contrary to the assumption that yohimbine's sexual effect is localized in the genitals, current research has shown that its dominant impact occurs in the brain (Clark, 1991; Clark & Smith, 1990). Although unexplored, this neural effect may be the critical source of its efficacy. In this respect, yohimbine may be useful as a supplement to pharmacologically-induced erections (PIE) in patients with low sexual desire.

Despite its ancient heritage, yohimbine remains a novel and unstudied chemical in pharmacological research. In our investigation of yohimbine's mechanism of action, we found it to have strong positive interactions with many of the new peptides that promote sexual responses, such as oxytocin, VIP, substance P, vasopressin, and ACTH. It also interacts with neurotransmitters such as acetylcholine and dopamine that are directly involved in the sexual response.

MECHANISMS OF ACTION

Daily use of yohimbine HCL (Yocon, Yohimex, Aphrodyne, 15 mg/day) or herbal yohimbine (YBRON) may facilitate normal ejaculation through increased sympathetic tone, while at the same time bolstering erection and decreasing neuropathy. There have been no published reports on the use of yohimbine for retrograde ejaculation, but it has been shown to facilitate other autonomic sympathetic actions (Goldberg & Robertson, 1983). It may be used at high doses (10–20 mg) or taken daily (5 mg, 3x/day). However, particularly if used acutely, it is likely to be less effective than specific alpha-1 adrenergic arousal with phenylpropanolamine or other such sympathomimetic drugs (yohimbine has yet to be identified as having a serotonergic effect, which conceivably would decrease its adrenergic effects). Taken daily, it may require six to eight weeks before any effects occur, but improvement should be maintained thereafter. There is no evidence that yohimbine causes premature ejaculation or penile supersensitivity. An interesting aspect of therapeutic dosage with yohimbine is that *less* is often *more*. Both higher and lower doses often have less effect on sexual function. Optimum therapeutic dosages appear to be moderate to low.

Facilitation of Lisuride Sexual Arousal

Yohimbine HCL has been shown to facilitate lisuride-induced mounting in male rats (Ferrari, Baggio, & Mangiafico, 1986). When lisuride was given in a dose too low to induce mounting, addition of a small dose (1 mg/kg) of yohimbine elicited mounting. The sexual effect of yohimbine with 200–400 micrograms of lisuride is as great as with 1,200 micrograms lisuride alone. Some of the sexual stimulation with ergots like lisuride and bromocriptine may be due to their considerable $alpha_2$ blocking property. The $alpha_2$ agonist clonidine inhibited lisuride-induced mounting.

Potentiation of ACTH Erection

Yohimbine HCL at low doses has been shown to potentiate ACTH-induced penile-erection in male rats (Poggioli, Vergoni, & Bertolini, 1985). ACTH is a brain peptide that stimulates the release of adrenal hormones. Though stimulated by stress, it improves attention and is considered a nootropic drug. A range of yohimbine doses (0.1–30 mg/kg) was tested for their effect on the ACTH-induced penile erection, yawning, and stretching syndrome. At all dose levels, yohimbine by itself did not induce any of the yawning/stretching symptoms. When injected before ACTH, low doses (0.1, 0.5, 1 mg/kg) strongly potentiated ACTH-induced penile erections (from 2.4 to 4.8). Yawning and stretching increased to a lesser extent. Higher doses (10–30 mg/kg) reduced ACTH-induced erections. The effect of 0.1 mg was as great as with 1 mg/kg. Only at this 0.1 mg/kg dose was yawning significantly increased. This finding, along with others noted in this sections, suggests that yohimbine can have a positive sexual effect at remarkably low doses. Furthermore, at doses above 1 mg/kg, yohimbine HCL is no longer selective for adrenergic $alpha_2$ receptor antagonism, so it may have more direct adrenergic actions that cause nervousness and are detrimental to sexual function and well-being.

Potentiation of Cholinergic Actions

Research has indicated that yohimbine facilitates cholinergic transmission in animals and humans (Goldberg & Robertson, 1983). $Alpha_2$ receptors are located on parasympathetic neurons, which inhibit cholinergic action. The $alpha_2$ agonist clonidine commonly reduces salivation (resulting in dry mouth) and cholinergic stimulation of the gut (resulting in constipation) (Thompson, Diamond, & Altiere, 1990). Since yohimbine blocks these $alpha_2$ receptors, it stimulates cholinergic parasympathetic activity. An oral dose (14 mg), has been shown to increase salivation in male and female subjects (Chatelut, Rispail, Berlan, & Montastruc, 1989) and diarrhea has been reported as an occasional cholinergic side effect of yohimbine in humans. This cholinergic potentiating action could contribute to the drug's facilitation of animal and human sexual responses.

Stimulation of Oxytocin and Vasopressin

Yohimbine has been shown to directly increase oxytocin and vasopressin release and activity. It can also potentiate oxytocin release indirectly by stimulating cholinergic and dopamine activity, while inhibiting opiate, GABA, and serotonin activity (Assenmacher, Szafarczyk, Alonso, Ixart, & Barbanel, 1987). Apparently, yohimbine directly stimulates oxytocin by removing tonic inhibition by $alpha_2$ receptors that act in tandem with opiate receptors. There is a relatively small increase of oxytocin release with yohimbine alone and a larger release with the opiate antagonist naloxone alone. With yohimbine and naloxone combined, there is mutual potentiation so that oxytocin release is nearly double compared to that found with yohimbine or naloxone alone (Zhao et al., 1988).

Effect on Serotonin

Yohimbine's action on serotonergic activity is complex and rarely investigated. Given our hypothesis that dopamine and serotonin exist on a polar axis, so that an increase of dopamine or a decrease of serotonin facilitates sex, we have searched for an explanation of yohimbine's sexual stimulation through actions on either dopamine or serotonin transmission. At this time, yohimbine does not seem to act through either substance. However, a few years ago a new serotonin receptor was discovered in humans—the 5-HT_{1D} receptor—and yohimbine was shown to have a strong affinity to it (Schoeffter & Hoyer, 1989). However, it is not yet known whether yohimbine is an agonist or antagonist of the 5-HT_{1D} receptor. This receptor appears to operate as an autoreceptor in the serotonin system, meaning that it may decrease serotonin release with an action similar to the $alpha_2$ receptor inhibition of norepinephrine release. Consequently, yohimbine's sexual action conceivably could be due to a reduction in serotonin activity or to a stimulation of serotonin receptors, such as 5-HT_{1A} receptors, with paradoxical positive sexual effects. Newer synthetic $alpha_2$ antagonists recently introduced into clinical research do not have this strong affinity to the 5-HT_{1D} receptor.

Prior pharmacological research on yohimbine has shown that it increases serotonin levels (Goldberg & Robertson, 1983). However, other research has shown that yohimbine blocks the vascular constricting action of serotonin (Lattimer et al., 1984), decreases serotonin release (Feuerstein, Hertting, & Jackisch, 1985), and even directly blocks 5-HT_2 receptors (Frenken & Kaumann, 1984). We expect that the contradictory actions of yohimbine on serotonin eventually will be understood and explained by its action on the various serotonin receptors. Conversely, actions of the newly discovered 5-HT_{1D} receptors could be clarified by investigating their contribution to yohimbine's sexual effects. The interaction of yohimbine with 5-HT_{1D} receptors should teach us much about the relation between anxiety and sexuality, because the anxiety-reducing action of buspirone (BuSpar) involves stimulation of both 5-HT_{1A} and $alpha_2$ adrenergic receptors.

YOHIMBINE COMBINATION FORMULATIONS

Patented and sponsored synthetic drugs with yohimbine's $alpha_2$ antagonist action have been introduced recently into clinical research: idazoxan, imiloxan, RS-15385 (delequamine), antipamezole, midaglizole, efaroxan, rilmenidine, CH-38083, and fluparoxan. Fluparoxan (from Glaxo) and delequamine (from Syntex) are currently being investigated for treatment of impotence in large controlled clinical trials, having completed promising pilot trials. Continuing interest in drugs with $alpha_2$ antagonist activity suggests that pharmaceutical companies believe this class of drugs has sufficient sexual potential to positively affect sexual function to invest in them. Except where otherwise specified, we will examine yohimbine first in its synthetic hydrochloride (HCL) form.

Potensan and Potensan Forte

These yohimbine preparations are described by Peter Taberner in his 1985 book *Aphrodisiacs*. Potensan, which contains 5 mg yohimbine HCL, 0.5 mg strychnine HCL, and 15 mg amylobarbitone, was targeted solely for the treatment of impotence. The inclusion of amylobarbitone is baffling, unless it was intended to suppress overexcitement (or prevent seizure due to the combination of yohimbine and strychnine!). Potensan Forte contains 5 mg yohimbine HCL, 5 mg methyltestosterone, 10 mg pemoline, and 0.5 mg strychnine HCL. Testosterone and pemoline (a mild dopaminergic stimulant used to treat hyperactive children) were added with the intention of treating loss of libido as well as erection. In 1973, Cooper, Smith, Ismael, and Lorraine tested Potensan Forte in impotent men with low testosterone levels. Intercourse with ejaculation increased significantly from 0.12 to 1.12 occurrences a week over four weeks of treatment (four pills a day). Placebo patients showed less improvement. Follow-up of the patients did not show long-term improvement.

Zumba

In its various manifestations, Zumba is probably the most widely sold yohimbine combination treatment. For many years in the United States this was the treatment kept "below the counter" for treatment of impotence. The most recent formulation we have found (in Tijuana) is Zumba Forte, a cafeteria mix of various herbal aphrodisiacs, including yohimbine bark, ginseng, damiana, lecithin, and 0.3 mg testosterone. The recommended dose is two tablets three times a day.

Tonaton

This yohimbine preparation was popular among urologists in Europe for many years. It contained natural yohimbine bark, strychnine, atropine, and ephedrine in an alcohol extract. It was recommended for hypotonic bladder, chronic prostatitis, and associated sexual dysfunction ("sexual neurasthenia"). Clinical reports showed improved bladder pressure and reduced residual urine in over 80% of patients (Bauer, 1956; Held, 1962). Held commented that patients were usually so pleased with the elimination of sexual neurasthenia and depression that they hardly noticed that micturition had improved until closely questioned. Tonaton was given in quite high doses for four to six weeks, with therapeutic effects apparent within 10 days.

Strychiomel

Strychiomel tablets contain 2.5 mg yohimbine HCL, 1.5 mg strychnine sulfate, and 10 mg thioridazine HCL. Thioridazine (Mellaril) was added presumably to enhance relaxation and reduce anxiety. It is interesting that both yohimbine and thioridazine are calcium channel antagonists, which (paradoxically) could relax penile blood vessels and smooth muscles. Savion, Segenreich, Kahan, and Servadio (1987) retrospectively evaluated 72 impotent patients treated for eight weeks with two tablets per day. Impotence was both psychogenic and organic in origin, and usually mixed. Twenty-six (36%) patients recovered normal, usable erections; 22 (31%) improved erection; and 24 (33%) showed no response. The 36% response rate is similar to recent reports of yohimbine treatment of organic impotence. Overall, 66.7% of the patients benefited. This figure is greater than the usual placebo response of 40% in impotence studies.

Pasuma

Pasuma was once distributed by the Merck Pharmaceuticals. Each tablet contained 5 mg methyltestosterone, 3 mg Vitamin E, 3 mg yohimbine HCL, 15 mg caffeine, and 1 mg ephedrine. The famous cardiologist Christian Barnard used it to treat four of his cardiac transplant patients who had become impotent (Wolpowitz & Barnard, 1978). Three to six pills per day were prescribed. Within one month, three of the four men recovered sexual function.

Afrodex

Afrodex was a prescription yohimbine combination pill marketed through doctors in the United States from the late 1950s until 1973. It was withdrawn by the Federal Drug Administration as an unproven and possibly unsafe combination drug. The pill was a combination of 5 mg yohimbine, 5 mg methyltestosterone, and 5 mg nux vomica extract (containing strychnine). Apparently, the presence of testosterone and a substantial amount of strychnine was the reason for FDR concern.

From surveillance studies and a placebo-controlled double-blind crossover trial, Afrodex appeared to have a beneficial effect in some impotent patients with few side effects. The surveillance trials were sponsored by its distributor. Doctors in private practice reporting on patients treated with Afrodex on a standard form subjectively rated the efficacy during the first 10 weeks of treatment as excellent, good, fair, or poor. The form also included patient age, duration of impotence, and the cause of impotence (if determined). Afrodex dose was one pill taken three times a day. The first author of the surveillance trial reports was Robert Margolis, a private practice physician in New York City. All reports appeared in *Current Therapeutic Research*, a legitimate but not stringently peer reviewed journal.

Margolis and Leslie (1966) reported on a total of 1,000 patients treated by 250 physicians who submitted review forms to the Afrodex distributor. Commonly noted causes of impotence included "neurasthenia, psychic factors, male climacteric, or hypogonadism." (Few diagnostic tests for organic pathology were available in 1966.) The number of patients decreased each week, reflecting either inefficacy, resolution of their impotence, lack of patient motivation and persistence, or failure of doctors to explain to patients that results might not occur until more than a month of daily use. By week 10, only 328 men remained in the study, of whom 50% were rated excellent, 36% good, and 14% fair or poor. For the patients who remained in the study, reports of excellent or good responses increased each week. In 721 patients who remained in the study for at least three weeks, the ratings of excellent or good increased from 26% at week 1, to 39% at week 2, to 56% at week 3. Men under 60 years of age responded more often than men over 60. Substantial therapeutic response was said to have occurred by the third week of daily treatment. Side effects reported were few (5% of patients), which is typical of surveillance studies. (Many of the dropouts may have experienced unrecorded side effects.) Most of the side effects were related to nervousness: palpitations, tachycardia, insomnia, nausea, gastric distress, headache, and dizziness.

Margolis, Sangree, Prieto, Stein, and Chinn (1967) updated the Afrodex surveillance with an additional 2,000 patients. Results were similar to the prior report. By week 8, more than half the patients had dropped out. Among patients remaining each week, 53% of 1,605 patients showed excellent or good responses at week 3, and 79% of 974 patients did so at week 8. Calculating from the figures available, the final week 10 response rate (excellent or good) was 734 of the original 2,000 patients, a response rate of 37% (17% for "excellent" responses, which probably represented consistently usable erections). Response rates were lower for men over 60 and for men on additional medications. Onset of action required one to three weeks. Side effects continued to be few and mild, consisting of the symptoms noted above. An update to 10,000 patients (Margolis, Prieto, Stein, & Chinn, 1971) reported essentially the same findings. Fifty-nine percent of patients dropped out by week 10.

Miller (1968) conducted a placebo-controlled, double-blind crossover study of 22 impotent patients on Afrodex (three times a day) or placebo for four weeks with a two-week washout between the four-week treatments. Response was judged by the number of weekly erections and ejaculation/orgasms. Men were aged 30 to 51 (perhaps an optimal age range for impotence treatment studies). Sixteen of the 22 patients showed psychogenic impotence, while six suggested organic impairment due to chronic prostatitis, back pain, or endocrine deficiencies. All patients completed the study. No side effects were reported, indicating superficial monitoring. During the first four weeks, erections increased with both Afrodex and placebo. Typically there is a large placebo effect in impotence treatment studies. Erection increases that first occurred on Afrodex were mostly sustained through the two-week washout of no medication, whereas the placebo response disappeared during the washout. In any event, no more than 50% of patients showed improvement and the overall change was nonsignificant.

Crossover studies are popular because all subjects receive the drug and the number of subjects is twice that of a non-crossover study. However, carry-over effects are often unexamined and discounted. The chief problem in impotence treatment trials is the large placebo effect (usually 30–40%). Carry-over effects make the placebo effect even larger, making it difficult to show any real effect.

Sobotka (1969) used the same crossover design as the 1968 Miller study. The only difference was that the washout period between trial phases was extended from two weeks to four weeks. Fifty impotent patients were treated. In most cases, impotence was either psychogenic or "hypogonadal." However, hypogonadal impotence was not defined. The term "male climacteric and/or hypogonadal impotence or neurasthenia," used for many patients, came from the *Physicians Desk Reference* labeling. The presence of many hypogonadal men makes it difficult to determine how much changes were due solely to the 15 mg/day oral dose of methyltestosterone rather than the yohimbine. (The recommended dose of methyltestosterone [Android] for treatment of low testosterone is 10–50 mg.) The results showed a clear increase in erections while on Afrodex in contrast to minimal improvement on initial placebo and loss of improvement when switched from Afrodex to placebo. With the four-week washout, the carry-over effect from Afrodex was very small. Changes in ejaculation were similar to the changes in erection. Unfortunately, there was no indication whether the increased erections on Afrodex involved successful intercourse (usable erection), masturbation, or nocturnal erections.

Evidence in the surveillance and controlled studies indicated some benefit from Afrodex. The Sobotka placebo-controlled trial showed that the improvement was greater than on placebo. However, lack of information on the nature of improvement and the lack of stringent peer review makes the evidence difficult to judge. The delay of improvement from one to three weeks and the continued improvement with further use was characteristic of later findings with yohimbine alone. However, the week-by-week results were not shown in these reports. The daily dose of yohimbine with Afrodex was 15 mg (5 mg three times a day), the same as current yohimbine HCL dosing. Even with the addition of methyltestosterone and strychnine, side effects appeared to be minor, although experience of the drop-outs was not well-described. There was no report of a toxic reaction to Afrodex in the literature. Nonetheless, removal from the market by the Federal Drug Administration in 1973 was probably wise, because the drugs combined with yohimbine were possibly of no benefit and were potentially toxic. Until the withdrawal of Afrodex in 1973, the Physicians Desk Reference entry included only a short note with no warning against higher doses, despite the large amount of strychnine.

The Margolis surveillance studies have been cited as establishing a greater response than they actually proved. For instance, Riley, Goodman, Kellett, and Orr (1989) stated that the 1971 Margolis surveillance summary (Margolis et al., 1971) reported "good to excellent results in 80%" of 10,000 cases of impotence. Morales, Surridge, Marshall, and Fenemore (1982) may have considered that their own 42.6% response rate in organically impotent patients was substantially lower than the highly positive figures reported in the Margolis studies. As we have shown, less than 40% of the patients started on Afrodex had an "excellent or good" response: 17% had excellent responses and 20% good responses. Since the duration and severity of impotence was not specified, and many of the patients were only psychogenically impotent, the impotence treated was probably less severe than in more stringent recent studies. Quoting 80% response rates on Afrodex in recent articles causes exaggerated expectations in patients and doctors, which are unlikely to be fulfilled. As noted, the response rate in the Afrodex surveillance studies was no higher than what may be expected by placebo alone.

LITERATURE REVIEW OF SYNTHETIC YOHIMBINE

With the FDA position against combination prescription medications established in the 1970s, urologists now use yohimbine alone (5 mg yohimbine HCL tablets, three times per day), but combination formulations with synthetic or natural yohimbine are still sold commercially, with unknown consequences. The total daily dose of yohimbine HCL is similar to that prescribed in the combinations. Recently, however, capsules of 250–500 mg yohimbine natural bark have appeared for over-the-counter sale in health food stores. Given the lack of legitimate research trials and chemical analysis of treatment with the natural bark, the putative huge doses in the capsules, and their questionnable safety and efficacy, such capsules should be removed from the market.

Without the addition of other drugs such as methyltestosterone and strychnine, yohimbine is very safe; toxic reactions have rarely been reported in the literature. In particular, we do not know of any cases of priapism due to yohimbine. Side effects of anxiety may prevent some patients from using yohimbine, but these unpleasant effects also discourage abuse. The FDA placement of yohimbine bark on a list of dangerous, toxic herbs has no literature support.

Therapeutic outcomes with yohimbine appear to be the same as with the combination pills. Though recent reports indicate increased use of yohimbine due to promising results, careful reading of these reports does not clearly differentiate yohimbine from placebo. A review of this literature follows.

Open Clinical Trials With Prescription Yohimbine HCL*

Macfarlane, Reynolds, and Rosencrantz (1983) reported a 50% (10/20) positive response, in which six patients returned to normal function and four were sometimes able to penetrate and ejaculate. Patients' impotence was not clearly organic or psychogenic. Three patients showed side effects of nausea, headaches, and skin flushing. Hanno and Charles (1986) similarly reported that 52% (22/42) of their patients regained normal function (erection, penetration, ejaculation, orgasm) on a routine combination treatment of yohimbine (15 mg/day), isoxsuprine (10 mg), and testosterone (200 mg weekly) enanthate injection (Delatestryl). In a follow-up study, Hanno, Wein, and Fletcher (1988) reported a 34%

*Unless noted otherwise, yohimbine dose was 5–6 mg tablets taken three times daily.

recovery rate (38/111) on the routine combination treatment used previously. Ninety percent of patients reporting recovery maintained it at a two-year-follow-up.

Morales et al. (1982) reported a 26% recovery rate (6/23) in patients with organic impotence due to diabetes and vascular disease. Three patients noted adverse effects of nausea, dizziness, or nervousness, and three diabetic patients noted disappearance of leg and feet paresthesia.

Chancellor, Bennett, Sonda, and Konnak (1987) reported improvement in 38% (87/231), with 6% (12) showing "complete" improvement. Three percent (7/231) had mild adverse effects. The authors suggested that better response might be achieved with higher than recommended doses.

Double-Blind Trials

In a 10-week double-blind trial with 100 patients on yohimbine or placebo, Morales et al. (1987) reported 21.3% *complete response* on yohimbine versus 13.8% on placebo; 21.3% *partial response* on yohimbine versus 13.8% on placebo; and 57.4% *no response* on yohimbine versus 72.4% on placebo. None of the differences was significant. Criterion for impotence was a minimum of three prior months with failure to obtain erection sufficient for penetration. There was no increase in nocturnal penile tumescence in complete responders, despite recovery of erection sufficient for intercourse (confirmed by sex partner). No side effects or drop-outs were noted.

Reid et al. (1987) reported a significant effect of yohimbine treatment. Total response (complete and partial) on yohimbine was 62% (18/29) versus 16% (3/19) on placebo. However, this finding was confounded by lack of response in placebo patients subsequently put on yohimbine on open basis (only one patient showed response), suggesting that the placebo group was invalid. Total response of both groups on yohimbine was 46%. No side effects or dropouts are reported.

Susset et al. (1989) reported that 10 of 71 patients (14%) recovered normal function in a double-blind partial crossover of four-week phases on yohimbine or placebo. Patients had a full range of impotence from very severe organic to very mild psychogenic. Higher than recommended doses of yohimbine were used: from one tablet four times a day (21.6 mg/day) up to two tablets four times a day (43.2 mg/day). Fifteen responders reported greatest improvement at maximum dose. Eight responders noted greatest response at 32.4 mg/day. Eight patients did not complete the study due to adverse effects at lowest doses and four of 15 patients with only partial responses discontinued yohimbine due to adverse effects (anxiety, nausea, dizziness, increased urination, chills, headaches, and vomiting). Positive response to yohimbine declined with more severe organic factors and duration of impotence. For mild psychogenic impotence, the positive response was over 60%. With the presence of organic factors, complete or partial responses ranged from 28% to 0%. Even at the high doses used in this study, yohimbine was quite safe. However, other studies have shown that severe panic and anxiety may occur at doses higher than 20 mg (Charney & Heninger, 1986).

Sonda, Mazo, and Chancellor (1990) reported no significant differences between yohimbine and placebo (16 of 33 [48%] responded to yohimbine versus 10 of 33 [30%] on placebo), although nine of the 11 patients responding only to yohimbine showed increased desire and four of 11 had improved orgasm. No change in penile blood pressure was observed on yohimbine despite restoration of usable erections in 16 patients (11 on yohimbine alone, five on yohimbine and placebo).

In summary, studies of the use of yohimbine in combination with other drugs have not been carefully monitored or reported. Success rates of up to 79% are corrected to much lower figures when dropouts are counted: about 37%, and only about 17% for "excellent" responses, which may represent true usable erections.

Studies of synthetic yohimbine have been carefully conducted and have shown response rates from 26% to 34% in organically impotent patients compared to about 15% on placebo. Once recovery occurred, it was well-maintained. Improvement rates of psychogenically impotent patients were better, ranging from 62% to 66%

versus about 20% placebo response. However, for both groups of patients, complete response indicating consistently usable erections was usually only half the total improvement rate. The 31% complete response rate shown by Reid et al. (1987) was probably a reliable figure. Placebo rates were usually less than half those with yohimbine, indicating a true drug effect. Synthetic yohimbine tablets seem to be remarkably safe, both initially and during long-term use. The well-controlled studies of Morales' and Susset's groups suggest an improvement rate of over 60% for psychogenic impotence, though response drops sharply when organic deficiency factors are present.

YOHIMBINE AND ANXIETY

Despite dysphoric anxiety symptoms usually seen with high doses of yohimbine, some subjects also reacted with erections unrelated to arousal. Holmberg and Gershon (1961) injected 0.5 mg/kg yohimbine into volunteer patients. The autonomic effects included facial flushing, perspiration, salivation, lachrymation, pupillary dilation, nausea, and micturition and defecation urgency. Yet, erection was seen in 10–20% of the patients. This early report was the first to recognize that the extent of these autonomic changes was related to pre-existing emotional reactivity in some subjects.

Many years later, during the 1980s, Dennis Charney and his colleagues at Yale University regarded these autonomic changes as indications of the presence of panic reactions in certain individuals (Charney, Heninger, & Breier, 1984). Panic reactivity is an emotional illness that has been differentiated from affective depression and generalized anxiety reactions. At higher doses (20 mg or higher, single oral dose) yohimbine can elicit panic reactions in people already prone to such responses, but persons not predisposed may feel nothing at all or mild nervousness and heart rate increases.

Redmond, Kosten, and Treiser (1983) noted the occurrence of spontaneous ejaculations during panic-anxiety and related such panic and perhaps phobia to premature ejaculation in anxious individuals. Yohimbine can also induce panic/anxiety states, so that sexual effects during these states may work through yohimbine-like action. Redmond (1985) described a similar effect in a 29-year-old woman with a panic disorder: She described an association between her anxiety and sexual arousal. Specifically, she reported that each time she experienced anxiety she concurrently experienced a physical sensation that involved an intense physical feeling in her genital area and down her legs and an urge to stretch her legs to relieve. She described the feelings as physically similar to "real" sexual feelings but different in that the cognitive and psychic components were minimal. This feeling had never led to an orgasm.

Jacobsen (1991) used yohimbine at a standard dose (5.4 mg, 3x/day) to treat 15 patients (six women, nine men) who were sexually dysfunctional due to fluoxetine treatment for depression. Eleven patients improved within two weeks of yohimbine supplementation. Jacobsen noted that additional positive responses to yohimbine had been found in a double-blind controlled trial in progress. Jacobsen's report contained the first indication that women could be treated for sexual dysfunction with yohimbine. A double-blind study by Jacobsen the following year (1992) confirmed the benefits.

Yohimbine can be expected to generate anxiety and cardiovascular side effects when combined with tricyclics. It should never be given with MAOIs, because excessive adrenergic stimulation could cause a hypertensive crisis or other severe side effects.

Charney and Heninger (1986) reported a more powerful sexual impact when yohimbine was combined with the opiate antagonist naloxone. They gave six 5 mg yohimbine tablets together with a 1 mg/kg injection of naloxone to six men and four women (mean age: 37). These subjects were healthy, free of mental illness, and not prone to panic reactions. All six men became fully erect five to 10 minutes after the addition of the naloxone injection, and the erections lasted at least 60 minutes. None of the men reported any increase in sexual drive. Following naloxone without yohimbine, only three of the six men reported partial erections that lasted no more than 30 minutes. No sexual changes occurred on yohimbine alone. Only one woman noted increased sexual drive starting 30 minutes after the naloxone injection and lasting 60 minutes. This woman reported neither an increase in lubrication nor orgasm. The surprising lack of genital responses in women suggests a differential effect of yohimbine in men and women.

Overall reactions to the yohimbine-naloxone combination were distinctively unpleasant. Increases occurred in nervousness, anxiety, nausea, palpitations, tremors, hot and cold flashes, and dysphoria. Charney and Heninger commented that the combination would only be helpful for treatment of impotence if it could be used at doses that would avoid these anxiety symptoms.

Routine opiate antagonist treatment for impotence would require that the oral opiate antagonist naltrexone (Trexan) be used instead of the injectable naloxone. Mendelson et al. (1979) found that the normal therapeutic dose of naltrexone (50 mg oral) produced recurrent spontaneous penile erections for one to three hours in three of seven healthy male subjects. However, all seven subjects reported dysphoric effects, including fatigue, sleepiness, light-headedness, faintness, nausea, sweating, and feelings of unreality. Even erection was considered unpleasant because it was "inappropriate in the research setting and inconsistent with their volitional attempts to control sexual ideation." Such dysphoric symptoms contraindicate the addition of naltrexone to yohimbine treatment of impotence. (In passing, it should be mentioned that when given the chance to control erection-inducing brain stimulation, rhesus monkeys usually press quickly to turn it off and hardly ever to turn it on [Robinson & Mishkin, 1968].)

YOHIMBINE AS ADJUNCTIVE MEDICATION

Price and Grunhaus (1990) reported a case study in which yohimbine reversed lack of orgasm/ejaculation in a 35-year-old man treated with clomipramine (Anafranil) for obsessive-compulsive and depressive disorders. Within two days of beginning treatment with clomipramine, the man experienced anorgasmia. The serotonin antagonist cyproheptadine (Periactin) was first used to restore orgasm. Not only did it fail to improve orgasm, it also caused suicidal thoughts, hypersomnia, and irritability. The man tried to decrease clomipramine dosage on his own because of his sexual problem but became more depressed. The authors prescribed yohimbine to be taken 90 minutes prior to intercourse and even ran a short placebo-controlled study to be sure that any effect of yohimbine was real. Orgasm occurred normally with 10 mg yohimbine, while lack of orgasm returned whenever placebo was used. When the dose of yohimbine was increased to 15 mg, the man even experienced premature ejaculation and requested to go back down to 10 mg.

Jacobsen (1991) prescribed 5 mg yohimbine three times a day to both men and women patients who experienced sexual dysfunction during long-term fluoxetine (Prozac) treatment. Of 160 patients successfully treated with fluoxetine (20–40 mg) for depression, 54 (34%) developed sexual dysfunction. Sixteen patients experienced decreased desire, 21 experienced decreased sexual response, and 17 experienced decreases in both desire and response. Fifteen patients (six woman, nine men) who had developed sexual dysfunction were prescribed yohimbine (5 mg/3x/day) while continuing on fluoxetine. Eleven of 15 patients (73%) reported complete or partial reversal of sexual dysfunction within two weeks on yohimbine. The other four patients reported no difference or discontinued yohimbine due to nausea and anxiety. Jacobsen (1992) has further reported favorable results in a placebo-controlled trial of yohimbine treatment of fluoxetine-induced sexual dysfunction. Adjunct yohimbine HCL is now used routinely in clinical practice to treat SSRI-induced sexual dysfunction.

Leonard, Morales, and Nickel (1988) reported the case of a patient treated for impotence due to hyperprolactinemia from a pituitary adenomata. Bromocriptine and supplemental testosterone had failed to reverse the impotence, but the addition of yohimbine led to complete recovery of sexual dysfunction. Quadraccia, Salvini, Cordani, and Pizzi (1988) used daily doses of oral yohimbine (0.30 mg/kg) together with weekly injections of papaverine-phentolamine to treat middle-aged men (30 to 60 years old) with mild to moderate organic arterial vasculogenic impotence (penile blood pressure index: 0.60–0.74). Thirteen men completely recovered erectile function, six showed partial improvement (more rigidity), and one man experienced no change.

HERBAL YOHIMBINE (YBRON)

During 1985–86, the Crenshaw Clinic was funded to test an herbal yohimbine (YBRON) extract for the treatment of psychogenic impotence. The solution was called *homeopathic* by the manufacturer and also said to contain a vasodilator in a very small concentration typical of homeopathic drugs. Since we were not trained in homeopathy, we viewed YBRON to be a very low dose alcohol extract of yohimbine bark, combined with an unmeasurable amount of vasodilator, and brewed by the manufacturer's "classified" process (intended to preserve freshness and potency).

Overview of Study

Prior to our studies we obtained an assay of the solution, which showed that yohimbine was the only active substance in the extract (besides alcohol). At the dose we prescribed in the study (2/3 of a CC stopper, 3x/day), the total daily dose of yohimbine from the extract was less than 1 mg when measured against a synthetic yohimbine HCL standard. The extract was taken sublingually so that minute amounts of drugs could be efficiently absorbed. The extract was brown in color and could be tasted (it stung like hot chili) when taken under the tongue.

We initially ran a small (10 patients) eight-week open pilot trial. Patients with mild to severe psychogenic impotence were screened for organic factors and depression. Noticeable improvement occurred in eight of 10 patients, and remarkable improvement was noted in several men, who regained full robust erectile function. Given our "eagle eye" for adverse effects, the total absence of such side effects was equally remarkable.

Due to limitations of funding, we were only able to conduct a small double-blind trial (25 men) of psychogenic impotence. The men had no evident physical or mental health problems. The results of the trial were similar to typical figures achieved in successful antidepressant studies: 69% (9/13) of the subjects improved "much" or "very much" on yohimbine versus 33% (4/12 subjects) on placebo. However, due to the low number of patients, the results were mostly nonsignificant. The investigator-rated overall CGI scores were significantly lower ($p < 0.05$) for yohimbine versus placebo over the last four weeks, but there were no significant differences in patient-rated improvement scores or in the erectile functioning improvement scale. There were no significant changes in weight, blood pressure, or pulse. Yohimbine did not generate anxiety, as it does at higher doses. The only side effects due to the drug were complaints by some subjects that the solution stained their teeth, but these subjects considered this effect mild and reversible with cleaning. There was a small but significant decrease in glucose levels in the yohimbine group (and not in the placebo group). Since subjects were not diabetic and had normal glucose levels on entry, the meaning of this effect was unclear. If yohimbine does lower glucose, this may be a benefit for diabetic men who may wish to try yohimbine for treatment of impotence.

For subjects 60 or older, there was no evident difference between yohimbine and placebo (33% [2/6] showed positive responses on both yohimbine and placebo). This may be due to the presence of insurmountable, unidentified, organic deficiencies in these older subjects. Overall improvement in sexual dysfunction appeared to be due to improvements in sexual desire as well as erectile function. There were no significant differences in erection improvement per se, however, suggesting that the erectile problems may have been due to desire deficits, or that improvements in sexual desire can lead to satisfactory erectile function in men with psychogenic impotence. Therefore, yohimbine may aid sexual function through improvements in desire. (Table 30.2 reproduces the patient-rated sexual desire inventory we created to determine changes in this area. It may prove useful to both physicians and therapists in questioning their patients regarding the more subtle areas of sexual function.) Differences between yohimbine and placebo on this sexual desire scale were apparent by week 4 and significant at week 6 ($p < 0.05$), but no longer significant at weeks 8 and 10, when change scores on placebo increased slightly (overall, between five and six of the desire-scale items were rated as improved by yohimbine-treated subjects versus one to two by placebo-treated subjects). The small number of study subjects reduced the chance of statistical signficance (a minimum of 60 subjects, 30 on drug and 30 on placebo, should be run). The most noteworthy changes in sexual desire occurred in the areas of sexual thoughts, physical sensations, touching and affectionate behavior, and receptiveness to and desire for sex.

There were no significant differences in the self-ratings of erection between yohimbine and placebo groups, but there was a clear though nonsignificant indication that yohimbine subjects showed greater improvement in achieving and sustaining a sufficient erection during intercourse. Over the course of the 10-week study, sufficient intercourse erections increased from 0.54/week to 1.50/week in yohimbine-treated patients versus an increase from 0.58/week to 1.00/week in placebo-treated patients. Changes in frequency of intercourse were no different between yohimbine and placebo. Surprisingly, there were no differences between yohimbine and placebo groups in the number and grade of waking erections (from sleep), and the placebo

Table 30.2 *Crenshaw-Goldberg Sexual Desire Inventory (CGSDI)**

Compared to the start of the study (the three months prior to the first week of medications), evaluate any changes in your sexual life during this week *only* by checking the appropriate column. Circle your mark if the change has been particularly great and noticeable.

	Increase	No Change	Decrease
1. Change in the number of erotic dreams?	_____	_____	_____
2. Change in the number of sexual thoughts or fantasies?	_____	_____	_____
3. Change in sexual ease or comfort?	_____	_____	_____
4. Change in sexual confidence?	_____	_____	_____
5. Change in how often you initiate sex?	_____	_____	_____
6. Change in your receptiveness to sex with your partner when he/she initiates?	_____	_____	_____
7. Change in touching and/or affectionate behavior with your partner?	_____	_____	_____
8. Change in enjoyment of sex?	_____	_____	_____
9. Change in desire for sex?	_____	_____	_____
10. Change in the intensity of sexual feelings?	_____	_____	_____
11. Change in physical sensations in your own body which changes your sexual desire?	_____	_____	_____
12. Change in intensity of your sex drive?	_____	_____	_____
13. Change in quality of physical sexual feelings?	_____	_____	_____

*Some items may seem redundant but are exploratory, to determine if terms such as *intensity of sexual feelings* (item 10) and *intensity of sex drive* (item 12) mean anything different. As yet, we do not know the best words to express what patients feel.

group showed higher a number and grade of waking erections throughout the study.

Discussion of Results

The response rate of 69% for yohimbine versus 33% for placebo was impressive. As noted, such a difference is characteristic of antidepressant trials that confirm efficacy. The large placebo rate of between 30–40% is typical of both impotence (Benkert, 1975) and antidepressant placebo-controlled trials. A placebo response is usually as "real" as a response to drug, except in short-term trials of four weeks or less, when the effect is not so sure. One benefit of a longer trial period, such as was used in the YBRON research, is that placebo responses have sufficient time to be tested. If there is no relapse over such a long period, then one can be relatively confident of the response. One of our placebo responders recovered and maintained normal erectile function, verified by his wife, for the first time in 30 years (he believed that traumatic experiences during the Korean War had caused his sexual dysfunction). Therefore, even ineffective drug treatment may allow recovery in a certain number of patients.

Since YBRON (sublingual herbal yohimbine extract) and synthetic yohimbine appear to have complex and often beneficial mental effects on sexual arousal, we are curious to evaluate its usefulness in treating sexual desire dysfunctions. Such dysfunctions often involve masked aversion, phobia, and depression. While SSRIs may be tried in such disorders, these drugs can reduce sexual drive and response themselves. The natural herbal nature of YBRON could encourage its use in patients who are reluctant to take non-organic synthetic medications. The herb itself may contain additional therapeutic elements and safeguards not present in synthetic medications. A drawback to herbal preparations is their questionable freshness and consistency of the product from batch to batch. The optimal results during our initial pilot trial of YBRON may have been due to the freshness of the solutions. Due to delays in initiating the double-blind trial, the YBRON medication sat on the shelf for a few months. Subsequent to the double-blind trial, we continued some subjects on open treatment with YBRON, which was not commercially available at that time. A few subjects reported that they experienced less benefit with the new open label YBRON. When we checked back with the manufacturer, it was learned that these supplemental bottles of YBRON were leftovers from the batch mixed for the earlier double-blind study. Consequently, the manufacturer was alerted that freshness of the solution may effect its potency. Subsequent to the double-blind study, we have treated patients both with YBRON and with yohimbine "mother tinctures" supplied by homeopathic companies and have found that the newer the preparation, the more likely it is to have a favorable effect.

During this subsequent treatment of patients with herbal yohimbine, a few patients switched over to the synthetic yohimbine (Yocon) and reported that this form was noticeably less effective than the herbal preparation. We have occasionally used homeopathic formulations of yohimbine (e.g., 2x, 3x, and 6x), which contain far less of the drug than the low dose (1x) found in YBRON. Though we have found no benefit from these true homeopathic preparations, we also have little experience with them or with homeopathic diagnosis. (We have also failed to find any benefit with other homeopathic drugs in minute-dose concentrations, including ginseng, ignatia, and cantharides [Spanish Fly].) The YBRON product containing significant amounts of yohimbine and a vasodilating herb at a minute homeopathic dose is the only preparation that has appeared effective in double-blind trials. Extended clinical experience has shown similar yohimbine 1X mother tincture extracts supplied by homeopathic manufacturers to be effective. Some of our patients have been on yohimbine 1X extracts for several years and still notice a decrease in drive and/or erection when they are not taking the herbal supplement. In our trial, improvement (separation from placebo) did not begin until the third week and increased consistently until the final measure, indicating a progressive improvement in sexual desire due to YBRON. The progressive nature of the improvement also suggested the possibility that clearer changes may have occurred with a longer trial period.

LONGEVITY

Although yohimbine has not been studied in regard to longevity at this time, it has a number of beneficial effects that may promote it: The specific action of yohimbine (antagonist of alpha$_2$ adrenergic neurons) may have an *antidepressant* effect; it can aid in the *control of glucose* and it also has a *synergistic action to insulin*; yohimbine has an *antiplatelet aggregation* effect (similar to effect of aspirin) and (in its herbal form) *antiarrythmic* effects; it can be used to treat *orthostatic hypotension* and *nerve degeneration* characteristic of diabetes and aging, and *Raynaud's disease* (constricted blood flow in fingers and toes); improve attention and *enhance learning and memory*; and indirectly affect *obesity* by antagonizing those chemical actions in the body that prevent fat breakdown.

CONCLUSIONS

Yohimbine began its modern history as a "combination" drug. Today, it appears to be returning in that direction, serving as an adjunctive or potentiating medication. With widespread use of SSRIs, such as fluoxetine (Prozac), paroxetine (Paxil), and sertraline (Zoloft), sexual dysfunction due to psychotropic medications may also become widespread. Suggested adjunct treatments such as bethanechol and cyproheptadine have unpleasant side effects which discourage their use. Cyproheptadine can even reverse therapeutic gains of SSRIs due to its serotonin-blocking action. Yohimbine itself has some antidepressant properties, so it would be an excellent adjunct for preserving sexual function.

Yohimbine could be a useful oral supplement to penile injection therapy. Penile injections do not increase sexual drive directly. Yohimbine's sexual effect appears to come from the brain, not the penis. Use of yohimbine could complement penile injection therapy by providing sufficient stimulation so that the injections were needed less often or not at all. Similarly, yohimbine might also be a valuable adjunct for men with penile prostheses who continue to experience sex drive disorders. Possibly new, potent alpha$_2$ antagonists, such as fluparoxan or delequamine, will prove to be efficacious and safe in current placebo-controlled trials, but these new drugs should also be compared to yohimbine, which has been used safely for many years.

The sexual facilitating action of yohimbine has been observed chiefly in men: we have used yohimbine to treat a few women experiencing low sex drive with no effect, but more research is needed. Jacobsen's (1991, 1992) reports of beneficial effects of adjunct yohimbine in fluoxetine-treated women are fascinating. It could be that the beneficial sexual effect of yohimbine is testosterone-dependent, so that it may be less likely to occur in women.

31

Vasodilators: Papaverine, Alpha Blockers, Vasoactive Intestinal Peptide, Topical Vasodilators

OBJECTIVES

- To identify the mechanisms involved in erection
- To evaluate the advantages, disadvantages, and diagnostic applications of pharmacological injection erection
- To explore alternatives to injections

The vascular mechanisms involved in achieving penile erection became clear only in the 1980s when erection was shown to be produced at will by injection of various adrenergic blocker drugs and vasodilators into the penile corpus cavernosum. The chief erectile mechanism has been identified as the relaxation of smooth muscle within the cavernosum, which allows blood to flow in and the tissue to expand against the cavernosum walls, thereby shutting off veins which drain the blood. The detailed inspection of this erectile mechanism showed that it was not a hormonal phenomenon (one can gain a rigid erection without testosterone), and not even primarily a cholinergic parasympathetic function. Instead, erection depends primarily upon the integrity of the actual penile tissue and simple hydraulic principles. We have come to appreciate additional dimensions from the cellular level to the complex dynamics of neurotransmitters.

Vasodilators are substances that dilate blood vessels in one part of the body or another. Many blood pressure medications operate by central vasodilation and peripheral vasoconstriction, resulting in conditions that inhibit erection. The last decade of research has introduced the initially questionable approach of injecting a variety of vasodilators directly into the penis in an effort to produce a lasting erection sufficient for sexual intercourse. Initial reservations among urologists and impotent patients seem to have been replaced in the 1990s with routine clinical use. Recently, topical vasodilators that do not require the psychological or physical discomfort of an injection have reached the research stage, as have patches. Unfortunately, none of the topical or transdermal techniques stimulate as firm and dependable an erection as the injections. In fact, they usually do not provide sufficient rigidity for penetration. In the meantime, researchers are exploring alternate technologies of administering the injections. As an extra dividend, vasodilators for penile injection have demonstrated tremendous usefulness in diagnosing the etiology of erection problems. They have illustrated new physiologic mechanisms for mediation of erection and ejaculation, and in some cases they have served as a catalyst for continued function.

PHYSIOLOGY OF ERECTION

Until the advent of induced erections via penile injections, the majority of urologists and experts in the field of human sexuality believed that erection was primarily a parasympathetic event mediated through acetylcholine. Investigation of adrenergic influences in men had chiefly involved the peripheral ejaculatory mechanism. The effect of vasodilators and further evaluation of the mechanisms of action involved made clear that the dynamics are more complex and that the sympathetic nervous system plays a more significant role than appreciated previously.

As noted, erection can be induced by injecting drugs into the corpus cavernosum. The mechanism of action of penile vasodilators operates by relaxing the circular smooth muscle fibers that fill the corpus cavernosum. Their vasodilating effect is achieved through varied chemical mechanisms, all of which counteract the tonic constricted state that characterizes the non-erect penile cavernosum smooth muscle tissue. This dynamic was first demonstrated in France by Virag (1982) using papaverine and more dramatically in England by Brindley (1983), who injected himself with phenoxybenzamine. Erection will fail to occur if blood flow into the cavernosum from arteries is insufficient, or if there is venous leakage so that blood is not held within the swollen cavernosum.

Both of these drugs, papaverine and phenoxybenzamine, block normal adrenergic (NE $alpha_1$ receptor) contraction of smooth muscle. With smooth muscle relaxation, blood flows into the corpus cavernosum like water into a sponge until the tissue expands maximally against the resistance of the tunica albuginea (which is tough, like an inner tube or a balloon). In hydraulic terms, all that is required to make a man potent is that significantly more blood flows *in* than *out*. However, biochemically and physiologically, an intricate system is involved that requires coordination among nerves, vessels, and tissues right down to the endothelial lining.

In fact, there are more than 30 mechanisms currently identified that influence sex (see Chapter 4). These mechanisms of action that affect the target organ are processed in various areas of the brain, particularly the limbic area, where thought and emotion are integrated into cognitions and attitudes. Thus these biochemical processes can be cancelled, short-circuited, interfered with, or enhanced by the brain. Injection of vasodilators directly into the penis bypasses many of these complex higher nervous system actions. Though normal erection may occur with the injection, the triggering sexual desire and stimulation factors mediating erection from the central nervous system are missing.

In recent years, several new sexually dynamic endogenous substances have been recognized. One is vasoactive intestinal peptide (VIP), which occurs naturally in the body and is localized in abundant quantities throughout the genitals (of both sexes), the uterus, and gastrointestinal tract. Since absence of sufficient quantities of vasointestinal polypeptide has been clearly implicated in some forms of impotence, VIP is one of the substances that has been injected directly into the penis. Prostaglandins (PGE1) were also identified as naturally occurring genital transmitters involved in erection. They have been used with consistent success for penile injections (e.g., Prostin), but have the disquieting side effect of causing persistent penile pain in up to 30% of patients. A new commercial preparation of PGE1, alprostadil (Caverject), recently FDA-approved and marketed, appears to cause less pain upon injection than Prostin.

Nitric oxide is another new discovery. It, too, is a naturally occurring substance involved in smooth muscle relaxation and specifically involved in promoting erection. Produced by the cells in the endothelial lining of the blood vessels, it mediates relaxation on a molecular level. It was interesting to observe the manner in which the medical community, with the help of the press, reacted to this particular discovery. Apparently overlooking the numerous mechanisms involved in erectile function, nitric oxide was initially labeled as "the cause" of erections and its absence responsible for any lack (Gibaldi, 1993). Again, a brief glance at Chapter 3 clearly indicates that nitric oxide levels are just one of many factors. At this time, we do not know whether there is any difference in penile nitric oxide levels between potent and impotent men, or whether the nature of nitric oxide release varies in functional compared to dysfunctional men.

PHARMACOLOGICAL INJECTION ERECTION

The drugs now being used for pharmacological injection erection (PIE) were already on the market though not indicated for this purpose. Therefore, penile injection with these drugs did not immediately require formal clinical testing and FDA approval. Doctors can legally use available drugs as they choose, but such use is not officially sanctioned. Clinical experience with a variety of these substances culminated in several published reports between 1986 and 1990 (Adaikan & Ratnam, 1988; Brindley, 1986a; Lue & Tanagho, 1987; Malloy & Wein, 1988; Tordjman, 1990) which have shown PIE to be generally safe and effective in selected patients—at least in the short term. Furthermore, freedom to explore various drugs has resulted in the discovery of more effective drugs, such as prostaglandin E1.

It is important to understand that PIE drugs are not considered "aphrodisiacs." They do not work by increasing sexual desire, although improvement in mechanical function can certainly improve desire, self-esteem, and activity-level indirectly. PIE drugs do not work through the brain; their mechanisms are neither psychological nor hormonal. A man can become erect through PIE when desire is totally absent and sex hormone levels are below normal. PIE drugs do not supply the emotional aspect of sex, but they may enhance it. Successful injection erections do not preclude the need for psychologically-oriented sex therapy. On the contrary, injections can be profoundly destructive to a woman's sexual enjoyment if a PIE-treated man eliminates romance and foreplay, thinking he does not need it anymore. Indeed, removing a mechanical problem of long standing may well aggravate relationship problems rather than resolve them if appropriate psychotherapy is not included.

Penile injections were discovered as the result of a fortuitous medical accident. During the 1970s, sexual revascularization surgery was successfully developed in Europe. Penile arterial blood flow was achieved by connecting abdominal arteries (from the hypogastric/pudendal arteries) to the penile arteries in the corpus cavernosum. During one such revascularization surgery, Michal, Kramer, and Pospichal (1977) accidently injected the muscle relaxant papaverine into the penile circulation. The patient's penis became erect and remained so for two hours. Over the next few years, Wagner and various colleagues performed surgical studies on penile vascular function during erection. During one of these studies (Wagner & Brindley, 1980), large doses (40–120 mg) of oral phenoxybenzamine (Dibenzyline) caused mild but noticeable penile tumescence in two of three subjects for 24 to 48 hours. From these studies, it became apparent that erection was more strongly affected by changes in adrenergic stimulation than by cholinergic activity in the parasympathetic system, as was formerly believed.

Subsequently, Brindley (1983) performed penile injections on himself with various adrenergic blocking agents and muscle relaxants, including phentolamine and phenoxybenzamine, to investigate their influence on erection. He found that an injection of phentolamine directly into the corpus cavernosum caused a firm erection for approximately eight minutes. Among many alternatives investigated, Brindley determined that phenoxybenzamine caused the most reliable and firm erection. He described phenoxybenzamine-induced erections for normal and impotent men in a 1983 article in the *British Journal of Psychiatry*. These erections lasted between 30 minutes to 30 hours. However, five of the 11 impotent men in the study failed to obtain full erections. A vigorous 56-year-old, Brindley presented his discovery at the 1983 meeting of the American Urological Association in Las Vegas. Wearing a jogging outfit rather than the usual business suit, Brindley described his studies with alpha adrenergic blockers and told the audience that, shortly before his talk, he had injected phenoxybenzamine into his own penis. At that point, he lowered his jogging pants and demonstrated his rigid erection!

Working independently in France, Virag (1982) also conducted a series of clinical studies on normal and impotent men. He performed penile injections with the muscle relaxant papaverine, which also indirectly blocks adrenergic $alpha_1$ receptor stimulation. Both normal and psychogenically impotent men experienced erections lasting one to four hours. Organically impotent patients frequently became erect, but their erections occurred less reliably, were less firm, and did not last as long as those in subjects without organic deficiencies. The advantage of papaverine injections over phenoxybenzamine was that erections did not last overly long, reducing the risk of priapism. With phenoxybenzamine, priapism was more common, ejaculation could be blocked, and other toxic effects could be expected.

Zorgniotti and Lefleur (1985) reported using a mixture of papaverine with a small amount of phentolamine. This combination increased rigidity when injection with papaverine alone did not generate a sufficiently firm erection. This mixture proved to be safe and effective for home injection. Patients were initially injected in the office to determine the effective dose and then taught how to inject themselves. Patients were routinely advised how to recognize and respond, should priapism occur.

After 1985, urologists throughout the world used papaverine and papaverine-phentolamine injections to diagnose as well as to treat impotent patients. Failure of the injection to cause a firm erection was reason to suspect a vascular problem – either insufficient arterial blood flow or venous leakage. Despite widespread caution among many urologists due to the lack of official testing with proper trials, clinical reports on the efficacy and safety of pharmacological injection erection during urological meetings in 1986 and 1987 were encouraging. When this clinical experience was documented in several articles published from 1988 to 1990, PIE became accepted clinical practice among some urologists. Many, however, remained skeptical about the merits of the injections and did not offer this option to patients. As confidence in the safety of pharmacological injection erection gradually increased, many urologists prescribed it for psychogenically impotent patients as well as physiologically impotent ones, bypassing therapy and risking long-term tissue complications from multiple injections over time.

In 1987, PIE research advanced the field of sexual pharmacology by introducing a new peptide, prostaglandin E1 (PGE1), into clinical practice. PGE1 (Prostin, Provastan, Alprostadil) is a vasodilating peptide found naturally in the penis. Problems with papaverine injections, such as priapism and local fibrosis, appear infrequently or not at all with prostaglandin injections. In addition, the use of a natural vasodilating erectile substance removes some of the stigma of artificiality from the injection procedure. Furthermore, PGE1 can generate a more "natural" erection than papaverine, and the corpus spongiosum and glans become firmer. The avoidance of priapism with PGE1 was reported by Ishii et al. in 1986 in Japanese trials with 88 patients and confirmed by Stackl, Loupal, and Holzmann (1988) in 112 patients. While papaverine-phentolamine mixtures are still the most commonly used preparations, PGE1 is becoming increasingly popular. Some urologists (Floth & Schramek, 1991) now use papaverine in combination with PGE1.

Side Effects

Numerous side effects limit the desirability of PIE-induced erections and the treatment population: Penile injections should not be used in cases of psychogenic impotence or to extend the duration of erection in men who ejaculate too quickly. Though documented dysfunctional toxicity is rare, tissue damage (scarring and fibrosis) from repeated injections can eventually cause obstruction of blood vessels, curvatures due to contractures, chronic pain from irritation, inflammation, and/or infection (chronic or acute). Priapism can be controlled or prevented if a patient is properly educated, but it can also cause irreversible damage if not corrected promptly and properly. In addition, there have been case reports of cerebrovascular accidents (strokes) associated with the systemic effects of the potent vasodilators used for PIE. The chemicals do not stay quarantined in the penis, but seep into the general circulation with the potential to affect other parts of the neurovascular system.

Short-term adverse effects include (Lue & Tanagho, 1987):

- bleeding at the injection site (sometimes requiring compression on the spot for one to two minutes)
- bruising (transient)
- facial flushing
- orthostatic hypotension (dizziness upon standing)
- pain at the penile glans during or after injection (may be brief or can persist for more than a day)
- priapism for more than six hours that may be painful
- retarded ejaculation/orgasm
- blood is shunted away from the cavernosum during pelvic movement (the "pelvic steal" syndrome)
- epinephrine flow due to nervousness competes with PIE-induced smooth muscle relaxants
- other concurrent medications may prevent effectiveness of PIE

Note that the possibility of priapism continues to be a drawback to treatment with papaverine, papaverine/phentolamine, and especially to phenoxybenzamine; persistent penile pain is the chief drawback of PGE1. (Hopefully, this will be minimized by availability of the alprostadil freeze-dried preparation [Caverject].)

Long-term adverse effects include:

- fibrosis and scar tissue in corpus cavernosum (may be worse in diabetics)
- angulation due to scar and plaque formation on the tunica albuginea
- smooth muscle hypertrophy within the corpus cavernosum (found in monkeys)
- increase in intracellular filaments
- abnormal liver function tests
- veins do not close down completely or leak
- there is decreased arterial blood inflow due to atherosclerosis or other artery disease
- penile expansion is prevented or restricted by Peyronie's disease plaques

These progressive changes may cause irreversible impotence over time, requiring a surgical implant for a return to sexual function. In addition, some women are disturbed by the notion of a chemically-induced erection, just as they are by the mechanical implant. Without therapy, couples are not likely to adjust to enjoy the revival of erectile function. Turner et al. (1992) reported that of 106 men starting self-injection therapy, only 42 completed 12 months; 64 (60%) dropped out before 12 months.

Pharmacological injection erection is contraindicated for the following populations:

- patients on neuroleptics
- patients on $alpha_1$ adrenergic blocking antihypertensives (such as prazosin)
- patients with coagulation defects and those on anticoagulant medication (such as coumadin)
- patients with sickle-cell anemia
- patients who are extremely nervous or anxious
- patients who cannot learn the injection technique
- patients prone to dizziness, flushing, or orthostatic hypotension after injections
- patients with active genital infections
- patients with current alcohol or drug-abuse problems
- patients with a history of stroke

One side effect *increases* the desirability of this procedure: PIE facilitation of spontaneous (non-PIE) erection. Several urologists outside the United States have noted that spontaneous erections adequate for intercourse may occur after one or more PIE erections (Aravena & Bustamente, 1986; Bahren, Scherb, Gall, Becker, & Holzki, 1989; Kiely, Blank, Bloom, & Williams, 1987; Kiely, Williams, & Goldie, 1987; Virag, Frydman, Legman, & Virag, 1984; Wagner, 1985; Watters et al., 1988). In some of Virag's patients (Virag, 1982), erection even improved at home between injections (which were given at the clinic, months apart), perhaps because the vascular pathways were opened by the forceful, chemically-induced circulation. This increase in spontaneous erection may last for a few days, weeks, or months. When the effect has faded, another single PIE injection can again trigger this response. Increased erection after and between injections occur in both organically and psychogenically impotent men, but are more frequent in psychogenic patients. Return of functional erections without need for injection, at least some of the time, was reported in the United States by Marshall, Breza, and Lue (1994) and Marshall and Lue (1993) in 35–40% of their subjects, indicating improved blood flow and smooth muscle function after long-term intracavernosal therapy.

Diagnostic Applications

During the past eight years, PIE research has provided greater understanding of erection physiology and it has become an invaluable diagnostic tool that is used for many purposes:

- to determine whether there are venous leaks preventing firm erections (Castillo, Barlog, Perfetto, Cartagena, & Sufrin, 1986)
- to inspect penile curvature and deformity in Peyronie's disease in the office setting
- to differentiate neurogenic from vascular organic impotence*
- to facilitate visualization (arteriography) of the pudendal artery system (Lue & Tanagho, 1987)
- to diagnose the "pelvic steal syndrome"

*If full, firm erection occurs within 10 minutes and lasts 30 minutes or more, one can assume that the vasculogenic system is not the cause of impotence: blood flow and venous closure are adequate. However, failure of erection does not necessarily identify a definite vascular problem; nervous patients who fear injection can defeat erection by sympathetic stimulation (epinephrine response).

AVAILABLE PIE DRUGS

Papaverine and Alpha-Adrenergic Blockers

Papaverine, an opium derivative, has been the mainstay of PIE therapy. It serves as a smooth muscle relaxant through phosphodiesterase inhibition, elevation of cyclic adenosine monophosphate, and attenuation of alpha-adrenergic receptor mediated contraction. Doses range from 5 mg for neurogenically impotent sensitive patients to 80–120 mg in patients with severe vasculogenic impotence. Urologists in the United States prescribe 15–30 mg papaverine mixed with 0.5–1 mg phentolamine (Regitine). This combination was first reported to be effective by Zorgniotti and Lefleur (1985). In a 15-patient study by Stief and Wetterauer (1988), 87% (13 patients) achieved full erection with a 15 mg papaverine and 0.5 mg phentolamine combination, compared to 40% (six patients) on papaverine alone; one patient responded to phentolamine alone.

Papaverine must be given in an acidic low PH (under 4) solution, because it precipitates out of solution when the PH factor is higher. Phentolamine requires only a slightly less acidic solution. In contrast, PGE1 comes in a moderate PH5 solution and remains stable when the solution is buffered to higher alkaline levels (Seidmon & Samaha, 1989). Overly acidic solutions can burn genital tissue. Monkeys given several papaverine injections have shown corporal fibrosis (Abozeid et al., 1987).

Sidi, Cameron, Duffy, and Lange (1986) and Allen and Brendler (1988) used the standard Zorgniotti combination of 25–30 mg papaverine with 0.5–1 mg phentolamine to show that vasculogenically impotent patients may fail to respond to PIE treatment. Sidi et al. found that 100% of neurogenically impotent patients showed adequate erection, compared to 66% of vasculogenically impotent patients. Similarly, Allen and Brendler found 100% response in neurogenic patients, compared to 60% in vasculogenic patients. Fifteen of 17 (88%) psychogenically impotent patients showed adequate erection in Allen and Brendler's study. The failure of psychogenically impotent men to respond to PIE injections may be due to anxiety during the procedure, which produces excessive adrenergic sympathetic activity (Granata, Carani, Del Rio, & Marrama, 1994).

In France, Virag, Shoukry, Floresco, Nollet, and Greco (1991) still use papaverine (20–40 mg) alone for the majority of cases of patients, particularly in the psychogenic impotence. The rest are treated with a mixture of papaverine and alpha-adrenergic blockers or vasodilators (ifenprodil or nicergoline) or a special mixture of papaverine with five other drugs (Ceritine). The Ceritine solution contains about 5 mg papaverine mixed with small amounts (0.006-.2 mg) of yohimbine, piribedil (a dopaminergic stimulant), ifenprodil, dipyridamole, and the anticholinergic drug atropine. Other mixtures of such drugs will no doubt be developed eventually by individual urologists and pharmaceutical companies.

Phenoxybenzamine (Dibenzyline) or Phentolamine

Although it has more adverse effects and has been found to be carcinogenic in animals, phenoxybenzamine can induce adequate erections when there is no response to high-dose papaverine or high-dose papaverine combined with phentolamine (Brindley, 1987). Phenoxybenzamine is not available in injectable form in the United States. In its oral formulation (Dibenzyline), it may cause increased tumescence but is apparently unable to generate a useful erection or treat erectile dysfunction. However, it has been used in selected patients as a treatment for premature ejaculation. (Papaverine does not generate or increase erection when taken orally.) Phentolamine taken orally or sublingually may also induce erections without direct injection (Gwinup, 1988; Zorgniotti, 1992).

Prostaglandin E1 (PGE1)

Prostaglandins are found naturally in the penis. PGE1 is well-known among health food users; it is metabolized in the body from gammalinolenic acid (GLA, evening primrose oil) supplements. In the United States, PGE1 is available as injectable alprostadil (Prostin VR pediatric). Its FDA-approved indication is to aid in the treatment of pediatric heart defects by keeping arterial ducts open until corrective surgery can be performed. As with other PIE drugs, it is not FDA-approved for use in erection injections and such use is discouraged by its manufacturer. However, clinical trials on a specially prepared PGE1 solution that minimizes pain and toxicity have been successfully completed by Upjohn, and this solution should be marketed in the United States during 1995.

After reports of PGE1 use in penile injection treatments appeared in Japan and Europe in 1987, American urologists began using Prostin as an alternative to papaverine and alpha-adrenergic blockers. Its initial appeal was the apparent lack of priapism as a side effect. Also, due to its natural presence in the penis, it was not expected to cause fibrosis during extended use (Stackl et al., 1988).

Human and rat penile tissue produces prostacylin, which is similar in action to PGE1 (Jeremy, Mikhailidis, & Dandona, 1987). Several findings have indicated a relationship of PGE1/prostacyclin to penile erection:

- Prostacyclin penile production is reduced in diabetic rats (Jeremy, Thompson, Mikhailidis, & Dandona, 1985).
- Cigarette smoke extracts inhibit penile prostacylin production (Jeremy, Mikhailidis, & Dandona, 1986).
- Cholinergic activity, which can trigger erection and vasodilation, also stimulates prostacyclin synthesis by penile tissue (Jeremy, Morgan, Mikhailidis, & Dandona, 1986).
- Papaverine has been shown to enhance prostaglandin responses in penile tissue (Virag & Adaikan, 1987).
- PGE1 directly relaxes penile CC muscle (Adaikan, 1979) and inhibits alpha-adrenergic action in CC muscle (Adaikan & Ratnam, 1987).
- Other forms of prostaglandin produced in human penile CC (Roy, Tan, Kottegoda, & Ratnam, 1984), such as PGF2a and PGE2 (at low doses), can contract penile

smooth muscle in contrast to PGE1's consistent vasodilatory action (Adaikan, 1979).

- In common with papaverine, PGE1 increases cyclic adenosine monophosphate in body tissue (Virag & Adaikan, 1987).

Ishii et al. (1986) first reported use of PGE1 in PIE treatment of organic impotence. In a larger study, Stackl et al. (1988) showed a 68% response rate (143/210); neither priapism nor fibrosis was observed. Subsequent double-blind trials showed equal or greater success with PGE1 in comparison to papaverine or the papaverine-phentolamine combination (Lee, Stevenson, & Szasz, 1989; Mahmoud, Dakhli, Fahmi, & Abdel-Aziz, 1992; Sarosdy, Hudnall, Erickson, Hardin, & Novicki, 1989).

Clinical experience has shown that some patients become erect with both drugs, neither drug, or with only one and not the other. Erection may have a slower onset with PGE1, but PGE1 erection may achieve greater fullness and blood flow than with papaverine (Chen, Hwang, & Yang, 1992; Hwang, Lue, Yang, & Chang, 1989). Stackl et al. (1988) found that length of erection was more closely related to PGE1 dose than had been found with papaverine. Consequently, dose could be adjusted flexibly and reliably for the desired degree of erection. Although the typical recommended dose for PGE1 injection is 10 to 40 μg, Godschalk, Chen, Katz, and Mulligan (1994) found that 70% of 17 patients injected required five μg or less for a rigid erection. They recommended a starting dose of 2.5 μg prostaglandin E1 (Alprostadil), with increments of 2.5 μg until rigidity occurs.

However, complications do occur with PGE1 injections that can be quite disturbing. Extended dull pain in the penis immediately following injections in about 10–30% of patients has caused many patients to prefer papaverine. This extended pain sensation may be unavoidable in certain patients due to the fact that prostaglandins naturally induce pain (aspirin and ibuprofen decrease pain by inhibiting prostaglandins). The new freeze-dried powder formulation of PGE1, aprostadil (Caverject), appears to cause less pain than prior prostaglandin formulations (Goldstein, 1994). Godschalk, Chen, Katz, and Mulligan (1994) observed pain with only 10% of injections of this new formulation, but used low doses of 10 μg or less. Erection adequate for intercourse was achieved in only 66% of 15 subjects, with an average rigidity of 59%.

Broderick and Lue (1989) found incidents of prolonged erection (four hours or longer) in 9% of patients (11/120) injected with PGE1. Priapism due to PGE1 injection has subsequently been noted by Stackl, Hasun, and Marberger (1990) in one of 550 men and by Schramek, Dorninger, Waldhauser, Konecny, and Porpaczy (1990) in four of 149 men. Prolonged erections due to PGE1 may spontaneously resolve without the damage that occasionally occurs with papaverine and papaverine-phentolamine erections.

PGE1 must be refrigerated and is more expensive than papaverine and alpha-blockers. Careful adjustment to the lowest necessary PGE1 dose could help reduce its expense. Many urologists have mixed papaverine-phentolamine and PGE1 together into a stock solution that often works better than any of them separately and allows lower doses of each (Floth & Schramek, 1991; Zorgniotti & Lizza, 1991).

Vasoactive Intestinal Peptide (VIP)

Vasoactive intestinal peptide (VIP) is a naturally occurring peptide neurotransmitter abundant in human genital tissue (Ottesen, Moller, Willis, & Fahrenkrug, 1982), in the human lumbosacral spinal cord (Anand et al., 1984), and in the gastrointestinal tract. Normally released during pelvic nerve stimulation of the corpus cavernosum, it stimulates local blood flow and is a potent smooth muscle relaxant in the corpus cavernosum. A deficiency of genital VIP has been identified in diabetic men with impotence secondary to neuropathy (Gu et al., 1984), indicating that this peptide may be partly responsible.

Vasoactive intestinal peptide seems to play a key role in mediating erections that is separate from the function of adrenergic neurotransmitters. Given its co-localization with acetylcholine in parasympathetic nerves, it is considered by many to be the noradrenergic, noncholinergic parasympathetic nerve transmitter that mediates vascular and smooth muscle relaxation previously associated solely with cholinergic action. Ottesen, Wagner, Virag, and Fahrenkrug (1984) found large increases of vasoactive intestinal peptide in eight of nine men stimulated to erection with PIE or visual sexual stimulation. Similarly, Dixson, Kendrick, Blank, and Bloom (1984) showed VIP elevation in the corpus cavernosum of rats following erection induced by touch stimulation, but not when erection was induced by electrical stimulation without touching. However, Kiely, Blank, Bloom, and Williams (1987) found no change in human genital VIP levels during PIE-induced erections or erections induced by touch or visual sexual stimulation.

As a pharmacological injection erection drug, VIP induces only moderate tumescence without producing sufficient rigidity for intercourse. Wagner and Gerstenberg (1988) failed to generate adequate PIE erections in patients, despite the use of doses up to 60 micrograms (doses of 2–4 micrograms are usually tested). However, VIP injections could induce adequate erections when augmented with sexual stimulation, including vibration of the penis. The authors concluded that VIP injections could "prime" the penis for sexual intercourse. Kiely, Bloom, and Williams (1989) reported tumescence without rigidity with VIP injections (2–4 micrograms) in both psychogenically and organically impotent men. However, inadequate erectile responses to papaverine or papaverine-phentolamine CC injections were improved to sufficient rigidity by addition of 2–4 micrograms VIP. Combination phentolamine-VIP injection yielded tumescence but not rigid, usable erection. The authors hypothesized that erections with phentolamine and VIP were inadequate because these drugs did not sufficiently increase arterial blood inflow. In contrast, aided by the sexual stimulation of partners adequately rigid erections for intercourse were reported by Gerstenberg, Metz, Ottesen, and Fahrenkrug (1992) with 30 μ VIP and 0.5–2.0 mg phentolamine combination injections. Roy, Petrone, and Said (1990) conducted a placebo-controlled double-blind study with VIP injections in 24 men (50–70 years old) with organic or psychogenic impotence. Penis length and diameter increased significantly with 400 pmol VIP compared to placebo, but rigidity was slight and not sufficient for intercourse.

The combination of VIP with PGE1 might be desirable, since both of these peptides are natural endogenous genital transmitters involved in erection. Unfortunately, PGE1 is expensive and VIP is even more expensive and commercially unavailable at this time. Furthermore, VIP is unstable in solution and difficult to handle and store (Roy et al., 1990). Consequently, VIP may remain a research tool rather than a clinical resource.

VIP has a fascinating association with oxytocin that makes it relevant to female sexual function. Oxytocin secretion during lactation releases VIP, and both oxytocin and VIP facilitate prolactin release (Stock & Uvnas-Moberg, 1985). During breast-feeding, oxytocin, VIP, and prolactin are released (Eriksson & Uvnas-Moberg, 1990; Ottesen, Schierup, Bardrum, & Fahrendrug, 1986) and, indeed, VIP is a potent releaser of prolactin (Ottesen et al., 1981; Rostene, 1984). In women, estrogen sensitizes responses to VIP, oxytocin, and prolactin. Palle, Bredkjaer, Fahrenkrug, and Ottesen (1991) have shown that VIP loses its ability to increase vaginal blood flow after menopause, but VIP-induced blood flow is restored by estrogen replacement. VIP could also be responsible for the brief genital increase in prolactin during coitus, which apparently is distinct from the prolactin elevation that decreases sexuality when chronically elevated (Drago & Scapagnini, 1983).

Given that coitus and nursing are both stimulated by the brain MPO active sex center, the mutual facilitation of VIP and oxytocin suggests an intimate physiological relation between reactions of the breasts and genital vasodilation. VIP is as abundant in the female genitals as in male genitals and greatly increases during vaginal and clitoral arousal (Ottesen, 1983). During coitus, VIP secreted in the vagina could conceivably stimulate VIP secretion in the inserted male penis, and vice-versa. Since VIP causes amnesia similar to oxytocin (Flood, Garland, & Morley, 1990), VIP and oxytocin together may contribute to the sweet forgetfulness characteristic of intensely affectionate sex.

It is not unusual to find that intercourse actually decreases when erection via pharmacological injection is available. With PIE, touching and communication are not as necessary for a man to achieve and sustain erection. In fact, PIE treatment from urologists can undermine sex therapy. Consideration of a common male and female genital action of VIP that is stimulated by touch and sexual activity could remove some of the mechanical coldness that "injected" sex connotes. When a man feels vulnerable and a woman feels obligated, romance can be ruined by a needle. Expert psychotherapy can help lighten the mood and bring perspective to preserve passion in the face of such intrusive treatment.

ALTERNATIVES

Tables 31.1 through 31.5 review the actions of drugs involved in pharmacological injection erection treatment. Some of these drugs have different effects when taken orally (for example, L-dopa) or injected systemically (for example, idazoxan). Drugs inducing non-rigid, unusable tumescence/erections (such as calcium channel blockers) are often misleadingly cited for their vasodilating PIE erectile properties. PIE with yohimbine has not been tested in humans, but research in animals indicates that yohimbine does not produce erection or tumescence when injected directly into the corpus cavernosum. Phenoxybenzamine is currently considered too strong and toxic. The most promising vasodilating substances available, but not yet tested in humans, are pinacidil (a potassium channel-opener antihypertensive) and adenosine (an endogenous sympathetic-inhibiting neurotransmitter). Peptide substances such as PGE1 and VIP appear to be the safest for extended use, but since they are not a clinically available combination, papaverine is still the most widely used PIE drug. None of these drugs directly increases sexual desire; their erectile effect is local and mechanical.

Nessel (1994) reports successful use over 10 weeks of daily oral yohimbine (5.4 mg t.i.d.) combined with oral pentoxifylline (400 mg t.i.d.) in seven of 10 men (40–63 years old) originally referred for injection therapy. No significant side effects were observed for this interesting combination of oral therapy.

TOPICAL VASODILATORS

Much of the information on topical vasodilators was learned by accident, sometimes in unorthodox ways. An amusing but important case study of erection induction by transdermal nitrate was reported by Talley and Crawley in 1985 in a brief letter to the editor.

A 53-year-old man treated with transdermal nitrate patches for atherosclerotic heart disease noticed that the side effect of headaches did not occur if he placed the patches lower than his chest. As a result, he experienced a semi-rigid erection and subsequently had intercourse. After intercourse, his wife experienced a severe headache that was attributed to absorption of nitrate from his ejaculate through her vagina.

Positive experiences with cavernosum-injected vasodilators during the early 1980s encouraged testing of topical nitroglycerin preparations to produce erection in impotent patients. Lue and Tanagho (1987) reported vasodilation after nitroglycerin injections in humans, monkeys, and dogs. An earlier article (Mudd, 1977) had reported use of sublingual glyceryl trinitrate nitroglycerin tablets to treat impotence in a 56-year-old depressed heart-disease patient. The patient had serendipitously noted the first spontaneous erections in more than two years while he was using sublingual glyceryl trinitate to treat acute chest pain. Erections continued to occur over several weeks soon after taking the sublingual nitrate, and the patient was able to have intercourse despite lack of sexual desire and occasional pain during erections.

Reports of erection induction in impotent patients were made by two urologists at the 1987 American Urological Association meetings (Godec, Narkhede, & Tomasula, 1987; Owen et al., 1987). Godec et al. (1987) compared erections induced through nitroglycerin 2% ointment (Nitrol Ointment) in 12 of 15 impotent patients to those produced by artificial erection by injection

Table 31.1 *PIE Resulting in Rigid and Usable Erection*

Drug	*Drug Type*	*Dose*	*Reference*	*Comment*
Phenoxybenzamine (Dibenzyline)	Non-selective alpha blocker	1–4 mg	Brindley, 1986a; Tordjman, 1990	Most rigid and long-lasting but toxic; some tumescence with systemic injection
PGE1	Prostaglandin	5–20 micrograms	Brindley, 1986a; Tordjman, 1990	Least toxic, most natural, but often painful
Papaverine	cAMP phosphodiesterase inhibitor	10–80 mg	Brindley, 1986a; Tordjman, 1990;Virag et al., 1991	Often supplemented with alpha-blockers like phentolamine
Ceritine	Combination: papaverine and five other drugs	12–40 units: 5–20 mg papaverine; minute doses of other drugs	Virag et al., 1991	Injection pen (Cerinjet) available)
Nitroglycerine	Vasodilator	Unknown	Lue & Tanagho, 1987	Used topically; mild effect as ointment
Adenosine	Endogenous antiarrhythmic	20–200 micrograms	Virag et al., 1991; Takahashi et al., 1990.	Weak human effect; strong relaxant effect in dogs
Ketanserin	$Alpha_1$ antagonist/$5\text{-}HT_2$ blocker	5 mg	Adaikan & Ratnam, 1988; Takahashi et al., 1990	

Table 31.2 *PIE Resulting in Briefly Rigid but Unusable Erection*

Drug	*Drug Type*	*Dose*	*Reference*	*Comment*
Phentolamine (Regitine)	Alpha-blocker (mainly NA-1)	5–10 mg	Brindley, 1986a; Gwinup, 1988; Tordjman, 1990	Rigid less than ten minutes; some effect taken orally
Thymaxomine	$Alpha_1$ blocker	5–10 mg	Brindley, 1986a	
Moxisylyte	$Alpha_1$ blocker	10–30 mg	Buvat, Lemaire, Buvat-Herbaut, & Marcolin, 1989	
Ifenprodil (Vadilex)	$Alpha_1$ blocker	5–20 mg	Virag et al., 1991	Used in France like phentolamine as papaverine adjunct
Verapamil (Calan)	Calcium channel-blocker/ $alpha_1$ blocker	1–5 mg	Brindley, 1986a	Rigid less than five minutes
Imipramine (Tofranil)	Tricyclic anti-depressant (also $alpha_1$ blocker)	5–10 mg	Brindley, 1986a	Initially rigid for few minutes, followed by shrinkage
Naftidrofuryl	Smooth muscle relaxant	20–25 mg	Brindley, 1986a	

Table 31.3 *PIE Resulting in Tumescence Only/Not Rigid*

Drug	*Drug Type*	*Dose*	*Reference*	*Comment*
Vasoactive intestinal peptide	Peptide neurotransmitter	2–4 microgram 200–400 pmol	Kieley et al., 1989	Effect increased by genital stimulation; augments papaverine
Adenosine	Antiarrhythmic	Unknown	Tordjman, 1990; Virag, 1989	Possible rigid effect in few patients
Dipyridamole (Persantine)	Antiarrhythmic/adenosine stimulate	Unknown	Tordjman, 1990	Anticholerinergic; some negative sexual effects when taken orally; augments adenosine CC erection
Lignocaine	Anesthetic	20–40 mg	Brindley, 1986a	
Salbutamol	$Beta_2$ agonist	0.4 mg	Brindley, 1986a; Tordjman 1990	
Moxisylyte	$Alpha_1$ blocker	10 mg	Buvat et al., 1989	Effect increased by genital stimulation
Nicergoline	$Alpha_1$ blocker	5 mg	Buvat, Lemaire, Marcolin, Dehaene, & Buvat-Herbault, 1986; Tordjman, 1990	
Nifedipine (Adalat)	Calcium channel-blocker	Not given	Tordjman, 1990	Minor or no effect
Bethanechol (Urecholine)	Cholinergic stimulant	Not given	Leyson, 1987	

Table 31.4 *Pie Resulting in No Erection*

Drug	*Drug Type*	*Dose*	*Reference*	*Comment*
Neostigmine	Cholinergic stimulant	0.25–5 mg	Brindley, 1986b	Tumescence with systemic injection (0.45 mg)
Atropine	Cholinergic blocker	0.3–0.6 mg	Brindley, 1986b	
Hydralazine (Apresoline)	Vasodilator antihypertensive	10–16 mg	Brindley, 1986a	
Propranolol (Inderal)	Beta-blocker antihypertensive	0.3–0.6 mg	Brindley, 1986a	
Idazoxan	$Alpha_2$ antagonist	0.5–2 mg	Brindley, 1986a	Tumescence with systemic injection

Table 31.5 *PIE Resulting in Prevention or Reduction of Erection*

Drug	*Drug Type*	*Dose*	*Reference*	*Comment*
Phenylephrine	Adrenergic/sympathetic stimulant	10 mg	Sidi, 1988; Zorgniotti & Lizza, 1991	
Epinephrine	Adrenergic/sympathetic stimulant	1 mg	Malloy & Wein, 1988	
Metaraminol	Adrenergic/sypathetic stimulant	0.6–4 mg	Brindley, 1986a	Possibly toxic, unpredictable duration of action
Ephedrine (Sudafed)	Adrenergic/sympathetic stimulant	50–100 mg	Lue & Tanagho, 1987; Zorgniotti & Lizza, 1991	Some erection reduction taken orally (30–60 mg)
Dopamine	Adrenergic/sympathetic stimulant	0.010 mg	Zorgniotti & Lizza, 1991	
L-Dopa	Adrenergic/sympathetic stimulant	Not given	Leyson, 1987	
Imipramine (Tofranil)	Adrenergic-uptake inhibitor	10 mg	Brindley, 1986a	Delayed effect; occurs one hour after initial erection
Guanethidine (Ismelin)	Adrenergic release/depletor	1–20 mg	Brindley, 1986a	Initial effect; later slight tumescence noted
Cigarette smoking	Nicotine stimulant	2 cigarettes prior to CC papaverine injection	Glina et al., 1988; Juenemann et al., 1987	Reduces CC rigidity acutely and chronically in dogs

of fluid. Nitroglycerin-induced erections showed a mean erection of 47% compared to the artificial erection.

The Kingston, Ontario research group of Morales, Owen, Surridge and their colleagues (Owen et al., 1987) tested nitroglycerin-2% ointment on the penis versus placebo on 30 impotent patients during erotic visual stimulation tests in which erection was measured by strain gauges. Twenty-six (85%) patients developed better erections with topical nitroglycerin ointment than with placebo ointment. In a published article on this study, Owen et al. (1989) noted equal response to topical nitroglycerin ointment in psychogenic and organic patients. Nitroglycerin erections were 36% of maximum artificial erection and 56% of maximum NPT erections. The authors noted that nitroglycerin must be applied directly to the penis.

In a later study of 140 impotent patients by the Kingston urological group (Heaton, Morales, Owen, Saunders, & Fenemore, 1990), topical glyceryl trinitrate applied to the penis produced a mean increase in penile arterial dilation of 47%. Six men requested prescriptions for self-administration of glyceryl trinitrate paste to treat impotence and reported "satisfactory results." Negelev (1990) reported that Nitroderm patches improved erection in both psychogenic and organically impotent patients. The patches were applied to the penile shaft for 24 hours and removed before intercourse. Results were best in psychogenic patients and those patients with sufficient sexual desire and at least borderline penile blood flow. Improved erection seldom occurred in diabetic patients. Successful treatment of impotence with nitroglycerin patches placed on the penis prior to intercourse has been reported in four of 10 patients (Meyhoff, Rosenkilde, & Bodker, 1992) and 21 of 26 patients (Claes & Baert, 1989).

Cavallini (1991) reported that a 2% minoxidil gel rubbed on the glans penis of impotent men during single laboratory trials produced significantly greater increases in penile circumference and rigidity than nitroglycerin ointment applied to the penile shaft. Both minoxidil and nitroglycerin produced better erections than a placebo ointment. However, the increase in penile rigidity averaged only 40% with minoxidil and 28% with nitroglycerin versus 13.6% with placebo. The failure to produce full erection by either topical minoxidil or nitroglycerin indicated that treatment with these topical substances is unlikely to produce usable erections in the majority of impotent patients. Informal discussions with other urologists who have tried to treat impotence with 2% minoxidil hair growth spray (Rogaine) have indicated that considerable tumescence frequently occurs, but sufficient rigidity for intercourse is far less likely. (Hair growth on the penis from Rogaine application is not a concern, because there are no hair follicles present for Rogaine to stimulate.)

Chancellor, Rivas, Panzer, Freedman, and Staas (1994) found some tumescence but no significant rigidity during treatment of 18 spinal-cord injured patients with a 2% minoxidil spray applied to the glans penis. In the same patients rigidity increased by 77% with papaverine injections. Similarly, Radomski, Herschorn, and Rangaswamy (1994) noted no significant erectile effect with topically applied 2% minoxidil in 20 patients.

Nitric oxide is a natural endothelium-derived-relaxant-factor (EDRF) involved in smooth muscle relaxation and subsequent production of erection (Andersson, Pascual, Persson, Forman, & Tottrup, 1992; Heaton, 1989; Rajfer, Aronson, Bush, Dorsey, and Ignarro, 1992). The conclusion that most impotence is caused by nitric oxide deficiency has been prematurely suggested in response to an article by Rajfer et al. (1992), which showed relaxation of strips of corpus cavernosum tissue taken from impotent men by nitric oxide. This study only suggested that nitric oxide is a *possible* penile vasodilatory substance released during erection. Direct proof that nitric oxide is the agent primarily responsible for erection, or that there is any difference in penile nitric oxide levels between potent and impotent men, does not yet exist.

Despite the illicit misuse of inhaled nitrous oxide (laughing gas) for sexual arousal, there is no evidence that this gas facilitates erection. In a laboratory visual erotic stimuli test, Gillman (1988) found decreased erection in five of seven male volunteer subjects. (The use of nitrous oxide, ether, and other inhalants for sexual arousal is a dangerous sexual practice and is best avoided.)

CONCLUSIONS

Vasodilators have added a fascinating new dimension to sexual pharmacology. We have known of their effects in medicine through the various antihypertensives, most of which cause peripheral vasoconstriction and associated sexual problems. With the exception of calcium channel blockers that seem to promote peripheral vasodilation, vasodilators per se had not been of any great value in the management of sexual dysfunction. It is of interest to note that phenoxybenzamine (Dibenzyline) has been used clinically from time to time by urologists in an effort to treat premature ejaculation with oral medication. It was never particularly effective, but in its role as a urinary tract antispasmodic, it reliably interfered with orgasm—to the distress of patients requiring the medication for other reasons. After a fortuitous and indeed accidental discovery, the advantages of injecting vasodilators directly into the penis became apparent.

There are several aspects of the penile injection that are not widely known. Although it sounds painful and forbidding to inject the penis, these injections occur with an exceedingly small needle near the base of the penis bilaterally. The shaft of the penis has very poor two-point discrimination and most men comment that they do not feel the insertion of the needle or the injection as long as it is infused slowly. The early vasodilators used for penile injection presented a difficulty with dose titration, resulting in serious conditions of priapism (with erections lasting 36 to 48 hours). With continued clinical use, the erections achievable with penile injections are now fairly predictable and can be monitored within a one-half hour to three-hour time-frame fairly easily. Because this approach to producing erections is relatively inexpensive (particularly compared to penile implant surgery), fairly convenient (now that patients are allowed to self-administer injections at home), and reproducible upon demand, urologists and their patients have been quick to use this technique for a broad range of problems.

One of the most important developments is the use of PIE as a diagnostic technique and as an adjunct to other diagnostic techniques requiring an erect penis. In conjunction with nocturnal penile tumescence monitoring, penile doppler studies, and laboratory evaluations of blood chemistry and hormones, injecting the penis with a vasodilator to determine the integrity of the circulatory mechanism within the penis has been of enormous value. We have also been able to better distinguish between neurological and vascular disorders affecting erection; a particular advantage exists with Peyronie's patients who formerly were limited to describing the shape and angulation of their erect penis or to taking Polaroid photographs for their physician in order to illustrate the nature and degree of defect. Today, during the diagnostic vasodilator injections, the physician can produce an erection to see for him- or herself the exact location of Peyronie's plaque, and whether the angulation is indeed secondary to Peyronie's or due to some other etiology causing penile curvature.

Penile injections are made easier by use of automated self-injection pens, which drive the injection needles in a specific length by pressing a button; or by needle-free injection guns, such as the adjustable Biojector 2000, which propels the solution inside the cavernosum by a "jet" spray powered by a CO_2, needle-free cartridge (Lemaire et al., 1990; Montorsi et al., 1993).

In spite of the benefits they have to offer, penile injections have been misused, overused, and misdirected, which is perhaps typical of new medications and discoveries. When antibiotics first became available, they were applied to just about everything until time and experience illustrated the advantages and disadvantages of their use. The potential consequences of penile injections are not benign. Men who pursue the use of penile injections as a solution to impotency are planning to use them repeatedly over the course of a lifetime. It is common sense to recognize that, if you repeatedly inject a localized area of your body, the tissue will eventually object. Diabetics carefully rotate their injections to minimize this effect. Those using penile injection do not have that degree of luxury. Scar tissue and fibrosis are inevitable to some degree and may disturb the integrity of the nerves, vessels, and tissue necessary for erection to materialize. A little known but most significant consideration is the incidence of cerebrovascular accident identified as a complication in a very small percentage of these patients.

For these and other reasons discussed in this chapter, it is taking considerable liberty to use these injections for psychological impotence or to promote enduring erections in an individual suffering from premature ejaculation. These two disorders can ordinarily be more effectively (although not as quickly) treated with appropriate sex therapy and relationship counseling. While less efficient, this approach is also considerably less toxic physiologically. I suspect that long-term studies will show that injections over the course of years inevitably sentence the patient to receiving an implant of one form or another at some point in the future. When alternative treatments are available that lack these long-term consequences, it is highly advisable to take advantage of them. Fortunately, a time is approaching when we will be able to bypass the physical trauma of injections through transdermal gels and other modern technologies.

Legitimate use of penile injection erection therapy should be differentiated from the widely advertised practice of penile "enlargement and lengthening" (enhancement phalloplasty). This cosmetic surgery is often grotesque, unreliable, and may interfere with normal erectile function. The penis is "lengthened" by cutting the suspensory and fundiform ligaments that hold it tethered at its base to the undersurface of the pubic bone. The operation releases the tethered part of the penis from the pubic bone so that it hangs at greater length "outside" the body (usually the length gain is one inch or less). Possible complications include loss of upward angle of the erect penis (leaving it pointing outward, downward, or sideways), penile pivoting, loss of stability in the erect state, external scars of the pubic skin incision, and hair on the newly exposed penis (Whitehead, 1994). The thickness or diameter of the penis is increased by injection of fat drawn from fat cells of the lower abdominal area of the patient (autobogous liposuction fat injection). Often the fat transferred to the penis is reabsorbed, so that additional fat injections are necessary within six months to a year and periodically thereafter. Reabsorption may be uneven, leaving an uneven penile contour and a bumpy surface. Additional complications that can occur are fibrosis, nodules, fat embolism, oil cyst formation, ecchymosis (bruising), edema (swelling), and infection (Whitehead, 1994). Penile erectile volume and function are not improved, because fat is not erectile tissue, but erection and penile sensation may be decreased due to the surgical changes. The cost ranges from about $4,000 to $6,000 (Gless & Overholser, 1994).

For men concerned with penis size, the mean erect penis length of 150 "potent" Caucasian males given papaverine-prostaglandin E1 penile injections was 14.5 cm (5.7 inches) with 76% ranging between 12 and 16 cm (4.7 to 6.3 inches), and the mean circumference was 11.05 to 11.92 cm (4.3 to 4.7 inches) with a range from 9 to 15 cm (3.5 to 5.9 inches) (Da Ros, Telöken, Sogari et al., 1994).

References

Abbasi, R., & Hodgen, G.D. (1986). Predicting the disposition to osteoporosis: Gonadotropin-releasing hormone antagonist for acute estrogen deficiency test. *Journal of the American Medical Association, 255,* 1600–1604.

Abber, J.C., Lue, T.F., Orvis, B.R., McClure, R.D., & Williams, R.D. (1986). Diagnostic tests for impotence: a comparison of papaverine injection with the penile-brachial index and nocturnal penile tumescence monitoring. *Journal of Urology, 135,* 923–925.

Abber, J.C., Luo, J.A., & Hinman, F. (1986). Pharmacology of drug-induced priapism. *Journal of Urology, 135,* 363A.

Abbey, A., Ross, L.T., & McDuffie, D. (1994). Alcohol's role in sexual assault. In R.R. Watson (Ed.), *Drug and alcohol abuse reviews. Vol. 5. Addictive behaviors in women* (pp. 97–124). Totowa, NJ: Humana Press.

Abbott, D.H., Holman, S.D., Berman, M., Neff, D.S., & Goy, R.W. (1984). Effects of opiate antagonists on hormones and behavior of male and female rhesus monkeys. *Archives of Sexual Behavior, 13,* 1–25.

Abel, E.L. (1981). Marijuana and sex: A critical survey. *Drug and Alcohol Dependence, 8,* 1–22.

Abel, E.L. (1984). Opiates and sex. *Journal of Psychoactive Drugs, 16,* 205–216.

Abel, E.L. (1985). *Psychoactive drugs and sex.* New York: Plenum Press.

Aboseif, S.R., Breza, J., Bosch, R.J., Benard, F., Stief, C.G., Stackl, W., Lue, T.F., & Tanagho, E.A. (1989). Local and systemic effects of chronic intracavernous injection of papaverine, prostaglandin El, and saline in primates. *Journal of Urology, 142,* 403–408.

Abozeid, M., Juenemann, K.P., Luo, J.A., Lue, T.F., Yen, T.S., & Tanagho, E.A. (1987). Chronic papaverine treatment: The effect of repeated injections on the simian erectile response and penile tissue. *Journal of Urology, 138,* 1263–1266.

Abplanalp, J., Rose, R., Donelly, A., & Livingston-Vaugh, L. (1979). Psychoendocrinology of the menstrual cycle: II. The relationship between enjoyment of activities, moods, and reproductive hormones. *Psychosomatic Medicine, 78,* 605–615.

Abraham, G.E. (1974). Ovarian and adrenal contribution to peripheral androgens during the menstrual cycle. *Journal of Clinical Endocrinology and Metabolism, 39,* 340–346.

Abraham, G.E., Manlimos, F.S., Solis, M., & Wichman, A.C. (1975). Combined radioimmunoassay of four steroids in one ml of plasma: II. Androgens. *Clinical Biochemistry, 8,* 374–378.

Abraham, G.E., & Maroulis, G.B. (1975). Effect of exogenous estrogen on serum pregnenolone, cortisol, and androgens in postmenopausal women. *Obstetrics and Gynecology, 45,* 271–274.

Abraham, S.F., Bendit, N., Mason, C., Mitchell, H., O'Connor, N., Ward, J., Young, S., & Llewellyn-Jones, D. (1985). The psychosexual histories of young women with bulimia. *Australian and New Zealand Journal of Psychiatry, 19,* 72–76.

Abrams, P. (1984). Bladder instability: Concept, clinical associations, and treatment. *Scandanavian Journal of Urology and Nephrology, Suppl. 87,* 7–12.

Adaikan, P.G. (1979). *Pharmacology of the human penis.* Master's thesis, University of Singapore.

Adaikan, P.G., & Ratnam, S.S. (1988). Pharmacological consideration of intracavernous drug injection in the treatment of impotence. *Acta Urologica Belgica, 56,* 149–153.

Adam, K., & Oswald, I. (1989). Effects of repeated ritanserin on middle-aged poor sleepers. *Psychopharmacology, 99,* 219–221.

Adam, S., Williams, V., & Vessey, M.P. (1981). Cardiovascular disease and hormone replacement treatment: A pilot case-control study. *British Medical Journal, 282,* 1277–1278.

Adams, D.B., Gold, A.R., & Burt, A.D. (1978). Rise in female-initiated sexual activity at ovulation and its suppression by oral contraceptives. *New England Journal of Medicine, 299,* 1145–1150.

Adashi, E.Y. (1991). The climacteric ovary: A viable endocrine organ. *Seminars in Reproductive Endocrinology, 9,* 200–205.

Adashi, E.Y. (1994). The climacteric ovary as a functional gonadotropin-driven androgen-producing gland. *Fertility and Sterility, 62,* 20–27.

Adler, S. (1974). Methyldopa-induced decrease in mental activity. *Journal of the American Medical Association, 230,* 1428–1429.

Aguirre, J.C., Del Arbol, J.L., Raya, J., Ruiz-Requena, M.E., & Irles, J.R. (1990). Plasma beta-endorphin levels in chronic alcoholics. *Alcohol, I,* 409–415.

Ahlenius, S., Carlsson, A., Hillegaart, V., Hjorth, S., & Larsson, K. (1987). Region-selective activation of brain monoamine synthesis by sexual activity in the male rat. *European Journal of Pharmacology, 144,* 77–82.

Ahlenius, S., Heimann, M., & Larsson, K. (1979). Prolongation of the ejaculation latency in the male rat by thioridazine and chlorimipramine. *Psychopharmacology, 65,* 137–140.

Ahlenius, S., & Larsson, K. (1984b). Lisuride, LY141865, and 8-OH-DPAT facilitate male rat sexual behavior via a non-dopaminergic mechanism. *Psychopharmacology, 83,* 330–334.

Ahlenius, S., & Larsson, K. (1984a). Failure to antagonize the 8-hydroxy-2(di-n-propylamino) tetralin-induced facilitation of male rat sexual behavior by administration of 5-HT receptor antagonists. *European Journal of Pharmacology, 99,* 279–286.

Ahlenius, S., Larsson, K., & Svensson, L. (1980). Stimulating effects of lisuride on masculine sexual behavior of rats. *European Journal of Pharmacology, 64,* 47–51.

Ahlenius, S., Larsson, K., Svensson, L., Hjorth, S., Carlsson, A., Lindberg, P. Wikstrom, H., Sanchez, D., Arvidsson, L.E., Hacksell, U., & Nilsson, J.L.G. (1981). Effects of a new type of 5-HT receptor agonist on male rat sexual behavior. *Pharmacology, Biochemistry, and Behavior, 15,* 785–792.

Ahmad, S. (1980). Disopyramide and impotence [Letter to the editor]. *Southern Medical Journal, 73,* 958.

Ahmad, S.A., Penhale, W.J., & Tatal, N. (1985). Sex hormones and autoimmune diseases: mechanisms of sex hormone action. *American Journal of Pathology, 121,* 531–559.

Aizenberg, D., Zemishlany, Z., Hermesh, H., Karp, L., & Weizman, A. (1991). Painful ejaculation associated with antidepressants in four patients. *Journal of Clinical Psychiatry, 52,* 461–463.

Aizenstein, M.L., Segal, D.S., & Kuczenski, R. (1990). Repeated amphetamine and fencamfamine: Sensitization and reciprocal cross-sensitization. *Neuropsychopharmacology, 3,* 283–290.

Albeck, D., Smock, T., Arnold, S., Raese, K., Paynter, K., & Colaprete, S. (1991). Peptidergic transmission in the brain. IV. Sex hormone dependence in the vasopressin/oxytocin system. *Peptides, 12,* 53–56.

Albert, D.J., Dyson, E.M., Walsh, M.L., & Wong, R. (1988). Defensive aggression and testosterone dependent intermale social aggression are each elicited by food competition. *Physiology and Behavior, 43,* 21–28.

Albert, D.J., Petrovic, D.M., & Walsh, M.L. (1989). Competitive experience activates testosterone-dependent social aggression toward unfamiliar males. *Physiology and Behavior, 45,* 723–727.

Albo, M., & Steers, W.D. (1993). Oral trazodone as initial therapy for management of impotence. *Journal of Urology, 149*(Suppl.), 344A.

Alderson, L.M., & Baum, M.J. (1981). Differential effects of gonadal steroids on dopamine metabolism in mesolimbic and nigrostriatal pathways of male rat brain. *Brain Research, 218,* 189–206.

Aldhous, P. (1994). A booster for contraceptive vaccines. *Science, 266,* 1484–1486.

Alexander, W.D., & Evans, J.I. (1975). Side effects of methyldopa [Letter to the editor]. *British Medical Journal, 2,* 501.

Allen, L.S., Richey, M.F., Chai, Y.M., & Gorski, R.A. (1991). Sex differences in the corpus callosum of the living human brain. *Journal of Neuroscience, 11,* 933–942.

Allen, M.H., & Frances, R.J. (1986). Varieties of psychopathology found in patients with addictive disorders: A review. In R. Meyer (Ed.), *Psychopathology and addictive disorders* (pp. 17–38). New York: Guilford Press.

Allen, R.E., Hosker, G.L., Smith, A.R., & Warrell, D.W. (1990). Pelvic floor damage and childbirth: A neurophysiological study. *British Journal of Obstetrics and Gynecology, 97,* 770–779.

Allen, R.P., & Brendler, C.B. (1988). Nocturnal penile tumescence predicting response to intracorporeal pharmacological erection testing. *Journal of Urology, 140,* 518–522.

Almeida, O.F., Nikolarakis, K.E., & Herz, A. (1987).

Significance of testosterone in regulating hypothalamic content and in vitro release of beta-endorphin and dynorphin. *Journal of Neurochemistry, 49,* 742–747.

Almeida, O.F., Nikolarakis, K.E., Sirinathsinghji, D.J., & Herz, A. (1989). Opioid-mediated inhibition of sexual behaviour and luteinizing hormone secretion by corticotropin-releasing hormone. In R.G. Dyer & R.J. Bicknell (Eds.), *Brain opioid systems in reproduction* (pp. 149–161). London: St. Edmundsbury Press.

Almeida, O.F., Nikolarakis, K.E., Sirinathsinghji, D.J., & Herz, A. (1989). Opioid-mediated inhibition of sexual behaviour and luteinizing hormone secretion by corticotropin-releasing hormone. In R.G. Dyer & R.J. Bickness (Eds.), *Brain opioid systems in reproduction* (pp. 149–161). Oxford: Oxford University Press.

Aloia, J.F. (1985). Calcitonin and osteoporosis. *Geriatric Medicine Today, 4*(No. II), 20–29.

Aloia, J.F., Vaswani, A., Ellis, K., Yuen, K., & Cohn, S.H. (1985). A model for involutional bone loss. *Journal of Laboratory and Clinical Medicine, 106,* 630–637.

Althof, S., Levine, S., Corty, E., Risen, C., & Stern, E. (1994). The role of clomipramine in the treatment of premature ejaculation. *Journal of Urology, 151*(Suppl.), 345A.

Altomonte, L., Zoli, A., Alessi, F., Ghirlanda, G., Manna, R., & Greco, A.V. (1987). Effect of fenfluramine on growth hormone and prolactin secretion in obese subjects. *Hormone Research, 27,* 190–194.

Alza Pharmaceuticals. (1994). Testoderm product monograph, Alza Pharmaceuticals, 950 Page Mill Road, P.O. Box 10950, Palo Alto, California 94303.

Aman, M.G., & Kern, R.A. (1989). Review of fenfluramine in the treatment of developmental disabilities. *Journal of the American Academy of Child and Adolescent Psychiatry, 28,* 549–565.

Ambrosi, B., Bara, R., & Faglia, G. (1977). Bromocriptine in impotence. *Lancet, 2,* 987.

Ambrosi, B., Bara, R., Travaglini, P., Weber, G., Beck Peccoz, P., Rondena, M., Elli, R., & Faglia, G. (1977). Study of the effects of bromocriptine on sexual impotence. *Clinical Endocrinology, 7,* 417–421.

American Medical Association drug evaluations annual 1991. Chicago: Author.

American Medical News. (1991, March 4). Top 20 prescription drugs dispensed in United States pharmacies (data summary table).

American Psychiatric Association. (1987). *Diagnostic and statistical manual of mental disorders—revised* (3rd ed.). Washington, DC: Author.

Amsterdam, J.D., Dunner, D.L., Fabre, L.F., Kiev, A., Rush, A.J., & Goodman, L.I. (1989). Double-blind placebo-controlled, fixed dose trial of minaprine in patients with major depression. *Pharmacopsychiatry, 22,* 137–143.

Anand, P., Gibson, S.J., Yiangou, Y., Christofides, N.D., Polak, J.M., & Bloom, S.R. (1984). PHI-like immunoreactivity co-locates with the VIP-containing system in human lumbosacral spinal cord. *Neuroscience Letters, 46,* 191–196.

Anand, S., & Van Thiel, D.H. (1982). Prenatal and neonatal exposure to cimetidine results in gonadal and sexual dysfunction in adult males. *Science, 218,* 493–494.

Anand, V.S. (1985). Clomipramine-induced galactorrhea and amenorrhea. *British Journal of Psychiatry, 147,* 87.

Anda, R.F., Williamson, D.F., Escobedo, L.G., Mast, E.E., Giovino, G.A., & Remington, P.L. (1990). Depression and the dynamics of smoking. *Journal of the American Medical Association, 264,* 1541–1545.

Anderson, I.M., Parry-Billings, M., Newsholme, E.A., Fairburn, C.G., & Cowen, P.J. (1990). Dieting reduces plasma tryptophan and alters brain 5-HT function in women. *Psychological Medicine, 20,* 785–791.

Anderson, R.A., Bancroft, J., & Wu, F.C.W. (1992). The effects of exogenous testosterone on sexuality and mood of normal men. *Journal of Clinical Endocrinology and Metabolism, 75,* 1503–1507.

Anderson, W.R., Simpkins, J.W., Brewster, M.E., & Bodor, N. (1987). Evidence for the reestablishment of copulatory behavior in castrated male rats with a brain-enhanced estradiol-chemical delivery system. *Pharmacology and Biochemistry, 27,* 265–271.

Anderson, W.R., Simpkins, J.W., Brewster, M.E., & Bodor, N. (1988). Effects of a brain-enhanced chemical delivery system for estradiol on body weight and serum hormones in middle-aged male rats. *Endocrine Research, 14,* 131–148.

Andersson, B., Zimmermann, M.E., Hedner, T., & Bjorntorp, P. (1991). Haemodynamic, metabolic, and endocrine effects of short-term dexfenfluramine treatment in young, obese women. *European Journal of Clinical Pharmacology, 40,* 249–254.

Andersson, K.E. (1988). Calcium antagonists and dysmenorrhea. In P.M. Vanhoutte, R. Raoletti, & S. Govoni (Eds.), *Calcium antagonists. Vol. 522. Annals of the New York Academy of Sciences* (pp. 747–755). New York: New York Academy of Sciences.

Andersson, K.E., Pascual, A.G., Persson, K., Forman, A., & Tottrup, A. (1992). Electrically-induced, nerve-mediated relaxation of rabbit urethra involves nitric oxide. *Journal of Urology, 147,* 253–259.

Ando, S., Rubens, R., & Rottiers, R. (1984). Androgen plasma levels in male diabetics. *Journal of Endocrinological Investigation, 7,* 21–24.

Ando, S., Rubens, R., & Rottiers, R. (1985). Endocrine testicular function in male diabetics. *Journal of Endocrinological Investigation, 8*(Suppl. 2), 103–109.

Andreyko, J.L., Marshall, L.A., Dumesic, D.A., & Jaffe, R.B. (1987). Therapeutic uses of gonadotropin-releasing hormone analogs. *Obstetrical and Gynecological Survey, 42,* 1–21.

Angrist, B. (1987). Clinical effects of central nervous system stimulants: A selective update. In J. Engel & L. Oreland (Eds.), *Brain reward systems and abuse* (pp. 109–127). New York: Raven Press.

Anokhina, I.P., Panchenko, L.F., Kogan, B.M., & Brusen, O.S. (1985). Catecholamine and opiate receptor systems in alcoholism. In H. Parvez (Ed.), *Progress in alcohol research. Vol. 1* (pp. 127–145). New York: VNU Science Press.

Ansari, J.M. (1976). Impotence: Prognosis (a controlled study). *British Journal of Psychiatry, 128,* 194–198.

Ansseau, M., Legros, J.J., Mormount, C., Cerfontaine, J.L., Gapart, P., Geenen, V., Adam, F., & Frank, G. (1988). Intranasal oxytocin in obsessive-compulsive disorder. *Parmaco-psychiatry, 21,* 57.

Antonicelli, R., Piani, M., & Paciaroni, E. (1989). Evaluation of the effectiveness and tolerability of captopril in the treatment of essential arterial hypertension in nine subjects with sexual impotence secondary to the use of beta-blockers. *Current Therapeutic Research, 46,* 837–841.

Antoniou, L.D., Shalhoub, R.J., Sudhaka, T., & Smith, J.C., Jr. (1977). Reversal of uralmic impotence by zinc. *Lancet, 2* (8042), 895–898.

Apgar, J. (1985). Zinc and reproduction. *Annual Review of Nutrition, 5,* 43–68.

Applegate, W.B., Borhani, N., DeQuattro, V., Kaihlanen, P.M., Oishi, S., Due, D.L., & Sirgo, M.A. (1991). Comparison of labetalol versus enalapril as monotherapy in elderly patients with hypertension: Results of a 24-hour ambulatory blood pressure monitoring. *American Journal of Medicine, 90,* 198–205.

Apter-Marsh, M. (1984). The sexual behavior of alcoholic women while drinking and during sobriety. In D.J. Powell (Ed.), *Alcoholism and sexual dysfunction: Issues in clinical management* (pp. 35–48). New York: Haworth Press.

Araki, H., Nojiri, M., Kimura, M., & Aihara, H. (1987). Effect of minaprine on "delayed neuronal death" in Mongolian gerbils with occluded common carotid arteries. *Journal of Pharmacology and Experimental Therapeutics, 242,* 686–691.

Aravena, E.P., & Bustamente, E.V. (1986). Treatment of psychogenic erectile impotence with intracavernous injection of papaverine (Abstract 11.20) *ISIR Proceedings 2d World Meeting on Impotence, Prague.*

Argiolas, A. (1989). Central dopamine-oxytocin link in the control of sexual behavior in male rats [Abstract]. *Abstracts of the 12th annual meeting of the European Neuroscience Association, 12,* 87.5.

Argiolas, A. (1992). Oxytocin stimulation of penile erection: Parmacology, site, and mechanism of action. In C.A. Pedersen, J.D. Caldwell, G.F. Jirikowskii, & T.R. Insel (Eds.), *Oxytocin in maternal, sexual, and social behaviors. Vol. 652. Annals of the New York Academy of Sciences,* 194–203.

Argiolas, A., Collu, M., Gessa, G.L., Melis, M.R., & Serra, G. (1988). The oxytocin antagonist $d(CH_2)_5$Tyr(Me)-Orn[8]vasotocin inhibits male copulatory behavior in rats. *European Journal of Pharmacology, 149,* 389–392.

Argiolas, A., & Gessa, G.L. (1987). Oxytocin: A powerful stimulant of penile erection and yawning in male rats. In D. Nerozzi, F.K. Goodwin, & E. Costa (Eds.), *Hypothalamic dysfunction in neuropsychiatric disorders* (pp. 153–163). New York: Raven Press.

Argiolas, A., & Melis, M.R. (1989). Oxytocin-induced penile erection and yawning: Role of calcium and prostaglandins. *Society for Neuroscience: 19th Meeting, 15*(1), 217.

Argiolas, A., Melis, M.R., & Gessa, G.L. (1985). Intraventricular oxytocin induces yawning and penile erection in rats. *European Journal of Pharmacology, 117,* 395–396.

Argiolas, A., Melis, M.R., & Gessa, G.L. (1988). Yawning and penile erection: Central dopamine-oxytocin-adrenocorticotropin connection. In D.L. Colbern & W.H. Gispen (Eds.), *Neural mechanisms and biological significance of grooming behavior Vol. 525. Annals of New York Academy of Sciences* (pp. 330–338). New York: New York Academy of Sciences.

Argiolas, A., Melis, M.R., Mauri, A., & Gessa, G.L. (1987). Paraventricular nucleus lesion prevents yawning and penile erection induced by apomorphine and oxytocin but not by ACTH in rats. *Brain Research, 421,* 349–352.

Argiolas, A., Melis, M.R., Stancampiano, R., & Gessa, G.L. (1989). Penile erection and yawning induced by oxytocin and related peptides: Structure-activity relationship. *Peptides, 10,* 559–563.

Argiolas, A., Melis, M.R., Stancampiano, R., & Gessa, G.L. (1990). W-Conotoxin prevents apomorphine- and oxytocin-induced penile erection and yawning in male rats. *Pharmacology, Biochemistry, and Behavior, 37,* 253–257.

Argiolas, A., Melis, M.R., Vargiu, L., & Gessa, G.L. (1987). $D(CH_2)_5$Tyr(Me)-[Orn[8]] Vasotocin, a potent oxytocin antagonist, antagonizes penile erection and yawning induced by oxytocin and apomorphine, but not by ACTH-(1-24). *European Journal of Pharmacology, 134,* 221-224.

Arletti, R., Bazzani, C., Castelli, M., & Bertolini, A. (1985). Oxytocin improves male copulatory performance in rats. *Hormones and Behavior, 19,* 14-20.

Arletti, R., Benelli, A., & Bertolini, A. (1990a). Sexual behavior of aging male rats is stimulated by oxytocin. *European Journal of Pharmacology, 179,* 377-381.

Arletti, R., Benelli, A., Luppi, P., Caroni, C., & Bertolini, A. (1990b). Testosterone modulation of the efffect of oxytocin on male sexual behavior. *Neuroscience, 39*(Suppl.).

Arnott, S., & Nutt, D. (1994). Successful treatment of fluvoxamine-induced anorgasmia by cyproheptadine. *British Journal of Psychiatry, 164,* 838-839.

Aronoff, G.M. (1984). Trazodone associated with priapism. *Lancet, 2,* 856.

Aronow, W.S. (1991). Digoxin or angiotensin converting enzyme inhibitors for congestive heart failure in geriatric patients. *Drugs and Aging, 1*(2), 98-103.

Askinazi, C., Weintraub, R.J., & Karamouz, N. (1986). Elderly depressed females as a possible subgroup of patients responsive to methylphenidate. *Journal of Clinical Psychiatry, 47,* 467-469.

Assalian, P. (1988). Clomipramine in the treatment of premature ejaculation. *Journal of Sex Research, 24,* 213-215.

Assenmacher, I., Szafarczyk, A., Alonso, G., Ixart, G., & Barbanel, G. (1987). *Physiology of the neural pathways affecting CRH secretion. Vol. 512. Annals of the New York Academy of Sciences* (pp. 149-161). New York: New York Academy of Sciences.

Athanasiou, R., Shaver, P., & Tavris, C. (1970). Sex. *Psychology Today, 4,* 37-44.

Auerbach K.G., & Schreiber, J.R. (1987). Beer and the breast-feeding mother. *Journal of the American Medical Association, 258,* 2126.

Austin, M.C., & Kalivas, P.W. (1991). Dopaminergic involvement in locomotion elicited from the ventral pallidum/substantia innominata. *Brain Research, 542,* 123-131.

Averette, H.E., Boike, G.M., & Jarrell, M.A. (1990). Effects of cancer chemotherapy on gonadal function and reproductive capacity. *CA-A Cancer Journal for Clinicians, 40,* 199-209.

Avorn, J., Everitt, D.E., & Weiss, S. (1986). Increased antidepressant use in patients prescribed beta-blockers. *Journal of the American Medical Association, 3,* 357-360.

Axon, A.T. (1994). The role of omeprazole and antibiotic combinations in the eradication of *Helicobacter pylori*—An update. *Scandinavian Journal of Gastroenterology, 29*(Suppl. 205), 31-37.

Ayd, F.J., Jr. (1985). Psychostimulant therapy for depressed medically ill patients. *Psychiatric Annals, 15,* 462-465.

Azadzoi, K.M., Payton, T., Krane, R.J., & Goldstein, I. (1990). Effects of intracavernosal trazodone hydrochloride: Animal and human studies. *Journal of Urology, 144,* 1277-1282.

Bachmann, G.A., Leiblum, S.R., Sandler, B., Ainsley, W., Narcessian, R., Shelden, R., & Hymans, H.N. (1985). Correlates of sexual desire in postmenopausal women. *Maturitas, 7,* 211-216.

Backstrom, T., Bixo, M., & Hammarback, S. (1985). Ovarian steroid hormones: Effects on mood, behavior, and brain excitability. *Acta Obstetrica et Gynecologica Scandinavica, 130* (Suppl.), 19-24.

Bagatell, C.J., Heiman, J.R., Rivier, J.E., & Bremmer, W.J. (1994). Effects of endogenous testosterone and estradiol on sexual behavior in normal young men. *Journal of Clinical Endocrinology and Metabolism, 78,* 711-716.

Bahren, W., Scherb, W., Gall, H., Becker, R., & Holzki, G. (1989). Effects of intracavernosal pharmacotherapy on self-esteem, performance anxiety, and partnership in patients with chronic erectile dysfunction. *European Urology, 16,* 175-180.

Bailey, P.E., & McKenna, P.J. (1990). Pharmacological approaches to the treatment of schizophrenia: The concept of "atypicality." *Triangle, 29,* 133-139.

Baker, E.R., Mathur, R.S., Kirk, R.F., Landgrebe, S.C., Moody, L.O., & Williamson, H.O. (1982). Plasma gonadotropins, prolactin, and steroid hormone concentrations in female runners immediately after a long-distance run. *Fertility and Sterility, 38,* 38-41.

Baker, R.W., Chengappa, K.N.R., Baird, J.W., Steingard, S., Christ, M.A.G., & Schooler, N.R. (1992). Emergence of obsessive-compulsive symptoms during treatment with clozapine. *Journal of Clinical Psychiatry, 53,* 439-442.

Balestrieri, M., Bragagnoli, N., & Bellantuong, C. (1991). Antidepressant drug prescribing in general practice: A 6-year study. *Journal of Affective Disorders, 21,* 45-55.

Ballenger, J.C. (1988). The clinical use of carbamazepine in affective disorders. *Journal of Clinical Psychiatry, 49*(Suppl. 4), 13-19.

Ballinger, C.B. (1975). Psychiatric morbidity and the menopause: Screening of the general population sample. *British Medical Journal, 3,* 344-346.

Ballinger, C.B. (1976). Psychiatric morbidity and

the menopause: Clinical features. *British Medical Journal, 15,* 1183–1185.

Ballinger, C.B., Browning, M.C., & Smith, A.H. (1987). Hormone profiles and psychological symptoms in peri-menopausal women. *Maturitas, 9,* 235–251.

Balogh, S., Hendricks, S.E., & Kang, J. (1992). Treatment of fluoxetine-induced anorgasmia with amantadine [Letter to the editor]. *Journal of Clinical Psychiatry, 53,* 212–213.

Balon, R., Yeragani, V.K., Pohl, R., & Ramesh, C. (1993). Sexual dysfunction during antidepressant treatment. *Journal of Clinical Psychiatry, 54,* 209–212.

Bancroft, J.H., Davidson, D.W., Warner, P., & Tyrer, G. (1980). Androgens and sexual behaviour in women using oral contraceptives. *Clinical Endocrinology, 12,* 327–340.

Bancroft, J.H., Dickerson, M., Fairburn, C.G., Gray, J., Greenwood, J., Stevenson, N., & Warner, P. (1986). Sex therapy outcome research: A reappraisal of methodology. I. A treatment study of male sexual dysfunction. *Psychological Medicine, 16,* 851–863.

Bancroft, J.H., O'Carroll, R., McNeilly, A., & Shaw, R.W. (1984). The effects of bromocriptine on the sexual behavior of hyperprolactinemic men: A controlled case study. *Clinical Endocrinology, 21,* 131–137.

Bancroft, J.H., Sanders, D., Davidson, D., & Warner, P. (1983). Mood, sexuality, hormones, and the menstrual cycle: III. Sexuality and the role of androgens. *Psychosomatic Medicine, 45,* 509–516.

Bancroft, J.H., & Sartorius, N. (1990). The effects of oral contraceptives on well-being and sexuality: A review. *Oxford Reviews in Reproductive Biology, 12,* 57–92.

Bancroft, J.H., Sherwin, B.B., Alexander, G.M., Davidson, D.W., & Walker, A. (1991). Oral contraceptives, androgens, and the sexuality of young women: II. The role of androgens. *Archives of Sexual Behavior, 20,* 121–135.

Bancroft, J.H., Tennent, T.G., Loucas, K., & Cass, J. (1974). Control of deviant sexual behavior by drugs: Behavioral effects of estrogens and antiandrogens. *British Journal of Psychiatry, 125,* 310–315.

Bancroft, J.H., & Wu, F.C. (1983). Changes in erectile responsiveness during androgen replacement therapy. *Archives of Sexual Behavior, 12,* 59–66.

Bannister, P., Handley, T., Chapman, C., & Losowsky, M.S. (1986). LH pulsatility following acute ethanol ingestion in men. *Clinical Endocrinology, 25,* 143–150.

Bansal, S. (1988). Sexual dysfunction in hypertensive men: A critical review of the literature. *Hypertension, 12,* 1–10.

Baraldi, M., Giberti, A., Caselgrandi, E., & Petraglia, F. (1986). Effects of zinc on ACTH secretion. In G. Biggio, P.F. Spano, G. Toffano, & G.L. Gessa (Eds.), *Modulation of central and peripheral transmitter function* (pp. 533–536). Pavoda: Liviana Press.

Barbeau, A. (1969). L-dopa therapy in Parkinson's disease: A critical review of nine years experience. *Journal of the Canadian Medical Association, 101,* 791–800.

Barber, S.G. (1979). Male sexual dysfunction and cimetidine. *British Medical Journal, 1,* 147.

Barber, S.G., & Hoare, A.M. (1979). Cimetidine effects on prolactin release and production. *Hormone and Metabolism Research, 11,* 220–221.

Barden, B., Merand, Y., Rouloux, D., Garon, M., & Dupont, A. (1981). Changes in beta-endorphin content of discrete hypothalamic nuclei during the estrous cycle of the rat. *Brain Research, 204,* 441–445.

Bardrum, B., Ottesen, B., Fahrenkrug, J., & Fuchs, A.R. (1988). Release of oxytocin and vasopressin by intracerebroventricular vasoactive intestinal polypeptide. *Endocrinology, 123,* 2249–2254.

Bardrum, B., Ottesen, B., & Fuchs, A.R. (1987). Preferential release of oxytocin in response to vasoactive intestinal polypeptide in rats. *Life Science, 40,* 169–173.

Barlow, D.H., Abdalla, H.I., Roberts, A.D., Al Azzawi, F., Leggate, I., & Hart, D.M. (1986). Long-term hormone implant therapy—hormonal and clinical effects. *Obstetrics and Gynecology, 67,* 321–325.

Barlow, D.H., Grosset, K.A., Hart, H., & Hart, D.M. (1989). A study of the experience of Glasgow women in the climacteric years. *British Journal of Obstetrics and Gynecology, 96,* 1192–1197.

Barlow, D.H., Sakeheim, D.K., & Beck, J.G. (1983). Anxiety increases sexual arousal. *Journal of Abnormal Psychology, 92,* 49–54.

Barnes, D.M., (1989). Neurotoxicity creates regulatory dilemma. *Science, 243,* 29–30.

Baron, J.A., Bulbrook, R.D., Wang, D.Y., & Kwa, H.G. (1986). Cigarette smoking and prolactin in women. *British Medical Journal, 293,* 482–483.

Barrett-Connor, E. (1986). Postmenopausal estrogen-current prescribing patterns of San Diego gynecologists. *Western Journal of Medicine, 144,* 620–621.

Barrett-Connor, E. (1988). Smoking and endogenous sex hormones in men and women. In N. Wald & J. Baron (Eds.), *Smoking and hormone-related disorders* (pp. 183–196). New York: Oxford University Press.

Barrett-Connor, E. (1989). Postmenopausal estrogen

replacement and breast cancer. *New England Journal of Medicine, 321,* 319–320.

Barrett-Connor, E., & Bush, T.L. (1991). Estrogen and coronary heart disease in women. *Journal of the American Medical Association, 265,* 1861–1867.

Barrett-Connor, E., & Khaw, K.T. (1987). Cigarette smoking and increased endogenous estrogen levels in men. *American Journal of Epidemiology, 126,* 187.

Barrett-Connor, E., Khaw, K.T., & Yen, S.C. (1986). A prospective study of dehydroepiandrosterone sulfate, mortality, and cardiovascular disease. *New England Journal of Medicine, 315,* 1519–1524.

Barrett-Connor, E., & Kritz-Silverstein, D. (1993). Estrogen replacement therapy and cognitive function in older women. *Journal of the American Medical Association, 269,* 2637–2641.

Bartels, D., Glasser, M., Wang, A., & Swanson, P. (1988). Association between depression and propranolol use in ambulatory patients. *Clinical Pharmacy, 7,* 146–150.

Bartke, A., Suare, B.B., Doherty, M.S., Smith, M.S., & Klemke, H.G. (1983). Effects of hyperprolactinemia on male reproductive functions. In A. Negro-Vilar (Ed.), *Reproduction and Andrology* (pp. 1–11). New York: Raven Press.

Barton, J. (1979). Orgasmic inhibition by phenelzine. *American Journal of Psychiatry, 136,* 1616–1617.

Bartova, D., Hajnova, R., Nahunek, K., & Svestka, J. (1981). Oxyprothepin decanoate in the treatment of deviant sexual behavior. *Activitas Nervosa Superior (Praha), 23,* 248.

Bartsch, W., Greeve, J., & Voigt, K.D. (1987). 17 beta-hydroxysteroid dehydrogenase in the human prostate: Properties and distribution between epithelium and stoma in benign hyperplastic tissue. *Journal of Steroid Biochemistry, 28,* 35–42.

Barwin, B.N. (1982). Mesterolone: A new androgen for the treatment of male infertility. In J. Bain, W.B. Schill, & L. Schwarzstein (Eds.), *Treatment of male infertility* (pp. 117–123). New York: Springer-Verlag.

Bassi, F., Pupi, A., Giannotti, P., Fiorelli, G., Forti, G., Pinchera, A., & Serio, M. (1980). Plasma dehydroepiandrosterone sulfate in hypothyroid premenopausal women. *Clinical Endocrinology (Oxford), 13,* 111–113.

Batra, S., Bjellin, L., Sjogen, C., Iosif, S., & Widmark, E. (1986). Increases in blood flow of the female rabbit urethra following low dose estrogens. *Journal of Urology, 136,* 1360–1362.

Bauer, G.E., Baker, J., Hunyor, S.N., & Marshall, P. (1978). Side effects of antihypertensive treatment: A placebo-controlled study. *Clinical Science and Molecular Medicine, 55,* 341s-344s.

Bauer, G.E., Hull, R.D., Stokes, G.S., & Raftos, J. (1973). The reversability of side effects of guanethidine therapy. *Medical Journal of Australia, 1,* 930–933.

Bauer, K.M. (1956). The hypotonic bladder: Simultaneously a contribution to cysto-sphincterometry. *Die Medizinische, 21,* 792–795.

Baulieu, E.E. (1994). RU 486: A compound that gets itself talked about. *Human Reproduction, 9* (Suppl. 1), 1–6.

Baulieu, E.E., Corpechot, C., Synguelakis, M., Groyer, A., Clarke, C., Schlegel, M.L., Brazeau, P., & Robel, P. (1984). 3 beta-hydroxysteroids in rat brain. In L. Martini, G.S. Gordan, & F. Sciarra (Eds.), *Steroid modulation of neuroendocrine function: Sterols, steroids, and bone metabolism* (pp. 89–99). New York: Elsevier Science Publishers.

Baulieu, E.E., Robel, P., Vatier, O., Haug, M., Le Goascogne, C., & Bourreau, E. (1987). Neurosteroids: Pregnenalone and dehydroepiandrosterone in the brain. In K. Fuxe & L.F. Agnati (Eds.), *Receptor-receptor interactions* (pp. 89–104). Basingstoke: MacMillan Press.

Bauman, J.E. (1980). Marijuana and the female reproductive system. Testimony before the subcommittee on criminal justice of the Committee on the Judiciary, United States Senate. In *Health consequences of marijuana use.* Washington DC: United States Government Printing Office.

Baumel, B., Eisner, L.S., Karukin, M., MacNamara, R., & Raphan, H. (1989). Nimodipine in the treatment of Alzheimer's disease. In M. Bergener & B. Reisberg (Eds.), *Diagnosis and treatment of senile dementia* (pp. 366–373). Berlin: Springer-Verlag.

Baumgarten, H.G., & Schlossberger, H.G. (1984). Anatomy and function of central serotonergic neurons. In H.L. Schlossberger (Ed.), *Progress in tryptophan and serotonin research* (pp. 173–188). New York: Walter de Gruyter & Co.

Bayliss, W.M., & Starling, E.H. (1904). The chemical regulation of the secretory process. Proceedings of the Royal Society of London, XXIII, 310–322.

Beach, F.A. (1976). Sexual attractivity, proceptivity, and receptivity in female mammals. *Hormones and Behavior, 7,* 105–138.

Beard, G.M., & Rockwell, A.D. (1906). *Sexual neurasthenia: Its hygiene, causes, symptoms, and treatment.* New York: E.B. Treat.

Beardsley, P.M., & Balster, R.L. (1987). Self-administration of minaprine in rhesus monkeys. *Drug and Alcohol Dependence, 19,* 121–129.

Beardwell, C., Hindley, A., Wilkinson, P., John, J., & Bu'Lock, D. (1985). Hormonal changes in postmenopausal women with breast cancer treated with trilostane and dexamethasone. *Clinical Endocrinology (Oxford), 23,* 413–421.

Beardwell, C., Hindley, A., Wilkinson, P., Todd, I.,

Ribeiro, G., & Bu'Lock, D. (1983). Trilostane in the treatment of advanced breast cancer. *Cancer Chemotherapy and Pharmacology, 10,* 158–160.

Beart, P.M., McDonald, D., Cincotta, M., de Vries, D., & Gundlach, A.L. (1986). Selectivity of some ergot derivatives for 5-HT_1 and 5-HT_2 receptors of rat cerebral cortex. *General Pharmacology, 17,* 57–62.

Beary, M.D., Lacey, J.H., & Merry, J. (1986). Alcoholism and eating disorders in women of fertile age. *British Journal of Addiction, 81,* 685–689.

Beatty, W.W. (1973). Effects of gonadectomy on sex differences in DRL behavior. *Physiology and Behavior, 10,* 177–178.

Beaumont, G. (1973). Sexual side effects of clomipramine (Anafranil). *Journal of Internal Medicine and Research, 1,* 469–472.

Beaumont, G. (1977). Sexual side effects of clomipramine (Anafranil). *Journal of International Medical Research, 5,* 37–44.

Beaumont, G. (1979). Side effects of toxicity of clomipramine *British Journal of Clinical Practice, (Suppl. 3),* 51–53.

Becker, G.J., & Hicks. M.E. (1986). Side effects of transdermal nitrate [Letter to the editor]. *Annals of Internal Medicine, 104,* 590.

Becker, R.E., & Dufresne, R.L. (1982). Perceptual changes with bupropion, a novel antidepressant. *American Journal of Psychiatry, 139,* 1200–1201.

Becker, U., Almdal, T., Christensen, E., Gluud, C., Farholt, S., Bennett, P., Svenstrup, B., & Hardt, F. (1991a). Sex hormones in postmenopausal women with primary biliary cirrhosis. *Journal of Hepatology, 13,* 865–869.

Becker, U., Gluud, C., Bennett, P., Micic, S., Svenstrup, B., Winkler, K., Christensen, N.J., & Hardt, F. (1988). Effect of alcohol and glucose infusion on pituitary-gonadal hormones in normal females. *Drug and Alcohol Dependence, 22,* 141–149.

Becker, U., Gluud, C., Farholt, S., Bennett, P., Micic, S., Svenstrup, B., & Hardt, F. (1991). Menopausal age and sex hormones in postmenopausal women with alcoholic and non-alcoholic liver disease. *Journal of Hepatology, 13,* 25–32.

Becker, U., Tonnesen, H., Kaas-Claesson, & Gluud, C. (1989). Menstrual disturbances and fertility in chronic alcoholic women. *Drug and Alcohol Dependence, 24,* 75–82.

Beckman, L.J. (1979). Reported effects of alcohol on the sexual feelings and behavior of women alcoholics and non-alcoholics. *Journal of Studies on Alcohol, 40,* 272–282.

Beckwith, B.E., Petros, T.V., Couk, D.I., & Tinius, T.P. (1990). The effects of vasopressin on memory in healthy young adult volunteers: Theoretical and methodological issues. In G.F. Koob, C.A. Sandman, & F.L. Strand (Eds.), A decade of neuropeptides: Past, present and future. Vol. 579. Annals of the New York Academy of Sciences, 215–226.

Becu, D., & Libertum, C. (1983). Serotonergic involvement in the cimetidine-induced prolactin release. *Endocrinology, 113,* 1980–1984.

Beer, N.A., Jakubowicz, D.J., Beer, R.M., Arocha, I.R., & Nestler, J.E. (1993). Effects of nitrendipine on glucose tolerance and serum insulin and dehydroepiandrosterone sulfate levels in insulin-resistant obese and hypertensive men. *Journal of Clinical Endocrinology and Metabolism, 76,* 178–183.

Beer, N.A., Jakubowicz, D.J., Beer, R.M., & Nestler, J.E. (1993). The calcium channel-blocker amlodipine raises serum dehydroepiandrosterone sulfate and androstenedione, but lowers serum cortisol, in insulin-resistant obese and hypertensive men. *Journal of Clinical Endocrinology and Metabolism, 76,* 1464–1469.

Beer, N.A., Jakubowicz, D.J., Beer, R.M., & Nestler, J.E. (1994). Disparate effects of insulin reduction with diltiazem on serum dehydroepiandrosterone sulfate levels in obese hypertensive men and women. *Journal of Clinical Endocrinology and Metabolism, 79,* 1077–1081.

Beevers, D.G., Blackwood, R.A., Garnham, S., Watson, M., Mehrzad, A.A., Admani, K., Angell-James, J.E., Feely, M., Kumar, S., Husaini, M.H., Mannering, D., Connett, C., & Long, C. (1991). Comparison of lisinopril versus atenolol for mild to moderate essential hypertension. *American Journal of Cardiology, 67,* 59–62.

Beghi, E., & Collaborative Group for Epidemiology of Epilepsy (1986). Adverse reactions to antiepileptic drugs: A multicenter survey of clinical practice. *Epilepsia, 27,* 323–330.

Beisland, H.O., Fossberg, E., Moer, A., & Sanders, S. (1984). Urethral sphincteric insufficiency in postmenopausal women. Treatment with phenylpropanolamine and estriol separately and in combination. A urodynamic and clinical evaluation. *Urologia Internationalis, 39,* 211–216.

Belanger, A., Candas, B., Dupont, A., Cusan, L., Diamond, P., Gomez, J.L., & Labrie, F. (1994). Changes in serum concentrations of conjugated and unconjugated steroids in 40- to 80-year-old men. *Journal of Clinical Endocrinology and Metabolism, 79,* 1086–1090.

Belanger, A., Labrie, F., Dupont, A., Brochu, M., & Cusan, L. (1988). Endocrine effects of combined treatment with an LHRH agonist in association with flutamide in metastatic prostatic carcinoma. *Clinical and Investigative Medicine, 11,* 321–326.

Belfer, M.L., Shader, R.I., Carroll, M., & Harmetz, J.S. (1971). Alcoholism in women. *Archives of General Psychiatry, 25,* 540–544.

Belisle, S., Patry, M., & Tetreault, L. (1982). Cimetidine and plasma levels of gonadotropins, prolactin, and gonadal steroids in women. *Canadian Medical Association Journal, 127,* 29-32.

Benard, F., Diederichs, W., Stief, C., Bosch, R.J., Aboseif, S.R., Lue, T.F., & Tanagho, E.A. (1989). The effect of epinephrine on erection. *Journal of Urology, 14,* 439A.

Benedek, T., & Rubinstein, B.B. (1939a). The correlations between ovarian activity and psychodynamic processes: The ovulative phase. *Psychosomatic Medicine, 1,* 245-270.

Benedek, T., & Rubenstein, B.B. (1939b). The correlations between ovarian activity and psychodynamic processes: II. The menstrual phase. *Psychosomatic Medicine,* 461-485.

Benelli, A., Zanoli, P., & Bertolini, A. (1990). Effect of clenbuterol on sexual behavior in male rats. *Physiology and Behavior, 47,* 373-376.

Benkert, O. (1972). L-dopa treatment of impotence: A clinical and experimental study. In S. Malitz (Ed.), *L-dopa and behavior* (pp. 73-85). New York: Raven Press.

Benkert, O. (1973). Pharmacological experiments to stimulate human sexual behavior. In T.A. Ban (Ed.), *Psychopharmacology, sexual disorders, and drug abuse* (pp. 489-495). London: North-Holland Publishing.

Benkert, O. (1975). Clinical studies of the effects of neurohormones on sexual behavior. In M. Sandler & G.L. Gessa (Eds.), *Social behavior: Pharmacology and biochemistry* (pp. 297-305). New York: Raven Press.

Benkert, O., Crombach, G., & Kockott, G. (1972). Effect of L-dopa on sexually impotent patients. *Psychopharmacologia, 23,* 91-95.

Benkert, O., Jordan, H.G., Dahlen, H.G., Schneider, H.P.G., & Gammel, G. (1975). Sexual impotence: A double-blind study of LHRH nasal spray versus placebo. *Neuropsychobiology, 1,* 203-210.

Benkert, O., Witt, W., Adam, W., & Leitz, A. (1979). Effects of testosterone undecanoate on sexual potency and the hypothalamic-pituitary-gonadal axis of impotent males. *Archives of Sexual Behavior, 8,* 471-479.

Bennett, A.H. (1991). Cost benefit of pharmacologic erection program. *Urology, 37,* 395.

Benwell, M.E., Balfour, D.J., & Anderson, J.M. (1990). Smoking-associated changes in serotonergic systems of discrete regions of human brain. *Psychopharmacology, 102,* 68-72.

Berendsen, H.H.G., & Broekkamp, C.L.E. (1987). Drug-induced penile erections in rats: Indications of serotonin receptor mediation. *European Journal of Pharmacology, 135,* 279-287.

Bergen, D., Daugherty, S., & Eckenfels, E. (1992). Reduction of sexual activities in females taking antiepileptic drugs. *Psychopathology, 25,* 1-4.

Bergkvist, L., Adami, H.O., Persson, I., Hoover, R., & Schairer, C. (1989). The risk of breast cancer after estrogen and estrogen-progestin replacement. *New England Journal of Medicine, 321,* 392-397.

Berken, G.H., Weinstein, D.O., & Stern, W.C. (1984). Weight gain: A side-effect of tricyclic antidepressants. *Journal of Affective Disorders, 7,* 133-138.

Berlin, F.S. (1981). Ethical use of antiandrogenic medications [Letter to the editor]. *American Journal of Psychiatry, 138,* 1515-1516.

Berlin, F.S., & Meinecke, C.F. (1981). Treatment of sex offenders with antiandrogenic medication: Conceptualization, review of treatment modalities, and preliminary findings. *American Journal of Psychiatry, 138,* 601-607.

Berlin, F.S., & Shaerf, F.W. (1985). Laboratory assessment of the paraphilias and their treatment with antiandrogenic medication. In R.C. Hall & T.P. Beresford (Eds.), *Handbook of psychiatric diagnostic procedures, Vol. 2* (pp. 273-305). New York: Spectrum.

Bernardi, M., Vergoni, A.V., Sandrini, M., Tagliavini, S., & Bertolini, A. (1989). Influence of ovarectomy, estradiol, and progesterone on the behavior of mice in an experimental model of depression. *Physiology and Behavior, 45,* 1067-1068.

Berry, M.D., Juorio, A.V., & Paterson, I.A. (1994). Possible mechanisms of action of (-) deprenyl and other MAO-B inhibitors in some neurologic and psychiatric disorders. Progress in Neurobiology, 44, 141-161.

Berta, L., Dusio, P., Fortunati, N., Fazzari, A., Crua, M.R., Frairia, R., & Gaidano, G. (1988). *Plasma sex steroid transport and histamine H2-receptor antagonists. Vol. 538. Annals of New York Academy of Science* (pp. 304-312). New York: New York Academy of Sciences.

Berta, L., Frairia, R., Fortunati, N., Fazzari, A., & Gaidano, G. (1992). Smoking effects on the hormonal balance of fertile women. *Hormone Research, 37,* 45-48.

Bertolini, A., Vergoni, W., Gessa, G.L., & Ferrari, W. (1969). Induction of sexual excitement by the action of adrenocorticotrophic hormone in brain. *Nature, 221,* 667-669.

Biaggioni, I., Paul, S., Puckett, A., & Arzubiaga, C. (1991). Caffeine and theophylline as adenosine receptor antagonists in humans. *Journal of Pharmacology and Experimental Therapeutics, 258,* 588-593.

Bicknell, R.J., & Leng, G. (1982). Endogenous opiates regulate oxytocin but not vasopressin secretion from the neurohypophysis. *Nature, 298,* 161-162.

Bicknell, R.J., Leng, G., & Russell, J.A. (1987). Oxytocin neurones: Tolerance to prolonged morphine exposure and hypersecretion following withdrawal. In N. Chalazonitis (Ed.), *Inactivation of hypersentive neurons* (pp. 187-194). New York: Alan R. Liss.

Bird, C.E., Masters, V., Sterns, E.E., & Clark, A.F. (1985). Effects of tamoxifen on testosterone metabolism in postmenopausal women with breast cancer. *Clinical and Investigative Medicine, 8,* 97-102.

Biriell, C., McEwen, J., & Sanz, E. (1989). Depression associated with diltiazem [Letter to the editor]. *British Medical Journal, 2,* 299.

Birkmayer, W., Riederer, P., Ambrozi, L., & Youdim, M.B. (1977). Implications of combined treatment with "Madopar" and L-deprenyl in Parkinson's disease. *Lancet, 8009,* 439-443.

Birkmayer, W., Riederer, P., Linauer, W., & Knoll, J. (1984). L-deprenyl plus l-phenylalanine in the treatment of depression. *Journal of Neural Transmission, 59,* 81-87.

Biron, P. (1979). Diminished libido with cimetidine therapy. *Canadian Medical Association Journal, 121,* 404-405.

Birt, D.F. (1989). Effects of the intake of selected vitamins and minerals on cancer prevention. *Magnesium, 8,* 17-30.

Biswas, N.M., Mazumder, R., Bhattacharya, S.K., & Das, T.K. (1985). Brain 5-hydroxytryptamine and plasma testosterone in L-tryptophan treated rats. *Endocrine Research, 11,* 131-137.

Bitran, D., & Hall, E.M. (1987). Pharmacological analysis of male rat sex behavior. *Neuroscience and Biobehavioral Reviews, 11,* 365-389.

Bittman, B.J. & Young, R.C. (1991). Mania in an elderly man treated with bupropion [Letter to the editor]. *American Journal of Psychiatry, 148*(4), 541.

Bixler, E.O., Kales, A., Brubaker, B.H., & Kales, J.D. (1987). Adverse reactions to benzodiazepine hypnotics: Spontaneous reporting system. *Pharmacology, 35,* 286-300.

Biziere, K., Kan, J.P., Souilhac, J., Muyard, J.P., & Roncucci, R. (1982). *Arzneim-Forsch/Drug Research, 32,* 824-830.

Blay, S.L., Ferraz, M.P., & Calil, H.M. (1982). Lithium-induced male sexual impairment: Two case reports. *Journal of Clinical Psychiatry, 43,* 497-498.

Bleumink, E. (1983). Antihistamines. In M.N.G. Dukes (Ed.), *Side effects of drugs (SED) annual 4* (pp. 111-119).

Blin, O., Schwertschlag, U.S., & Serratrice, G. (1991). Painful clitoral tumescence during bromocriptine therapy. *Lancet, 337,* 1231-1232.

Bliwise, D.L., Bliwise, N.G., Partinen, M., Pursley, A.M., & Dement, W.C. (1988). Sleep apnea and mortality in an aged cohort. *American Journal of Public Health, 78,* 544-547.

Bloch, G.J., & Davidson, J.M. (1968). Effects of adrenalectomy and experience on postcastration sex behavior in the male rat. *Physiology and Behavior, 3,* 461-465.

Block, A.J., Cohn, M.A., Conway, W.A., Hudgel, D.W., Powles, A.C.P., Sanders, M.H., & Smith, P.L. (1985). Indications and standards for cardiopulmonary sleep studies. *Sleep, 8,* 371-379.

Block, R.I., Farinpour, R., & Schlechte, J.A. (1991). Effects of chronic marijuana use on testosterone, luteinizing hormone, follicle stimulating hormone, prolactin, and cortisol in men and women. *Drug and Alcohol Dependence, 28,* 121-128.

Blum, K. (1984). *Handbook of abusable drugs.* New York: Gardner Press.

Blumberg, M.S., & Moltz, H. (1988). How the nose cools the brain during copulation in the male rat. *Physiology and Behavior, 43,* 173-176.

Blumer, D., & Migeon, C. (1975). Hormone and hormonal agents in the treatment of aggression. *Journal of Nervous and Mental Diseases, 160,* 127-137.

Bo, P., Patrucco, M., & Savoldi, F. (1984). Behavioral and EEG graphic changes induced by dopaminergic antidepressants in rabbits. *Il Farmaco, 40,* 608-616.

Bodor, N., & Farag, H. (1984). Improved delivery through biological membranes XIV: Brain specific, sustained delivery of testosterone using a redox chemical delivery system. *Journal of Pharmacological Science, 73,* 385-389.

Bogden, J.D., Oleski, J.M., Lavenhar, M.A., Munves, E.M., Kemp, F.W., Bruening, K.S., Holding, K.J., Denny, T.N., Guarino, M.A., & Holland, B.K. (1990). Effects of one year of supplementation with zinc and other micronutrients on cellular immunity in the elderly. *Journal of the American College of Nutrition, 9,* 214-225.

Bohnet, H.G., Greiwe, W.M., Hanker, J.P., Aragona, C., & Schneider, H.P. (1978). Effects of cimetidine on prolactin, LH, and sex steroid secretion in male and female volunteers. *Acta Endocrinologica, 88,* 428-434.

Bohus, B., & Koolhaas, J.M. (1985). Neuropeptides, neurotransmitters and memory: Sociosexual aspects. *Biological processes and theoretical issues* (pp. 3-16). North Holland: Elsevier Science Publishers.

Bohus, B., Urban, I., van Wimersma Greidanus, TjB, & de Wied, D. (1978). Opposite effects of oxytocin and arginine vasopressin on avoidance behavior and hippocampal theta rhythm in the rat. *Neuropharmacology, 17,* 239-247.

Bolzano, K., et al. (1987). The antihypertensive effect of lisinopril compared to atenolol in patients with mild to moderate hypertension. *Journal of Cardiovascular Pharmacology, 9*(Suppl. 3), S43-S47.

Bondy, C. A., Gainer, H., & Russell, J.T. (1988). Dynorphin A inhibits and naloxone increases the electrically stimulated release of oxytocin but not vasopressin from the terminals of the neural lobe. *Endocrinology, 122,* 1321-1327.

Bonnet, J.J, Chagraoui, A., Protais, P., & Costentin, J. (1987). Interactions of amineptine with the neuronal dopamine uptake system. *Journal of Neural Transmission, 69,* 211-220.

Bonnet, M.H., Dexter, J.R., & Arand, D.L. (1990). The effect of triazolam on arousal and respiration in central sleep apnea patients. *Sleep, 13,* 31-41.

Booher, D.L. (1990). Estrogen supplements in menopause. *Cleveland Clinic Journal of Medicine, 57,* 154-160.

Borison, R.L., & Diamond, B.I. (1987). Neuropharmacology of the extrapyramidal system. *Journal of Clinical Psychiatry, 48*(Suppl. 9), 7-12.

Bos, R.V.D., & Cools, A.R. (1989). The involvement of the nucleus accumbens in the ability of rats to switch to cue-directed behaviours. *Life Sciences, 44,* 1697-1704.

Bostick, R.M., Luepker, R.V., Kofron, P.M., & Pirie, P.L. (1991). Changes in physician practice for the prevention of cardiovascular disease. *Archives of Internal Medicine, 151,* 478-484.

Bowers, M.B., Van Woert, M., & Davis, L. (1971). Sexual behavior during L-dopa treatment for Parkinsonism. *American Journal of Psychiatry, 127,* 1691-1693.

Bowker, L.H. (1978). The relationship between sex, drugs, and sexual behavior on a college campus. *Drug Forum, 7,* 69-80.

Boyce, A., Schwartz, D., & David, G. (1976). Smoking and genitourinary infection [Letter to the editor]. *British Medical Journal,* 1013.

Bozarth, M.A. (1986). Neural basis of psychomotor stimulant and opiate reward: Evidence suggesting the involvement of a common dopaminergic system. *Behavioral Brain Research, 22,* 107-116.

Bradford, J.M. (1988). Organic treatment for the male sexual offender. In R.A. Prentky & V.L. Quinsey, *Human sexual aggression: Current perspectives. Vol. 528. Annals of the New York Academy of Sciences* (pp. 193-202). New York: New York Academy of Sciences.

Bradford, J.M., & Pawlak, A. (1993). Double-blind placebo crossover study of cyproterone acetate in the treatment of the paraphilias. *Archives of Sexual Behavior, 22,* 383-402.

Bradford, R.H., Shear, C.L., Chremos, A.N., Dujovne, C., Downton, M., Franklin, F., Gould, A.L., Hesney, M., Higgins, J., Hurley, D.P., Langendorfer, A., Nash, D.T., Pool, J.L., & Schnaper, H. (1991). Expanded clinical evaluation of lovastatin (EXCEL) study results. *Archives of Internal Medicine, 151,* 43-49.

Brady, K.T., Lydiard, R.B., & Kellner, C. (1991). Tranylcypromine abuse [Letter to the editor]. *American Journal of Psychiatry, 148,* 1268-1269.

Brahams, D. (1990). Benzodiazepine sex fantasies: Acquittal of dentist. *Lancet, 335,* 403-404.

Bramanti, P., Bianchi, L., Benedetto, M., Ricci, R.M., Cribano, M.A., & Di Perri, R. (1985). Study of the hypnic effect of amineptine evaluation by means of polygraphy and tests. *Progress in Neuro-Psychopharmacology and Biological Psychiatry, 9,* 157-165.

Branconnier, R.T., & Cole, J.O. (1980). The therapeutic role of methylphenidate in senile organic brain syndrome. In J.O. Cole & J.E. Barrett (Eds.), *Psychopathology of aging* (pp. 183-196). New York: Raven Press.

Braunwald, E., Isselbacher, K.J., Petersdorf, R.G., Wilson, J.D., Martin, J.B., & Fauci, A.S. (Eds.). (1987). *Harrison's principles of internal medicine (11th ed.).* New York: McGraw-Hill.

Brautbar, N., Roy, A.T., Hom, P., & Lee, D.B. (1988). Hypomagnesemia and hypermagnesemia. In H. Sigel & A. Sigel (Eds.), *Compendium on magnesium and its role in biology, nutrition, and physiology* (pp. 285-320) New York: Dekker.

Bray, G.A. (1985). Current status of drug therapy in obesity. In J.P. Morgan, D.V. Kagan, & J.S. Brody (Eds.), *Phenylpropanolamine: Risks, benefits, and controversies* (pp. 94-131). New York: Praeger Publishers.

Brazell, M.P., Mitchell, S.N., Joseph, M.H., & Gray, J.A. (1990). Acute administration of nicotine increases the in vivo extracellular levels of dopamine, 3, 4-dihydroxyphenylacetic acid, and ascorbic acid preferentially in the nucleus accumbens of the rat: Comparison with caudate-putamen. *Neuropharmacology, 29,* 1177-1185.

Breslau, N., Kilbey, M.M., & Andreski, P. (1993a). Nicotine dependence and major depression. *Archives of General Psychiatry, 50,* 31-35.

Breslau, N., Kilbey, M.M., & Andreski, P. (1993b). Vulnerability to psychopathology in nicotine-dependent smokers: An epidemiologic study of young adults. *American Journal of Psychiatry, 150,* 941-946.

Briddel, D.W., & Wilson, G.T. (1976). The effects of alcohol and expectancy set on male sexual arousal. *Journal of Abnormal Psychology, 85,* 225-234.

Briddel, D.W., Rimm, D., Caddy, G., Kravitz, G., Sholis, D., & Wunderlin, R. (1978). The effects of alcohol and cognitive set on sexual arousal to deviant stimuli. *Journal of Abnormal Psychology, 87,* 418–430.

Bridges, R.S., & Mann, P.E. (1990). Central beta-endorphin administration disrupts maternal behavior in lactating rats. *Neuroendocrinology, 52*(Suppl. 1), 46.

Brier, A., Ginsberg, E.M., & Charney, D.S. (1984). Seminal emission induced by tricyclic antidepressant. *American Journal of Psychiatry, 141,* 610–611.

Briggs, M.H. (1973). Cigarette smoking and infertility in men. *Medical Journal of Australia, 1,* 616–617.

Brinblecombe, R.W., & Duncan, W.A. (1977). The relevance to man of pre-clinical data for cimetidine. In W.L. Burland & M.A. Simkins (Eds.), *Cimetidine: Proceedings of the Second International Symposium on histamine H2-receptor antagonists* (pp. 54–65). Amsterdam-Oxford: Excerpta Medica.

Brincat, M., & Studd, J.W. (1988). Skin and the menopause. In J.W. Studd & I.M. Whitehead (Eds.), *The menopause* (pp. 85–101). London: Blackwell Scientific.

Brincat, M., Studd, J.W., O'Dowd, T., Magas, A., Cordoza, L.D., & Cooper, D. (1984). Subcutaneous hormone implants for the control of climacteric symptoms. *Lancet, 1,* 16–18.

Brincat, M., Versi, E. Moniz, C.F., Magos, A., de Trafford, J., & Studd, J.W. (1987). Skin collagen changes in postmenopausal women receiving different regimens of estrogen therapy. *Obstetrics and Gynecology, 70,* 123–127.

Brindley, G.S. (1983). Cavernosal alpha-blockade: A new technique for investigating and treating erectile impotence. *British Journal of Psychiatry, 143,* 332–337.

Brindley, G.S. (1986a). Pilot experiments on the action of drugs injected into the human corpus cavernosum penis. *British Journal of Pharmacology, 87,* 495–500.

Brindley, G.S. (1986b). Sacral root and hypogastric plexus stimulators and what these models tell us about autonomic actions on the bladder and urethra. *Clinical Science, 70*(Suppl. 14), 41s-44s.

Brindley, G.S. (1987). Treatment of erectile impotence by intracavemosal injection. In W.F. Henry (Ed.), *Recent advances in urology/andrology: Number 4* (pp. 263–267). New York: Churchill Livingstone.

Brisson, G.R., Quirion, A., Ledoux, M., Raiotte, D., & Pellerin-Massicotte, J. (1984). Influence of long-distance swimming on serum androgens in males. *Hormone and Metabolism Research, 16,* 160.

British Medical Journal (1979). Drugs and male sexual function [editorial]. *British Medical Journal, 4,* 883–884.

Brittain, R.T., Daly, M.J., Jack, D., Martin, L.E., Stables, R., & Sutherland, M. (1982). The outline of the animal pharmacology of ranitidine. In J.J. Misiewicz & K.G. Wormsley (Eds.), *The clinical use of ranitidine,* (pp. 1–10). Oxford: Medicine Publishing Foundation.

Broderick, G.A., & Lue, T.F. (1989). Penile blood flow study and the diagnostic use of prostaglandin E1: A review of 120 patients. *Journal of Urology, 141,* 288A.

Broekman, C.P., Haensel, S.M., Van de Ven, L.L., & Slob, A.K. (1992). Bisoprolol and hypertension: Effects on sexual functioning in men. *Journal of Sex and Marital Therapy, 18,* 325–331.

Bronson, F.H., & Rissman, E.F. (1989). Epinephrine release in response to sexual activity in male versus female rats. *Physiology and Behavior, 45,* 185–189.

Bronzo, M.R., & Stahl, S.M. (1993). Galactorrhea induced by sertraline [Letter to the editor]. *American Journal of Psychiatry, 150,* 1269–1270.

Broverman, D.M., Klaiber, E.L., Vogel, W., & Kobayashi, Y. (1974). Short-term versus long-term effects of adrenal hormones on behaviors. *Psychological Bulletin, 81,* 672–694.

Brown, R.G., Jahanshahi, M., Quinn, N., & Marsden, C.D. (1990). Sexual function in patients with Parkinson's disease and their partners. *Journal of Neurology, Neurosurgery, and Psychiatry, 53,* 480–486.

Brubaker, L.T., & Sand, P.K. (1989). Urinary frequency and urgency. *Obstetrics and Gynecology Clinics of North America, 16,* 883–896.

Bruchovsky, N. (1971). Comparison of the metabolites formed in rat prostate following the in vivo administration of seven natural androgens. *Endocrinology, 89,* 1212–1216.

Brun, L.D., Bielmann, P., Gagne, C., Moorjani, S., Nadeau, A., & Lupien, P.J. (1988). Effects of fenfluramine in hypertriglyceridemic obese subjects. *International Journal of Obesity, 12,* 423–431.

Brysson, P.D. (1989). *Comprehensive review in toxicology* (2nd ed.). Rockville, MD: Aspen Publishers.

Brzek, A. (1987). Alcohol and male fertility (preliminary report). *Andrologia, 19,* 32–36.

Buchanan, N. (1985). Epilepsy and weight reduction [Letter to the editor]. *Medical Journal of Australia, 143,* 428.

Buena, F., Serdloff, R.S., Steiner, B.S., Lutohmansingh, P., Peterson, M.A., Pandian, M.R., Galmarini, M., & Bhasin, S. (1993). Sexual function does not change when serum testosterone levels are pharmacologically varied within the normal male range. *Fertility and Sterility, 59,* 1118–1123.

Buffington, C.K. (1991). Opposing actions of DHEA and testosterone on insulin sensitivity: In vivo and in vitro studies of hyperandrogenic females. *Diabetes, 40,* 693-700.

Buffum, J. (1982). Pharmacosexology: The effect of drugs on sexual function: A review. *Journal of Psychoactive Drugs, 14,* 5-44.

Buffum, J. (1986). Pharmacosexology update: Prescription drugs and sexual function. *Journal of Psychoactive Drugs, 18*(2), 97-106.

Buglass, D., Clarke, J., Henderson, A.S., Kreitman, N., & Presley, A.S. (1977). A study of agoraphobic housewives. *Psychological Medicine, 7,* 73-86.

Buigues, J., & Vallejo, J. (1987). Therapeutic response to phenelzine in patients with panic disorders and agoraphobia with panic attacks. *Journal of Clinical Psychiatry, 48,* 55-59.

Bulbrook, R.D., Hayward, J.L., & Spicer, C.C. (1971). Urinary androgen and corticoid excretion and subsequent breast cancer. *Lancet, 2,* 395-398.

Bulpitt, C.J., & Dollery, C.T. (1973). Side effects of hypotensive agents evaluated by a self-administered questionnaire. *British Medical Journal, 3,* 485-490.

Bulpitt, C.J., Dollery, C.T., & Carne, S. (1974). A symptom questionnaire for hypertensive patients. *Journal of Chronic Disease, 27,* 309-323.

Bulpitt, C.J., Dollery, C.T., & Carne, S. (1976). Change in symptoms of hypertensive patients after referral to hospital clinic. *British Heart Journal, 38,* 121-128.

Bulpitt, C.J., & Fletcher, A.E. (1990). The measurement of quality of life in hypertensive patients: A practical approach *British Journal of Clinical Pharmacology, 30,* 353-364.

Bump, R.C., & McClish, D.M. (1992). Cigarette smoking and urinary incontinence in women. *American Journal of Obstetrics and Gynecology, 167,* 1213-1218.

Bump, R.C., & McClish, D.M. (1994). Cigarette smoking and pure genuine stress incontinence of urine: A comparison of risk factors and determinants between smokers and nonsmokers. *American Journal of Obstetrics and Gynecology, 170,* 579-582.

Burch, J.C., Byrd, B.F., & Vaughn, W.K. (1974). The effects of long-term estrogen on hysterectomized women. *American Journal of Obstetrics and Gynecology, 118,* 778-782.

Burch, P.R. (1986). Postmenopausal estrogen use and heart disease. *New England Journal of Medicine, 315,* 134.

Burger, H.G., Hailes, J., & Nelson, J. (1987). Effect of combined implants of oestradiol and testosterone on libido in postmenopausal women. *British Medical Journal, 294,* 936-937.

Burger, H.G., Hailes, J., Menelaus, M., Nelson, J., Hudson, B., & Balazo, W. (1984). The management of persistent menopausal symptoms with oestradiol-testosterone implants: Clinical lipid and hormone results. *Maturitas, 6,* 351-358.

Burgio, K.L., Matthews, K.A., & Engel, B.T. (1991). Prevalence, incidence, and correlates of urinary incontinence in healthy, middle-aged women. *Journal of Urology, 146,* 1255-1259.

Burnish, T.G., Meyerowitz, B.E., Carey, M.P., & Morrow, G.R. (1987). The stressful effects of cancer in adults. In A. Baum & T.E. Singer (Eds.), *Handbook of psychology and health, Vol. 5: Stress* (pp. 137-158).

Burns, D.A. (1980). *Feeling good.* New York: William Morrow & Company.

Burris, A.S., Banks, S.M., Carter, C.S., Davidson, J.M., & Sherins, R.J. (1992). A long-term prospective study of the physiologic and behavioral effects of hormone replacement in untreated hypogonadal men. *Journal of Andrology, 13,* 297-304.

Burris, A.S., Gracely, R.H., Carter, C.S., Sherins, J., & Davidson, J.M. (1991). Testosterone therapy is associated with reduced tactile sensitivity in human males. *Hormones and Behavior, 25,* 195-205.

Bush, T.L. (1986). Postmenopausal estrogen use and heart disease. *New England Journal of Medicine, 315,* 131-136.

Bush, T.L., Barrett-Connor, E., Cowan, L.D., Criqui, M.H., Wallace, R.B., Suchindran, C.M., Tyroler, H.A., & Rifkind, B.M. (1987). Cardiovascular mortality and noncontraceptive use of estrogen in women: Results from the Lipid Research Clinics Program Follow-up Study. *Circulation, 75,* 1102-1109.

Buvat, J., Lemaire, A., Buvat-Herbaut, M., Fourlinnie, J.C., Racadot, A., & Fossati, P. (1985). Hyperprolactemia and sexual function in men. *Hormone Research, 22,* 196-203.

Buvat, J., Lemaire, A., Buvat-Herbaut, M., Guieu, J.D., Bailleul, J.P., & Fossati, P. (1985). Comparative investigations of 26 impotent and 26 nonimpotent diabetic patients. *Journal of Urology, 133,* 34-38.

Buvat, J., Lemaire, A., Buvat-Herbaut, M., & Marcolin, G. (1989). Safety of intracavernous injections using an alpha-blocking agent. *Journal of Urology, 141,* 1364-1367.

Buvat, J., Lemaire, A., Marcolin, G., Dehaene, J.L., Buvat-Herbaut, M. (1986). Injections intracaverneuses de drogues vaso-actives. *Journal d'Urologie, 92,* 111-116.

Byyny, R.L., & Speroff, L. (1990). *A clinical guide for the care of older women.* Baltimore, MD: Williams & Wilkins.

Caballeria, J., Baraona, E., Rodamilans, M., & Lieber, C.S. (1987). Effects of cimetidine on gastric alcohol dehydrogenase activity and blood ethanol levels. *Gastroenterology, 92,* 1169–1173.

Caballeria, J., Baraona, E., Rodamilans, M., & Lieber, C.S. (1989b). Reply: Cimetidine and alcohol absorption. *Gastroenterology, 97,* 1067–1068.

Caballeria, J., Baraona, E., Rodamilans, M., & Lieber, C.S. (1989a). Effects of cimetidine on gastric alcohol dehydrogenase activity and blood ethanol levels. *Gastroenterology, 96,* 388–392.

Caldwell, J.D., Jirikowski, G.D., Greer, E.R., & Pedersen, C.A. (1987). Medial preoptic area oxytocin and female sexual receptivity. *Behavioral Neuroscience, 103*(3), 655–662.

Caldwell, J.D., Jirikowski, G.F., Greer, E.R., Stumpf, W.E., & Pedersen, C.A. (1988). Ovarian steroids and sexual interaction alter oxytocinergic content and distribution in the basal forebrain. *Brain Research, 446*(2), 236–244.

Caldwell, J.D., Prange, A.J., & Pedersen, C.A. (1986). Oxytocin facilitates the sexual receptivity of estrogen-treated female rats. *Neuropeptides, 7,* 175–189.

Cameron, O.G., Modell, J.G., & Hariharan, M. (1990). Caffeine and human cerebral blood flow: A positron emission tomography study. *Life Sciences, 47,* 1141–1146.

Campbell, S. (1976). Double-blind psychometric studies on the effects of natural estrogens on postmenopausal women. In S. Campbell (Ed.), *The management of the menopause and post-menopausal years* (pp. 149–158). Lancaster, England: MTP Press.

Campbell, S., & Whitehead, M. (1977). Oestrogen therapy and the menopausal syndrome. *Clinics in Obstetrics and Gynaecology, 42,* 31–47.

Campos, J.L. (1972). Continuous positive aging in Hodgkin's disease. *British Journal of Radiology, 45,* 917–922.

Cannavo, S., Granata, A., Sobbrio, G.A., Aragona, A., & Trimarchi, F. (1989). Serum 17-hydroxyprogesterone, DHEAS, and free testosterone level decrease following loperamide in women with late onset 21-hydroxylase deficiency and with idiopathic hirsutism. *Journal of Endocrinological Investigation, 12*(Suppl. 1), 198.

Canterbury, R.J., Haskins, B., Kahn, N., Saathoff, G., & Yazel, J. (1987). Postpartum psychosis induced by bromocriptine. *Southern Medical Journal, 80,* 1463–1464.

Cantrill, J.A., Dewis, P., Large, D.M., Newman, M., & Anderson, D.C. (1984). Which testosterone replacement therapy? *Clinical Endocrinology, 21,* 97–107.

Carani, C., Zini, D., Baldini, A., Della Casa, L., Ghizzarni, A., & Marrama, P. (1990). Effects of androgen treatment in impotent men with normal and low levels of free testosterone. *Archives of Sex Behavior, 19,* 223–234.

Carette, B., & Poulain, P. (1984). Excitatory effect of dehydroepiandrosterone, its sulphate ester and pregnenolone sulfate, applied by iontophoresis and pressure, on single neurones in the septopreoptic area of the guinea pig. *Neuroscience Letters, 45,* 205–210.

Carlson, H.E. (1981). Gynecomastia. *New England Journal of Medicine, 303,* 795–799.

Carlson, H.E., & Ippoliti, A.F. (1977). Cimetidine, an H-2-antihistamine, stimulates prolactin secretion in man. *Journal of Clinical Endocrinology and Metabolism, 45,* 367–370.

Carlsson, M., & Carlsson, A. (1988). A regional study of sex differences in rat brain serotonin. *Progress in Neuro-Psychopharmacology and Biological Psychiatry, 12,* 53–61.

Carlsson, M., Svensson, K., Eriksson, E., & Carlsson, A. (1985). Rat brain serotonin: Biochemical and functional evidence for a sex difference. *Journal of Neural Transmission, 63,* 297–313.

Carmichael, M.S., Humbert, R., Dixen, J., Palmisano, G., Greenleaf, W., & Davidson, J.M. (1987). Plasma oxytocin increases in the human sexual response. *Journal of Clinical Endocrinology and Metabolism, 64,* 27–31.

Carnes, P. (1989). *Contrary to love.* Minneapolis, MN: CompCare Publishers.

Carney, A., Bancroft, J., & Mathews, A. (1978). Combination of hormonal and psychological treatments for female sexual unresponsiveness: A comparative study. *British Journal of Psychiatry, 133,* 339–346.

Carney, M.W.P. (1988). Diethylpropion and psychosis. *Clinical Neuropharmacology, 11,* 183–188.

Carney, R.M., Rich, M.W., teVelde, A., Saini, J., Clark, K., & Freedland, K.E. (1987). Prevalence of major depressive disorder in patients receiving beta-blocker therapy versus other medication. *American Journal of Medicine, 83,* 223–226.

Carroll, M., & Gallo, G. (1985). *Quaaludes: The quest for oblivion.* New York: Chelsea House Publishers.

Carroll, M.E., & Meisch, R.A. (1984). Increased drug-reinforced behavior due to food deprivation. In T. Thompson, P.B. Dews, & J. E. Barrett (Eds.), *Advances in behavioral pharmacology. Vol. 4* (pp. 47–88). Hillsdale, NJ: Lawrence Erlbaum Associates.

Carruba, M.O., Coen, E., Pizzi, M., Memo, M., Missale, C., Spano, P.F., & Mantegazza, P. (1986). Mechanism of action of anorectic drugs: An overview. In M.O. Carruba & J.E. Blundell (Eds.), *Pharmacology of eating disorders: Theoretical and clinical developments* (pp. 1-27). New York: Raven Press.

Carruba, M.O., Garosi, V.L., Pizzi, M., Memo, M., Missale, C., Spano, P.F., & Mantegazza, P. (1986b). Long-term treatment with anorectic drugs. In E. Ferrari & F. Brambilla (Eds.), *Disorders of eating behavior: A psychoneuroendocrine approach* (pp. 305-311). New York: Pergamon Press.

Carruba, M.O., Zambotti, F., Vicentini, L., Picotti, B., & Mantegazza, P. (1978). Pharmacology and biochemical profile of a new anorectic drug: Mazindol. In S. Garattini & R. Samanin (Eds.), *Central mechanisms of anorectic drugs* (pp. 145-164). New York: Raven Press.

Carter, J.N., Tyson, J.E., Tolis, G., Van Vliet, S., Fairman, C., & Friesen, H.G. (1978). Prolactin secreting tumors and hypogonadism in 22 men. *New England Journal of Medicine, 299,* 847-852.

Carver, J.R., & Oaks, W.W. (1976). Sex and hypertension. In W.W. Oaks, G.A. Melchiode, & I. Ficher (Eds.), *Sex and the life cycle* (pp. 175-178). New York: Grune & Stratton.

Casper, R.C., Redmond, D.E., Katz, M.M., Schaffer, C.B., Davis, J.M., & Koslow, S.H. (1985). Somatic symptoms in primary affective disorder. *Archives of General Psychiatry, 42,* 1098-1104.

Casson, P.R., Andersen, R.N., Herrod, H.G., Stentz, F.B., Straughn, A.B., Abraham, G.E., & Buster, J.E. (1993). Oral dehydroepiandrosterone in physiologic doses modulates immune function in postmenopausal women. *American Journal of Obstetrics and Gynecology, 169,* 1536-1539.

Castelo-Branco, C., Pons, F., Gratacós, E., Fortuny, A., Vanrell, J.A., & González-Merlo, J. (1994). Relationship between skin collagen and bone changes during aging. *Maturitas, 38,* 199-206.

Castillo, J., Barlog, K., Perfetto, C., Cartagena, R., & Sufrin, G. (1986). Erection cavernosography—A new diagnostic tool. *Journal of Urology, 135,* 307A.

Castot, A., Benzaken, C., Wagniart, F., & Efthymiou, M.L. (1990). Surconsommation d'amineptine. *Therape, 45,* 399-405.

Cauley, J.A., Cummings, S.R., Black, D.M., Mascioli, S.R., & Seeley, D.G. (1990). Relevance and determinants of estrogen replacement therapy in elderly women. *American Journal of Obstetrics and Gynecology, 163,* 1438-1444.

Cauley, J.A., Gutai, J.P., Kuller, L.H., LeDonne, D., Sandler, R.B., Sashin, D., & Powell, J.G. (1988). Endogenous estrogen levels and calcium intakes in postmenopausal women: Relationships with cortical bone mass. *Journal of the American Medical Association, 260,* 3150-3155.

Cavallini, G. (1991). Minoxidil versus nitroglycerin: A prospective double-blind controlled trial in transcutaneous erection facilitation for organic impotence. *Journal of Urology, 146,* 50-53.

Cavanaugh, D.J., & Cann, C.E. (1988). Brisk walking does not stop bone loss in postmenopausal women. *Annals of Internal Medicine, 9,* 201-204.

Ceci, A., Garattini, S., Gobbi, M., & Mennini, T. (1986). Effect of long-term amineptine treatment on pre and postsynaptic mechanisms in rat brain. *British Journal of Pharmacology, 88,* 269-275.

Cecio, A., & Vittoria, A. (1989). Urogenital paraneurons in several mammals. *Archives of Histology and Cytology, 52*(Suppl.), 403-413.

Chait, L.D., Uhlenhuth, E.D., & Johanson, C.E. (1986). The discriminative stimulus and subjective effects of phenylpropanolamine, mazindol, and d-amphetamine in humans. *Pharmacology, Biochemistry, and Behavior, 24,* 1665-1672.

Chait, L.D., Uhlenhuth, E.H., & Johanson, C.E. (1987). Reinforcing and subjective effects of several anorectics in normal human volunteers. *Journal of Pharmacology and Experimental Therapeutics, 242,* 777-782.

Chait, L.D., Uhlenhuth, E.H., & Johanson, C.E. (1988). Phenylpropanolamine: Reinforcing and subjective effects in normal human volunteers. *Psychopharmacology, 96,* 212-217.

Chaki, S., Usuki-Ito, C., Muramatsu, M., & Otomo, S. (1990). Differentiation of the active site of minaprine from that of phencyclidine in rat hippocampus. *Research Communications in Chemical Pathology and Pharmacology, 69,* 85-97.

Chambers, K.C., & Phoenix, C.H. (1989). Apomorphine, deprenyl, and yohimbine fail to increase sexual behavior in rhesus males. *Behavioral Neuroscience, 103,* 816-823.

Chambon, M., Grizard, G., & Boucher, D. (1985). Bromocriptine, a dopamine agonist, directly inhibits testosterone production by rat Leydig cells. *Andrologia, 17,* 172-177.

Chan, A.F., Mortola, J.F., Wood, S.H., & Yen, S.S.C. (1994). Persistence of premenstrual syndrome during low-dose administration of progesterone antagonist RU 486. *Obstetrics and Gynecology, 84,* 1001-1005.

Chancellor, M.B., Bennett, C.J., Sonda, L.P., & Konnak, J.W. (1987). Effectiveness of yohimbine in the treatment of erectile impotence: Retropsective analysis. *Journal of Urology, 139,* 310A.

Chancellor, M.B., Rivas, D.A., Panzer, D.E., Freedman, M.K., & Staas, W.E., Jr. (1994). Prospective comparison of topical minoxidil to vacuum constriction device and intracorporeal papaverine injection in treatment of erectile dysfunction due to spinal-cord injury. *Urology, 43,* 365-369.

Chang, S.W., Fine, R., Siegel, D., Chesney, M., Black, D., & Hulley, S.B. (1991). The impact of diuretic therapy on reported sexual function. *Archives of Internal Medicine, 151,* 2402–2408.

Chapman, R.M. (1982). Effects of cytotoxic therapy on sexuality and gonadal function. *Seminars in Oncology, 9,* 84–94.

Chapman, R.M. (1984). Effect of cytotoxic therapy on sexuality and gonadal function. In M.C. Perry & J.W. Yarbro (Eds.), *Toxicity of chemotherapy* (pp. 343–363). New York: Grume & Stratton.

Chapman, R.M., Sutcliffe, S.B., & Malpas, J.S. (1979). Cytoxic-induced ovarian failure in women with Hodgkin's disease: I. Hormone function. *Journal of the American Medical Association, 242,* 1877–1881.

Chapman, R.M., Sutcliffe, S.B., & Malpas, J.S. (1981). Male gonadal dysfunction in Hodgkin's disease. *Journal of the American Medical Association, 245,* 1323–1328.

Chard, T. (1985). Oxytocin: Physiology and pathophysiology. In: P.H. Baylis & P.L. Padfield (Eds.), *The posterior pituitary,* (pp. 361–389). New York: Marcel Dekker.

Charney, D.S, & Heninger, R.G. (1986). $Alpha_2$ adrenergic and opiate receptor blockade. *Archives of General Psychiatry, 43,* 1037–1041.

Charney, D.S., Heninger, R.G., & Breier, A. (1984). Noradrenergic function in panic anxiety. *Archives of General Psychiatry, 41,* 751–763.

Chatelut, E., Rispail, Y., Berlan, M., & Montastruc, J.L. (1989). Yohimbine increases human salivary secretion. *British Journal of Clinical Pharmacology, 28,* 366–368.

Chen, J.K., Godschalk, M., Katz, P.G., & Mulligan, T. (1995). The lowest effective dose of prostaglandin E1 as treatment for erectile dysfunction. *Journal of Urology, 153,* 80–81.

Chen, J.K., Hwang, T.I., & Yang, C.R. (1992). Comparison of effects following the intracorporeal injection of papaverine and prostaglandin E1. *British Journal of Urology, 69,* 404–407.

Cheramy, A., Barbeito, L., Godeheu, G., Desce, J.M., Pittaluga, A., Galli, T., Artaud, F., & Glowinski, J. (1990). Respective contributions of neuronal activity and presynaptic mechanisms in the control of the in vivo release of dopamine. *Journal of Neural Transmission, 29*(Suppl.), 183–193.

Chessick, R.D. (1960). The "pharmacogenic orgasm" in the drug addict. *Archives of General Psychiatry, 3,* 545–556.

Cheung, D., Timmers, M.C., Zwinderman, A.H., Bel, E.H., Dijkman, J.H., & Sterk, P.J. (1992). Long-term effects of a long-acting beta-adrenoceptor agonist, salmeterol, on airway hyperresponsiveness in patients with mild asthma. *New England Journal of Medicine, 327,* 1198–1203.

Chez, R.A. (1989). Clinical aspects of the three new progestogens: Desogestrel, gestodene, and norgestimate. *American Journal of Obstetrics and Gynecology, 160,* 1296–1300.

Chiao, Y., Johnston, D., Gavaler, J., & Van Thiel, D. (1981). Effect of chronic ethanol feeding on testicular content of enzymes required for testosteroneogenesis. *Alcoholism: Clinical and Experimental Research, 5,* 230–236.

Chiarello, R.J., & Cole, J.O. (1987). The use of psychostimulants in general psychiatry: A reconsideration. *Archives of General Psychiatry, 44,* 286–295.

Childress, C.H., & Katz, V.L. (1994). Nifedipine and its indications in obstetrics and gynecology. *Obstetrics and Gynecology, 83,* 616–624.

Chiodera, P., & Coiro, V. (1990). Inhibition by dexamethasone of arginine vasopressin and ACTH responses to insulin-induced hypoglycemia and cigarette smoking in normal men. *Acta Endocrinologica, 123,* 487–492.

Choi, N.G., Maayani, S., & Melman, A. (1988). Modification of sexual behavior by drugs acting on serotonin receptors. *Journal of Urology, 139,* 253a.

Chopra, I.J., Tulchinsky, D., & Greenway, F.L. (1973). Estrogen-androgen imbalance in hepatic cirrhosis: Studies in 13 male patients. *Annals of Internal Medicine, 79,* 198–203.

Christiansen, C., & Riis, B.J. (1989). Sex steroids and bone. In M. L'Hermite (Ed.), *Update on hormonal treatment in the menopause* (pp. 16–28). Basel: Karger.

Christiansen, C., Riis, B.J., Johansen, J.S., & Podenphant, J. (1988). The effect of nasal calcitonin on postmenopausal osteoporosis. *Gynecological Endocrinology, 2*(Suppl. 2), 21.

Chung, S.K., McVary, K.T., & McKenna, K.E. (1988). Sexual reflexes in male and female rats. *Neuroscience Letters, 94,* 343–348.

Chuong, C.J., & Hsi, B.P. (1994). Effect of naloxone on luteinizing hormone secretion in premenstrual syndrome. *Fertility and Sterility, 61,* 1039–1044.

Cicero, T.J. (1980). Common mechanisms underlying the effects of ethanol and narcotics on neuroendocrine function. In N.K. Mello (Ed.), *Advances in substance abuse, behavioral and biological research. Vol. 1* (pp. 201–254). Greenwich, CT: JAI Press.

Cicero, T.J., Bell, R.D., Meyer, E.R., & Badger, T. (1980). Ethanol and acetaldehyde directly inhibit testicular steroidogenesis. *Journal of Pharmacology and Experimental Therapeutics, 213,* 228–233.

Cicero, T.J., Meyer, E.R., Gabriel, S.M., Bell, R.D., & Wilcox, C.E. (1980). Morphine exerts testosterone-like effects in the hypothalamus of the castrated male rat. *Brain Research, 202,* 151–164.

Cicero, T.J., Wilcox, C.E., Bell, R.D., & Meyer, E.R. (1980). Naloxone-induced increases in serum luteinizing hormone in the male: Mechanisms of action. *Journal of Pharmacology and Experimental Therapeutics, 212,* 573–578.

Claes, H., & Baert, L. (1989). Transcutaneous nitroglycerin therapy in the treatment of impotence. *Urologia Internationalis, 44,* 309–312.

Claghorn, J.L. (1992). A double-blind comparison of paroxetine and placebo in the treatment of depressed outpatients. *International Clinical Psychopharmacology, 6,* 212.

Clark, D.B., & Agras, W.S. (1991). The assessment and treatment of performance anxiety in musicians. *American Journal of Psychiatry, 148,* 598–605.

Clark, J.T. (1991). Suppression of copulatory behavior in male rats following central administration of clonidine. *Neuropharmacology, 30,* 373–382.

Clark, J.T., Kalra, S.P., & Kalra P.S. (1987). Effects of a selective $alpha_1$-adrenoceptor agonist, methoxamine, on sexual behavior and penile reflexes. *Physiology and Behavior, 40,* 747–753.

Clark, J.T., & Smith, E.R. (1990). Clonidine suppresses copulatory behavior and erectile reflexes in male rats: Lack of effect of naloxone pretreatment. *Neuroendocrinology, 51,* 357–364.

Clark, J.T., Smith, E.R., & Davidson, J.M. (1984). Enhancement of sexual motivation in male rats by yohimbine. *Science, 225,* 847–849.

Clark, J.T., Smith, E.R., & Davidson, J.M. (1985a). Evidence for the modulation of sexual behavior by alpha-adrenoceptors in male rats. *Neuroendocrinology, 41,* 36–43.

Clark, J.T., Smith, E.R., & Davidson, J.M. (1985b). Testosterone is not required for the enhancement of sexual motivation by yohimbine. *Physiology and Behavior, 35,* 517–521.

Clark, R.W., Schmidt, H.S., Schaal, S.F., Bondoulas, H., & Schuller, D.E. (1979). Sleep apnea: Treatment with protriptyline. *Neurology, 29,* 1287–1292.

Clarke, E.A., Hatcher, J., McKeown-Eyssen, G.E., & Lickrish, G.M. (1985). Cervical dysplasia: Association with sexual behavior, smoking, and contraceptive use? *American Journal of Obstetrics and Gynecology, 151,* 612–616.

Clarke, P.B.S. (1990). Dopaminergic mechanisms in the locomotor stimulant effects of nicotine. *Biochemical Pharmacology, 40,* 1427–1432.

Clarke, R.J. (1991). Indapamide: A diuretic of choice for the treatment of hypertension? *American Journal of the Medical Sciences, 301,* 215–220.

Claus, G., Kling, A., & Bolander, K. (1981). Effects of methaqualone on social-sexual behavior in monkeys (*M. mulatta*). *Brain, Behavior, and Evolution, 18,* 105–113.

Clayton, R.R., Voss, H.L., Robbins, C., & Skinner, W.F. (1986). Gender differences in drug use: An epidemiological perspective. In B.A. Ray & M.C. Brande (Eds.), *Women and drugs: National Institute of Drug Abuse Research Monograph, 65,* 80–99.

Cleary, M.P. (1991). The antiobesity effect of dehydroepiandrosterone in rats. *Proceedings of the Society for Experimental Biology and Medicine, 196,* 8–16.

Cleary, M.P., Shepherd, A., & Jenks, B. (1984). Effect of dehydroepiandrosterone on growth in lean and obese Zucker rats. *Journal of Nutrition, 114,* 1242–1251.

Cleary, M.P., & Zisk, J.F. (1986). Antiobesity effect of two different levels of dehydroepiandrosterone in lean and obese middle-aged female Zucker rats. *International Journal of Obesity, 10,* 193–204.

Cleeves, L., & Findley, L.J. (1987). Bromocriptine-induced impotence in Parkinson's disease. *British Medical Journal, 295,* 367.

Clone, C.A. (1986). Unilateral gynecomastia and nifedipine. *British Medical Journal, 292,* 380.

Cloninger, C.R. (1988). Neurogenetic adaptive mechanisms in alcoholism. *Science, 236,* 410–416.

Clopper, R.R., Voorhess, M.L., MacGillivray, M.H., Lee, P.A., & Mills, B. (1993). Psychosexual behavior in hypopituitary men: A controlled comparison of gonadotropin and testosterone replacement. *Psychoneuroendocrinology, 18,* 149–161.

Cloud, M.L. (1987). Safety of nizatidine in clinical trials conducted in the United States and Europe. *Scandinavian Journal of Gastroenterology, 22,* (Suppl. 136), 29–36.

Clozel, M., Kuhn, H., & Hefti, F. (1990). Effects of angiotensin converting enzyme inhibitors and of hydralazine on endothelial function in hypertensive rats. *Hypertension, 16,* 532–540.

Cohen, A.J. (1992). Fluoxetine-induced yawning and anorgasmia reversed by cyproheptadine treatment. *Journal of Clinical Psychiatry, 53,* 174.

Cohen, A.S., Rosen, R.C., & Goldstein, L. (1985). EEG hemispheric asymmetry during sexual arousal: Psychophysiological patterns in responsive, unresponsive, and dysfunctional men. *Journal of Abnormal Psychology, 94,* 580–590.

Cohen, B.M., & Zubenko, G.S. (1988). Captopril in the treatment of recurrent major depression [Letter to the editor]. *Journal of Clinical Psychopharmacology, 8,* 143–144.

Cohen, H.D., Rosen, R.C., & Goldstein, L. (1976). Electroencephalographic laterality changes during the human sexual orgasm. *Archives of Sexual Behavior, 5,* 189–199.

Cohen, L.J. (1994). Evaluation of new drugs: Risperidone. *Pharmacotherapy, 14,* 253–265.

Cohen, M.E., Robins, E., Purtell, J.J., Altmann, M.W., & Reid, D.E. (1953). Excessive surgery in hysteria. *Journal of the American Medical Association, 151,* 977–986.

Cohen, M.G., & Prowse, M.V. (1989). Drug-induced rheumatic syndromes: Diagnosis, clinical features, and management. *Medical Toxicology and Adverse Drug Experience, 4,* 199–218.

Cohen, S. (1977). Diethylpropion (Tenuate): An infrequently abused anorectic. *Psychosomatics, 18,* 28–33.

Cohen, S. (1985, January). Marijuana and reproductive functions. *Drug Abuse and Alcoholism Newsletter: Vista Hill Foundation, 13*(10), 1–3.

Cohn, C.K., Shrivastava, R., Mendels, J., Cohn, J.B., Fabre, L.F., Claghorn, J.L., Dessain, E.C., Itil, T.M., & Lautin, A. (1990). Double-blind, multicenter comparison of sertraline and amitriptyline in elderly depressed patients. *Journal of Clinical Psychiatry, 51*(12) (Suppl. B), 28–33.

Colditz, G.A., Egan, K.M., & Stampfer, M.J. (1993). Hormone replacement therapy and risk of breast cancer: Results from epidemiologic studies. *American Journal of Obstetrics and Gynecology, 168,* 1473–1480.

Colditz, G.A., Stampfer, M.J., Willett, W.C., Hennekens, C.H., Rosner, B., & Speizer, F.E. (1990). Prospective study of estrogen replacement therapy and risk of breast cancer in postmenopausal women. *Journal of the American Medical Association, 264,* 2648–2653.

Cole, E.N., Groom, G.V., Link, J., O'Flanagan, P.M., & Seldrup, J. (1976). Plasma prolactin concentrations in patients on clomipramine. *Postgraduate Medical Journal, 52*(Suppl. 3), 93–100.

Cole, J., & Bodkin, J.A. (1990). Antidepressant drug side effects. *Journal of Clinical Psychiatry, 51*(1) (Suppl.), 21–26.

Colin-Jones, D.G., Langman, M.J., Lawson, D.H., & Vessey, P. (1985). Post-marketing surveillance of the safety of cimetidine: 12-month morbidity report. *Quarterly Journal of Medicine, 54,* 253–268.

Collins, J. (1990, January). Research highlights. *Research Resources Reporter: Information Exchange,* 1.

Colomes, M., Rispail, Y., Berlan, M., Pous, J., & Montastruc, J.L. (1990). Consommation medicamenteuse d'une population de retraites. *Therapie, 45,* 321–324.

Colpi, G.M., Fanciullacci, F., Aydos, K., & Grugnetti, C. (1991). Effectiveness mechanism of chlomipramine by neurophysiological tests in subjects with true premature ejaculation. *Andrologia, 23,* 45–47.

Comhaire, F. (1976). Treatment of oligospermia with tamoxifen. *International Journal of Fertility, 21,* 232–238.

Condra, M., Surridge, D.H., Morales, A., Fenemore, J., & Owen, J.A. (1986). Prevalence and significance of tobacco smoking in impotence. *Urology, 27,* 495–498.

Connell, J.M., Rapeport, W.G., Beastall, G.H., & Brodie, M.J. (1984). Changes in circulating androgens during short-term carbamazepine therapy. *British Journal of Clinical Pharmacology, 17,* 347–351.

Contrera, J.F., Battaglia, G., Zaczek, R., & DeSouza, E.B. (1988). Fenfluramine neurotoxicity: Selective degeneration and recovery of brain serotonin neurons. *Society for Neuroscience Abstracts: 18th Meeting, 14 (pt. 1),* 556.

Cooke, C.W., & Dworkin, S. (1979). *The Ms. guide to a woman's health.* New York: Doubleday & Co.

Coombes, R.C., Powles, T.J., Muindi, J., Hunt, J., Ward, M., Perez, D., & Neville, A.M. (1985). Trilostane therapy for advanced breast cancer. *Cancer Treatment Reports, 69,* 351–354.

Cooper, A.J. (1977). Bromocriptine in impotence [Letter to the editor]. *Lancet, 2,* 567.

Cooper, A.J. (1986). Progestogens in the treatment of male sexual offenders: A review. *Canadian Journal of Psychiatry, 31,* 73–79.

Cooper, A.J. (1988). Medroxyprogesterone acetate as a treatment for sexual acting out in organic brain syndrome [Letter to the editor]. *American Journal of Psychiatry, 145,* 1179–1180.

Cooper, A.J., Smith, C.G., Ismail, A.A., & Loraine, J.A. (1973). A controlled trial of Potensan Forte ("aphrodisiac" and testosterone combined) in impotence. *Irish Journal of Medical Science, 142,* 155–161.

Cooper, B.R., Hester, T.J., & Maxwell, R.A. (1980). Behavioral and biochemical effects of the antidepressant bupropion (Wellbutrin): Evidence for selective blockade of dopamine uptake in vivo. *Journal of Pharmacology and Experimental Therapeutics, 215,* 127–134.

Cooper, R.L., Seppala, M., & Linnoila, M. (1984). Effect of luteinizing hormone-releasing hormone antiserum on sexual behavior in the female rat. *Pharmacology, Biochemistry, and Behavior, 20,* 527–530.

Coopland, A.T. (1989). Geriatric urogynecology. *Obstetrics and Gynecology Clinics of North America, 16,* 931–937.

Coplen, S.E., Antman, E.M., Berlin, J.A., Hewitt, P., & Chalmers, T.C. (1990). Efficacy and safety of quinidine therapy for maintenance of sinus rhythm after cardioversion. A meta-analysis of randomized control trials. *Circulation, 82,* 1106-1116.

Corby, J.C., Roth, W.T., Zarcone, V.P., & Kopell, B.S. (1978). Psychophysiological correlates of the practice of tantric yoga meditation. *Archives of General Psychiatry, 35,* 571-577.

Cordoba, O.A., & Chapel, J.L. (1983). Medroxyprogesterone acetate antiandrogen treatment of hypersexuality in a pedophiliac sex offender. *American Journal of Psychiatry, 140,* 1036-1039.

Corinaldesi, R., Pasquali, R., Capelli, M., Galassi, A., Plate, L., Melchionda, N., & Barbara, L. (1982). Effect of acute oral and intravenous administration of ranitidine on prolactin, thyrotropin, and gonadotropin serum levels. *Hepatogastroenterology, 29,* 120-123.

Corpas, E., Harman, S.M., & Blackman, M.R. (1993). Human growth hormone and human aging. *Endocrine Reviews, 14,* 20-39.

Costall, B., Naylor, R.J., Marsden, C.D., & Pycock, C. J. (1976). Serotonergic modulation of the dopamine response from the nucleus accumbens. *Journal of Pharmacy and Pharmacology, 28,* 523-526.

Cotariu, D., & Zaidman, J.L. (1991). Minireview: Developmental toxicity of valproic acid. *Life Sciences, 48,* 1341-1350.

Cotton, N.S. (1979). The familial incidence of alcoholism: A review. *Journal of Studies on Alcohol, 40,* 89-116.

Couper-Smartt, J.D., & Rodham, R. (1973). A technique for surveying side effects of tricyclic drugs with reference to reported sexual effects. *Journal of International Medical Research, 1,* 473-476.

Couwenbergs, C.J.T. (1988). Acute effects of drinking beer or wine on the steroid hormones of healthy men. *Journal of Steroid Biochemistry, 31,* 467-473.

Coward, D.M. (1992). General pharmacology of clozapine. *British Journal of Psychiatry, 160* (Suppl. 17), 5-11.

Cowart, V. (1988a). In reply: Behavior disorders and the Ritalin controversy [Letter to the editor]. *Journal of the American Medical Association, 260,* 2219.

Cowart, V. (1988b). The Ritalin controversy: What's made this drug's opponents hyperactive. *Journal of the American Medical Association, 259,* 2521-2523.

Cowdry, R.W., & Gardner, D.L. (1988). Pharmacology of borderline personality disorder. *Archives of General Psychiatry, 45,* 184-188.

Cox, H.M., & Cuthbert, A.W. (1989). Antisecretory activity of the alpha$_2$-adrenoceptor agonist, xylazine, in rat jejunal epithelium. *Naunyn-Schmiedeberg's Archives of Pharmacology, 339,* 669-674.

Creed, K.E. (1989). Effect of castration on penile erection in the dog. *Neurourology and Urodynamics, 8,* 607-614.

Crenshaw, R. (1992). Treatment of premature ejaculation with fluoxetine. Paper presented at American Psychiatric Association Meeting, May.

Crenshaw, T.L. (1983). *Bedside manners: Your guide to better sex.* New York: McGraw-Hill Book Co.

Crenshaw, T.L., Goldberg, J.P., & Stern, W.C. (1987). Pharmacologic modification of psychosexual dysfunction. *Journal of Sex and Marital Therapy, 13,* 239-252.

Crews, D. (1988). The problem with gender. *Psychobiology, 16,* 321-334.

Criqui, M.H., Suarez, L., Barrett-Connor, E., McPhillips, J., Wingard, D.L., & Garland, C. (1988). Postmenopausal estrogen use and mortality. *American Journal of Epidemiology, 128,* 606-614.

Critchley, P., Perez, F.G., Quinn, N., Coleman, R., Parkes, D., & Marsden, C.D. (1986). Psychosis and the lisuride pump. *Lancet, 2,* 349.

Croog, S.H., Elias, M.F., Colton, T., Baume, R.M., Leiblum, S.R., Jenkins, C.D., Perry, H.M., & Hall, W.D. (1994). Effects of antihypertensive medications on quality of life in elderly hypertensive women. *American Journal of Hypertension, 7,* 329-339.

Croog, S.H., Kong, W., Levine, S., Weir, M.R., Baume, R.M., & Saunders, E. (1990). Hypertensive black men and women: Quality of life and effects of antihypertensive medications. *Archives of Internal Medicine, 150,* 1733-1741.

Croog, S.H., Levine, S., Sudilovsky, A., Baume, R.M., & Clive, J. (1988). Sexual symptoms in hypertensive patients: A clinical trial of antihypertensive medications. *Archives of Internal Medicine, 148,* 788-794.

Croog, S.H., Levine, S., Testa, M.A., Brown, B., Bulpitt, C.J., Jenkins, C.D., Klerman, G., & Williams, G.H. (1986). The effects of antihypertensive therapy on quality of life. *New England Journal of Medicine, 314,* 1657-1664.

Crooij, M.J., de Nooyer, C.C., Rao, B.R., Berends, G.T., Gooren, L.J., & Janssens, J. (1988). Termination of early pregnancy by the 3-beta-hydroxysteroid dehydrogenase inhibitor epostane. *New England Journal of Medicine, 319,* 813-817.

Crowley, T.J., Hydinger, M., Stynes, A.J., & Feiger, A. (1975). Monkey motor stimulation and altered social behavior during chronic methadone administration. *Psychopharmacologia, 43,* 135-144.

Cullberg, J. (1972). Mood changes and menstrual symptoms with different gestagen/estrogen combinations. A double-blind comparison with a placebo. *Acta Psychiatrica Scandanavica, 236* (Suppl. 1), 1-86.

Cumming, D.C., Rebar, R.W., Hopper, B.R., &

Yen, S.S. (1982). Evidence for an influence of the ovary on circulating dehydroepiandrosterone sulfate levels. *Journal of Clinical Endocrinology and Metabolism, 54,* 1069–1071.

Cummings, S.R., Black, D.M., & Rubin, S.M. (1989). Lifetime risk of hip, Colles', or vertebral fracture and coronary heart disease among white postmenopausal women. *Archives of Internal Medicine, 149,* 2445–2448.

Cundy, T., Evans, M., Roberts, H., Wattie, D., Ames, R., & Reid, T.R. (1991). Bone density in women receiving depot medroxyprogesterone acetate for contraception. *British Medical Journal, 303,* 13–16.

Cunningham, G.R., Cordero, E., & Thornby, J.I. (1989). Testosterone replacement with transdermal therapeutic systems. *Journal of the American Medical Association, 261,* 2525–2530.

Curb, J.D., Borhani, N.O., Blaszkowski, T.P., Zimbaldi, N., Fotiu, S., & Williams, W. (1985). Long-term surveillance for adverse effects of antihypertensive drugs. *Journal of the American Medical Association, 253,* 3263–3268.

Curb, J.D., Maxwell, M.H., Schneider, K.A., Taylor, J.O., & Shulman, N.B. (1986). Adverse effects of antihypertensive medications in the Hypertension Detection and Follow-up Program (HDFP). *Progress in Cardiovascular Diseases, 29* (3) (Suppl. 1), 73–88.

Curran, H.V. (1986). Tranquilizing memories: A review of the effects of benzodiazepines on human memory. *Biological Psychology, 23,* 179–213.

Currie, D., Lewis, R.V., McLay, J., Tregaskis, B., & McDevitt, D.G. (1988). Relative effects of digoxin and diltiazem upon memory and psychomotor performance in patients with AF. *Proceedings of British Pharmacological Society (BPS). British Journal of Clinical Pharmacology, 27,* 652P.

Currier, K.D., & Aponte, J.F. (1991). Sexual dysfunction in female adult children of alcoholics. *International Journal of the Addictions, 26,* 195–201.

Cushman, P. (1975). Plasma testosterone levels in healthy male marijuana smokers. *American Journal of Drug and Alcohol Abuse, 2,* 269–275.

Cutler, W.B., & Garcia, C.R. (1984). *The medical management of menopause and premenopause.* Philadelphia: J.B. Lippincott.

Cutler, W.B., & Garcia, C.R. (1992). *Menopause: A guide for women and the men who love them.* (Rev. ed.). New York: W.W. Norton.

Cutler, W.B., Garcia, C.R., & Krieger A.M., (1979). Sexual behavior frequency and menstrual cycle length in mature premenopausal women. *Psychoneuroendocrinology, 4,* 297–309.

Cutler, W.B., Garcia, C.R., & McCoy, N. (1987). Perimenopausal sexuality. *Archives of Sexual Behavior, 16,* 225–234.

Cutolo, M., Balleari, E., Accardo, S., Samanta, E., Cimmino, M.A., Giusti, M., Monachesi, M., & Lomeo, A. (1984). Preliminary results of serum androgen level testing in men with rheumatoid arthritis. *Arthritis and Rheumatism, 27,* 958–959.

Cutolo, M., Balleari, E., Giusti, M., Intra, E., & Accardo, S. (1991). Androgen replacement therapy in male patients with rheumatoid arthritis. *Arthritis & Rheumatism, 34,* 1–5.

Cutolo, M., Balleari, E., Giusti, M., Monachesi, M., & Accardo, S. (1986). Sex hormone in women suffering from rheumatoid arthritis. *Journal of Rheumatology, 13,* 1019–1023.

Dabbs, J.M., & de la Rue, D. (1991). Salivary testosterone measurements among women: relative magnitude of circadian and menstrual cycles. *Hormone Research, 35,* 182–184.

Dackis, C.A., & Gold, M.S. (1985). New concepts in cocaine addiction: The dopamine depletion hypothesis. *Neuroscience and Biobehavioral Review, 9,* 469–477.

Dager, S.R., & Heritch, A.J. (1990). A case of bupropion-associated delirium. *Journal of Clinical Psychiatry, 51*(7), 307–308.

Dahlof, C. (1991). Well-being (quality of life) in connection with hypertensive treatment. *Clinical Cardiology, 14,* 97–103.

Dallo, J., & Knoll, J. (1992). Effect of (-)-para-fluorodeprenyl on survival and copulation in male rats. *Acta Physiologica Hungarica, 79,* 125–129.

Dallo, J., Lekka, N., & Knoll, J. (1986). The ejaculatory behavior of sexually sluggish male rats treated with (-) deprenyl, apomorphine, bromocriptine and amphetamine. *Polish Journal of Pharmacology and Pharmacy, 38,* 251–255.

Dallo, J., Yen, T.T., Farago, I., & Knoll, J. (1988). The aphrodisiac effect of (-) deprenyl in non-copulator males rats. *Pharmacological Research Communications, 20*(Suppl.), 25–26.

Dallob, A.L., Sadick, N.S., Unger, W., Lipert, S., Geissler, L.A., Gregoire, S.L., Nguyen, H.H., Moore, E.C., & Tanaka, W.K. (1994). The effect of finasteride, a 5-alpha-reductase inhibitor, on scalp-skin testosterone and dihydrotestosterone concentrations in patients with male-pattern baldness. *Journal of Clinical Endocrinology and Metabolism, 79,* 703–706.

Dalton, K. (1990). *Once a month: The original premenstrual syndrome handbook.* (4th ed.). Claremont, CA: Hunter House.

Dalton, K., & Dalton, M.J. (1991). DMPA and bone density [Letter to the editor]. *British Medical Journal, 303,* 855.

Damsma, G., Day, J., & Fibiger, H.C. (1989). Lack

of tolerance to nicotine-induced dopamine release in the nucleus accumbens. *European Journal of Pharmacology, 168,* 363-368.

Dana-Haeri, J., Oxley, J., & Richens, A. (1982). Reduction of free testosterone by antiepileptic drugs. *British Medical Journal, 284,* 85-86.

Danguir, J. (1983). Sleep deficits in rats with hereditary diabetes insipidus. *Nature (London), 304,* 163-164.

Daniel, D.G., Mathew, R.J., & Wilson, W.H. (1988). Sex roles and regional cerebral blood flow. *Psychiatry Research, 27,* 55-64.

DaPrada, M., Bonetti, E.P., & Keller, H.H. (1977). Induction of mounting behavior in female and male rats by lisuride. *Neuroscience Letters, 6,* 349-353.

DaPrada, M., Bonetti, E.P., Scherschlicht, R., & Bondiolotti, G.P. (1985). Serotonin involvement in lisuride-induced mounting and in sleep. *Pharmaco-psychiatry, 18,* 202-208.

DaPrada, M., Carruba, M., Saner, A., O'Brien, A., & Pletscher, A. (1973). The action of 5, 6-dihydroxytryptamine and L-dopa on sexual behavior of male rats. *Brain Research, 55,* 383-389.

Da Ros, C., Telöken, C., Sogari, P., Bacelos, M., Silva, F., & Sonto, C. (1994). Caucasian penis: What is the normal size? [abstract] *Journal of Urology, 151,* 323A.

Davidson, J. (1989). Seizures and bupropion: A review, *Journal of Clinical Psychiatry, 50,* 256-261.

Davidson, J. (1990). Reply to: "bupropion dose, seizures, women, and age" [Letter to the editor] *Journal of Clinical Psychiatry, 51,* 389.

Davidson, J.M. (1986a). Androgen replacement therapy in a wider context: Clinical and basic aspects. In L. Dennerstein & I. Fraser (Eds.), *Hormones and behavior* (pp. 433-441). New York: Elsevier Science Publishers.

Davidson, J.M. (1986b). Menopause, sexuality and hormones: A critical survey. In L. Dennerstein & I. Fraser (Eds.), *Hormones and behavior* (pp. 561-572). New York: Elsevier Science Publishers.

Davidson, J.M., Camargo, C., & Smith, E.R. (1979). Effects of androgen on sexual behavior in hypogonadal men. *Journal of Clinical Endocrinology and Metabolism, 48,* 955-958.

Davidson, J.M., Chen, J.J., Crapo, L., Gray, G.D., Greenleaf, W.J., & Catania, J.A. (1983). Hormonal changes and sexual function in aging men. *Journal of Clinical Endocrinology and Metabolism, 57,* 71-77.

Davidson, J.M., & Levine, S. (1972). Endocrine regulation of behavior. *Annual Review of Physiology, 34,* 375-408.

Davidson, J.M., & Rosen, R.C. (1992). Hormonal determinants of erectile function. In R.C. Rosen & S.R. Leiblum (Eds.), *Erectile disorders: Assessment and treatment* (pp. 72-95). New York: Guilford Press.

Davidson, J.M., Stefanick, M.L., Sachs, B.D., & Smith, E.R. (1978). Role of androgen in sexual reflexes of the male rat. *Physiology and Behavior, 21,* 141-146.

Davies, R.H., Harris, B., Thomas, D.R., Cook, N., Read, G., & Riad-Fahmy, D. (1992). Salivary testosterone levels and major depressive illness in men. *British Journal of Psychiatry, 161,* 629-632.

Davies, T.F., Gomez-Pan, A., Watson, M.J., Mountjoy, C.Q., Hanker, J.P., Besser, G.M., & Hall, R. (1977). Reduced gonadotrophin: Response to releasing hormone after chronic administration to impotent men. *Clinical Endocrinology, 5,* 6.

Davis, B.R., Ford, C.E., Remington, R.D., Stamler, R., & Hawkins, C.M. (1986). The Hypertension Detection and Follow-up Program design, methods, and baseline characteristics and blood pressure response of the study population. *Progress in Cardiovascular Diseases, 29*(Suppl. 1), 11-28.

Davis, G.A., Goy, R.W., Baum, S., & Johnson, J. (1988). Facilitation of sexual arousal in male and female rhesus monkeys *(Macaca mulatta)* by the dopamine (D2) agonist LY163502. *Society for Neuroscience Abstracts, 14,* 808.

Davis, M.R. (1987). Screening for postmenopausal osteoporosis. *American Journal of Obstetrics and Gynecology, 156,* 1-5.

Dawson-Hughes, B., Dallal, G.E., Krall, E.A., Sadowski, L., Sahyoun, N., & Tannenbaum, S. (1990). A controlled trial of the effect of calcium supplementation on bone density in postmenopausal women. *New England Journal of Medicine, 323,* 878-883.

Daynes, R.A., Araneo, B.A., Ershler, W.B., Maloney, C., Li, G.Z., & Ryu, S.Y. (1993). Altered regulation of IL-6 production with normal aging: Possible linkage to the age-associated decline in dehydroepiandrosterone and its sulfate derivative. *Journal of Immunology, 150,* 5219-5230.

Deandrea, D., Walker, N., Mehlmauer, M., & White, K. (1982). Dermatological reactions to lithium: A critical review of the literature. *Journal of Clinical Psychopharmacology, 2,* 199-204.

de Beaurepaire, R., & Freed, W.J. (1987). Anatomical mapping of the rat hypothalamus for calcitonin-induced anorexia. *Pharmacology, Biochemistry, and Behavior, 27,* 177-182.

DeBruyne, F.M., Denis, L., Lunglmayer, G., Mahler, C., Newling, D.W., Richards, B., Robinson, M.R., Smith, P.H., Weil, E.H., & Whelan, P. (1988). Long-term therapy with a depot luteinizing hormone-releasing hormone analogue (Zoladex) in patients with advanced prostatic carcinoma. *Journal of Urology, 140,* 775-777.

De Castro, R.M. (1985). Reversal of MAOI-induced anorgasmia with cyproheptadine [Letter to the editor]. *American Journal of Psychiatry, 142,* 783.

Decensi, A.U., Guarneri, D., Marroni, P., Di Cristina, L., Paganuzzi, M., & Boccardo, F. (1989). Evidence for testicular impairment after long-term treatment with a luteinizing hormone-releasing hormone agonist in elderly men. *Journal of Urology, 142,* 1235–1238.

Dechant, K.L., & Clissold, S.P. (1991). Paroxetine: A review of its pharmacodynamic and pharmacokinetic properties and therapeutic potential in depressive illness. *Drugs, 41,* 225–253.

Decina, P., Caracci, G., Harrison, K., & Sandyk, R. (1990). Do neuroleptics cause pain? *American Psychiatric Association Meeting Abstracts, 1990,* 149.

De Feo, M.L., Maggi, M., Guardabasso, V., Rodbard, D., Delitala, G., Fazzi, V., Genazzani, A.D., Facchinetti, F., & Forti, G. (1986). Naloxone administration does not affect gonadotropin secretion in agonadal men either basally or during testosterone treatment. *Journal of Clinical Endocrinology and Metabolism, 63,* 257–261.

DeFreitas, B., & Schwartz, G. (1979). Effects of caffeine in chronic psychiatric patients. *American Journal of Psychiatry, 136,* 1337–1338.

Degen, K. (1982). Sexual dysfunction in women using major tranquilizers. *Psychosomatics, 23,* 959–961.

Deicken, R.F. (1986). Captopril treatment of depression. *Biological Psychiatry, 21,* 1425–1428.

Deicken, R.F., & Carr, R.E. (1987). Testicular swelling associated with desipramine. *Journal of Clinical Psychiatry, 48,* 251–252.

De Labry, L.O., Glynn, R.J., Levenson, M.R., Hermos, J.A., LoCastro, J.S., & Vokonas, P.S. (1992). Alcohol consumption and mortality in an American male population: Recovering the U-shaped curve—findings from a normative aging study. *Journal of Studies on Alcohol, 53,* 25–32.

De Leo, D., Dalla Barba, G., & Dalla Barba, G. (1986). Amineptine versus amitriptyline: Effects on depression, sex drive, and prolactin levels. *Current Therapeutic Research, 40,* 124–132.

Delgado, J.M.R. (1973). Antiaggressive effects of chlordiazepoxides. In S. Garattini, E. Mussini, & L.O. Randall (Eds.), *The benzodiazepines* (pp. 419–432). New York: Raven Press.

DeLisi, L.E., Dauphinais, I.D., & Hauser, P. (1989). Gender differences in the brain: Are they relevant to the pathogenesis of schizophrenia? *Comprehensive Psychiatry, 30,* 197–208.

DeLisi, L.E., Murphy, D.L., Karoum, F., Mueller, E., Targum, S., & Wyatt, R.J. (1984). Phenylethylamine excretion in depression. *Psychiatry Research, 13,* 193–201.

Delitala, G., Devilla, L., Pende, A., & Canessa, A. (1982). Effects of the H2-receptor antagonist ranitidine on anterior pituitary hormone secretion in man. *European Journal of Clinical Pharmacology, 22,* 207–211.

Delitala, G., Devilla, L., Pende, A., & Lotti, G. (1980). Stimulation of prolactin induced by ranitidine, an antagonist of H2-receptors in man. *Journal of Endocrinological Investigation, 3,* 112.

Delitala, G., Giusti, M., Mazzocchi, G., Granziera, L., Tarditi, W., & Giordano, G. (1983). Participation of endogenous opiates in regulation of the hypothalamic-pituitary testicular axis in normal men. *Journal of Clinical Endocrinology and Metabolism, 57,* 1277–1281.

Delle Fave, G.F., Tamburrano, G., DeMagistris, L., Natoli, C., Santoro, M.L., Carratu, R., & Torsoli, A. (1977). Gynaecomastia with cimetidine. *Lancet, 1,* 1319.

Del Pozo, E., Caro, G., & Baeyens, J.M. (1987). Analgesic effects of several calcium channel-blockers in mice. *European Journal of Pharmacology, 137,* 155–160.

Demers, R., Lukesh, R., & Prichard, J. (1970). Convulsions during lithium therapy. *Lancet, 2,* 315–316.

Deminiere, J.M., Piazza, P.V., Le Moal, M., & Simon, H. (1989). Experimental approach to individual vulnerability to psychostimulant addiction. *Neuroscience and Biobehavioral Reviews, 13,* 141–147.

De Moraes, S., & Capaz, F.R. (1983). The effects of ethanol dependence on drug responsiveness of mouse isolated vas deferens. *Journal of Pharmacy and Pharmacology, 36,* 70–72.

Dencker, S.J., & Johansson, G. (1990). Benzodiazepine-like substances in mother's milk. *Lancet, 335,* 413.

Dencker, S.J., Johansson, G., & Milsom, I. (1992). Quantification of naturally occurring benzodiazepine-like substances in human breast milk. *Psychopharmacology, 107,* 69–72.

Denis, L.J., Carneiro de Moura, J.L., Bono, A., Sylvester, R., Whelan, P., Newling, D., Depauw, M., & members of the EORTC GU Group and EORTC Data Center. (1993). Goserelin acetate and flutamide versus bilateral orchidectomy and a phase-III EORTC trail (30853). *Urology, 42,* 119–130.

Dennerstein, L., & Burrows, G. (1986). Psychological effects of progestogens in the postmenopausal years. *Maturitas, 8,* 101–106.

Dennerstein, L., Burrows, G.D., Wood, C., & Hyman, G. (1980). Hormones and sexuality: Effect of estrogen and progestogen. *Obstetrics and Gynecology, 56,* 316–322.

Dennerstein, L., Gotts, G., Brown, J.B., Morse, C.A., Farley, T.M., & Pinol, A. (1994). The relationship between the menstrual cycle and female sexual interest in women with PMS complaints and volunteers. *Psychoneuroendocrinology, 19,* 293-304.

Dennerstein, L., Spencer-Gardner, C., Gotts, G., Brown, J.B., Smith, M.A., & Burrows, G.D. (1985). Progesterone and the premenstrual syndrome: A double-blind crossover trial. *British Medical Journal, 290,* 1617-1621.

Dequeker, J. (1988). Calcified tissues: Structure-function relationships. In B.E. Nordin (Ed.), *Calcium in human biology* (pp. 209-240). New York: Springer-Verlag.

Dequeker, J., & Geusens, P. (1990). Treatment of established osteoporosis and rehabilitation: Current practice and possibilities. *Maturitas, 12,* 1-36.

Deslypere, J.P., Verdonck, L., & Vermeulen, A. (1985). Fat tissue: A steroid reservoir and site of steroid metabolism. *Journal of Clinical Endocrinology and Metabolism, 61,* 564-570.

Deslypere, J.P., & Vermeulen, A. (1984). Leydig cell function in normal men: Effect of age, life-style, residence, diet, and activity. *Journal of Clinical Endocrinology and Metabolism, 59,* 955-962.

Deslypere, J.P., & Vermeulen, A. (1985). Influence of age on steroid concentrations in skin and striated muscle in women and in cardiac muscle and lung tissue in men. *Journal of Clinical Endocrinology and Metabolism, 61,* 648-653.

Deutsch, S.I., Kaushik, M., Huntzinger, J.A., Novitzki, M.R., & Mastropaolo, J. (1991). Potentiation of ethanol via interference with calcium channels. *Pharmacology, Biochemistry, and Behavior, 38,* 665 668.

DeVeaugh-Geiss, J., Landau, P., & Katz, R. (1989). Preliminary results from a multi-center trial of clomipramine in obsessive-compulsive disorder. *Psychopharmacology Bulletin, 25,* 36-40.

De Vries, G.J., Buijs, R.M., & Sluiter, A.A. (1984). Gonadal hormone actions on the morphology of the vasopressinergic innervation of the adult rat brain. *Brain Research, 298,* 141-145.

De Vries, G.J., Buijs, R.M., & Van Leeuwen, F.W. (1984). Sex differences in vasopressin and other neurotransmitter systems in the brain. *Progress in Brain Research, 61,* 185-203.

De Vries, G.J., Buijs, R.M., Van Leeuwen, F.W., Caffe, A.R., & Swaab, D.F. (1985). The vasopressinergic innervation of the brain in normal and castrated rats. *Journal of Comparative Neurology, 233,* 236-254.

De Vries, J., Van de Merwe, S.A., & Jan de Heer, L. (1989). From timolol to betaxolol [Letter to the editor]. *Archives of Ophthalmology, 107,* 634.

Dewar, J.A., Horobin, J.M., Preece, P.E., Tavendale, R., Tunstall-Pedoe, H., & Wood, R.A. (1992). Long-term effects of tamoxifen on blood lipid values in breast cancer. *British Medical Journal, 305,* 225-226.

Dews, P.B. (1982). Caffeine. *Annual Review of Nutrition, 2,* 323-341.

Dewsbury, D.A. (1967). Effects of alcohol ingestion on copulatory behavior of male rats. *Psychopharmacologia (Berlin), 11,* 276-281.

Diamond, M. (1970). Intromission pattern and species vaginal code in relation to induction of pseudopregnancy. *Science, 169,* 995-997.

Diamond, M.P., Grainger, D.A., Laudano, A.J., Starick-Zych, K., & DeFronzo, R.A. (1991). Effect of acute physiological elevations of insulin on circulating androgen levels in nonobese women. *Journal of Clinical Endocrinology and Metabolism, 72,* 883-887.

Di Chiara, G., & Imperato, A. (1985). Ethanol preferentially stimulates dopamine release in the nucleus accumbens of freely moving rats. *European Journal of Pharmacology, 115,* 131-132.

Di Chiara, G., & Imperato, A. (1986). Alcohol and barbiturates preferentially stimulate dopamine release in the nucleus accumbens of freely moving rats. In G. Biggio, P.F. Spano, G. Toffano, & G.L. Gessa (Eds.), *Modulation of central and peripheral transmitter function* (pp. 89-95). New York: Springer-Verlag.

Diederichs, W., Stief, C.G., Benard, F., Bosch, R., Lue, T.F., & Tanagho, E.A. (1991). The sympathetic role as an antagonist of erection *Urological Research, 19,* 123-126.

Diederichs, W., Stief, C.G., Lue, T.F., & Tanagho, E.A. (1990). Norepinephrine involvement in penile detumescence. *Journal of Urology, 143,* 1264-1266.

Dienstfrey, H. (1991). *Where the mind meets the body.* New York: Harper Collins.

Dietch, J.T., & Jennings, R.K. (1988). Aggressive dyscontrol in patients treated with benzodiazepines. *Journal of Clinical Psychiatry, 49,* 184-188.

DiMascio, A. (1973). The effects of benzodiazepines on aggression: Reduced or increased? *Psychopharmacologia, 30*(2), 95-110.

Dimenas, E.S., Wiklund, J.K., Dahlof, C.G., Lindvall, K.G., Olofsson, B.K., & De Faire, U. H. (1989). Differences in the subjective well-being and symptoms of normotensives, borderline hypertensives, and hypertensives. *Journal of Hypertension, 7,* 885-890.

DiPaolo, T., Masson, S., Daigle, M., & Belanger, A. (1987). Effect of a combined physiological dose of 17B-estradiol and progesterone on male and female rat striatum dopamine and serotonin metabolism. *Journal of Neurochemistry, 48* (Suppl.), S126.

Ditkoff, E.C., Crary, W., Cristo, M., & Lobo, R.A. (1991). Estrogen improves psychological function in asymptomatic postmenopausal women. *Obstetrics and Gynecology, 78,* 991-995.

Dixson, A.F. (1987). Effects of adrenalectomy upon proceptivity, receptivity, and sexual attractiveness in ovariectomized marmosets (*Callithrix jacchus*). *Physiology and Behavior, 39,* 495-499.

Dixson, A.F., Kendrick, K.M., Blank, M.A., & Bloom, S.R. (1984). Effects of tactile and electrical stimuli upon release of vasoactive intestinal polypeptide in the mammalian penis. *Journal of Endocrinology, 100,* 249-252.

Doelle, G.C., Alexander, A.N., Evans, R.M., Linde, R., Rivier, J., Vale, W., & Rabin, D. (1983). Combined treatment with a LHRH agonist and testosterone in man: Reversible oligozoospermia without impotence. *Journal of Andrology, 4,* 298-302.

Dolecek, R. (1980). Endocrine studies with mazindol in obese patients. *Pharmatherapeutica, 2,* 309-316.

Dollery, C.T. (1987). An update on the Medical Research Council hypertenstion trial. *Journal of Hypertension, 5*(Suppl. 3), S75-S78.

Dollery, C.T., & Harington, M. (1962). Methyldopa in hypertension. Clinical and pharmacological studies. *Lancet, 1,* 759-763.

Donkervoort, T., Zinner, N.R., Sterling, A.M., Donker, P.J., Van Ness, J., & Ritter, R.C. (1975). Megestrol acetate in treatment of benign prostatic hypertrophy. *Urology, 6,* 580-587.

Doogan, D.P., & Caillard, V. (1988). Sertraline: A new antidepressant. *Journal of Clinical Psychiatry, 49* (Suppl. 8), 46-51.

Doren, M., & Schneider, H.P.G. (1989). Overall rationale for hormonal substitution therapy after the menopause. In M. L'Hermite (Ed.), *Update on hormonal treatment in the menopause* (pp. 1-15). Basel: Karger.

Dorevitch, A., & Davis, H. (1994). Fluvoxamine-associated sexual dysfunction. *Annals of Pharmacotherapy, 28,* 872-874.

Dornbush, R.L., Kolodny, R.C., Bauman, J.E., & Webster, S.K. (1978). Human female chronic marijuana use and endocrine functioning. *Society for Neuroscience Abstracts, 4,* 490.

Dorner, G., Docke, F., Gotz, F., Rohde, W., Stahl, F., & Tonjes, R. (1987). Sexual differentiation of gonadotrophin secretion, sexual orientation, and gender role behavior. *Journal of Steroid Biochemistry, 27,* 1081-1087.

Dow, A. (1993). Deprenyl: The anti-aging drug. Delavan, WI: Hallberg Publishing.

Dow, M.G., Hart, D.M., & Forrest, C.A. (1983). Hormonal treatments of sexual unresponsiveness in postmenopausal women: A comparative study. *British Journal of Obstetrics and Gynecology, 90,* 361-366.

Dow, M.G.T. (1983). A controlled comparative evaluation of conjoint counseling and self-help behavioral treatment for sexual dysfunction. Unpublished Ph.D. dissertation: University of Glasgow.

Downie, J.W., & Bialik, G.J. (1988). Evidence for a spinal site of action of clonidine on somatic and viscerosomatic reflex activity evoked on the pudendal nerve in cats. *Journal of Pharmacology and Experimental Therapeutics, 246,* 352-358.

Downie, J.W., Espey, M.J., & Gajewski, J.B. (1991). Alpha$_2$-adrenoceptors not imidazole receptors mediate depression of a sacral spinal reflex in the cat. *European Journal of Pharmacology, 195,* 301-304.

Drago, F., & Scapagnini, U. (1983). Prolactin and behavior: A neurochemical substrate. In R. D'Agata, M.B. Lipsett, P. Polosa, & H.J. van der Molen (Eds.), *Recent advances in male reproduction: Molecular basis and clinical implications.* (pp. 299-303). New York: Raven Press.

Driscoll, R., & Thompson, C. (1993). Salivary testosterone levels and major depressive illness in men [Letter to the editor]. *British Journal of Psychiatry, 163,* 122-123.

Duch, S., Duch, C., Pasto, L., & Ferrer, P. (1992). Changes in depressive status associated with topical beta-blockers. *International Ophthalmology, 16,* 331-335.

Duffy, J.D., & Campbell, J. (1994). Bupropion for the treatment of fatigue associated with multiple sclerosis. *Psychosomatics, 35,* 170-171.

Dufresne, R.L., Kass, D.J., & Becker, R.E. (1988). Bupropion and thiothixene versus placebo and thiothixene in the treatment of depression in schizophrenia. *Drug Dev. Res., 12,* 259-266.

Dukes, M.N. (1988). *Meyler's side effects of drugs. Vol. 11.* New York: Excerpta Medica.

Dundee, J.W. (1990). Fantasies during benzodiazepine sedation in women. Proceedings of British Pharmacological Society. *British Journal of Clinical Pharmacology, 30,* 311P.

Dupont, W.D., & Page, D.L. (1991). Menopausal estrogen replacement therapy and breast cancer. *Archives of Internal Medicine, 151,* 67-72.

Durden-Smith, J., & deSimone, D. (1983). *Sex and the brain.* New York: Arbor House.

Durst, N., & Maoz, B. (1979). Psychology of the menopause. In P.A. van Keep, D.M. Serr, & R.B. Greenblatt (Eds.), *Female and male climacteric* (pp. 9-16). Baltimore: Universtiy Park Press.

Duvoisin, R.C., & Yahr, M.D. (1972). Behavioral abnormalities occurring in Parkinsonism during treatment with L-dopa. In S. Malitz (Ed.), *L-dopa and behavior* (pp. 57–72). New York: Raven Press.

Dux, S., Grosskopf, I., Boner, G., & Rosenfeld, J.B. (1986). Labetalol in the treatment of essential hypertension: A single-blind dose ranging study. *Journal of Clinical Pharmacology, 26,* 346–350.

Dyner, T.S., Lang, W., Geaga, J., Golub, A., Stites, D., Winger, E., Galmarini, M., Masterson, J., & Jacobson, M.A. (1993). An open-label dose-escalation trial of oral dehydroepiandrosterone tolerance and pharmacokinetics in patients with HIV disease. *Journal of Acquired Immune Deficiency Syndromes, 6,* 459–465.

Eaker, E.D., & Castelli, W.P. (1987). Differential risk for coronary heart disease among women in the Framingham Study. In E. Eaker, B. Packar, N. Wenger, T. Clarkson, & H.A. Tyroler (Eds.), *Coronary heart disease in women* (pp. 122–130). New York: Haymarket Doyma.

Early Breast Cancer Trialists' Collaborative Group. (1992). Systemic treatment of early breast cancer by hormonal, cytotoxic, or immune therapy. *Lancet, 339,* 1–15, 71–85.

Eaton, H. (1973). Clomipramine (Anafranil) in the treatment of premature ejaculation. *Journal of International Medical Research, 1,* 432–434.

Eaton, R.C., Markowski, V.P., Lumley, L.A., Thompson, J.T., Moses, J., & Hull, E.M. (1991). D2 receptors in the paraventricular nucleus regulate genital responses and copulation in male rats. *Pharmacology, Biochemistry & Behavior, 39,* 177–188.

Eccleston, D., & Cole, A.J. (1990). Calcium-channel blockade and depressive illness. *British Journal of Psychiatry, 156,* 889–891.

Echenhofer, F.G., & Coombs, M.M. (1987). A brief review of research and controversies in EEG biofeedback and meditation. *Journal of Transpersonal Psychology, 19,* 161–170.

Edmonds, D., Vetter, H., & Vetter, W. (1987). Angiotensin converting enzyme inhibitors in the clinic: Quality of life. *Journal of Hypertension, 5*(Suppl. 3), S31-S35.

Edwards, C.R., & Padfield, P.L. (1985). Angiotensin-converting enzyme inhibitors: Past, present, and bright future. *Lancet, 1,* 30–35.

Egan, G.P., & Hammad, G.E.M. (1976). Sexual disinhibition with L-tryptophan. *British Medical Journal, 2,* 701.

Ehlers, C.L., Chaplin, R.I., & Koob, G.F. (1990). EEG effects of Ro-15-4513 and FG 7142 alone and in combination with ethanol. *Pharmacology, Biochemistry and Behavior, 36,* 607–611.

Ehlers, C.L., Rickler, K.C., & Hovey, J.E. (1980). A possible relationship between plasma testosterone and aggressive behavior in a female outpatient population. In M. Girgis & L.G. Kiloh (Eds.), *Limbic epilepsy and the dyscontrol syndrome* (pp. 183–194). New York: Elsevier/North-Holland Biomedical Press.

Ehrensing, R.H., & Kastin, A.J. (1976). Clinical investigations for emotional effects of neuropeptide hormones. *Pharmacology, Biochemistry, and Behavior, 5,* 89–93.

Ehrinpreis, M.N., Dhar, R., & Narula, A. (1989). Cimetidine-induced galactorrhea. *American Journal of Gastroenterology, 84,* 563–565.

Eison, A.S., Eison, M.S., Torrente, J.R., Wright, R.N., & Yocca, F.D. (1990). Nefazodone: Preclinical pharmacology of a new antidepressant. *Psychopharmacology Bulletin, 26,* 311–315.

Elands, J., van Doremalen, E., Spruyt, B., & de Kloet, E.R. (1991). Oxytocin receptors in the rat hypothalamic ventromedial nucleus: A study of possible mediators of female sexual behavior. In S. Jard & R. Jamison (Eds.), *Vasopressin* (pp. 311–319). London: John Libbey Eurotext.

Elia, G., & Bergman, A. (1993). Estrogen effects on the urethra: Beneficial effects in women with genuine stress incontinence. *Obstetrical and Gynecological Survey, 48,* 509–517.

Elist, J., Jarman, W.D., & Edson, M. (1984). Evaluating medical treatment of impotence. *Urology, 23,* 374.

Elixhauser, A., McMenamin, P., & Witsberger, C. (1991). A study of gastroenterologists in the United States. *American Journal of Gastroenterology, 86,* 406–411.

Elkayam, U., Amin, J., Mehra, A., Vasquez, J., Weber, L., & Rahimtoola, S.H. (1990). A prospective, randomized, double-blind crossover study to compare the efficacy and safety of chronic nifedipine therapy with that of isosorbide dinitrate and their combination in the treatment of chronic congestive heart failure. *Circulation, 82,* 1954–1961.

Ellertsen, B., Johnsen, T.B., & Ursin, H. (1978). Relationship between the hormonal responses to activation and coping. In H. Ursin, E. Baade, & S. Levine (Eds.), *Psychobiology of stress: A study of coping men* (pp. 105–122). New York: Academic Press.

Ellinwood, E.H., & Rockwell, W.J.K. (1975, March). Effect of drug use on sexual behavior. *Medical Aspects of Human Sexuality, 9,* 10–23.

Ellis, W.J., & Grayhack, J.T. (1963). Sexual function in aging males after orchiectomy and estrogen therapy. *Journal of Urology, 89,* 895–899.

Emeriau, J.P., Descamps, A., Dechelotte, P., Poch, B., Harribey, B., Alla, P., & Colle, M. (1988). Zolpidem and flunitrazepam: A multicenter trial in elderly hospitalized patients. In J.P. Sauvanet,

S.Z. Langer, & P.L. Morselli (Eds.), *Imidazopyridines in sleep disorders* (pp. 317-326). New York: Raven Press.

Engelhardt, H., Gore-Langton, R.E., & Armstrong, D.T. (1988). Mevinolin (lovastatin) inhibits androstenedione production by porcine ovarian thecal cells at the level of the 17 alpha-hydroxylase: C-17, 20-lyase complex. *Endocrinology, 124*(5), 2297-2304.

Erickson, J., & Fisher, A. (1983). Myalgia associated with trazodone. *American Journal of Psychiatry, 140,* 1256-1257.

Eriksson, M., & Uvnas-Moberg, K. (1990). Plasma levels of vasoactive intestinal polypeptide and oxytocin in response to suckling, electrical stimulation of the mammary nerve, and oxytocin infusion in rats. *Neuroendocrinology, 51,* 237-240.

Ernster, V.L., Bush, T.L., Huggins, G.R., Hulka, B.S., Kelsey, J.L., & Schottenfeld, D. (1988). Clinical perspectives: Benefits and risks of menopausal estrogen and/or progestin hormone use. *Preventative Medicine, 17,* 201-223.

Eskin, B.A. (1984). Current approaches in endocrinology. In M. Ficher, R.E. Fishkin, & J.A. Jacobs (Eds.), *Sexual arousal* (pp. 116-141). Springfield, Illinois: Charles C. Thomas.

Espinel, C.H., Williams, J.L., & Coughlin, S.S. (1990). Enalapril and lisinopril in the treatment of mild to moderate essential hypertension. *Clinical Therapeutics, 12,* 181-190.

Estes, K.S., Brewster, M.E., Simpkins, J.W., & Bodor, N. (1987). A novel redox system for CNS-directed delivery of estradiol causes sustained LH suppression in castrated rats. *Life Sciences, 40,* 1327-1334.

Etgen, A.M. (1990). Intrahypothalamic implants of noradrenergic antagonists disrupt lordosis behavior in female rats. *Physiology and Behavior, 48,* 31-36.

Ettinger, B. (1987). Overview of the efficacy of hormonal replacement therapy. *American Journal of Obstetrics and Gynecology, 156,* 1298-1303.

Evans, C.M. (1986). Alcohol and violence: Problems relating to methodology, statistics, and causation. In P.F. Brain (Ed.), *Alcohol and aggression* (pp. 138-160). Dover, NH: Croom Helm.

Evans, H.J., Fletcher, J., Torrance, M., & Hargreave, T.B. (1981). Sperm abnormalities and cigarette smoking. *Lancet, 1,* 627.

Evans, I.M., & Distiller, L.A. (1979). Effects of luteinizing hormone-releasing hormone on sexual arousal in normal men. *Archives of Sexual Behavior, 8,* 385-395.

Everett, H.C. (1975). The use of bethanechol chloride with tricyclic antidepressant. *American Journal of Psychiatry, 132,* 1202-1204.

Everitt, B.J. (1977). Effects of clomipramine and other inhibitors of monoamine uptake on the sexual behavior of female rats and rhesus monkeys. *Postgraduate Medical Journal, 53*(Suppl. 4), 202-210.

Everitt, B.J. (1978). Monoamines and sexual behavior in non-human primates. In R. Porter & J. Whelan (Eds.), *Sex, hormones, and behavior: Ciba Foundation symposium* (pp. 329-358). New York: Excerpta Medica.

Everitt, B.J. (1980). Alterations in sexual behavior and 5-hydroxyindoleacetic acid in the cerebrospinal fluid of female rhesus monkeys treated with clomipramine. *Postgraduate Medical Journal, 56* (Suppl. 1), 53-57.

Everitt, B.J. (1990). Sexual motivation: A neural and behavioral analysis of the mechanisms underlying appetitive and copulatory responses of male rats. *Neuroscience and Biobehavioral Reviews, 14,* 217-232.

Everitt, B.J., Cador, M., & Robbins, T.W. (1989). Interactions between the amygdala and ventral striatum in stimulus-reward associations: Studies using a second-order schedule of sexual reinforcement. *Neuroscience, 30,* 63-75.

Everitt, B.J., & Fuxe, K. (1977). Dopamine and sexual behavior in female rats: Effects of dopamine receptor agonists and sulpiride. *Neuroscience Letters, 4,* 209-213.

Everitt, B.J., Fuxe, K., & Hokfelt, T. (1974). Inhibitory role of dopamine and 5-hydroxytryptamine in the sexual behavior of female rats. *European Journal of Pharmacology, 29,* 187-193.

Everitt, B.J., Fuxe, K., Hokfelt, T., & Jonsson, G. (1975). Role of monoamines in the control by hormones of sexual receptivity in the female rat. *Journal of Comparative and Physiological Psychology, 89,* 556-572.

Everitt, B.J., & Hansen, S. (1983). Catecholamines and hypothalamic mechanisms. In D. Wheatley (Ed.), *Psychopharmacology and sexual disorders* (pp. 3-14). New York: Oxford University Press.

Everitt, B.J., & Herbert, J. (1971). The effects of dexamethasone and androgens on sexual receptivity in female rhesus monkeys. *Journal of Endocrinology, 51,* 575-588.

Everitt, B.J., Herbert, J., & Hamer, J.D. (1972). Sexual receptivity of bilaterally adrenalectomized female rhesus monkeys. *Physiology and Behavior, 8,* 409-415.

Everitt, D.E., Avorn, J., & Baker, M.W. (1990). Clinical decision-making in the evaluation and treatment of insomnia. *American Journal of Medicine, 89,* 357-362.

Ewertz, M. (1988). Influence of noncontraceptive exogenous and endogenous sex hormones on breast cancer risk in Denmark. *International Journal of Cancer, 42,* 832-838.

Eyal, A., Ish-Shalom, S., Hoch, Z., & Hochberg, Z. (1988). Androgen therapy in hypogonadotrophic hypogonadism: Time course of erotosexual functions. *Archives of Andrology, 20,* 163-169.

Ezzaher, A., Bouanani, N., Su, J.B., Hittinger, L., & Crozatier, B. (1991). Increased negative inotropic effect of calcium channel-blockers in hypertrophied and failing rabbit heart. *Journal of Pharmacology and Experimental Therapeutics, 257,* 466-471.

Fabbri, A., Jannini, E.A., Gnessi, L., Moretti, C., Ulisse, S., Franzese, A., Lazzari, R., Fraioli, F., Frajese, G., & Isidori, A. (1989). Endorphins in male impotence: Evidence for naltrexone stimulation of erectile activity in patient therapy. *Psychoneuroendocrinology, 14,* 103-111.

Fabbri, A., Ulisse, S., Bolotti, M., Ridolfi, M., Spera, G., Dufau, M.L., & Isidori, A. (1989). Opioid regulation of testicular function. In M. Serio (Ed.), *Perspectives in andrology* (pp. 203-212). New York: Raven Press.

Facchinetti, F., Martignoni, E., Petraglia, F., Sances, M., Nappi, G., & Genazzani, A.R. (1987). Premenstrual fall of plasma beta-endorphin in patients with premenstrual syndrome. *Fertility and Sterility, 47,* 570-573.

Fadem, B.H., Barfield, R.J., & Whalen, R.E. (1979). Dose-response and time-response relationships between progesterone and the display of patterns of receptive and proceptive behavior in the female rat. *Hormones and Behavior, 13,* 40-48.

Fahraeus, L., Larsson-Cohn, U., & Wallentin, L. (1983). L-norgestrel and progesterone have different influences on plasma lipoproteins. *European Journal of Clinical Investigation, 13,* 447-453.

Fahrback, S.E., Morrell, J.I., & Pfaff, D.W. (1985). Role of oxytocin in the onset of estrogen-facilitated maternal behavior. In J.S. Amico & A.G. Robinson (Eds.), *Oxytocin: Clinical and laboratory studies* (pp. 372-388). New York: Elsevier Science Publishers.

Fairweather, D.B., Kerr, J.S., & Hindmarch, I. (1993). Psychopharmacological profiles of antidepressants with particular reference to moclobemide and the elderly. In M. Bergener, R.H. Belmaker, & M.S. Trapper (Eds.), *Psychopharmacology for the elderly: Research and clinical implications* (pp. 344-364). New York: Springer.

Falch, J.A., Oftebro, H., & Haug, E. (1987). Early postmenopausal bone loss is not associated with a decrease in circulating levels of 25-hydroxyvitamin D, 1-25-dihydroxyvitamin D, or vitamin D-binding protein. *Journal of Clinical Endocrinology and Metabolism, 64,* 836-841.

Falconer, C., Ekman, G., Malmström, A., & Ulmsten, U. (1994). Decreased collagen synthesis in stress-incontinent women. *Obstetrics and Gynecology, 84,* 583-586.

Falduto, M.T., Czerwinski, S.M., & Hickson, R.C. (1990). Glucocorticoid-induced muscle atrophy prevention by exercise in fast-twitch fibers. *Journal of Applied Physiology, 69,* 1058-1062.

Fan, A.M., & Kizer, K.W. (1990). Selenium—nutritional, toxicologic, and clinical aspects. *Western Journal of Medicine, 153,* 160-167.

Farkas, G.M., & Rosen, R.C. (1976). Effect of alcohol on elicited male sexual response. *Journal of Studies on Alcohol, 37,* 265-272.

Farnsworth, W.E., Cavanaugh, A.H., Brown, J.R., Alvarez, I., & Lewandowski, L.M. (1978). Factors underlying infertility in the alcoholic. *Archives of Andrology, 1,* 193-195.

Farquhar, C.M., Rogers, V., Franks, S., Pearce, S., Wadsworth, J., & Beard, R.W. (1989). A randomized controlled trial of medroxyprogesterone acetate and psychotherapy for the treatment of pelvic congestion. *British Journal of Obstetrics and Gynecology, 96,* 1153-1162.

Fava, G.A., Fava, M., Kellner, R., Serafini, E., & Mastrogiacomo, I. (1981). Depression, hostility and anxiety in hyperprolactinemic amenorrhea. *Psychotherapy and Psychosomatics, 36,* 122-128.

Fava, M., & Borofsky, G.F. (1991). Sexual disinhibition during treatment with a benzodiazepine: A case report. *International Journal of Psychiatry in Medicine, 21,* 99-104.

Fava, M., Fava, G.A., Kellner, R., Serafini, E., & Mastrogiacomo, I. (1982). Depression and hostility in hyperprolactinemia. *Progress in Neuropsychopharmacology and Biological Psychiatry, 6,* 479-482.

Fave, G.F.D., Tamburrano, G., Magistris, L.D., Natoli, C., Santoro, M.L., Carratu, R., & Torsoli, A. (1977). Gynecomastia with cimetidine. *Lancet, i,* 1319.

Feder, R. (1991). Reversal of antidepressant activity of fluoxetine by cyproheptadine in three patients. *Journal of Clinical Psychiatry, 52,* 163-164.

Fedor-Freyburgh, P. (1977). The influence of estrogens on the well being and mental performance in climacteric and postmenopausal women *Acta Obstetricia et Gynecologica Scandinavica, 47* (Suppl. 64), 1-64.

Fedoroff, J.P. (1992). Buspirone hydrochloride in the treatment of an atypical paraphilia. *Archives of Sexual Behavior, 21,* 401-406.

Feher, K., & Feher, T. (1984). Plasma dehydroepiandrosterone, dehydroepiandrosterone sulfate, and androsterone sulfate levels and their interaction with plasma proteins in rheumatoid arthritis. *Ex-*

perimental and Clinical Endocrinology, 84, 197–202.

Feher, T., Szalay, K.S., & Szilagyi, G. (1985). Effect of ACTH and prolactin on dehydroepiandrosterone, its sulfate ester and cortisol production by normal and tumorous human adrenocortical cells. *Journal of Steroid Biochemistry, 23,* 153–157.

Fehm-Wolfsdorf, G., Bachholz, G., Born, J., Voigt, K., & Fehm, H.L. (1988). Vasopressin but not oxytocin enhances cortical arousal: An integrative hypothesis on behavioral effects of neurohypophyseal hormones. *Psychopharmacology, 94,* 496–500.

Fehm-Wolfsdorf, G., Born, J., Voigt, K.H., & Fehm, H.L. (1984). Human memory and neurohypophyseal hormones: Opposite effects of vasopressin and oxytocin. *Psychoneuroendocrinology, 9*(3), 285–292.

Feighner, J.P., Gardner, E.A., Johnston, A., Batey, S.R., Khayrallah, M.A., Ascher, J.A., & Lineberry, C.G. (1991). Double-blind comparison of bupropion and fluoxetine in depressed outpatients. *Journal of Clinical Psychiatry, 52,* 329–335.

Feinstein, A. (1988). Scientific standards in epidemiologic studies of the menace of daily life. *Science, 242,* 1257–1263.

Felding, C., Jensen, L.M., & Tonnesen, H. (1992). Influence of alcohol intake on postoperative morbidity after hysterectomy. *American Journal of Obstetrics and Gynecology, 166,* 667–670.

Feldman, P.E. (1962). An analysis of the efficacy of diazepam. *Journal of Neuropsychiatry, 3*(Suppl.), S62–S67.

Fenster, L., Eskenazi, B., Windham, G.C., & Swan, S.H. (1991). Caffeine consumption during pregnancy and fetal growth. *American Journal of Public Health, 81,* 458–461.

Fentiman, I.S. (1986). Tamoxifen and mastalgia: An emerging indication. *Drugs, 32,* 477–480.

Fentiman, I.S., Caleffi, M., Rodin, A., Murphy, B., & Fogelman, I. (1989). Bone mineral content of women receiving tamoxifen for mastalgia. *British Journal of Cancer, 60,* 262–264.

Fentiman, I.S., & Powles, T.J. (1987). Tamoxifen and benign breast problems. *Lancet, ii,* 1070–1072.

Ferder, L., Inserra, F., & Medina, F. (1987). Safety aspects of long-term antihypertensive therapy (10 years) with clonidine. *Journal of Cardiovascular Pharmacology, 10*(Suppl. 12), S104-S108.

Ferguson, J., Henrickson, S., Cohen, H., Mitchell, G., Barohas, J., & Dement, W. (1970). Hypersexuality and behavioral changes in cats caused by administration of p-chlorophenylalanine. *Science, 168,* 499–501.

Ferguson, K.J., Hoegh, C., & Johnson, S. (1989). Estrogen replacement therapy: A survey of women's knowledge and attitudes. *Archives of Internal Medicine, 149,* 133–136.

Ferkin, M.H., Sorokin, E.S., Renfroe, M.W., & Johnston, R.E. (1994). Attractiveness of male odors to females varies directly with plasma testosterone concentration in meadow voles. *Physiology and Behavior, 55,* 347–353.

Fernandez, F., Adams, F., Holmes, V.F., Levy, J.K., & Neidhart, M. (1987). Methylphenidate for depressive disorders in cancer patients. *Psychosomatics, 28,* 455–461.

Fernandez-Guasti, A., Escalante, A., & Agmo, A. (1989). Inhibitory action of various 5-HT_{1B} receptor agonists on rat masculine sexual behavior. *Pharmacology, Biochemistry, and Behavior, 34,* 811–816.

Ferrari, F. (1984). Cimetidine, but not ranitidine, inhibits penile erections in rats. *Lancet, 1,* 112.

Ferrari, F., & Baggio, G. (1985). Influence of cimetidine, ranitidine, and imidazole on the behavioral effects of (+/−) N-n-propylnorapomorphine in male rats. *Psychopharmacology, 85,* 197–200.

Ferrari, F., Baggio, G., & Mangiafico, V. (1986). Lisuride-induced mounting and its modification by drugs active on adrenergic and dopaminergic receptors. *Pharmacological Research Communications, 18,* 1159–1168.

Ferrari, F., Baggio, G., & Martinelli, R. (1986). Similarities between the behavioral effects of imidazole and those of yohimbine on four animal models. In G. Biggio, P.F. Sparo, G. Toffano, & G.L. Gessa (Eds.), *Modulation of central and peripheral transmitter function* (pp. 519–525). Padova: Liviana Press.

Ferrari, F., Martinelli, R., & Baggio, G. (1986). Imidazole has similar behavioral effects to yohimbine. *Psychopharmacology (Berlin), 88,* 58–62.

Ferreira, S.H. (1985). History of the development of inhibitors of angiotensin I conversion. *Drugs, 30*(Suppl. 1), 1–5.

Ferretti, P., Algeri, S., Benfenati, F., Cimino, M., Ferretti, C., Garattini, S., & Lipartiti, M. (1984). Biochemical effects of minaprine on striatal dopaminergic neurons in rats. *Journal of Pharmacy and Pharmacology, 36,* 48–50.

Ferris, C.F., Pollock, J., Albers, H.E., & Leeman, S.E. (1985). Inhibition of flank marking behavior in golden hamsters by microinjection of a vasopressin antagonist into the hypothalamus. *Neuroscience Letters, 55,* 239–243.

Ferris, R.M., Cooper, B.R., & Maxwell, R.A. (1983). Studies of bupropion's mechanism of antidepressant activity. *Journal of Clinical Psychiatry, 44,* 74–78.

Ferris, R.M., Russell, A., & Topham, P. (1987). Pharmacological studies suggest that sigma receptors labelled in vivo with (+)-[H3]-SKF 10,0047 are predominantly of the high affinity type. In E.F. Domino & J.M. Rameaka (Eds.), *Sigma opioid phenacyclamine-like compounds as molecular probes in biology* (pp. 315-325). Ann Arbor: NPP Books.

Feuerstein, T.J., Hertting, G., & Jackisch, R. (1985). Endogenous noradrenaline as modulator of hippocampal serotonin (5-HT) release: Dual effects of yohimbine, rauwolscine, and corynanthine as alpha-adrenoceptor antagonists and 5-HT-receptor agonists. *Naunyn-Schmiedeberg's Archives of Pharmacology, 329,* 216-221.

Fichtner, C.G., & Braun, B.G. (1992). Bupropion-associated mania in a patient with HIV infection. *Journal of Clinical Psychopharmacology, 12,* 366-367.

Figiel, G.S., & Jarvis, M.R. (1990). Electroconvulsive therapy in a depressed patient receiving bupropion [Letter to the editor]. *Journal of Clinical Psychopharmacology, 10,* 376.

File, S.E., & Guardiola-Lemaitre, B.J. (1988). L-fenfluramine in tests of dominance and anxiety in the rat. *Neuropsychobiology, 20,* 205-211.

File, S.E., & Pellow, S. (1987). Behavioral pharmacology of minor tranquilizers. *Pharmacology and Therapeutics, 35,* 265-290.

Filicori, M., & Crowley, W.F., Jr. (1983). Hypothalamic regulation of gonadotropin secretion in women. In R.L. Norman (Ed.), *Neuroendocrine aspects of reproduction* (pp. 285-294). New York: Academic Press.

Finkelstein, J., Klibanski, A., Neer, R., Greenspan, S., Rosenthal, D., & Crowley, W. (1987). Osteoporosis in men with idiopathic hypogonadotropic hypogonadism. *Annals of Internal Medicine, 106,* 354-361.

Finn, P.R., Kleinman, I., & Pihl, R.O. (1990). The lifetime prevalence of psychopathology in men with multigenerational family histories of alcoholism. *Journal of Nervous and Mental Disease, 178,* 500-504.

Finn, P.R., & Pihl, R.O. (1987). Men at high risk for alcoholism: The effect of alcohol on cardiovascular response to unavoidable shock. *Journal of Abnormal Psychology, 96,* 230-236.

Finn, P.R., & Pihl, R.O. (1988). Risk for alcoholism: A comparison between two different groups of sons of alcoholics on cardiovascular reactivity and sensitivity to alcohol. *Alcoholism: Clinical and Experimental Research, 12,* 742-747.

Finn, S.E., Bailey, J.M., Schultz, R.T., & Faber, R. (1990). Subjective utility ratings of neuroleptics in treating schizophrenia. *Psychological Medicine, 20,* 843-848.

Fioretti, P., Corsini, G.U., Murru, S., Medda, F., Romagnino, F., & Genazzani, A.R. (1978). Psychoneuroendocrinological effects of 2-alfa-bromocriptine therapy in cases of hyperprolactinemic amenorrhea. In L. Carenza, P. Pancheri, & L. Zichella (Eds.), *Clinical psychoneuroendocrinology in reproduction* (pp. 83-106). New York: Academic Press.

Fisher, G., & Steckler, A. (1974). Psychological effects, personality and behavioral changes attributed to marijuana use. *International Journal of the Addictions, 9,* 101-126.

Fisher, S. (1973). *The female orgasm.* New York: Basic Books.

Fisher, S., Bryant, S.G., & Kent, T.A. (1993). Postmarketing surveillance by patient self-monitoring: Trazodone versus fluoxetine. *Journal of Clinical Psychopharmacology, 13,* 235-242.

Fitzgerald, C.T., Elstein, M., & Mansel, R.E. (1993). Hormone replacement therapy and malignancy. *British Journal of Obstetrics and Gynecology, 100,* 408-410.

Flamenbaum, W., Weber, M.A., McMahon, F.G., Materson, B.J., Carr, A.A., & Poland, M. (1985). Monotherapy with labetalol compared with propranolol: Differential effects by race. *Journal of Clinical Hypertension, 1,* 56-69.

Fleischhacker, W.W., Hummer, M., Kurz, M., Kurzthaler, I., Lieberman, J.A., Pollack, S., Safferman, A.Z., & Kane, J.M. (1994). Clozapine dose in the United States and Europe: Implications for therapeutic and adverse effects. *Journal of Clinical Psychiatry, 55*(9: Suppl. B), 78-81.

Fleischmann, J.D., Huntley, H.N., Shingleton, W.B., & Wentworth, D.B. (1991). Clinical and immunological response to nifedipine for the treatment of interstitial cystitis. *Journal of Urology, 146,* 1235-1239.

Fletcher, A.P. (1991). Spontaneous adverse drug reaction reporting versus event monitoring: A comparison. *Journal of the Royal Society of Medicine, 84,* 341-344.

Fletcher, A.E., Bulpitt, C.J., Hawkins, C.M., Havinga, T.K., ten Berge, B.S., May, J.F., Schuurman, F.H., van der Veur, E., & Wesseling, H. (1990). Quality of life on antihypertensive therapy: A randomized double-blind controlled trial of captopril and atenolol. *Journal of Hypertension, 8,* 463-466.

Flood, J.F., Garland, J.S., & Morley, J.E. (1990). Vasoactive intestinal peptide (VIP): An amnestic neuropeptide. *Peptides, 11,* 933-938.

Floth, A., & Schramek, P. (1991). Intracavernous injection of prostaglandin E1 in combination with papaverine: Enhanced effectiveness in comparison with papaverine plus phentolamine and prostaglandin E1 alone. *Journal of Urology, 145,* 56-59.

Fluoxetine Bulimia Nervosa Collaborative Study Group (1992). Fluoxetine in the treatment of bulimia nervosa. *Archives of General Psychiatry, 49,* 139–147.

Fogelman, J. (1988). Verapamil caused depression, confusion, and impotence [Letter to the editor]. *American Journal of Psychiatry, 145,* 380.

Fogelson, D.L., Bystritsky, A., & Pasnau, R. (1992). Bupropion in the treatment of bipolar disorders: The same old story? *Journal of Clinical Psychiatry, 53,* 443–446.

Fontaine, R., & Chouinard, G. (1989). Fluoxetine in the long-term maintenance treatment of obsessive compulsive disorder. *Psychiatric Annals, 19,* 88–91.

Foreman, M.M., Fuller, R.W., Nelson, D.L., Calligaro, D.O., Kurz, K.D., Misner, J.W., Garbrecht, W.L., & Parli, C.J. (1992). Preclinical studies of LY237733, a potent and selective serotonergic antagonist. *Journal of Pharmacology and Experimental Therapeutics, 260,* 51–57.

Foreman, M.M, & Hall, J.L. (1987a). Effects of D-2-dopaminergic receptor stimulation on male rat sexual behavior. *Journal of Neural Transmission, 68,* 153–170.

Foreman, M.M., & Hall, J.L. (1987b). Effects of D-2-dopaminergic receptor stimulation on the lordotic response of female rats. *Psychopharmacology, 91,* 96–100.

Forrest, G. (1983). *Alcoholism and human sexuality.* Springfield, IL: Charles C. Thomas.

Forsberg, L., Gustavii, B., Hojerback, T., & Olsson, A.M. (1979). Impotence, smoking, and beta-blocking drugs. *Fertility and Sterility, 31,* 589–591.

Fossey, M.D., & Hamner, M.B. (1994). Male sexual dysfunction induced by bupropion-sustained release. Paper presented at the Annual Meeting of the American Psychiatric Association. Philadephia, May 21–26.

Fowlie, S., & Burton, J. (1987). Hyperprolactianemia and nonpuerperal lactation associated with clomipramine. *Scottish Medical Journal, 32,* 52.

Fox, C.A., Ismail, A.A., Love, D.N., Kirkham, K.E., & Loraine, J.A. (1972). Studies on the relationship between plasma testosterone levels and human sexual activity. *Journal of Endocrinology, 52,* 51–58.

Fox, C.A., & Knaggs, G.S. (1969). Milk-ejection activity (oxytocin) in peripheral venous blood in man during lactation and in association with coitus. *Journal of Endocrinology, 45,* 145–146.

Frajese, G. (1989). Impotency and replacement therapy. In G. Frajese, E. Steinberger, & L.J. Rodriguez-Rigau (Eds.), *Reproductive medicine: Medical therapy* (pp. 247-263). New York: Elsevier Science Publishers.

Franceschi, M., Perego, L., Cavagnini, F., Cattaneo, A.G., Invitti, C., Caviezel, F., Strambi, L.F., & Smirne, S. (1984). Effects of long-term antiepileptic therapy on the hypothalamic-pituitary axis in man. *Epilepsia, 25,* 46–52.

Frank, E., Anderson, C., & Rubinstein, D. (1978). Frequency of sexual dysfunction in normal couples. *New England Journal of Medicine, 299,* 111–115.

Frankenhaeuser, M. (1983). The sympathetic-adrenal and pituitary-adrenal response to challenge: Comparison between the sexes. In T.M. Dembroski, T.H., Schmidt, & G. Blumchen (Eds.), *Biobehavioral bases of coronary heart disease* (pp. 91–105). Basel: Karger.

Frankenhaeuser, M. (1986). A psychobiological framework for research on human stress and coping. In N.H. Appley & R. Trumbull (Eds.), *Dynamics of stress* (pp. 101–116). New York: Plenum Press.

Franks, A.L., Kendrick, J.S., & Tyler, C.W. (1987). Postmenopausal smoking, estrogen replacement therapy, and the risk of endometrial cancer. *American Journal of Obstetrics and Gynecology, 156,* 20–23.

Fraser, A.R. (1984). Sexual dysfunction following antidepressant drug therapy [Letter to the editor]. *Journal of Clinical Psychopharmacology, 4,* 62–63.

Fraser, D.I., Padwick, M.L., Whitehead, M.I., White, J., Ryder, T.A., & Pryse-Davies, J. (1989). The effects of the addition of nomegesterol acetate to post-menopausal estrogen therapy. *Maturitas, 11,* 21–34.

Fraser, D.I., Whitehead, M.I., Endacott, J., Morton, J., Ryder, T.A., & Pryse-Davies, J. (1989). Are fixed-dose estrogen/progestogen combinations ideal for all HRT users? *British Journal of Obstetrics and Gynecology, 96,* 776–782.

Fraunfelder, F.T., & Meyer, S.M. (1985). Sexual dysfunction secondary to topical ophthalmic timolol [Letter to the editor]. *Journal of the American Medical Association, 253,* 3092–3093.

Frcka, G., & Lader, M. (1988). Psychotropic effects of repeated doses of enalapril, propranolol, and atenolol in normal subjects. *British Journal of Clinical Pharmacology, 25,* 67–73.

Freed, E. (1983). Increased sexual function with nomifensine. *Medical Journal of Australia, 1,* 551.

Freedman, R.R., Sabharwal, S.C., & Desai, N. (1986). Sex differences in peripheral vascular adrenergic receptors. *Circulation Research, 61*(4), 581–585.

Freeman, B.S. (1973, September). Stretch marks on the breast. *Medical Aspects of Human Sexuality,* 263.

Freeman, C.P., Barry, F., Dunkeld-Turnbull, J.D., & Henderson, A. (1988). Controlled trial of psychotherapy for bulimia nervosa. *British Medical Journal, 296,* 521-525.

Freeman, C.P., Trimble, M.R., Deakin, J.F., Stokes, T.M., & Ashford, J.J. (1994). Fluvoxamine versus clomipramine in the treatment of obsessive-compulsive disorder: A multicenter, randomized, double-blind, parallel group comparison. *Journal of Clinical Psychiatry, 55,* 301-305.

Freeman, E., Rickels, K., Sondheimer, S.J., & Polansky, M. (1990). Ineffectiveness of progesterone suppository treatment for premenstrual syndrome. *Journal of the American Medical Association, 264,* 349-353.

Freishtat, H.W. (1988). View from the nation's courts. *Journal of Clinical Psychopharmacology, 8,* 434-436.

Frenken, M., & Kaumann, A.J. (1984). Interaction of ketanserin and its metabolite ketanserinol with 5-HT_2 receptors in pulmonary and coronary arteries of calf. *Naunyn-Schmiedeberg's Archives of Pharmacology, 326,* 334-339.

Frew, A.J., & Holgate, S.T. (1993). Clinical pharmacology of asthma. *Drugs, 46,* 847-862.

Fried, P.A. (1982). Marijuana use by pregnant women and effects on offspring: An update. *Neurobehavioral Toxicology and Teratology, 4,* 451.

Friedman, G.D., & Klatsky, A.L. (1993). Is alcohol good for your health? [Editorial]. *New England Journal of Medicine, 329,* 1882-1883.

Friedman, H.S., Abramowitz, I., Nguyen, T., Babb, B., Stern, M., Farrer, S.M., & Tricomi, V. (1987). Urinary digoxin-like immunoreactive substance in pregnancy. *American Journal of Medicine, 83,* 261-264.

Friedman, S., Kantor, I., Sobel, S., & Miller, R. (1978). A follow-up study of the chemotherapy of neurodermatitis with a monoamine oxidase inhibitor. *Journal of Nervous and Mental Diseases, 166,* 349-357.

Friel, P.N., Logan, B.K., & Fligner, C.L. (1993). Three fatal drug overdoses involving bupropion. *Journal of Analytical Toxicology, 17*(7), 436-438.

Friesen, L.V.C. (1976). Aphrodisia with mazindol. *Lancet, 2,* 974.

Frishman, W.H., Shapiro, W., & Charlap, S. (1989). Labetolol compared with propranolol in patients with both angina pectoris and systemic hypertension: A double-blind study. *Journal of Clinical Pharmacology, 29,* 504-511.

Froehlich, J.C., Harts, J., Lumeng, L., & Li, T.K. (1986). Opioid involvement in ethanol consumption. *Alcohol and Alcoholism, 21,* A107.

Fuchs, A.R. (1985). Oxytocin in animal parturation. In J. Amica & A.G. Robinson (Eds.), *Oxytocin: Clinical and laboratory studies* (pp. 207-235). New York: Elsevier Science Publishers.

Fuller, R.W., Snoddy, H.D., & Robertson, D.W. (1988). Mechanisms of effects of d-fenfluramine on brain serotonin metabolism in rats: Uptake inhibition versus release. *Pharmacology, Biochemistry, and Behavior, 30,* 715-721.

Fuxe, K., Andersson, K., Eneroth, P., Harfstrand, A., & Agnati, L.F. (1989). Neuroendocrine actions of nicotine and of exposure to cigarette smoke: Medical implications. *Psychoneuroendocrinology, 14,* 19-41.

Gaggi, R., & Gianni, A.M. (1990). Effects of calcium antagonists on biogenic amines in discrete brain areas. *European Journal of Pharmacology, 181,* 187-197.

Galanter, M. (Ed.) (1987). *Recent developments in alcoholism: Vol. 7: Treatment research.* New York: Plenum Press.

Galbraith, R.A., & Jellinck, P.H. (1989a). Decreased estrogen hydroxylation in male rat liver following cimetidine treatment. *Biochemical Pharmacology, 38,* 313-319.

Galbraith, R.A., & Jellinck, P.H. (1989b). Differential effects of cimetidine, ranitidine, and famotidine on the hepatic metabolism of estrogen and testosterone in male rats. *Biochemical Pharmacology, 38,* 2046-2049.

Galbraith, R.A., & Michnovicz, J.J. (1989). The effects of cimetidine on the oxidative metabolism of estradiol. *New England Journal of Medicine, 321,* 269-274.

Galeone, M., Moise, G., Ferrante, F., Cacioli, D., Casula, P.L., & Bignamini, A.A. (1978). Double-blind clinical comparison between a gastrin-receptor antagonist, proglumide, and a histamine-H2 blocker, cimetidine. *Current Medical Research and Opinion, 5,* 376-382.

Galeano, C., Corcos, J., Carmel, M., & Jubelin, B. (1989). Action of clonidine on micturitional reflexes in decerebrate cats. *Brain Research, 491,* 45-56.

Galina, Z.H., & Kastin, A.J. (1987). Tyr-MIF-1 attenuates antinociceptive responses induced by three models of stress-analgesia. *British Journal of Pharmacology, 90,* 669-674.

Gambacciani, M., Spinetti, A., Taponeco, F., Cappagli, B., Maffei, S., Manetti, P., Piaggesi, L., & Fioretti, P. (1994). Bone loss in perimenopausal women: A longitudinal study. *Maturitas, 18,* 191-197.

Gambrell, R.D. (1989). Sex steroids and the breast. In M. L'Hermite (Ed.), *Update on hormonal treatment in the menopause* (pp. 49-62). Basel: Karger.

Gambrell, R.D. (1992). Progestogen therapy. In W.F. Rayburn & F.P. Zuspan (Eds.), *Drug therapy in obstetrics and gynecology* (3rd Ed.) (pp. 542-555). St. Louis, MO: Mosby-Year Book.

Gammon, G.D. (1981). Neuroleptics and decreased bone density in women. *American Journal of Psychiatry, 138,* 1517.

Garattini, S., Bizzi, A., Caccia, S., Mennini, T., & Samanin, R. (1988). Progress in assessing the role of serotonin in the control of food intake. *Clinical Neuropharmacology, 11,* S8–S32.

Garattini, S., Borroni, T., Mennini, T., & Samanin, R. (1978). Differences and similarities among anorectic agents. In S. Garattini & R. Samanin (Eds.), *Central mechanisms of anorectic drugs* (pp. 127–143). New York: Raven Press.

Garcia, G., Crismon, M.L., & Dorson, P.G. (1994). Seizures in two patients after the addition of lithium to a clozapine regimen [Letter to the editor]. *Journal of Clinical Psychopharmacology, 14,* 426–428.

Garcia-Ruiz, P.J., de Yébenes, J.G., Jiménez-Jiménez, F.J., Vázquez, A., Urra, D.G., & Morales, B. (1992). Parkinsonism associated with calcium channel-blockers: A prospective follow-up study. *Clinical Neuropharmacology, 15,* 19–26.

Gardner, E.A. (1983). Long-term preventative care in depression: The use of bupropion in patients intolerant of other antidepressants. *Journal of Clinical Psychiatry, 44,* 157–162.

Gardner, E.A. (1984). Effects of bupropion on weight in patients intolerant to previous antidepressants. *Current Therapeutic Research, 35,* 188–199.

Gardner, E.A., & Johnston, J.A. (1985). Bupropion—an antidepressant without sexual pathophysiological action. *Journal of Clinical Psychopharmacology, 5,* 24–29.

Garnett, T., Mitchell, A., & Studd, J. (1991). Patterns of referral to a menopause clinic. *Journal of the Royal Society of Medicine, 84,* 128–130.

Gartrell, N. (1986). Increased libido in women receiving trazodone. *American Journal of Psychiatry, 143,* 781–782.

Gaspard, U.J., Dubois, M., Gillain, D., Franchimont P., & Duvivier, J. (1984). Ovarian function is effectively inhibited by a low-dose triphasic oral contraceptive containing ethinylestradiol and levonorgestrel. *Contraception, 29,* 305–318.

Gastaut, H., & Collomb, H. (1954). Etude du comportement sexuel chez les epileptiques psychomoteurs. *Annales Medico-Psychologiques, 112* (Pt. 2), 657–696.

Gavaler, J.S., & Rosenblum, E.R. (1994). Alcohol effects in postmenopausal women. In R.R. Watson (Ed.), *Drug and alcohol abuse reviews. Vol. 5. Addictive behaviors in women* (pp. 195–214). Totowa, NJ: Humana Press.

Gavras, H., & Gavras, I. (1991). Cardioprotective potential of angiotensin converting enzyme inhibitors. *Journal of Hypertension, 9,* 385–392.

Gawin, F., Compton, M., & Byck, R. (1989). Buspirone reduces smoking [Letter to the editor]. *Archives of General Psychiatry, 46,* 288–289.

Gay, G.R., Newmeyer, J.A., Perry, M., Johnson, G., & Kurland, M. (1982). Love and Haight: The sensuous hippie revisited. Drug/sex practices in San Francisco 1980–1981. *Journal of Psychoactive Drugs, 14,* 111–123.

Gay, G.R., & Sheppard, C.W. (1972). Sex in the "drug culture." *Medical Aspects of Human Sexuality, 6,* 28–47.

Gay, G.R., & Sheppard, C.W. (1973). Sex-crazed dope fiends—myth or reality? *Drug Forum, 2,* 125–140.

Gaziano, J.M., Buring, J.E., Breslow, J.L., Goldhaber, S.Z., Rosner, B., VanDenburgh, M., Willett, W., & Hennekens, C.H. (1993). Moderate alcohol intake increased levels of high-density lipoprotein and its subfractions, and decreased risk of myocardial infarction. *New England Journal of Medicine, 329,* 1829–1834.

Geissler, A.H., Turnlund, J.R., & Cohen, R.D. (1986). Effect of chlorthalidone on zinc levels, testosterone, and sexual function in man. *Drug-Nutrient Interactions, 4,* 275–283.

Gelenberg, A.J. (1991). Valproate in acute mania. *Biological Therapies in Psychiatry Newsletter, 14*(5), 8.

Geller, I., & Seifter, J. (1960). The effects of meprobamate, barbiturates, d-amphetamine, and promazine on experimentally induced conflict in the rat. *Psychopharmacologia, 1,* 482–492.

Geller, J., Nelson, C.G., Albert, J.D., & Pratt, C. (1979). Effect of megestrol acetate on uroflow rates in patients with benign prostatic hypertrophy: Double-blind study. *Urology, 14,* 467–474.

Genazzani, A.R., DeVoto, M., Cianchetti, C., Pintor, C., Facchinetti, F., Mangoni, A., & Fioretti, P. (1978). Possible correlation between plasma androgen variations during the menstrual cycle and sexual behavior in the human female. In P. Carenza, P. Pancheri, & L. Zichella (Eds.), *Clinical psychoneuroendocrinology in reproduction* (pp. 419–436). New York: Academic Press.

Genazzani, A.R., Gastaldi, M., Bidzinska, B., Mercuri, N., Genazzani, A.D., Nappi, R.E., Segre, A., & Petraglia, F. (1992). The brain as a target organ of gonadal steroids. *Psychoneuroendocrinology, 17,* 385–390.

Genazzani, A.R., Petraglia, F., Cleva, M., Brilli, G., Mercuri, N., De Ramundo, B.M., & Volpe, A. (1989). Norgestimate increases pituitary and hypothalamic concentrations of immunoreactive beta-endorphin. *Contraception, 40,* 605–613.

Genazzani, A.R., Petraglia, F., Facchinetti, F., D'Ambrogio, G., Cocchi, D., & Muler, E.E.

(1984). Effects of sex steroids on peripheral and pituitary endorphins. In P. Pancheri, L. Zichella, & P. Falaschi (Eds.), *Endorphins, neuroregulators, and behavior in human reproduction* (pp. 148–152). Princeton: Excerpta Medica.

Genazzani, A.R., Petraglia, F., Facchinetti, F., Grasso, A., Alessandrini, G., & Volpe, A. (1988). Steroid replacement treatment increases beta-endorphin and beta-lipotropin plasma levels in postmenopausal women. *Gynecologic and Obstetric Investigation, 26,* 153–159.

Geneve, J., Larrey, D., Amouyal, G., Belghiti, J., & Pessayre, D. (1987). Metabolic activation of the tricyclic antidepressant amineptine by human liver cytochrome P-450. *Biochemical Pharmacology, 36,* 2421–2424.

Gennaro, A. (Ed.). (1990). *Remington's pharmaceutical sciences (18th ed.).* Easton, PA: Maok Publishing.

George, N.J., & Reading, C. (1986). Sympathetic nervous system and dysfunction of the lower urinary tract. *Clinical Science, 70*(Suppl. 14), 69s–76s.

George, W.H., Gournic, S.J., & McAfee, M.P. (1988). Perceptions of postdrinking female sexuality: Effects of gender, beverage choice, and drink payment. *Journal of Applied Social Psychology, 18,* 1295–1317.

George, W.H., & Marlatt, G.A. (1986). The effects of alcohol and anger on interest in violence, erotica, and deviance. *Journal of Abnormal Psychology, 95,* 150–158.

Gerald, M.C., & Schwirian, P.M. (1973). Nonmedical use of methaqualone. *Archives of General Psychiatry, 28,* 627–631.

Geraldini, C., Faedda, M.T., & Sideri, G. (1984). Anticonvulsant therapy and its possible consequences on peripheral nervous system: A neurographic study. *Epilepsia, 25,* 502–505.

Gerber, J.G. (1983). The role of prostaglandins in the hemodynamic and tubular effects of furosemide. *Federation Proceedings, 42,* 1707–1710.

Gerlach, J., & Peacock, L. (1994). Motor and mental side effects of clozapine. *Journal of Clinical Psychiatry, 55*(9: Suppl B), 107–109.

Germain, L., & Chouinard, G. (1989). Open-label study of captopril in the treatment of major unipolar recurrent depression. *Biological Psychiatry, 25,* 81A.

Gerner, R.H., & Stanton, A. (1992). Algorithm for patient management of acute manic states: Lithium, valproate, or carbamazepine. *Journal of Clinical Psychopharmacology, 12,* 575–635.

Gerris, J., Peeters, K., Comhaire, F., Schoonjans, F., & Hellemans, P. (1991). Placebo-controlled trial of high-dose mesterolone treatment of idiopathic male infertility. *Fertility and Sterility, 55,* 603–607.

Gerstenberg, T.C., Metz, P., Ottesen, B., & Fahrenkrug, J. (1992). Intracavernous self-injection with vasoactive intestinal polypeptide and phentolamine in the management of erectile failure. *Journal of Urology, 147,* 1277–1279.

Gerster, J.C., Charhon, S.A., Jaeger, P., Boivin, G., Briancon, D., Rostan, A., Baud, C.A., & Meunier, P.J. (1983). Bilateral fractures of femoral neck in patients with moderate renal failure receiving fluoride for spinal osteoporosis. *British Medical Journal, 287,* 723–725.

Geschwind, N., Shader, R., Bear, D., North, B., Levin, K., & Chetham, D. (1980). Behavioral changes with temporal lobe epilepsy: Assessment and treatment. *Journal of Clinical Psychiatry, 41,* 89–95.

Gessa, G.L., & Napoli-Farris, L. (1983). Dopamine receptors and premature ejaculation. In D. Wheatley (Ed.), *Psychopharmacology and sexual disorders* (pp. 15–21). London: Oxford University Press.

Gessa, G.L., & Tagliamonte, A. (1974a). Possible role of brain serotonin and dopamine in controlling male sexual behavior. In E. Costa, G.L. Gessa, & M. Sandler (Eds.), *Serotonin: New vistas. Vol. 11. Advances in biochemical psychopharmacology* (pp. 217–228). New York: Raven Press.

Gessa, G.L., & Tagliamonte, A. (1974b). Role of brain monoamines in male sexual behavior. *Life Sciences, 14,* 425–436.

Gessa, G.L., & Tagliamonte, A. (1975). Role of brain serotonin and dopamine in male sexual behavior. In M. Sandler & G.L. Gessa (Eds.), *Sexual behavior: Pharmacology and biochemistry* (pp. 117–128). New York: Raven Press.

Gessa, G.L., Tagliamonte, A., & Brodie, B.B. (1970). Essential role of testosterone in the sexual stimulation induced by p-chlorophenylalanine in male animals. *Nature, 227,* 616–617.

Ghadirian, A.M., Annable, L., & Belanger, M.C. (1992). Lithium, benzodiazepines, and sexual function in bipolar patients. *American Journal of Psychiatry, 149,* 801–805.

Ghadirian, A.M., Chouinard, G., & Annable, L. (1982). Sexual dysfunction and plasma prolactin levels in neuroleptic-treated schizophrenic outpatients. *Journal of Nervous and Mental Diseases, 170,* 463–467.

Giannini, A.J., Folts, D.J., Feather, J.N., & Sullivan, B.S. (1989). Bromocriptine and amantadine in cocaine detoxification. *Psychiatry Research, 29,* 11–16.

Gianoulakis, C., & Barcomb, A. (1987). Effect of acute ethanol in vivo and in vitro on the beta-endorphin system in the rat. *Life Sciences, 40,* 19–28.

Gibaldi, M. (1993). What is nitric oxide and why are so many people studying it? *Journal of Clinical Pharmacology, 33,* 488–496.

Gibb, W.E., Turner, P., Malpas, J.S., & White, R.J. (1970). Comparison of bethanidine, alpha-methyldopa, and reserpine in essential hypertension. *Lancet, 2,* 275–277.

Gibbs, E.L., Gibbs, F.A., & Fuster, B. (1948). Psychomotor epilepsy. *Archives of Neurology and Psychiatry, 60,* 331–339.

Gibson, G.T., Baghurst, P.A., & Colley, D.P. (1983). Maternal alcohol, tobacco, and cannabis consumption and the outcome of pregnancy. *Australia and New Zealand Journal of Obstetrics and Gynecology, 23,* 15.

Gifford, L.M., Aeugle, M.E., Myerson, R.M., & Tannenbaum, P.J. (1980). Cimetidine postmarket outpatient surveillance program. *Journal of the American Medical Association, 243,* 1532–1535.

Gilbar, O. (1991). The quality of life of cancer patients who refuse chemotherapy. *Social Science and Medicine, 32*(12), 1337.

Gilbeau, P.M., Almirez, R.G., Holaday, J.W., & Smith, C.G. (1984). The role of endogenous opioid peptides in the control of androgen levels in the male nonhuman primate. *Journal of Andrology, 5,* 339–343.

Gilbert, D.G., Hagen, R.L., & D'Agostino, J.A. (1986). The effects of cigarette smoking on human sexual potency. *Addictive Behaviors, 11,* 431–434.

Gilbert, F., Dourish, C.T., Brazell, C., McClue, S., & Stahl, S.M. (1988). Relationship of increased food intake and plasma ACTH levels to 5-HT_{1A} receptor activation in rats. *Psychoneuroendocrinology, 13,* 471–478.

Gilbert, R.M. (1984). Caffeine consumption. *Methylxanthine beverages, and food: Chemistry consumption and health effects.* New York: Liss.

Gilbert, R.N., Graham, C.W., & Regan, J.B. (1992). Double-blind, crossover trial of testosterone enanthate in impotent men with low or low-normal serum testosterone levels. *Journal of Urology, 147,* [Annual meeting program supplement], 264A.

Gill, K., & Amit, Z. (1987). Serotonin uptake blockers and voluntary alcohol consumption: A review of recent studies. In M. Galanter (Ed.), *Recent developments in alcoholism. Vol. 7. Treatment research* (pp. 225–248). New York: Plenum Press.

Gillman, M.A. (1988). Assessment of the effects of analgesic concentrations of nitrous oxide on human sexual response. *International Journal of Neuroscience, 43,* 27–33.

Gilman, A.G., Rall, T.W., Nies, A.S., & Taylor, P. (Eds.). (1990). *Goodman and Gilman's The pharmacological basis of therapeutics (8th ed.).* New York: Pergamon.

Ginestet, D., Cazas, O., & Branciard, M. (1984). Deux cas de dependance a l'amineptine. *L'Encephale, X,* 189–191.

Girgis, S.M., El-Haggar, S., & El-Hermouzy, S. (1982). A double-blind trial of clomipramine in premature ejaculation. *Andrologia, 14,* 364–368.

Gitlin, M.I. (1994). Psychotropic medications and their effects on sexual function: Diagnosis, biology, and treatment approaches. *Journal of Clinical Psychiatry, 55,* 406–413.

Glaser, J.L., Brind, J.L., Eisner, M., & Wallace, R.K. (1986). Elevated serum dehydroepiandrosterone sulfate levels in older experienced practitioners of the transcendental meditation and TM-Sidhi programs. *Society for Neuroscience Abstracts, 12,* 1481.

Glass, R.M. (1981). Ejaculatory impairment from both phenelzine and imipramine with tinnitus from phenelzine. *Journal of Clinical Psychopharmacology, 1,* 152–154.

Glassman, A., Helzer, J., Covey, L., Cottler, L., Stetner, F., Tipp, J., & Johnson, J. (1990). Smoking, smoking cessation, and major depression. *Journal of the American Medical Association, 264,* 1546–1549.

Gless, K., & Overholser, L. (1994). If size really matters: Penile enlargements are plastic surgery's latest controversial trend! *Health and Money: Living Better,* July, 4–7.

Glick, I.D., & Bennett, S.E. (1981). Psychiatric complications of progesterone and oral contraceptives. *Journal of Clinical Psychopharmacology, 1,* 350–367.

Glick, S.D., Hinds, P.A., & Shapiro, R.M. (1983). Cocaine-induced rotation: Sex-dependent differences between left- and right-sided rats. *Science, 221,* 775–777.

Glina, S., Reichelt, A.C., Leao, P.P., & Dos Reis, J.M. (1988). Impact of cigarette smoking on papaverine-induced erection. *Journal of Urology, 140,* 523–524.

Glue, P.W., Cowen, P.J., Nutt, D.J., Kolakowska, T., & Grahame-Smith, D.G. (1986). The effect of lithium on 5-HT-mediated neuroendocrine responses and platelet 5-HT receptors. *Psychopharmacology, 90,* 398–402.

Glue, P.W., Nutt, D.J., Cowen, P.J., & Broadbent, D. (1987). Selective effect of lithium on cognitive performance in man. *Psychoparmacology, 91,* 109–111.

Glueck, C.J., Tieger, M., Kunkel, R., Hamer, T., Tracy, T., & Speirs, J. (1994). Hypocholesterolemia and affective disorders. *American Journal of Medical Sciences, 308,* 218–225.

Godec, C.J., Narkhede, N., & Tomasula, J.J. (1987). The use of nitroglycerine in impotent patients (abstract). *Journal of Urology,* part 2, *137*: 184A, abstract 323.

Godfraind, T., & Govoni, S. (1989). Increasing complexity revealed in regulation of Ca^{2+} antagonist receptor. *Trends in Pharmacological Sciences, 10,* 297-301.

Godfrey, B. (1981). Sperm morphology in smokers. *Lancet, 1,* 948.

Godschalk, M.F., Chen, J., Katz, P.G., & Mulligan, T. (1994). Treatment of erectile failure with prostaglandin E1: A double-blind, placebo-controlled, dose-response study. *Journal of Urology, 151,* 1530-1532.

Goff, D.C. (1985). Two cases of hypomania following the addition of L-tryptophan to a monoamine oxidase inhibitor. *American Journal of Psychiatry, 142,* 1487-1488.

Goldberg, J.P. (1990). Bupropion dose, seizures, women, and age [Letter to the editor]. *Journal of Clinical Pharmacology, 51,* 388-389.

Goldberg, J.P., & Crenshaw, T.L. (1992). Bupropion treatment of sexual dysfunction. *Journal of Psychopharmacology Abstract Book: British Association for Psychopharmacology Meeting,* A11.

Goldberg, M.R., & Robertson, D. (1983). Yohimbine: A pharmacological probe for the study of the $alpha_2$ adrenoceptor. *Pharmacological Reviews, 35,* 143-180.

Goldberg, M.R., Sushak, C.S., Rockhold, F.W., Thompson, W.L., & the Pinacidil Vs. Prazosin Multicenter Investigator Group (1988). Vasodilator monotherapy in the treatment of hypertension: Comparative efficacy and safety of pinacidil, a potassium channel opener, and prazosin. *Clinical Pharmacology and Therapeutics, 44,* 78-92.

Goldberg, R.L. (1984). Sustained yawning as a side effect of imipramine. *International Journal of Psychiatry in Medicine, 13,* 277-280.

Goldbloom, D.S., & Kennedy, S.H. (1991). Adverse interaction of fluoxetine and cyproheptadine in two patients with bulimia nervosa. *Journal of Clinical Psychiatry, 52,* 261-262.

Golden, J.S. (1987, August). Embarrassment caused by unusual form of stimulation. *Medical Aspects of Human Sexuality,* 20.

Golden, R.N., DeVane, C.L., Laizure, S.C., Rudorfer, M.V., Sherer, M.A., & Potter, W.Z. (1988). Bupropion in depression: II. The role of metabolites in clinical outcome. *Archives of General Psychiatry, 45,* 145-149.

Golden, R.N., Hsiao, J., Lane, E., Hicks, R., Rogers, S., & Potter, W.Z. (1989). The effects of intravenous clomipramine on neurohormones in normal subjects. *Journal of Clinical Endocrinology and Metabolism, 68,* 632-637.

Golden, R.N., James, S.P., Sherer, M.A., Rudorfer, M.V., Sack, D.A., & Potter, W.Z. (1985). Psychoses associated with bupropion treatment. *American Journal of Psychiatry, 142,* 1459-1462.

Golden, R.N., Rudorfer, M.V., Sherer, M.A., Linnoila, M., & Potter, W.Z. (1988). Bupropion in depression: I. Biochemical effects and clinical response. *Archives of General Psychiatry, 45,* 139-144.

Golditch, J.M., & Price, V.H. (1990). Treatment of hirsutism with cimetidine. *Obstetrics and Gynecology, 75,* 911-913.

Goldman, L., & Tosteson, A.N. (1991). Uncertainty about postmenopausal estrogen. *New England Journal of Medicine, 325,* 800-802.

Goldstein, I. (1991, March 21). Trazodone may alleviate impotence. *Medical Tribune, 32*(6).

Goldstein, I. (1994). Editorial: Impotence. *Journal of Urology, 151,* 1533-1534.

Goldstein, J.A. (1986). Erectile function and naltrexone. *Annals of Internal Medicine, 105,* 799.

Goldzieher, J.W. (1993). Pharmacology of contraceptive steroids. In D. Shoupe & F.P. Haseltine (Eds.), *Contraception* (pp. 17-24). New York: Springer-Verlag.

Gomez, G., & Phillips, L.A. (1980). Labetalol ("Trandate") in hypertension: A multicenter study in general practice. *Current Medical Research and Opinion, 6,* 677-684.

Goodare, H. (1992). Adjuvant treatment in breast cancer [Letter to the editor]. *Lancet, 339,* 424.

Goode, D.J., & Manning, A.A. (1983). Comparison of bupropion alone and with haloperidol in schizo-affective disorder, depressed type. *Journal of Clinical Psychiatry, 44,* 253-255.

Goode, E. (1972). Drug use and sexual activity on a college campus. *American Journal of Psychiatry, 128,* 1272-1276.

Goodman, R.E. (1980). An assessment of clomipramine (Anafranil) in the treatment of premature ejaculation. *Journal of International Medical Research, 8*(Suppl. 3), 53-59.

Goodnick, P.J., (1990). Bupropion in chronic fatigue syndrome. *American Journal of Psychiatry, 147,* 1091.

Goodnick, P.J., & Extein, I.L. (1989). Bupropion and fluoxetine in depressive subtypes. *Annals of Clinical Psychiatry, 1,* 119-122.

Goodwin, D.W. (1979a). Alcoholism and heredity: A review and hypothesis. *Archives of General Psychiatry, 36,* 57-61.

Goodwin, D.W. (1979b). Genetic determinants of alcoholism. In J.H. Mendelson & N.K. Mello (Eds.), *The diagnosis and treatment of alcoholism* (pp. 59-82). New York: McGraw Hill.

Goodwin, F., & Jamison, K. (1986). NIMH researcher gives update on lithium to clinicians. *Psychiatric News*, December 5, p. 15.

Goodwin, G.M., De Souza, R.J., Wood, A.J., & Green, A.R. (1986). Lithium decreases 5-HT_{1A} and 5-HT_2 receptor and $alpha_2$ adrenoceptor mediated function in mice. *Psychopharmacology, 90,* 482-487.

Goodwin, G.M., Fairburn, C.G., & Cowen, P.J. (1987). The effects of dieting and weight loss on neuroendocrine responses to tryptophan, clonidine, and apomorphine in volunteers. *Archives of General Psychiatry, 44,* 952-957.

Gooren, L.J. (1985). Human male sexual functions do not require aromatization of testosterone: A study using tamoxifen, testolactone, and dihydrotestosterone. *Archives of Sexual Behavior, 14,* 539-548.

Gordon, G.G., Altman, K., Southren, A.L., Rubin, E., & Lieber, C.S. (1976). Effect of alcohol (ethanol) administration on sex-hormone metabolism in normal men. *New England Journal of Medicine, 295,* 793-797.

Gordon, G.G., Southren, A.L., & Lieber, C.S. (1979). Hypogonadism and feminization in the male: A triple effect of alcohol. *Alcoholism: Clinical and Experimental Research, 3,* 210-212.

Gorelick, D.A. (1987). Serotonin uptake blockers and the treatment of alcoholism. In M. Galanter (Ed.), *Recent developments in alcoholism. Vol. 7. Treatment research* (pp. 267-282). New York: Plenum Press.

Gorski, R.A. (1976). The possible neural sites of hormonal facilitation of sexual behavior in the female rat. *Psychoneuroendocrinology, 1,* 371-387.

Gorski, R.A. (1985). Gonadal hormones as putative neurotrophic substances. In C.W. Cotman (Ed.), *Synaptic plasticity* (pp. 287-310). New York: Guilford Press.

Gorski, R.A. (1987). Sex differences in the rodent brain: Their nature and origin. In J.M. Reinisch, L.A. Rosenblum, & S.A. Sanders (Eds.), *Masculinity/femininity: Basic perspectives* (pp. 37-67). New York: Oxford University Press.

Gorsky, R.D., Koplan, J.P., Peterson, H.B., & Thacker, S.B. (1994). Relative risks and benefits of long-term estrogen replacement therapy: A decision analysis. *Obstetrics and Gynecology, 83,* 161-166.

Gorzalka, B.B., Luck, K.A., & Tanco, S.A. (1991). Effects of the oxytocin fragment prolyl-leucylglycinamide on sexual behavior in the rat. *Pharmacology, Biochemistry, and Behavior, 38,* 273-279.

Gorzalka, B.B., & Whalen, R.E. (1975). Inhibition not facilitation of sexual behavior by PCPA. *Pharmacology, Biochemistry, and Behavior, 3,* 511-513.

Gottesman, H.G., & Schubert, D.S. (1993). Low-dose oral medroxyprogesterone acetate in the management of the paraphilias. *Journal of Clinical Psychiatry, 54,* 182-188.

Goudsmit, E., Feenstra, M.G.P., & Swaab, D.F. (1990). Central monoamine metabolism in the male brown-Norway rat in relation to aging and testosterone. *Brain Research Bulletin, 25,* 755-763.

Gough, K.R., Bardhan, K.D., Crowe, J.P., Korman, M.G., Lee, F.I., & Reed, P.I. (1984). Ranitidine and cimetidine in prevention of duodenal ulcer relapse. *Lancet, 2,* 659-662.

Gould, R.J., Murphy, K.M., Reynolds, I.J., & Snyder, S.H. (1984). Calcium channel blockade: Possible explanation for thioridazine's peripheral side effects. *American Journal of Psychiatry, 141,* 352-357.

Govoni, S., Bossio, A., DiMonda, D., Fazzari, G., Spano, P.F., & Trabucchi, M. (1983). Immunoreactive metenkephaline plasma concentrations in chronic alcoholics and in children born from alcoholic mothers. *Life Sciences, 33,* 1581-1586.

Govoni, S., Goss, I., DiGiovine, S., Battaini, F., & Trabucchi, M. (1990). Calcium antagonists inhibit met-enkephalin immunoreactive material release: In vitro and ex vivo experiments. *Journal of Neural Transmission, 80,* 1-8.

Gower, A.J., Berendsen, H.G., Princen, M.M., & Broekkamp, C.L. (1984). The yawning-penile erection syndrome as a model for putative dopamine autoreceptor activity. *European Journal of Pharmacology, 103,* 81-89.

Grady, D., Rubin, S.M., Petitti, D.B., Fox, C.S., Black, D., Ettinger, B., Ernster, V.L., & Cummings, S.R. (1992). Hormone therapy to prevent disease and prolong life in postmenopausal women. *Annals of Internal Medicine, 117,* 1016-1037.

Graedon, J. (1985). *The people's pharmacy: New and revised.* New York: St. Martin's Press.

Graedon, J., & Graedon, T. (1991). *Graedon's best medicine.* New York: Bantam Books.

Grafeille, N., Joutard, J.C., & Ruffle, A. (1984). Plasma prolactin levels in 300 cases of sexual disorders. In R.T. Segraves & E.J. Haeberle (Eds.), *Emerging dimensions of sexology* (pp. 261-275). New York: Praeger.

Graham, D.Y., Malaty, H.M., & Go, M.F. (1994). Are there susceptible hosts to *Helicobacter pylori* infection? *Scandinavian Journal of Gastroenterology, 29* (Suppl. 205), 6-10.

Gralla, E.J., & McIlhenny, H.M. (1972). Studies in pregnant rats, rabbits, and monkeys with lithium carbonate. *Toxicology and Applied Pharmacology, 21,* 428-433.

Granata, A.R., Carani, C., Del Rio, G., & Marrama, P. (1994). The influence of anxiety on the penile response to intracavernosal drug injection. *Journal of Endocrinological Investigation, 17* (Suppl. 1-2), 28.

Grant, E.C., & Pryse-Davies, J. (1968). Effect of oral contraceptives on depressive mood changes and on endometrial monoamine oxidase and phosphates. *British Medical Journal, 3,* 777-780.

Graves, N.M., & Leppik, I.E. (1991). Antiepileptic medications in development. *The Annals of Pharmacotherapy, 25,* 978-986.

Gray, A., Feldman, H.A., McKinlay, J.B., & Longcope, C. (1991). Age, disease, and changing sex hormone levels in middle-aged men: Results of the Massachusetts Male Aging Study. *Journal of Clinical Endocrinology and Metabolism, 73,* 1016-1025.

Gray, G.D., Davis, H.N., & Dewsbury, D.A. (1974). Effects of L-dopa on the heterosexual copulatory behavior of male rats. *European Journal of Pharmacology, 27,* 367-370.

Greenberg, C., Kukreja, S.C., Bowser, E.N., Hargis, G.K., Henderson, W.J., & Williams, G.A. (1986). Effects of estradiol and progesterone on calcitonin secretion. *Endocrinology, 118,* 2594-2598.

Greenberg, H.R. (1965). Erectile impotence during the course of Tofranil therapy. *American Journal of Psychiatry, 121,* 1021.

Greenberg, H.R. (1971). Inhibition of ejaculation by chlorpromazine. *Journal of Nervous and Mental Disease, 152,* 364-366.

Greenblatt, D.J., & Koch-Weser, J. (1973). Gynecomastia and impotence: Complications of spironolactone therapy [Letter to the editor]. *Journal of the American Medical Association, 223,* 82.

Greenblatt, R.B. (1943). Testosterone propionate pellet implantation in gynecic disorders. *Journal of the American Medical Association, 121,* 17-24.

Greenblatt, R.B. (1987). The use of androgens in the menopause and other gynecic disorders. *Obstetrics and Gynecology Clinics of North America, 14,* 251-268.

Greenblatt, R.B., Barfield, W.E., Garner, J.F., Calk, G.L., & Harrod, J.P. (1950). Evaluation of an estrogen, androgen, estrogen-androgen combination and a placebo in the treatment of the menopause. *Journal of Clinical Endocrinology, 10,* 1547-1558.

Greenblatt, R.B., Jungck, E.C., & Blum, H. (1972, January). Endocrinology of sexual behavior. *Medical Aspects of Human Sexuality,* 110-130.

Greenblatt, R.B., & Karpas, A. (1983). Hormone therapy for sexual dysfunction. *Postgraduate Medicine, 74,* 78-89.

Greenblatt, R.B., Mortara, F., & Torpin, R. (1942). Sexual libido in the female. *American Journal of Obstetrics and Gynecology, 44,* 658-663.

Greer, M. (1988). Carrier drugs. *Neurology, 38,* 628-632.

Grenhoff, J., & Svensson, T.H. (1987). Regularization of nigral dopamine cell activity by clonidine. *Neuroscience, 22,* S352.

Grenhoff, J., & Svensson, T.H. (1988). Selective stimulation of limbic dopamine activity by nicotine. *Acta Physiologica Scandanavica, 133,* 595-596.

Grenhoff, J., & Svensson, T.H. (1989). Clonidine modulates dopamine cell firing in rat ventral tegmental area. *European Journal of Pharmacology, 165,* 11-18.

Griffith, S.R., & Zil, J.S. (1984). Priapism in a patient receiving antipsychotic therapy. *Psychosomatics, 25,* 629-631.

Griffiths, R.R., & Woodson, P.P. (1988). Reinforcing properties of caffeine: Studies in humans and laboratory animals. *Pharmacology, Biochemistry, and Behavior, 29,* 419-427.

Grimsley, S.R., & Jann, M.W. (1992). Paroxetine, sertraline, and fluvoxamine: New selective serotonin reuptake inhibitors. *Clinical Pharmacy, 11,* 930-957.

Gripon, E.B. (1985). General discussion. In E.B. Gripon (Ed.), *Hypnotics: A symposium, October 16, 1984* (pp. 43-48). Princeton: Excerpta Medica.

Grisso, J.A., Baum, C.R., & Turner, B.J. (1990). "What do physicians in practice do to prevent osteoporosis?" *Journal of Bone and Mineral Research, 5,* 213-219.

Grob, C., Bravo, G., & Walsh, R. (1990). Second thoughts on 3.4-methylenedioxymethamphetamine (MDMA) neurotoxicity [Letter to the editor]. *Archives of General Psychiatry, 47,* 288.

Gross, M.D. (1982). Reversal by bethanechol of sexual dysfunction caused by anticholinergic antidepressants. *American Journal of Psychiatry, 139,* 1193-1194.

Grow, D.R., & Wiczyk, H.P. (1994). Mifepristone (RU 486) and other anti-progestins: A review of their clinical applications. *Assisted Reproduction Reviews, 4,* 101-109.

Gruchow, H.W., Anderson, A.J., Barboriak, J.J., & Sobocinski, K.A. (1988). Postmenopausal use of estrogen and occlusion of coronary arteries. *American Heart Journal, 115,* 954-963.

Gu, J., Polak, J.M., Lazarides, M., Morgan, R., Pryor, J.P., Marangos, P.J., Blank, M.A., & Bloom, S.R. (1984). Decrease of vasoactive intestinal polypeptide (VIP) in the penises from impotent men. *Lancet, 2,* 315-318.

Guez, D., Crocq, L., Safavian, A., & Labardens, P.

(1988). Effects of indapamide on the quality of life in hypertensive patients. *American Journal of Medicine, 84*(Suppl. 1B), 53–58.

Guilleminault, C. (1985). Drug-induced sleep disorders. In K. Blum & L. Manzo (Eds.), *Neurotoxicity* (pp. 101–110). New York: Marcel Dekker.

Guilleminault, C., Carskadon, M., & Dement, W.C. (1974). On the treatment of rapid eye movement narcolepsy. *Archives of Neurology, 30,* 90–93.

Gustavson, C.R., Gustavson, J.C., Young, J.K., Pumariega, A.J., Nicholas, L.K. (1989). Estrogen-induced malaise. In J.M. Lakoski (Ed.), *Neural control of reproductive function* (pp. 501–523). New York: Alan R. Liss.

Gwinup, G. (1988). Oral phentolamine in nonspecific erectile insufficiency. *Annals of Internal Medicine, 109,* 162–163.

Haldar, J., Hoffman, D.L., & Zimmerman, E.A. (1982). Morphine, beta-endorphin, and [D-ala^2] met-enkephalin inhibit oxytocin release by acetylcholine and suckling. *Peptides, 3,* 663–668.

Halikas, J., Weller, R., & Morse, C. (1982). Effects of regular marijuana use on sexual performance. *Journal of Psychoactive Drugs, 14,* 59–70.

Hall, M.J. (1994). Breast tenderness and enlargement induced by sertraline [Letter to the editor]. *American Journal of Psychiatry, 151,* 1395–1396.

Hall, R.C.W., & Joffe, J.R. (1972). Aberrant response to diazepam: A new syndrome. *American Journal of Psychiatry, 129,* 738.

Hall, S.M., Tunstall, C.D., Vila, K.L., & Duffy, J. (1992). Weight gain prevention and smoking cessation: Cautionary findings. *American Journal of Public Health, 82,* 799–803.

Hall, W.H. (1976). Breast changes in males on cimetidine. *New England Journal of Medicine, 295,* 841.

Halliday, A., Bush, B., Cleary, P., Aronson, M., & Delbanco, T. (1986). Alcohol abuse in women seeking gynecologic care. *Obstetrics and Gynecology, 68,* 322–326.

Hamlet, M.A., Rorie, D.K., & Tyce, G.M. (1980). Effects of estradiol on release and disposition of norepinephrine from nerve endings. *American Journal of Physiology, 239,* H450.

Hammond, E.C. (1991). Smoking in relation to physical complaints. *Archives of Environmental Health, 3,* 28.

Handelsman, D.J., Conway, A.J., Boylan, L.M., & Turtle, J.R. (1984). Testicular function in potential sperm donors: Normal ranges and the effects of smoking and varicocele. *International Journal of Andrology, 7,* 369–382.

Hanno, P.M., & Charles, R. (1986). Initial pharmacologic treatment of erectile dysfunction. *Journal of Urology, 135,* 362A.

Hanno, P.M., Wein, A., & Fletcher, S. (1988). Long-term follow up of initial pharmacologic treatment of erectile dysfunction. *Journal of Urology, 139,* 253A.

Hanson, J.W., & Smith, D.W. (1975). The fetal hydantoin syndrome. *Journal of Pediatrics, 87,* 285–290.

Harrison, W.M. (1987). Response to Dr. Cooper: Antidepressant medication and sexual function [Letter to the editor]. *Journal of Clinical Psychopharmacology, 7,* 120–121.

Harrison, W.M., Rabkin, J.G., Ehrhardt, A.A., Stewart, J.W., McGrath, P.J., Ross, D., & Quitkin, F.M. (1986). Effects of antidepressant medication on sexual function: A controlled study. *Journal of Clinical Psychopharmacology, 6,* 144–149.

Harrison, W.M., Stewart, J., Ehrhardt, A.A., Rabkin, J., McGrath, P., Liebowitz, M., & Quitkin, F.M. (1985). A controlled study of the effects of antidepressants on sexual function. *Psychopharmacology Bulletin, 21,* 85–85.

Harsing, L.G., & Yang, H.Y.T. (1984). Serotonergic regulation of hypothalamic met^5-enkephalin content. In I. Hanin (Ed.), *Dynamics of neurotransmitter function* (pp. 169–176). New York: Raven Press.

Hart, B.L. (1969). Effects of alcohol on sexual reflexes and mating behavior in the male dog. *Quarterly Journal of Studies on Alcohol, 29,* 839–844.

Hartman, E. (1978). *The sleeping pill.* New Haven: Yale University Press.

Harto-Truax, N., Miller, L.L., Cato, A.E., Stern, W.C., & Sato, T.L. (1983). Effects of bupropion on body weight. *Journal of Clinical Psychiatry, 44*(5), 183–186.

Harvey, J.A., & McMaster, S.E. (1977). Fenfluramine: Cumulative neurotoxicity after chronic treatment with low dosages in the rat. *Communications in Psychopharmacology, 1,* 3–17.

Harvey, S.M. (1987). Female sexual behavior: Fluctuations during the menstrual cycle. *Journal of Psychosomatic Research, 31,* 101–110.

Harvey, S.M., & Beckman, L.J. (1986). Alcohol consumption, female sexual behavior, and contraceptive use. *Journal of Studies on Alcohol, 47,* 327–332.

Haspels, A.A., Bennink, H.J., van Keep, P.A., & Schreurs, W.H. (1975). Estrogens and vitamin B_6. *Frontiers in Hormone Research, 3,* 199–207.

Hatsukami, D., Mitchell, J.E., Eckert, E.D., & Pyle, R. (1986). Characteristics of patients with bulimia only, bulimia with affective disorder, and bulimia with substance abuse problems. *Addictive Behaviors, 11,* 399–406.

Hauger, R.L., Hulihan-Giblin, B., Janowsky, A., Angel, I., Berger, P., Luu, M.D., Schweri, M.M.,

Skolnick, P., & Paul, S.M. (1986). Central recognition sites for psychomotor stimulants: Methylphenidate and amphetamine. In R. O'Brien (Ed.), *Receptor binding in drug research* (pp. 167–182). New York: Marcel Dekker.

Hawkes, C.H. (1992). Endorphins: The basis of pleasure? *Journal of Neurology, Neurosurgery, and Psychiatry, 55,* 247–250.

Haykal, R.F., & Akiskal, H.S. (1990). Bupropion as a promising approach to rapid cycling bipolar II patients. *Journal of Clinical Psychiatry, 51,* 450–455.

Heath, R.G., (1963). Electrical self-stimulation of the brain in man. *American Journal of Psychiatry, 120,* 571–577.

Heath, R.G. (1964a). Correlation of brain function with emotional behavior. *Biological Psychiatry, 11,* 463–480.

Heath, R.G. (1964b). Pleasure response of human subjects to direct stimulation of the brain. In R.G. Heath (Ed.), *The role of pleasure in behavior* (pp. 219–243). New York: Harper and Row.

Heath, R.G. (1972). Pleasure and brain activity in man. *Journal of Nervous and Mental Diseases, 154,* 3–18.

Heath, R.G., & Hodes, R. (1952). Induction of sleep by stimulation of the caudate nucleus in *Macacus rhesus* and man. *Transactions of the American Neurological Association, 77,* 204–210.

Heaton, J.P.W. (1989). Preliminary studies in rabbit penile cavernosal tissue, of the role of synthetic nitrovasodilators in erectile response. *Current Therapeutic Research, 45,* 278–284.

Heaton, J.P.W., Morales, A., Owen, J., Saunders, F.W., & Fenemore, J. (1990). Topical glyceryltrinitrate causes measurable penile arterial dilation in impotent men. *Journal of Urology, 143,* 729–731.

Hedricks, C., Piccinino, L.J., Udry, J.R., & Chimbira, T.H. (1987). Peak coital rate coincides with onset of luteinizing hormone surge. *Fertility and Sterility, 48,* 234–238.

Heinonen, P.K., Koivula, T., & Pystynen, P. (1987). Decreased serum level of dehydroepiandrosterone sulfate in postmenopausal women with ovarian cancer. *Gynecologic and Obstetric Investigation, 23,* 271–274.

Heinsbroek, R.P.W., van Haaren, F., Zantvoord, F., & van de Poll, N. (1987). Sex differences in response rates during random ratio acquisition: Effects of gonadectomy. *Physiology and Behavior, 39,* 269–272.

Hekimian, L.J., Friedhoff, A.J., & Deever, E. (1978). A comparison of the onset of action and therapeutic efficacy of amoxapine and amitriptyline. *Journal of Clinical Psychaitry, 39,* 633–637.

Held, H.G. (1962). Experience in the treatment of chronic prostatitis. *Fortschritte der Medizin, 80,* 187–190.

Held, P.H., & Yusuf, S. (1994). Impact of calcium channel-blockers on mortality. In B.N. Singh, V.J. Dzau, P.M. Vanhoutte, & R.L. Woosley (Eds.), *Cardiovascular pharmacology and therapeutics* (pp. 525–533). New York: Churchill Livingstone.

Helgeland, A., Hagelund, C.H., Strommen, R., & Tretli, S. (1986). Enalapril, atenolol, and hydrochlorothiazide in mild to moderate hypertension. *Lancet, 1,* 872–875.

Hembree, W.C., Nahas, G.G., & Huang, H.F. (1979). Changes in human spermatozoa associated with high dose marijuana smoking. In G.G. Nahas & W.D. Paton (Eds.), *Marijuana: Biological effects* (pp. 429–440). New York: Pergamon.

Hembree, W.C., Zeidenberg, P., & Nahas, G.G. (1976). Marijuana effects upon human gonadal function. In G.G. Nahas (Ed.), *Marijuana: Chemistry, biochemistry, and cellular effects* (pp. 521–532). New York: Springer-Verlag.

Hemenway, D., Colditz, G.A., Willett, W.C., Stampfer, M.J., & Speizer, F.E. (1988). Fractures and lifestyle: Effect of cigarette smoking, alcohol intake, and relative weight on the risk of hip and forearm fractures in middle-aged women. *American Journal of Public Health, 78,* 1554–1558.

Henderson, B.E., Paganini-Hill, A., & Ross, R.K., (1991). Decreased mortality in users of estrogen replacement therapy. *Archives of Internal Medicine, 151,* 75–78.

Henderson, B.E., Ross, R.K., Paganini-Hill, A., & Mack, T.M. (1986). Estrogen use and cardiovascular disease. *American Journal of Obstetrics and Gynecology, 154,* 1181–1186.

Henzl, M.R. (1993) Evolution of steroids and their contraceptive and therapeutic use. In D. Shoupe & F.P. Haseltine (Eds.), *Contraception* (pp. 1–16). New York: Springer-Verlag.

Herbert, T. (1989). Specific roles for beta-endorphin in reproduction and sexual behavior. In R.G. Dyer & R.J. Bickness (Eds.), *Brain opioid systems in reproduction* (pp. 167–186). Oxford: Oxford University Press.

Herman, J.B., Brotman, A.W., Pollack, M.H., Falk, W.E., Biederman, J., & Rosenbaum, J. (1990). Fluoxetine-induced sexual dysfunction. *Journal of Clinical Psychiatry, 51,* 25–27.

Hermes, M.L., Buijs, R.M., Masson-Pevet, M., van der Woude, T.P., Pevet, P., Brenkle, R., & Kirsch, R. (1989). Hibernation requires the absence of central vasopressin release. *European Journal of Neuroscience, 1*(Suppl. 2), 287.

Hernandez, L., & Hoebel, B.G. (1988). Food reward and cocaine increase extra cellular dopamine in the nucleus accumbens as measured by microdialysis. *Life Sciences, 42,* 1705–1712.

Herrick, A.L., Waller, P., Berkin, K., Pringle, S.D., Callender, J.S., Robertson, M.P., Findlay, J.G., Murray, G.D., Reid, J.L., Lorimer, A.R., Weir, R.J., Carmichael, H.A., Robertson, J.I.S., Ball, S.G., & McInness, G.T. (1989). Comparison of enalapril and atenolol in mild to moderate hypertension. *American Journal of Medicine, 86,* 421-426.

Herridge, P., & Gold, M.S. (1988). Pharmacological adjuncts in the treatment of opioid and cocaine addicts. *Journal of Psychoactive Drugs, 20,* 233-242.

Herrling, P.L. (1991). Mechanism of action of atypical antipsychotics. *Pharmacopsychiatry, 24,* 48-49.

Herzog, A.G., Seibel, M.M., Schomer, D.L., Vaitukaitis, J.L., & Geschwind, N. (1986a). Reproductive endocrine disorders in men with partial seizures of temporal lobe origin. *Archives of Neurology, 43,* 347-350.

Herzog, A.G., Seibel, M.M., Schomer, D.L., Vaitukaitis, J.L., & Geschwind, N. (1986b). Reproductive endocrine disorders in women with partial seizures of temporal lobe origin. *Archives of Neurology, 43,* 341-346.

Hesselbrock, M.N., Meyer, R.E., & Keener, J.J. (1985). Psychopathology in hospitalized alcoholics. *Archives of General Psychiatry, 42,* 1050-1055.

Hiatt, R.A., Bawol, R., Friedman, G.D., & Hoover, R. (1984). Exogenous estrogen and breast cancer after bilateral oophorectomy. *Cancer, 54,* 139-144.

Hidvegi, T., Feher, G., Feher, T., Koo, E., & Fust, G. (1984). Inhibition of the complement activation by an adrenal androgen, DHA. *Complement, 1,* 201-204.

Hiilesmaa, V.K. (1992). Pregnancy and birth in women with epilepsy. *Neurology, 42*(Suppl. 5), 8-11.

Hill, D., Falconer, M.A., Pampiglione, G., & Liddell, D.W. (1953). Discussion on the surgery of temporal lobe epilepsy. *Proceedings of the Royal Society of Medicine (London), 46,* 965-976.

Hill, D.A., Wallace, R.K., Walton, K.G., & Meyerson, L.R. (1989). Acute decreased platelet serotonin and attenuation of autonomic activity in the transcendental meditation program (TM). *Society for Neuroscience Abstracts: 19th Meeting, 15,* 1281.

Hilton, P., & Stanton, S.L. (1983). The use of intravaginal estrogen creme in genuine stress incontinence. *British Journal of Obstetrics and Gynecology, 90,* 940-944.

Hindmarch, I., Sherwood, N., & Kerr, J.S. (1993). Amnestic effects of triazolam and other hypnotics. *Progress in Neuro-Psychopharmacology and Biological Psychiatry, 17,* 407-413.

Hines, M., & Gorski, R.A. (1985). Hormonal influences on the development of neural asymmetrics. In D.F. Benson & E. Zaidel (Eds.), *The dual brain* (pp. 75-96). New York: Guilford Press.

Hingson, R., Alpert, J.J., Day, N., Dooling, E.Z., Kayne, H., Morelock, S., Oppenheimer, E., & Zuckerman, B. (1982). Effects of maternal drinking and marijuana use on fetal growth and development. *Pediatrics, 70,* 539-546.

Hirate, K., & Kuribara, H. (1991). Characteristics of the ambulation-increasing effect of GBR-12909, a selective dopamine uptake inhibitor, in mice. *Japanese Journal of Pharmacology, 55,* 501-511.

Hirsh, L.S. (1939). Controlling appetite in obesity. *Journal of Medicine, 20,* 84-86.

Hirshkowitz, M., Arcasoy, M.O., Karacan, I., Williams, R.L., & Howell, J.W. (1992). Nocturnal penile tumescence in cigarette smokers with erectile dysfunction. *Urology, 39,* 101-107.

Hirvonen, E., Malkonen, M., & Manninen, V. (1981). Effects of different progestogens on lipoproteins during postmenopausal replacement therapy. *New England Journal of Medicine, 304*(10), 560-563.

Hite, S. (1976). *The Hite report.* New York: Macmillan and Co.

Hlinak, Z. (1987). Lisuride temporarily inhibits sexual behavior in female rats. *Pharmacology, Biochemistry, and Behavior, 27,* 211-215.

Hocman, G. (1988). Chemoprevention of cancer: Selenium. *International Journal of Biochemistry, 20,* 123-132.

Hodgson, B.T., Dumas, S., Bolling, D.R., & Heesch, C.M. (1978). Effect of estrogen on sensitivity of rabbit bladder and urethra to phenylephrine. *Investigative Urology, 16,* 67-69.

Hodsman, G.P., Brown, J.J., Cumming, A.M., Davies, D.L., East, B.W., Lever, A.F., Morton, J.J., Murray, G.D., & Robertson, J.I.S. (1983). Enalapril (MK421) in the treatment of hypertension with renal artery stenosis. *Journal of Hypertension, 1*(Suppl. 1), 109-117.

Hoehn-Saric, R., Lipsey, J.R., & McLeod, D.R. (1990). Apathy and indifference in patients on fluvoxamine and fluoxetine. *Journal of Clinical Psychopharmacology, 10,* 343-345.

Hoekenga, M.T., Dillon, R.H., & Leyland, H.M. (1978). A comprehensive review of diethylpropion hydrochloride. In S. Garattini & R. Samanin (Eds.), *Central mechanisms of anorectic drugs* (pp. 391-404). New York: Raven Press.

Hoensch, H.P., Hutzel, H., Kirch, W., & Ohnhaus, E.E. (1985). Isolation of human hepatic microsomes and their inhibition by cimetidine and ranitidine. *European Journal of Clinical Pharmacology, 29,* 199-206.

Hoffman, A.R., & Crowley, W.F., Jr. (1983). Chronic low-dose pulsatile gonadotropin-releasing hormone treatment of idiopathic hypogonadotropic hypogonadism in men. In R. D'Agata, M.B. Litsett, P. Polosa, & H.J. van der Molen (Eds.), *Recent advances in male reproduction: Molecular basis and clinical implications* (pp. 249-256). New York: Raven Press.

Hogan, M.J., Wallin, J.D., & Baer, R.M. (1980). Antihypertensive therapy and male sexual dysfunction. *Psychosomatics, 21,* 234-237.

Holden, K.L., McLaughlin, E.J., Reilly, E.L., & Overall, J.E. (1988). Accelerated mental aging in alcoholic patients. *Journal of Clinical Psychology, 44,* 286-292.

Hollander, E., & McCarley, A. (1992). Yohimbine treatment of sexual side effects induced by serotonin reuptake blockers. *Journal of Clinical Psychiatry, 53,* 207-209.

Hollander, E., Liebowitz, M.R., DeCaria, C., Fairbanks, J., Fallon, B., & Klein, D. (1990). Treatment of depersonalization with serotonin reuptake blockers. *Journal of Clinical Psychopharmacology, 10,* 200-203.

Hollenberg, N.K. (1987). Initial therapy in hypertension: Quality-of-life considerations. *Journal of Hypertension, 5*(Suppl. 1), S3-S7.

Hollister, L.E. (1990). Commentary on Noyes et al. In L. E. Hollister & L. Lasagna (Eds.), *Yearbook of drug therapy—1990* (p. 221). Chicago: Year Book Medical Publishers.

Holmberg, G., & Gershon, S. (1961). Autonomic and psychic effects of yohimbine hydrochloride. *Psychopharmacologia, 2,* 93-98.

Holme, J.B., Christensen, M.M., Rasmussen, P.C., Jacobsen, F., Nielsen, J., Nørgaard, J.P., Olesen, S., Noer, I., Wolf, H., & Husted, S.E. (1994). 29-week doxazosin treatment in patients with symptomatic benign prostatic hyperplasia. *Scandanavian Journal of Urology and Nephrology, 28,* 77-82.

Holmes, B., & Sorkin, E.M. (1986). Indoramin: A review of its pharmacodynamic and pharmacokinetic properties, and therapeutic efficacy in hypertension and related vascular, cardiovascular, and airway diseases. *Drugs, 31,* 467-499.

Holmquist, F., Hedlund, H., & Andersson, K.E. (1990). Effects of the alpha-adrenoceptor antagonist R-(-)-YM12617 on isolated human penile erectile tissue and vas deferens. *European Journal of Pharmacology, 186,* 87-93.

Holsboen, F., Benkert, O., Meier L., & Kreuz-Kersting, A. (1985). Combined estradiol and vitamin B_6 treatment in women with major depression. *American Journal of Psychiatry, 142,* 658.

Holst, J., Backstrom, T., Hammarback, S., & von Schoultz, B. (1989). Progestogen addition during estrogen replacement therapy—effects on vasomotor symptoms and mood. *Maturitas, 11,* 13-20.

Holt, S. (1990). Alcohol and H2 receptor antagonists: Over the counter, under the table? *American Journal of Gastroenterology, 85,* 516-517.

Holt, S. (1991). Response to Dr. Palmer [Letter to the editor]. *American Journal of Gastroenterology, 86,* 113-116.

Holt, S., Skinner, H.A., & Israel, Y. (1981). Early identification of alcohol abuse. II. Clinical and laboratory indicators. *Canadian Medical Association Journal, 124,* 1279-1295.

Holzki, G., Gall, H., & Hermann, J. (1991). Cigarette smoking and sperm quality. *Andrologia, 23,* 141-144.

Honer, W.G., Thompson, C., Lightman, S.L., Williams, T.D., & Checkley, S.A. (1986). No effect of naloxone on plasma oxytocin in normal men. *Psychoneuroendocrinology, 11,* 245-248.

Hoon, P.W., Bruce, K., & Kinchloe, B. (1982). Does the menstrual cycle play a role in sexual arousal? *Psychophysiology, 19,* 21-27.

Hoover, R., Glass, A., Finkle, W.D., Azevedo, D., & Milne, K. (1981). Conjugated estrogens and breast cancer risk in women. *Journal of the National Cancer Institute, 67,* 815-820.

Hopkins, R.J., & Morris, J.G., Jr. (1994). *Helicobacter pylori:* The missing link in perspective. *American Journal of Medicine, 97,* 265-276.

Horne, R.L., Ferguson, J.M., Pope, H.G., Hudson, J.I., Lineberry, C.G., Ascher, J., & Cato, A. (1988). Treatment of bulimia with bupropion: A multicenter controlled trial. *Journal of Clinical Psychiatry, 49,* 262-266.

Horrobin, D.F. (1989). Lipid-lowering drugs and violence [Letter to the editor]. *British Journal of Psychiatry, 154,* 882-883.

Horton, R., & Lobo, R. (1986). Peripheral androgens and the role of androstanediol glucuronide. *Clinics in Endocrinology and Metabolism, 15,* 293-306.

Hoschl, C. (1983). Verapamil for depression? [Letter to the editor]. *American Journal of Psychiatry, 140,* 1100.

Hoyland, V.J., Shillito, E.E., & Vogt, M. (1970). The effect of parachlorophenylalanine on the behavior of cats. *British Journal of Pharmacology, 40,* 659-667.

Hucker, S., Langevin, R., & Bain, J. (1988). A double-blind trial of sex drive reducing medication in pedophiles. *Annals of Sex Research, 1,* 227-242.

Hudson, R., Gonzalez-Mariscal, G., & Beyer, C. (1990). Chin marking behavior, sexual receptivity, and pheromone emission in steroid-treated, ovarectomized rabbits. *Hormones and Behavior, 24,* 1-13.

Hughes, A.M., Everitt, B.J., & Herbert, J. (1987). Selective effects of beta-endorphin infused into the hypothalamus, preoptic area, and bed nucleus of the stria terminalis on the sexual and ingestive behavior of male rats. *Neuroscience, 23,* 1063-1073.

Hughes, A.M., Everitt, B.J., Lightman, S.L., & Todd, K.T. (1987). Oxytocin in the central nervous system and sexual behavior in male rats. *Brain Research, 414,* 133-137.

Hughes, J.M. (1964). Failure to ejaculate with chlordiazepoxide. *American Journal of Psychiatry, 121,* 610-611.

Hughes, J.R., Amorie, G., & Hatsukami, B.L. (1988). A survey of physician's advice about caffeine. *Journal of Substance Abuse, 1,* 67-70.

Hughes, J.R., Hunt, W.K., Higgins, S.T., Bickel, W.K., Fenwick, J.W., & Pepper, S.L. (1992). Effect of dose on the ability of caffeine to serve as a reinforcer in humans. *Behavioral Pharmacology, 3,* 211-218.

Hugues, J.N., Coste, T., Perret, G., Jayle, M.F., Sebaoun, J., & Modigliani, E. (1980). Hypothalamo-pituitary ovarian function in 31 women with chronic alcoholism. *Clinical Endocrinology, 12,* 543-551.

Hulka, B.S., Chambless, L.E., Deubner, D.C., & Wilkinson, W.E. (1982). Breast cancer and estrogen replacement therapy. *American Journal of Obstetrics and Gynecology, 143,* 638-644.

Hull, E.M., Warner, R.K., Bazzett, T.J., Eaton, R.C., Thompson, J.T., & Scaletta, L.L. (1989). D2/D1 ratio in the medial preoptic area affects copulation of male rats. *Journal of Pharmacology and Experimental Therapeutics, 251,* 422-427.

Humphries, T.J., Myerson, R.M., Gifford, L.M., Aeugle, M.E., Josie, M.E., Wood, S.L., & Tannenbaum, P.J. (1984). A unique postmarket outpatient surveillance program of cimetidine: Report on phase II and final summary. *American Journal of Gastroenterology, 79,* 593-596.

Hunt, K., & Vessey, M. (1989). Mortality from cancer and cardiovascular disease and hormonal substitution therapy. In M. L'Hermite (Ed.), *Update on hormonal treatment in the menopause* (pp. 63-71). Basel: Karger.

Hunt, K., Vessey, M., McPherson, K., & Coleman, M. (1987). Long-term surveillance of mortality and cancer incidence in women receiving hormone replacement therapy. *British Journal of Obstetrics and Gynecology, 94,* 620-635.

Husain, S., & Lame, M.W. (1984). Possible mechanism for the cellular effects of marijuana on male reproductive function. In S. Agurell, W.L., Dewey, & R.E. Willette (Eds.), *The cannabinoids: chemical, pharmacologic, and therapeutic aspects* (pp. 453-470). New York: Academic Press.

Husserl, F.E., & Messerli, F.H. (1981). Adverse effects of antihypertensive drugs. *Drugs, 22,* 188-210.

Hutchinson, T.A., Polansky, S.M., & Feinstein, A.R. (1979). Post-menopausal estrogens protect against fractures of the hip and distal radius-A case-control study. *Lancet, 2,* 705-709.

Huttunen, M.O., Harkonen, M., Niskanen, P., Leino, T., & Ylikahri, R. (1976). Plasma testosterone concentrations in alcoholics. *Journal of Studies on Alcohol, 37,* 1165-1177.

Hwang, T.I.S., Lue, T.F., Yang, C., & Chang, C. (1989). Drug-induced penile blood flow study: Effect of papaverine versus prostaglandin E1. *Journal of Urology, 141,* 261A.

Hyyppa, M.T., Falck, S.C., & Rinne, V.K. (1975). Is L-dopa an aphrodisiac in patients with Parkinson's disease? In M. Sandler & G.L. Gessa (Eds), *Sexual behavior: Pharmacology and biochemistry.* New York: Raven Press.

Hyyppa, M.T., Lehtinen, P., & Rinne, U.K. (1971). Effect of L-dopa on the hypothalamic, pineal, and striatal monoamines and on the sexual behavior of the rat. *Brain Research, 30,* 265-272.

Hyyppa, M.T., Rinne, U.K., & Sonninen, V. (1970). The activating effect of L-dopa treatment on sexual functions and its experimental background. *Acta Neurologica Scandinavica, 46* (Suppl. 43), 223-224.

Ikeda, Y., Tanaka, I., Oki, Y., Morita, H., Komatsu, K., & Yoshimi, T. (1990). Testosterone or GnRH treatment improves impaired response of plasma vasopressin to osmotic stimuli in men with hypogonadism. *Endocrine Society 72nd Meeting Abstracts,* 148.

Imperato, A., Honore, T., & Jensen, L.H. (1990). Dopamine release in the nucleus caudatus and in the nucleus accumbens is under glutamatergic control through non-NMDA receptors: A study in freely moving rats. *Brain Research, 530,* 223-228.

Imperato, A., Mulas, A., & DiChiara, G. (1986). Nicotine preferentially stimulates dopamine release in the limbic system of freely moving rats. *European Journal of Pharmacology, 132,* 337-338.

Ingram, I.M., & Timbury, G.C. (1960). Side effects of librium [Letter to the editor]. *Lancet, 2,* 766.

Insel, T.R. (1992). Oxytocin – a neuropeptide for affiliation: Evidence from behavioral, receptor autoradiographic, and comparative studies. *Psychoneuroendocrinology, 17,* 3-35.

Insel, T.R., & Shapiro, L.E. (1992). Oxytocin receptors and maternal behavior. In C.A. Pedersen, J.D. Caldwell, G.F. Jirikowski, & T.R. Insel (Eds.), *Oxytocin in maternal, sexual, and social behaviors. Vol. 652. Annals of the New York Academy of Sciences,* pp. 122-141.

Invernizzi, R., Bertorelli, R., Consolo, S., Garattini, S., & Samanin, R. (1989). Effects of the l-isomer of fenfluramine on dopamine mechanisms in rat brain: Further studies. *European Journal of Pharmacology, 164,* 241–248.

Iodice, M., Lombardi, G., Tommaselli, A.P., Rossi, R., & Minozzi, M. (1981). Inhibition of cimetidine-induced hyperprolactinemia by pretreatment with metergoline. *Journal of Endocrinological Investigation, 4,* 111–113.

Ionescu-Pioggia, M., Bird, M., & Cole, J.O. (1989). Subjective effects of methaqualone. *Nida Research Monograph, 95,* 455.

Ishii, N., Watanabe, H., Irisawa, C., Kikuchi, Y., Kawamura, S., Suzuki, K., Chiba, R., Tokiwa, M., & Shirai, M. (1986). Studies on male sexual impotence. Report 18. Therapeutic trial with prostaglandin E1 for organic impotence. *Japanese Journal of Urology, 77,* 954–962.

Isojarvi, J.I.T. (1990). Serum steroid hormones and pituitary function in female epileptic patients during carbamazepine therapy. *Epilepsia, 31,* 438–445.

Isojarvi, J.I., Pakarinen, A.J., Ylipalosaari, P.J., & Myllyla, V.V. (1990). Serum hormones in male epileptic patients receiving anticonvulsant medication. *Archives of Neurology, 47,* 670–676.

Issidorides, M.R. (1980). Observations in chronic hashish users: Nuclear observations in blood and sperm and abnormal acrosomes in spermatozoa. In G.G. Nahas & W.D. Paton (Eds.), *Marijuana: Biological effects* (pp. 377–387). Oxford: Pergamon Press.

Ivkovic, L., & Dulic, S. (1988). Biological and clinical results on the use of salmon calcitonin nasal spray in treatment of postmenopausal osteoporosis. *Gynecological Endocrinology, 2*(Suppl. 2), 241.

Jachuck, S.J., Brierley, H., Jachuck, S., & Willcox, P.M. (1982). The effects of hypotensive drugs on quality of life. *Journal of the Royal College of General Practitioners, 32,* 103–105.

Jacob, T., & Bremer, D.A. (1986). Assortative mating among men and women alcoholics. *Journal of Studies on Alcohol, 47,* 219–222.

Jacobsen, F.M. (1991). Fluoxetine-induced sexual dysfunction: Open and placebo-controlled trials of treatment with yohimbine. *Biological Psychiatry, 29,* 150A-151A.

Jacobsen, F.M. (1992). Fluoxetine-induced sexual dysfunction and an open trial of yohimbine. *Journal of Clinical Psychiatry, 53,* 119–122.

Jacobsen, F.M. (1993). Low-dose valproate: A new treatment for cyclothymia, mild rapid cycling disorders, and premenstrual syndrome. *Journal of Clinical Psychiatry, 54,* 229–234.

Jaffe, B.J., Haitas, B., & Seftel, H.C. (1987). Hormonal and metabolic effects of commonly used antihypertensive agents. In J.B. Puschett & A. Greenberg (Eds.), *Diuretics II: Chemistry, pharmacology clinical applications* (pp. 526–537). New York: Elsevier Science Publishers.

Jasonni, V.M., Bulletti, C., Bolelli, G.F., Franceschetti, F., Bonavia, M., Ciotti, P., & Flamigni, C. (1983). Estrone sulfate, estrone, and estradiol concentrations in normal and cirrhotic postmenopausal women. *Steroids, 41,* 569–573.

Jeffcoate, W.J., Herbert, M., Cullen, M.H., Hastings, A.G., & Walder, C.P. (1979). Prevention of effects of alcohol intoxication by naloxone. *Lancet, 2,* 1157–1159.

Jefferson, J.W. (1992). Is tranylcypromine really metabolized to amphetamine? [Letter to the editor]. *Journal of Clinical Psychiatry, 53,* 450–451.

Jeffreys, D.B., Flanagan, R.J., & Volans, G.N. (1980). Reversal of ethanol-induced coma with naloxone. *Lancet, 1,* 308–309.

Jenike, M.A. (1990). Managing sexual side effects of antiobsessional drugs. *OCD Newsletter, 4,* 2.

Jenike, M.A., Baer, L., Summergrad, P., Minichiello, W.E., Holland, A., & Seymour, R. (1990). Sertraline in obsessive-compulsive disorder: A double-blind comparison with placebo. *American Journal of Psychiatry, 147,* 923–928.

Jennings, B.H., Andersson, K.E., & Johansson, S.A. (1991). Assessment of systemic effects of inhaled glucocorticosteroids: Comparison of the effects of inhaled budesonide and oral prednisolone on adrenal function and markers of bone turnover. *European Journal of Clinical Pharmacology, 40,* 77–82

Jensen, H., & Madsen, J.L. (1988). Diet and cancer. *Acta Medica Scandinavica, 223,* 293–304.

Jensen, R.T., Collen, M.J., McArthur, K.E., Howard, J.M., Maton, P.N., Cherner, G., & Gardner, J.D. (1984). Comparison of the effectiveness of ranitidine and cimetidine in inhibiting acid secretion in patients with gastric hypersecretory states. *American Journal of Medicine, 77,* 90–105.

Jensen, R.T., Collen, M.J., Pandol, S.J., Allende, H.D., Raufman, J.P., Bissonnette, B.M., Duncan, W.C., Durgin, P.L., Gillin, J.C., & Gardner, J.D. (1983). Cimetidine-induced impotence and breast changes in patients with gastric hypersecretory states. *New England Journal of Medicine, 308,* 883–887.

Jensen, S.B. (1984). Sexual function and dysfunction in younger married alcoholics. *Acta Psychiatrica Scandanavica, 69,* 543–549.

Jensen, S.B., & Gluud, C. (1985). Sexual dysfunction in men with alcoholic liver cirrhosis: A comparative study. *Liver, 5,* 94–100.

Jeremy, J.Y., Mikhailidis, D.P., & Dandona, P. (1985). Cigarette smoke extracts inhibit prostacyclin synthesis in the rat urinary bladder. *British Journal of Cancer, 51,* 837–842.

Jeremy, J.Y., Mikhailidis, D.P., & Dandona, P. (1986). Muscarinic stimulation of prostacyclin synthesis by the rat penis. *European Journal of Pharmacology, 123,* 67–71.

Jeremy, J.Y., Mikhailidis, D.P., & Dandona, P. (1987). RE: Effects of prostaglandin E1 on penile erection and erectile failure [Letter to the editor]. *Journal of Urology, 140,* 1556.

Jeremy, J.Y., Morgan, R.J., Mikhailidis, D.P., & Dandona, P. (1986). Prostacyclin synthesis by the corpora cavernosa of the human penis: Evidence for muscarinic control and pathological implications. *Prostaglandins, Leukotrienes and Medicine, 23,* 211–216.

Jeremy, J.Y., Thompson, C.S., Mikhailidis, D.P., & Dandona, P. (1985). Experimental diabetes mellitus inhibits prostacyclin synthesis by the rat penis: Pathological implications. *Diabetologia, 28,* 365–368.

Jerie, P. (1986). Long-term evaluations of therapeutic efficacy and safety of guanfacine. *American Journal of Cardiology, 57,* 55E-59E.

Jirikowski, G.F., Caldwell, J.D., Pilgrim, C., Stumpf, W.E., & Pedersen, C.A. (1989). Changes in immunostaining for oxytocin in the forebrain of the female rat during late pregnancy, parturition and early lactation. *Cell and Tissue Research, 256*(2), 411–417.

Jirikowski, G.F., Caldwell, J.D., Stumpf, W.E., & Pedersen, C.A. (1988). Estradiol influences oxytocin immunoreactive brain systems. *Neuroscience, 25,* 237–248.

Johanson, C.E. (1986). Stimulant depressant report. In L.S. Harris (Ed.), *NIDA Research Monograph No. 67* (pp. 98–104). Rockville, MD: United States Government Printing Office.

Johanson, C.E. (1990). The evaluation of the abuse liability of drugs. *Drug Safety, 5*(Suppl. 1), 46–57.

Johanson, C.E., & Schuster, C.R. (1975, November). *A comparison of cocaine and diethylpropion under two different schedules of drug presentation.* Paper at presented at conference on contemporary issues in stimulant research, Duke University Medical Center.

Johansson, C.E., & Meyerson, B.J. (1991). The effects of long-term treatment with 8-OHDPAT on the lordosis response and hypothermia in female rats. *European Journal of Pharmacology, 196,* 143–147.

Johnson, A.E., Ball, G.F., Coirini, H., Harbaugh, C.R., McEwen, B.S., & Insel, T.R. (1989). Time course of the estradiol-dependent induction of oxytocin receptor binding in the ventromedial hypothalamic nucleus of the rat. *Endocrinology, 125,* 1414–1419.

Johnson, A.E., Coirini, H., McEwen, B.S., & Insel, T.R. (1989). Testosterone modulates oxytocin binding in the hypothalamus of castrated male rats. *Neuroendocrinology, 50,* 199–203.

Johnson, A.R., & Jarow, J.P. (1992). Is routine endocrine testing of impotent men necessary? *Journal of Urology, 147,* 1542–1544.

Johnson, D.F., & Phoenix, C.H. (1976). Hormonal control of female sexual attractiveness, proceptivity, and receptivity in rhesus monkeys. *Journal of Comparative and Physiological Psychology, 90,* 473–483.

Johnson, D.N, & Diamond, M. (1969). Yohimbine and sexual stimulation in the male rat. *Physiology and Behavior, 4,* 411–413.

Johnson, G.T., & Goldfinger, S.E. (1981). *The Harvard Medical School health letter book.* Cambridge, MA: Harvard University Press.

Johnson, P., Kitchin, A.H., Lowther, C.P., & Turner, R.W. (1966). Treatment of hypertension with methyldopa. *British Medical Journal, S480,* 133–137.

Johnston, C.A., Lopez, F., Samson, W.K., & Negro-Vilar, A. (1990). Physiologically important role for central oxytocin in the preovulatory release of luteinizing hormone. *Neuroscience Letters, 120,* 256–258.

Johnston, C.A., & Negro-Vilar, A. (1988). Role of oxytocin on prolactin secretion during proestrus and in different physiological or pharmacological paradigms. *Endocrinology, 122,* 341–350.

Johnston, D.E., Chiao, Y.B., Gavaler, J.S., & Van Thiel, D.H. (1981). Inhibition of testosterone synthesis by ethanol and acetaldehyde. *Biochemical Pharmacology, 30,* 1827–1831.

Jonas, J.M. (1990). Do substance abuses, including alcoholism and bulimia, covary? In L.D. Reid (Ed.), *Opioids, bulimia, and alcoholism* (pp. 247–258). New York: Springer-Verlag.

Jonas, J.M., Coleman, B.S., Sheridan, A.Q., & Kalinske, R.W. (1992). Comparative clinical profiles of triazolam versus other shorter-acting hypnotics. *Journal of Clinical Psychiatry, 53* (Suppl. 12), 19–31.

Jonas, J.M., Gold, M.S., Sweeney, D., & Pottash, A.L.C. (1987). Eating disorders and cocaine abuse: A survey of 259 cocaine abuses. *Journal of Clinical Psychiatry, 48,* 47–50.

Jones, B.M., & Jones, M.K. (1976). Women and alcohol: Intoxication, metabolism, and the menstrual cycle. In M. Greenblatt & M.A. Schuckit (Eds.), *Alcoholism problems in women and children* (pp. 103–136). New York: Grune & Stratton.

Jones, C.N., Howard, J.L., & McBennett, S.T. (1980). Stimulus properties of antidepressants in the rat. *Psychopharmacology (Berlin), 67,* 111-118.

Jones, G.H., Neill, D.B., & Justice, J.B. (1990). Nucleus accumbens, dopamine, and anticipatory behavior. *Society for Neuroscience: 20th Meeting, 16* (Pt. 1), 437.

Jones, R.B., Luscombe, D.K., & Groom, G.V. (1977). Plasma prolactin concentration in normal subjects and depressive patients following oral clomipramine. *Postgraduate Medical Journal, 53* (Suppl. 4), 166-171.

Jones, S. (1984). Ejaculatory inhibition with trazodone. *Journal of Clinical Psychopharmacology, 4,* 279-281.

Jordan, V.C. (1992). Overview from the International Conference on Long-Term Tamoxifen Therapy for Breast Cancer. *Journal of the National Cancer Institute, 84,* 231-234.

Jorgensen, H.A., & Hole, K. (1986). Evidence from behavioral and in vitro receptor-binding studies that the enkephalinergic system does not mediate acute ethanol effects. *European Journal of Pharmacology, 125,* 249-256.

Judd, L.L. (1979). Effect of lithium on mood, cognition, and personality function in normal subjects. *Archives of General Psychiatry, 36,* 860-866.

Juenemann, K.P., Lue, T.F., Luo, J.A., Benowitz, N.L., Abozeid, M.T., & Tanagho, E.A. (1987). The effect of cigarette smoking on penile erection. *Journal of Urology, 138*(2), 438-441.

Jungers, P., Nahoul, K., Pelissier, C., Dougados, M., Tron, F., & Bach, J. (1982). Low plasma androgens in women with active and quiescent systemic lupus erythematosus. *Arthritis and Rheumatism, 25,* 454-457.

Jung-Hoffman, C., & Kuhl, H. (1987). Divergent effects of two low-dose oral contraceptives on sex hormone-binding globulin and free testosterone. *American Journal of Obstetrics and Gynecology, 156,* 199-203.

Jurcovicova, J., Le, T., & Krulich, L. (1989). The paradox of alpha$_2$ adrenergic regulation of prolactin (PRL) secretion. II. PRL-releasing action of the alpha$_2$ receptor antagonists. *Brain Research Bulletin, 23,* 425-432.

Kahn, C. (1985). *Beyond the helix: DNA and the quest for longevity.* New York: Times Books.

Kahn, C. (1990, December). An anti-aging aphrodisiac. *Longevity,* 42-48.

Kahn, D.A. (1987). Possible toxic interaction between cyproheptadine and phenelzine [Letter to the editor]. *American Journal of Psychiatry, 144,* 1242-1243.

Kaiser, E., Kies, N., Maass, G., Schmidt, H., Beach, R.C., Bormacher, K., Herrmann, W.M., & Richter, E. (1978). The measurement of the psychotropic effects of an androgen in aging males with psychovegetative symptomatology: A controlled double blind study of mesterolone versus placebo. *Progress in Neuro-Psychopharmacology, 2,* 505-515.

Kaiser, F.E., & Morley, J.E. (1994). Gonadotropins, testosterone, and the aging male. *Neurobiology of Aging, 15,* 559-563.

Kales, A. (1985). Therapeutic index/side effects of long half-life versus short and intermediate half-life benzodiazepine hypnotics. In E.B. Gripon (Ed.), *Hypnotics. A clinical update: Proceedings of a symposium October 16, 1984* (pp. 8-18). Princeton: Excerpta Medica.

Kamien, J.B., & Woolverton, W.L. (1989). A pharmacological analysis of the discriminative stimulus properties of d-amphetamine in rhesus monkeys. *Journal of Pharmacology and Experimental Therapeutics, 248,* 938-945.

Kampen, D.L., & Sherwin, B.B. (1994). Estrogen use and verbal memory in healthy postmenopausal women. *Obstetrics and Gynecology, 83,* 979-983.

Kane, J.M., & Freeman, H.L. (1994). Toward more effective antipsychotic treatment. *British Journal of Psychiatry, 165*(Suppl. 25), 22-31.

Kaneko, S., Fukushima, Y., Sato, T., Nomura, Y., Ogawa, Y., Saito, M., Shinagawa, S., & Yamazaki, S. (1984). Hazards of fetal exposure to antiepileptic drugs: A preliminary report. In T. Sato & S. Shinagawa, S. (Eds.), *Antiepileptic drugs and pregnancy* (pp. 132-138). Amsterdam: Excerpta Medica.

Kaplan, H.S. (1974). *The new sex therapy: Active treatment of sexual dysfunction.* New York: Brunner/Mazel.

Kaplan, H.S. (1987). *Sexual aversion, sexual phobias, and panic disorder.* New York: Brunner/Mazel.

Kaplan, H.S. (1992a). Adjuvant treatment in breast cancer [Letter to the editor]. *Lancet, 339,* 424.

Kaplan, H.S. (1992b). A neglected issue: The sexual side effects of current treatments for breast cancer. *Journal of Sex and Marital Therapy, 18,* 3-19.

Kaplan, H.S., & Owett, T. (1993). The female androgen deficiency syndrome. *Journal of Sex and Marital Therapy, 19,* 3-24.

Kaplan, N.M. (1991). Dredging the data on antihypertensive therapy. *American Journal of Hypertension, 4,* 195-197.

Kaplitz, S.E. (1975). Withdrawn, apathetic geriatric patients responsive to methylphenidate. *Journal of the American Geriatric Society, 23,* 271-276.

Karacan, I. (1986). Erectile dysfunction in narcoleptic patients. *Sleep, 9,* 227-231.

Karacan, I., Salis, P.J., Hirshkowitz, M., Borreson, R.E., Narter, E., & Williams, R.L. (1990). Erectile dysfunction in hypertensive men: Sleep-related erections, penile blood flow, and musculovascular events. *Journal of Urology, 142,* 56–61.

Karacan, I., Salis, P.J., & Williams, R.L. (1978). The role of the sleep laboratory in the diagnosis and treatment of impotence. In R.L. Williams and I. Karacan (Eds.), *Sleep disorders: Diagnosis and treatment* (pp. 353-382). New York: Wiley.

Karacan, I., Snyder, S., Salis, P.J., Williams, R.L., & Derman, S. (1980). Sexual dysfunction in male alcoholics and its objective evaluation. In W.E. Fann, I. Karacan, A.D. Pokorny & R.L. Williams (Eds.), *Phenomenology and treatment of alcoholism* (pp. 259-268). New York: Spectrum.

Karaki, H., Ahn, H.Y., & Urakawa, N. (1987). Caffeine-induced contraction in vascular smooth muscle. *Archives of Internationales de Pharmacodyam et de Therapie, 285,* 60–71.

Karram, M.M., & Bhatia, N.N. (1989). Management of coexistent stress and urge urinary incontinence. *Obstetrics and Gynecology, 73,* 4–7.

Karram, M.M., Yeko, T.R., Sauer, M.V., & Bhatia, N.N. (1989). Urodynamic changes following hormonal replacement therapy in women with premature ovarian failure. *Obstetrics and Gynecology, 74,* 208–211.

Kastin, A.J., Ehrensing, R.H., Banks, W.A., & Zadina, J.E. (1987). Possible therapeutic implications of the effects of some peptides on the brain. In E.R. de Kloet, V.M. Wiegant, & D. deWied (Eds.), *Neuropeptides and brain function: Progress in brain research, Vol. 72* (pp. 223-234). New York: Elsevier Science Publishers.

Kastin, A.J., Ehrensing, R.H., Coy, D.H., Schally, A.V., & Kostrzewa, R.M. (1979). Behavioral effects of brain peptides, including LH-RH. In L. Zichella & P. Pancheri (Eds.), *Psychoneuroendocrinology in reproduction* (pp. 69–80). North Holland: Elsevier Science Publishers.

Katz, E., Schran, H.F., & Adashi, E.Y. (1989). Successful treatment of a prolactin-producing pituitary macro-adenoma with intravaginal bromocriptine mesylate: A novel approach to intolerance of oral therapy. *Obstetrics and Gynecology, 73*(3 pt 2), 517–520.

Katz, J.M. (1986). Sexual dysfunction and ocular timolol [Letter to the editor]. *Journal of the American Medical Association, 255,* 37–38.

Katz, R., & Rosenthal, M. (1994). Adverse interaction of cyproheptadine with serotonergic antidepressants [Letter to the editor]. *Journal of Clinical Psychiatry, 55,* 314–315.

Katz, R.J., DeVeaugh-Geiss, J., & Landau, P. (1990). Clomipramine in obsessive-compulsive disorder. *Biological Psychiatry, 28,* 401–414.

Kaufman, D.W., Miller, D.R., Rosenberg, L., Helmrich, S.P., Stolley, P., Schottenfeld, D., & Shapiro, S. (1984). Noncontraceptive estrogen use and the risk of breast cancer. *Journal of the American Medical Association, 252,* 63–67.

Kaufman, D.W., Slone, D., Rosenberg, L., Miettinen, O.S., & Shapiro, S. (1980). Cigarette smoking and age at natural menopause. *American Journal of Public Health, 70,* 420.

Kavaliers, M. (1987). Stimulatory influences of calcium channel antagonists on stress-induced opioid analgesia and locomotor activity. *Brain Research, 408,* 403–407.

Kawakami, M., & Sawyer, C.H. (1959). Induction of behavioral and electroencephalographic changes in the rabbit by hormone administration or brain stimulation. *Endocrinology, 65,* 631–643.

Kay, C.R. (1984). The Royal College of General Practitioners' oral contraception study: Some recent observations. *Clinical Obstetrics and Gynecology, 11,* 759–786.

Kaye, N.S., & Dancu, C. (1994). Paroxetine and obsessive-compulsive disorder [Letter to the editor]. *American Journal of Psychiatry, 151,* 1523.

Keck, P.E., McElroy, S.L., & Friedman, L.M. (1992). Valproate and carbamazepine in the treatment of panic and post-traumatic stress disorders, withdrawal states, and behavioral dyscontrol syndromes. *Journal of Clinical Psychopharmacology, 12,* 36S–41S.

Kedia, K.R., & Markland, C. (1975). The effect of pharmacological agents on ejaculation. *Journal of Urology, 114,* 569–573.

Kedia, K.R., & Persky, L. (1984). Effects of phenoxybenzamine (Dibenzyline) on sexual function in men. *Urology, 18,* 620–621.

Keeler, M.H., Taylor, C.I., & Miller, W.C. (1979). Are all recently detoxified alcoholics depressed? *American Journal of Psychiatry, 136,* 586–588.

Keitner, G.I., & Selub, S. (1983). Spontaneous ejaculations and neuroleptics. *Journal of Clinical Psychopharmacology, 3,* 34–36.

Keller, H.H., Bonetti, E.P., Pieri, L., & DaPrada, M. (1983). Lisuride-induced mounting behavior and effects on the monaminergic system in rat brain. In D.B. Calne, R. Horowski, R. McDonald, & W. Wuttke (Eds.), *Lisuride and other dopamine agonists* (pp. 79–87). New York: Raven Press.

Kelley, A.E., & Delfs, J.M. (1991). Dopamine and conditioned reinforcement. II: Contrasting effects of amphetamine microinjection into the nucleus accumbens with peptide microinjection into the ventral tegmental area. *Psychopharmacology, 103,* 197–203.

Kellner, R., Buckman, M.T., Fava, G.A., & Pathak, D. (1984). Hyperprolactinemia, distress, and hostility. *American Journal of Psychiatry, 141,* 759–763.

Kelly, D. (1980). *Anxiety and emotion*. Springfield, IL: Charles C. Thomas.

Kelly, M.P., Strassbert, D.S., & Kircher, J.R. (1990). Attitudinal and experiential correlates of anorgasmia. *Archives of Sexual Behavior, 19,* 165–177.

Kelly, M.W., & Myers, C.W. (1990). Clomipramine: A tricyclic antidepressant effective in obsessive compulsive disorder. *DICP: The Annals of Pharmacotherapy, 24,* 739–743.

Kemnitz, J.W., Goy, R.W., Flitsch, T.J., Lohmiller, J.J., & Robinson, J.A. (1989). Obesity in male and female rhesus monkeys: Fat distribution, glucoregulation, and serum androgen levels. *Journal of Clinical Endocrinology and Metabolism, 69,* 287–292.

Kemper, T.D. (1990). *Social structure and testosterone: Explorations of the socio-biosocial chain*. New Brunswick: Rutgers University Press.

Kendrick, K.M., & Dixson, A.F. (1985). Luteinizing hormone releasing hormone enhances proceptivity in a primate. *Neuroendocrinology, 41,* 449–453.

Kertesz, E., Somoza, G.M., D'Erano, J.L., & Libertus, C. (1987). Further evidence for endogenous hypothalamic serotonergic neurons involved in the cimetidine-induced prolactin release in the rat. *Brain Research, 413,* 10–14.

Keverne, E.B. (1979). Sexual and aggressive behavior in social groups of talapoin monkeys. *In Ciba Foundation Symposium. Vol. 62. Symposium on sex, hormones, and behavior, London* (pp. 291–297). Amsterdam: Excerpta Medica.

Kewitz, H., Jesdinsky, H.J., Schroter, P.M., & Lindtner, E. (1977). Reserpine and breast cancer in women in Germany. *European Journal of Clinical Pharmacology, 11,* 79–83.

Key, T.J., Pike, M.C., Wang, D.Y., & Moore, J.W. (1990). Long-term effects of first pregnancy on serum concentrations of dehydroepiandrosterone sulfate and dehydroepiandrosterone. *Journal of Clinical Endocrinology and Metabolism, 70,* 1651–1653.

Key, T.J., Pike, M.C., Baron, J.A., Moore, J.W., Wang, D.Y., Thomas, B.S., & Bulbrook, R.D. (1991). Cigarette smoking and steroid hormones in women. *Journal of Steroid Biochemistry and Molecular Biology, 39,* 529–534.

Khan, M.A. (1975). Side effects of amitriptyline. *British Medical Journal, 3,* 708.

Khan, S.A., Spiegel, D.A., & Jobe, P.C. (1987). Psychotomimetic effects of anorectic drugs. *American Family Physician, 36*(2), 107–112.

Khandelwal, S.K. (1988). Complete loss of libido with short-term use of lorazepam. *American Journal of Psychiatry, 145,* 1313–1314.

Khaw, K.T., Tazuke, S., & Barrett-Connor, E. (1988). Cigarette smoking and levels of adrenal androgens in postmenopausal women. *New England Journal of Medicine, 318,* 1705–1709.

Kiel, D.P., Baron, J.A., Anderson, J.J., Hannan, M.T., & Felson, D.T. (1992). Smoking eliminates the protective effect of oral estrogens on the risk for hip fracture among women. *Annals of Internal Medicine, 116,* 716–721.

Kiel, D.P., Felson, D.T., Anderson, J.J., Wilson, P.W., & Moskowitz, M.A. (1987). Hip fracture and the use of estrogens in postmenopausal women: The Framingham study. *New England Journal of Medicine, 317,* 1169–1174.

Kiely, E.A., Blank, M.A., Bloom, S.R., & Williams, G. (1987). Studies of intracavernosal VIP levels during pharmacologically induced penile erections. *British Journal of Urology, 59,* 334–339.

Kiely, E.A., Bloom, S.R., & Williams, G. (1989). Penile response to intracavernosal vasoactive intestinal polypeptide alone and in combination with other vasoactive agents. *British Journal of Urology, 64,* 191–194.

Kiely, E.A., Williams, G., & Goldie, L. (1987). Assessment of the immediate and long-term effects of pharmacologically induced penile erections in the treatment of psychogenic and organic impotence. *British Journal of Urology, 59,* 164–169.

Kilkku, P., Gronroos, M., Hirvonen, T., & Rauramo, L. (1983). Supravaginal uterine amputation versus hysterectomy: Effects on libido and orgasm. *Acta Obstetrica et Gynecologica Scandinavica, 62,* 147–152.

Kim, Y.M., Tejani, N., Chayen, B., & Verma, U.L. (1986). Management of third-stage labor with nipple stimulation. *Journal of Reproductive Medicine, 31,* 1033–1034.

King, V.L., Jr., & Horowitz, I.R. (1993). Vaginal anesthesia associated with fluoxetine use [Letter to the editor]. *American Journal of Psychiatry, 150,* 984–985.

Kinsey, A.C., Pomeroy, W.B., & Martin, C.E. (1948). *Sexual behavior in the human male*. Philadelphia: W.B. Saunders.

Kinsey, A.C., Pomeroy, W.B., Martin, C.E., & Gebhard, P.H. (1953). *Sexual behavior in the human female*. Philadelphia: W.B. Saunders.

Kissin, B. (1986). *Conscious and unconscious programs in the brain*. New York: Plenum Medical.

Klaiber, E.L., Broverman, D.M., Vogel, W., Kobayashi, Y., & Moriarty, D. (1972). Effects of estrogen therapy on plasma MAO activity and EEG driving responses of depressed women. *American Journal of Psychiatry, 128*(12), 1492–1495.

Klassen, A.D., & Wilsnack, S.C. (1986). Sexual experience and drinking among women in a United States national survey. *Archives of Sexual Behavior, 15,* 363–392.

Klein, K.B., Mendels, J., Lief, H.I., & Phillips, J. (1987). Drug treatment of inhibited sexual desire: A controlled clinical trial. Paper presented at the 1987 Society for Sex Therapy and Research Annual Meeting, New Orleans.

Kleven, M.S., Schuster, C.R., & Seiden, L.S. (1988). Effect of depletion of brain serotonin by repeated fenfluramine on neurochemical and anorectic effects of acute fenfluramine. *Journal of Pharmacology and Experimental Therapeutics, 246,* 822-828.

Kleven, M.S., & Seiden, L.S. (1989). D-, L-, and DL-fenfluramine cause long-lasting depletions of serotonin in rat brain. *Brain Research, 505,* 351-353.

Kline, M.D. (1989). Fluoxetine and anorgasmia [Letter to the editor]. *American Journal of Psychiatry, 146,* 804.

Kling, A., Steklis, H.D., & Deutsch, S. (1979). Radiotelemetered activity from the amygdala during social interactions in the monkey. *Experimental Neurology, 66,* 88-96.

Klove, K.L., Roy, S., & Lobo, R.A. (1984). The effect of different contraceptive treatments on the serum concentration of dehydroepiandrosterone sulfate. *Contraception, 29,* 319-324.

Kluver, H., & Bucy, P.C. (1938). An analysis of certain effects of bilateral temporal lobectomy in the rhesus monkey, with special reference to "psychic blindness." *Journal of Psychology, 5,* 33-54.

Knarr, J.W. (1976). Impotence from propranolol [Letter to the editor]. *Annals of Internal Medicine, 85,* 259.

Knigge, U., Thuesen, B., & Christiansen, P.M. (1986). Histaminergic regulation of prolactin secretion: Dose-response relationship and possible involvement of the dopaminergic system. *Journal of Clinical Endocrinology and Metabolism, 62,* 491-496.

Knobil, E. (1980). The neuroendocrine control of the menstrual cycle. *Recent Progress in Hormone Research, 36,* 53-88.

Knoll, J. (1981). The pharmacology of selective MAO inhibitors. In M.B. Youdim & E.S. Paykel (Eds.), *Monoamine oxidase inhibitors: The state of the art* (pp. 45-61). New York: John Wiley & Sons.

Knoll, J. (1985). The facilitation of dopaminergic activity in the aged brain by (-) deprenyl. A proposal for a strategy to improve the quality of life in senescence. *Mechanisms of Aging and Development, 30,* 109-122.

Knoll, J. (1988). Extension of life span of rats by long-term (-) deprenyl treatment. *Mount Sinai Journal of Medicine, 55,* 67-74.

Knoll, J., Dallo, J., & Yen, T.T. (1989). Striatal dopamine, sexual activity, and lifespan. Longevity of rats treated with (-) deprenyl. *Life Sciences, 45,* 525-531.

Knoll, J., Yen, T.T., & Dallo, J. (1983). Long-lasting, true aphrodisiac effect of (-) deprenyl in sexually sluggish old male rats. *Modern Problems in Pharmacopsychiatry, 19,* 135-153.

Knussmann, R., Christiansen, K., & Couwenbergs, C. (1986). Relations between sex hormone levels and sexual behavior in men. *Archives of Sexual Behavior, 15,* 429-445.

Kochansky, G.E., Salzman, C., Shader, R.I., Harmatz, J.S., & Ogeltree, A.M. (1975). The differential effects of chlordiazepoxide and oxazepam on hostility in a small group setting. *American Journal of Psychiatry, 132,* 861-863.

Koe, B.K., Lebel, A., Burkhart, C.A., & Schmidt, A.W. (1989). Sertraline: A potent inhibitor of (+) [^{3}H]3-PPP binding to brain sigma (o-) receptors. *Society for Neuroscience Abstracts: 19th Meeting, 15,* (Pt. 2), 1235.

Koene, P., Prinssen, E., & Cools, A.R. (1990). Involvement of the nucleus accumbens in orofacial behavior in the rat. *Psychopharmacology, 101*(Suppl), 530.

Koff, W.C. (1974). Marijuana and sexual activity. *Journal of Sex Research, 10,* 194-204.

Koller, W.C., Vetere-Overfield, B., Williamson, A., Busenbark, K., Nash, J., & Parrish, D. (1990). Sexual dysfunction in Parkinson's disease. *Clinical Neuropharmacology, 13,* 461-463.

Kolodny, R.C., Lessin, P., Toro, G., Masters, W.H., & Cohen, S. (1976). Depression of plasma testosterone with acute marijuana administration. In M.C. Braude & S. Szara (Eds.), *The pharmacology of marijuana, Vol. 1* (pp. 217-225). New York: Raven Press.

Kolodny, R.C., Masters, W.H., & Johnson, V.E. (1979). *Textbook of sexual medicine*. Boston: Little Brown & Co.

Kolodny, R.C., Masters, W.H., Kolodner, R.M., & Toro, G. (1974). Depression of plasma testosterone levels after chronic intensive marijuana use. *New England Journal of Medicine, 290,* 872-874.

Komanicky, P., Spark, R.F., & Melby, J.C. (1978). Treatment of Cushing's syndrome with trilostane (WIN 24,540), an inhibitor of adrenal steroid biosynthesis. *Journal of Clinical Endocrinology and Metabolism, 47,* 1042-1051.

Komisaruk, B.R. (1982). Neural-hormonal interactions in reproductive behavior in animals with reference to human studies. In Z. Hoch & H. Lief (Eds.), *Sexology* (pp. 62-66).

Komisaruk, B., Ciofalo, V., & Latranyi, M. (1976). Stimulation of the vaginal cervix is more effective than morphine in suppressing a nociceptive response in rats. In J. Bonica & D. Albe-Fessard (Eds.), *Advances in pain research and therapy* (pp. 439–443). New York: Raven Press.

Koppelman, M.C.S., Parry, B.L., Hamilton, J.A., Alagna, S.W., & Loriaux, D.L. (1987). Effect of bromocriptine on affect and libido in hyperprolactinemia. *American Journal of Psychiatry, 144,* 1037–1041.

Korenman, S.G. (1980). Estrogen window hypothesis of the etiology of breast cancer. *Lancet, 1,* 700–701.

Kotin, J., Wilbert, D.E., Verburg, D., & Soldinger, S.M. (1976). Thioridazine and sexual dysfunction. *American Journal of Psychiatry, 133,* 82–85.

Kovacs, G.L., Sarnyai, Z., Izbeki, F., Szabo, G., Telegdy, G., Barth, T., Jost, K., & Brtnik, F. (1987). Effects of oxytocin-related peptides on acute morphine tolerance: Opposite actions by oxytocin and its receptor antagonists. *Journal of Pharmacology and Experimental Therapeutics, 241,* 569–573.

Kowalski, A., Stanley, R.O., Dennerstein, L., Burrows, G., & Maguire, K.P. (1985). The sexual side effects of antidepressant medication: A double-blind comparison of two antidepressants in a non-psychiatric population. *British Journal of Psychaitry, 147,* 413–418.

Krahn, D.D., Gosnell, B., & Kurth, C. (1994). Dieting and alcohol use in women. In R.R. Watson (Ed.), *Drug and alcohol abuse reviews. Vol. 5. Addictive behaviors in women* (pp. 177–194). Totowa, NJ: Humana Press.

Kramer, P. (1993). *Listening to Prozac.* New York: Viking.

Kranzler, H.R., Burleson, J.A., Del Boca, F.K., Babor, T.F., Korner, P., Brown, J., & Bohn, M.J. (1994). Buspirone treatment of anxious alcoholics. *Archives of General Psychiatry, 51,* 720–731.

Kraupl-Taylor, F. (1972). Loss of libido in depression. *British Medical Journal, 1,* 305.

Kraus, J.F., Curb, J.D., Cutter, G., Daugherty, S.A., Neill, K.C., & Wassertheil-Smoller, S. (1983). Baseline medical history characteristics of the hypertensive participants. *Hypertension, 5*(6:II), IV51-IV91.

Kreuz, L., Rose, R.M., & Jennings, J.R. (1972). Suppression of plasma testosterone levels and psychological stress. *Archives of General Psychiatry, 26,* 479–482.

Kripke, D.F. (1985). Chronic hypnotic use: The neglected problem. In W.P. Koella, E. Ruther, & H. Schultz (Eds.), *Sleep '84* (pp. 338–340). New York: Gustav Fischer Verlag.

Kristensen, E., & Jorgensen, P. (1987). Sexual function in lithium-treated manic-depressive patients. *Pharmacopsychiatry, 20,* 165–167.

Kroner, B.A., Mulligan, T., & Briggs, G.C. (1993). Effect of frequently prescribed cardiovascular medications on sexual function: A pilot study. *Annals of Pharmacotherapy, 27,* 1329–1332.

Krupp, P., & Barnes, P. (1992). Clozapine-associated agranulocytosis: Risk and etiology. *British Journal of Psychiatry, 160*(Suppl. 17), 38–40.

Kryger, M.H., Steljes, D., Pouliot, Z., Neufeld, H., & Odynski, T. (1991). Subjective versus objective evaluation of hypnotic efficacy: Experience with zolpidem. *Sleep, 14,* 399–407.

Kuhl, H., Gahn, G., Romberg, G., März, W., & Taubert, H.D. (1985). A randomized crossover comparison of two low-dose oral contraceptives upon hormonal and metabolic parameters: I. Effects upon sexual hormone levels. *Contraception, 31,* 583–592.

Kuhnz, W., Sostarek, D., Gansau, C., Louton, T., & Mahler, M. (1991). Single and multiple administration of a new triphasic oral contraceptive to women: Pharmacokinetics of ethinyl estradiol and free and total testosterone levels in serum. *American Journal of Obstetrics and Gynecology, 165,* 596–602.

Kurumaji, A., Mitsushio, H., Ichikawa, H., & Shibuya, H. (1986). Effects of chronic treatment with antidepressants on opioid peptides in rat brain. *Japanese Journal of Psychiatry and Neurology, 40,* 542–543.

Kwan, M., Greenleaf, W.J., Mann, J., Crapo, L., & Davidson, J.M. (1983). The nature of androgen action on male sexuality: A combined laboratory self-report study on hypogonadal men. *Journal of Clinical Endocrinology and Metabolism, 57,* 557–562.

Kwong, L.L., Smith, E.R., Davidson, J.M., & Peroutka, S.J. (1986). Differential interactions of "prosexual" drugs with 5-hydroxytryptamine-1A and alpha$_2$-adrenergic receptors. *Behavioral Neuroscience, 100,* 664–668.

Labenz, J., Leverkus, F., & Börsch, G. (1994). Omeprazole plus amoxicillin for cure of *Helicobacter pylori* infection. *Scandinavian Journal of Gastroenterology, 29,* 1070–1075.

Laborit, H., Brunaud, M., Savy, J.M., Baron, C., Vallee, E., Lamothe, C., Thuret, F., Muyard, J.P., & Calvino, B. (1972). Etude biochimique et pharmacologique du 3-(2-morpholino-ethyl-amino) 4-methy 6-phenyl pyridazine, dichlorhydrate (Agr 1240). *Aggressologie, 13,* 291–318.

Labrie, C., Simard, J., Zhao, H.F., Belanger, A., Pelletier, G., & Labrie, F. (1989). Stimulation of androgen-dependent gene expression by the adrenal precursors dehydroepiandrosterone and androstenedione in the rat ventral prostate. *Endocrinology, 124,* 2745–2754.

Labrie, C., Simard, J., Zhao, H.F., Belanger, A.,

Pelletier, G., & Labrie, F. (1990). Stimulation of androgen-dependent gene expression by the adrenal precursors dehydroepiandrosterone and androstenedione in the rat ventral prostate. In L. Castagnetta, S. D'Aguino, F. Labrie & H.L. Bradlow (Eds.), *Steroid formation, degradation, and the action in peripheral tissues. Vol. 595. Annals of the New York Academy of Sciences* (pp. 395-398). New York: New York Academy of Sciences.

Labrie, F., Dupont, A., Cusan, L., Belanger, A., Giguere, M., Labrie, C., Lacourciere, Y., Monfette, G., & Emond, J. (1988). Combination therapy with flutamide and [D-Trp[6], DES-GLY-NH_{210}] LHRH ethylamide in stage C and D prostate cancer: Today's therapy of choice-rationale and five-year clinical experience. In W.D. Hankins (Ed.), *Hormones, cell biology, and cancer: Perspectives and potentials* (pp. 11-63). New York: Alan R. Liss.

Lacourciere, Y. (1988). Analysis of well-being and 24-hour blood pressure recording in a comparative study between indapamide and captopril. *American Journal of Medicine, 84,* 47-52.

LaCroix, A.Z., Mead, L.A., Liang, K., Thomas, C.B., & Pearson, T.A. (1986). Coffee consumption and the incidence of coronary heart disease. *New England Journal of Medicine, 315,* 977-982.

LaCroix, A.Z., Wienpahl, J., White, L.R., Wallace, R.B., Scherr, P.A., George, L.K., Cornoni-Huntley, J., & Ostfeld, A.M. (1990). Thiazide diuretic agents and the incidence of hip fracture. *New England Journal of Medicine, 322,* 286-290.

Ladisich, W. (1977). Influence of progesterone on serotonin metabolism: A possible causal factor for mood changes. *Psychoneuroendocrinology, 2,* 257-266.

LaFerla, J.J., Anderson, D.L., & Schalch, D.S. (1978). Psychoendocrine response to sexual arousal in human males. *Psychosomatic Medicine, 40,* 166-172.

LaFerla, J.J., Labrum, H., & Tang, K. (1982). Psychoendocrine response to sexual arousal in human females. In H.J. Prill & M. Stauber (Eds.), *Advances in psychosomatic obstetrics* (p. 20). Berlin: Springer-Verlag.

Laganière, S., Biron, P., & Robert, P. (1986). Opinion of 679 general practitioners on subjective side effects of antihypertensive drugs. *Current Therapeutic Research, 39,* 970-978.

Lahita, R., Bradlow, H., Ginzler, E., Pang, S., & New, M. (1987). Low plasma androgens in women with systemic lupus erythematosus. *Arthritis and Rheumatism, 30,* 241-248.

Lai, K.H., Cho, C.H., Ogle, C.W., & Wang, J.Y. (1986). Effects of eight-week treatment with histamine H2-antagonists or an antacid on plasma levels of histamine and serotonin in duodenal ulcer patients. *Pharmacological Research Communications, 18,* 807-812.

Lake, C.R., Reid, A., Martin, C., & Chernow, B. (1987). Cyclothymic disorder and bromocriptine: Predisposing factors for postpartum mania. *Canadian Journal of Psychiatry, 32,* 693-694.

Lakoski, J.M., Aghajanian, G.K., & Gallager, D.W. (1983). Interaction of histamine H2-receptor antagonists with GABA and benzodiazepine binding sites in the CNS. *European Journal of Pharmacology, 88,* 241-245.

Lal, S. (1988). Apomorphine in the evaluation of dopaminergic function in man. *Progress in Neuropsychopharmacology and Biological Psychiatry, 12,* 117-164.

Lal, S., Ackman, D., Thavundayil, J.X., Kiely, M.E., & Etienne, P.C. (1984). Effect of apomorphine, a dopamine receptor agonist, on penile tumescence in normal subjects. *Progress in Neuropsychopharmacology and Biological Psychiatry, 8,* 695-699.

Lal, S., Rios, O., & Thavundayil, J.X. (1990). Treatment of impotence with trazodone: A case report. *Journal of Urology, 143,* 819-820.

Lamb, R.J., & Griffiths, R.R. (1990). Self-administration in baboons and the discriminative stimulus effects in rats of bupropion, nomifensine, diclofensine, and imipramine. *Psychopharmacology, 102,* 183-190.

Lamb, R.J., Sannerud, C.A., & Griffiths, R.R. (1987). An examination of the intravenous self-administration of phenylpropanolamine using a cocaine substitution procedure in the baboon. *Pharmacology, Biochemistry, and Behavior, 28,* 389-392.

Lambert, A., Mitchell, R., & Robertson, W.R. (1987). Biopotency and site of action of drugs affecting testicular steroidogenesis. *Journal of Endocrinology, 113,* 457-461.

Lamberti, J.S., Bellnier, T., & Schwarzkopf, S.B. (1992). Weight gain among schizophrenic patients treated with clozapine. *American Journal of Psychiatry, 149*(5), 689-690.

Lamberts, S.W.J. (1983). Neuroendocrine aspects of centrally acting hypotensive drugs. *British Journal of Clinical Pharmacology, 15,* 5255-5285.

Lampl, Y., Eshel, Y., Rapaport, A., & Sarova-Pinchas, I. (1991). Weight gain, increased appetite, and excessive food intake induced by carbamazepine. *Clinical Neuropharmacology, 14,* 251-255.

Lancet. (1991). Editorial: Teratogenesis with carbamazepine. *Lancet, 337,* 1316-1317.

Lancon, C., Valle, M., & Jadot, G. (1990). Utilisation des inhibiteurs calciques en pathologie neuropsychiatrique. *Therapie, 45,* 131-137.

Lang, A.R. (1981). Drinking and disinhibition: Contributions from psychological research. In R.

Room & G. Collins (Eds.), *Alcohol and disinhibition: Nature and meaning of the link. United States Department of Health and Human Services Research. Monograph No. 12* (pp. 48-90). Rockville, MD: United States Government Printing Office.

Lang, A.R., Goeckner, D., Adesso, V., & Marlatt, A. (1975). Effects of alcohol on aggression in male social drinkers. *Journal of Abnormal Psychology, 84,* 508-518.

Lang, A.R., Searles, J., Lauerman, R., & Adesso, V. (1980). Expectancy, alcohol, and sex guilt as determinants of interest in and reaction to sexual stimuli. *Journal of Abnormal Psychology, 89,* 644-653.

Langer, S.Z., Arbilla, S., Scatton, B., Niddam, R., & Dubois, A. (1988). Receptors involved in the mechanism of action of zolpidem. In J.P. Sauvanet, S.Z. Langer, & P.L. Morselli (Eds.), *Imidazopyridines in sleep disorders* (pp. 55-70). New York: Raven Press.

Langer, G., Schonbeck, G., Koinig, G., Reiter, H., Schussler, M., Aschauer, H., & Lesch, O. (1980). Evidence for neuroendocrine involvement in the therapeutic effects of antidepressant drugs. In F. Brambilla, G. Racagni, & D. deWied (Eds.), *Progress in psychoneuroendocrinology* (pp. 197-211). Amsterdam: Elsevier/North-Holland Biomedical Press.

Langevin, R., Ben-Aron, M.H., Coulthard, R., Hucker, S.J., Purins, J.E., Russon, A.E., Day, D., Roper, V., & Webster, C.D. (1985). The effect of alcohol on penile erection. In R. Langevin (Ed.), *Erotic preference, gender identity, and aggression in men: New research studies* (pp. 101-111). Hillsdale, NJ: Lawrence Erlbaum Associates.

Langley, M.S, & Heel, R.C. (1988). Transdermal clonidine: A preliminary review of its pharmacodynamic properties and therapeutic efficacy. *Drugs, 35,* 123-142.

Langley, W.F., & Mann, D.J. (1991). Skeletal buffer function and symptomatic magnesium deficiency. *Medical Hypotheses, 34,* 62-65.

Lansky, D., & Wilson, G.T. (1981). Alcohol, expectations, and sexual arousal in males: An information processing analysis. *Journal of Abnormal Psychology, 90,* 35-45.

Lanthier, A., & Patwardhan, V.V. (1986). Sex steroids and 5-3 beta-hydroxysteroids in specific regions of the human brain and cranial nerves. *Journal of Steroid Biochemistry, 25,* 445-449.

Lardinois, C.K., & Mazzaferri, E.L. (1985). Cimetidine blocks testosterone synthesis. *Archives of Internal Medicine, 145,* 920-922.

Larsson, B., Andersson, K.E., Batra, S., Mattiasson, A., & Sjogren, C. (1984). Effects of estradiol on norepinephrine-induced contraction, alpha adrenoceptor number and norepinephrine content in the female rabbit urethra. *Journal of Pharmacology and Experimental Therapeutics, 229,* 557-563.

Larsson, K., & Ahlenius, S. (1986). Masculine sexual behavior and brain monoamines. In M. Segal (Ed.), *Psychopharmacology of sexual disorders* (pp. 15-32). London: John Libbey & Co.

Lasaga, M., Duvilanski, B.H., Seilicovich, A., Afione, S., & Debeljuk, L. (1988). Effect of sex steroids on GABA receptors in the rat hypothalamus and anterior pituitary gland. *European Journal of Pharmacology, 155,* 163-166.

Lattimer, N., McAdams, R.P., Rhodes, K.F., Sharma, S., Turner, S.J., & Waterfall, J.F. (1984). Alpha$_2$-adrenoceptor antagonism and other pharmacological antagonist properties of some substituted benzoquinolizines and yohimbine in vitro. *Nauyn-Schmiedeberg's Archives of Pharmacology, 327,* 312-318.

Lauritzen, C.H. (1973). The management of the premenopausal and the postmenopausal patient. *Frontiers in Hormone Research, 2,* 2-21.

Lauritzen, C.H. (1976). The female climacteric syndrome: Significance, problems, and treatment. *Acta Obstetrica et Gynecologica Scandinavica, 51* (Suppl.), 47-61.

Lauritzen, C.H., & Meier, F. (1984). Risks of endometrial and mammary cancer morbidity and mortality in long-term estrogen treatment. In H. van Herendael, F.E. Riphagen, & L. Goosens (Eds.), *The climacteric: An update* (pp. 207-221). Lancaster, England: MTP Press.

Lauritzen, C.H. (1986) Cost-benefit-risk analysis of estrogen treatment in the climacteric. *Gynakologe, 4,* 266-275.

Leadem, C.A., & Yagenova, S.V. (1987). Effects of specific activation of mu-, delta-, and kappa-opioid receptors on the secretion of luteinizing hormone and prolactin in the ovariectomized rat. *Neuroendocrinology, 45,* 109-117.

Lee, F., Stafford, I., & Hoebel, B.G. (1989). Similarities between the stimulus properties of phenylpropanolamine and amphetamine. *Psychopharmacology, 97,* 410-412.

Lee, L.M., Stevenson, R.W.D., & Szasz, G. (1989). Prostaglandin E1 versus phentolamine/papaverine for the treatment of erectile impotence: A double-blind comparison. *Journal of Urology, 141,* 549-550.

Le Feuvre, R.A., Aisenthal, L., & Rothwell, N.J. (1991). Involvement of corticotrophin releasing factor (CRF) in the thermogenic and anorexic actions of serotonin (5-HT) and related compounds. *Brain Research, 555,* 245-250.

Legros, J.J., Chiodera, P., Mormont, C., & Servais, J. (1980). A psychoneuroendocrinological study of sexual impotence in patients with abnormal reaction to a glucose tolerance test. In J. Mendlewicz & H.M van Praag (Eds.), *Psychoneuroendocrinology and abnormal behavior* (pp. 117–124). Basel: S. Karger.

Lehmann, J., Koenig-Berard, E., & Vitou, P. (1989). The imidazoline-preferring receptor. *Life Sciences, 45,* 1609–1615.

Leiblum, S.R., Bachmann, G.A., Kemmann, E., Colburn, D., & Swartzman, L. (1983). Vaginal atrophy in the postmenopausal woman. *Journal of the American Medical Association, 249,* 2195–2198.

Leiblum, S.R., & Rosen, R.C. (1984). Alcohol and human sexual response. In D.J. Powell (Ed.), *Alcoholism and sexual dysfunction: Issues in clinical management* (pp. 113–128). New York: Haworth Press.

Leiblum, S.R., & Swartzman, L.C. (1986). Women's attitudes toward the menopause: An update. *Maturitas, 8,* 47–56.

Leigh, B. (1990). The relationship of sex-related alcohol expectancies to alcohol consumption and sexual behavior. *British Journal of Addiction, 85,* 919–928.

Le Jeunne, C.L., Hugues, F.C., Munera, Y., & Ozanne, H. (1991). Dizziness in the elderly and calcium channel antagonists. *Biomedicine and Pharmacotherapy, 45,* 33–36.

Lemaire, A., Bailleul, J.P., Sister, M.P., Demaine, J.L., & Buvat, J. (1990). Subcutaneous injections of the penis without needle can induce erection: An alternative for those patients refusing intracavernous injections. *International Journal of Impotence Research, 2*(Suppl. 2), 319–320.

Lemere, F., & Smith, J.W. (1973). Alcohol-induced sexual impotence. *American Journal of Psychiatry, 130,* 212–213.

Leng, G., & Russell, J.A. (1988). Opioid control of oxytocin secretion. In S. Yoshida & L. Share (Eds.), *Recent progress in posterior pituitary hormones* (pp. 89–96). Amsterdam: Elsevier Science Publishers.

Leonard, M.A., Morales, A., & Nickel, J.C. (1988). The revelance of hyperprolactemia in impotence. *Journal of Urology, 139,* 1988.

Leonard, M.P., Nickel, C.J., & Morales, A. (1989). Hyperprolactinemia and impotence: Why, when, and how to investigate. *Journal of Urology, 142,* 992–994.

Lephart, E.D., Baxter, C.R., & Parker, C.R. (1987). Effect of burn trauma on adrenal and testicular steroid hormone production. *Journal of Clinical Endocrinology and Metabolism, 64,* 842–848.

Lesko, L.M., Stotland, N.L., & Segraves, R.T. (1982). Three cases of female anorgasmia associated with MAOIs. *American Journal of Psychiatry, 139,* 1353–1354.

Lesley, G.B., & Walker, T.F. (1977). A toxilogical profile of cimetidine. In W.L. Bruland & M.A. Simkins (Eds.), *Cimetidine: Proceedings of the Second International Symposium on histamine H_2-receptor antagonists* (pp. 24–33). Amsterdam: Excerpta Medica.

Lesniewska, B., Nowak, M., & Malendowicz, K. (1990). Sex differences in adrenocortical structure and function. *Hormone and Metabolism Research, 22,* 378–381.

LeVay, S. (1991). A difference in hypothalamic structure between heterosexual and homosexual men. *Science, 253,* 1034–1037.

Levesque, L.A., Herzog, A.G., & Seibel, M.M. (1986). The effect of phenytoin and carbamazepine on serum dehydroepiandrosterone sulfate in men and women who have partial seizures with temporal lobe involvement. *Journal of Clinical Endocrinology and Metabolism, 63,* 243–245.

Levin, R.M. (1991). The prevention of osteoporosis. *Hospital Practice, 26*(5), 77–97.

Levitt, A.J., & Joffe, R.T. (1988). Total and free testosterone in depressed men. *Acta Psychiatrica Scandinavica, 77,* 346–348.

Levitt, N., Vinik, A., Sive, A., Klaff, L., & Phillips, C. (1980). Synthetic luteinizing hormone-releasing hormone in impotent male diabetics. *South African Medical Journal, 57,* 701–704.

LeWinn, E.B. (1984). The steroidal actions of digitalis. *Perspectives in Biology and Medicine, 27,* 183–199.

Lewis, D.A., & Sherman, B.M. (1984). Serotonergic stimulation of adrenocorticotropin secretion in man. *Journal of Clinical Endocrinology and Metabolism, 58,* 458–462.

Lewis, J., Braganza, J., & Williams, T. (1993). Psychomotor retardation and semistuporous state with paroxetine [Letter to the editor]. *British Medical Journal, 306,* 1169.

Lewis-Jones, D.I., Lynch, R.V., Machin, D.C., & Desmond, A.D. (1987). Improvement in semen quality in infertile males after treatment with tamoxifen. *Andrologia, 19,* 86–90.

Lex, B. (1994). Women and substance abuse. In R.R. Watson (Ed.), *Drug and alcohol abuse reviews. Vol. 5: Addictive behaviors in women* (pp. 279–327). Totawa, NJ: Humana Press.

Leyson, J.F.J. (1987). Comparative study between oral and intrapenile vasoactive drugs in the management of impotence in neurologically impaired patients. *Journal of Urology, 138,* 185A.

Libanati, C.R., Schulz, E.E., Shook, J.E., Bock, M., & Baylink, D.J. (1992). Hip mineral density in females with a recent hip fracture. *Journal of*

Clinical Endocrinology and Metabolism, 74, 351-356.

Liberzon, I., Dequardo, J.R., & Silk, K.R. (1990). Bupropion and delirium [Letter to the editor]. *American Journal of Psychiatry, 147*(12), 1689-1690.

Lichtenstein, M.J., Yarnell, J.W., Elwood, P.C., Beswick, A.D., Sweetnam, P.M., Marks, V., Teale, D., & Riad-Fahmy, D. (1987). Sex hormones, insulin, lipids, and prevalent ischemic heart disease. *American Journal of Epidemiology, 126,* 647-657.

Lichtigfeld, F.J., & Gillman, M.A. (1992). Tranylcypromine abuse: Cause for concern? [Letter to the editor]. *American Journal of Psychiatry, 149,* 989.

Lichtman, R., & Papera, S. (1990). *Gynecology: Well-woman care.* Englewood Clifts, NJ: Appleton & Lange.

Lidberg, L., & Sternthal, V. (1977). A new approach to the hormonal treatment of impotentia erectionis. *Pharmacopsychiatric, 10,* 21-25.

Liebowitz, M.R. (1983). *The chemistry of love.* Boston: Little, Brown & Company.

Liebowitz, M.R., Hollander, E., Schneier, F., Campeas, R., Hatterer, J., Papp, L. Fairbanks, J., Sandberg, D., Davies, S., & Stein, M. (1989). Fluoxetine treatment of obsessive-compulsive disorder: An open clinical trial. *Journal of Clinical Psychopharmacology, 9,* 423-427.

Liebowitz, M.R., Karoum, F., Quitkin, F.M., Davies, S.O., Schwartz, D., Levitt, M., & Linnoila, M. (1985). Biochemical effects of l-deprenyl in atypical depressives. *Biological Psychiatry, 20,* 558-565.

Liegel, J.M., Fabre, L.F., Howard, P.Y., & Farmer, R.W. (1972). Plasma testosterone and sex hormone binding globulin (SHBG) in alcoholic subjects. *The Physiologist, 15,* 198.

Limouzin-Lamothe, M.A., Mairon, N., Joyce, C.R.B., & Le Gal, M. (1994). Quality of life after the menopause: Influence of hormonal replacement therapy. *American Journal of Obstetrics and Gynecology, 170,* 618-624.

Lin, S.N., Yu, P.C., Yang, M.C., Chang, L.S., Chiang, B.N., & Kuo, J.S. (1988). Local suppressive effect of clonidine on penile erection in the dog. *Journal of Urology, 139,* 849-852.

Linden, C.H., Vellman, W.P., & Rumack, B. (1985). Yohimbine: A new street drug. *Annals of Emergency Medicine, 14,* 1002-1004.

Lindenmayer, J.P. (1994). Risperidone: Efficacy and side effects. *Journal of Clinical Psychiatry Monograph, 12,* 53-60.

Lindheim, S.R., Notelovitz, M., Feldman, E.B., Larsen, S., Khan, F.Y., & Lobo, R.A. (1994). The independent effects of exercise and estrogen on lipids and lipoproteins in postmenopausal women. *Obstetrics and Gynecology, 83,* 167-172.

Lindholm, J., Fabricius-Bjerre, N., Bahnsen, M., Boiesen, P., Bangstrup, L., Lau Perdersen, M., & Hagen, C. (1978a). Pituitary-testicular function in patients with chronic alcoholism. *European Journal of Clinical Investigation, 8,* 269-272.

Lindholm, J., Fabricius-Bjerre, N., Bahnsen, M., Boiesen, P., Hagen, C., & Christensen, T. (1978b). Sex steroids and sex-hormone binding globulin in males with chronic alcoholism. *European Journal of Clinical Investigation, 8,* 273-276.

Lindsay, R. (1986a, September Suppl.). Estrogen replacement for osteoporosis. *Hospital Practice,* 25-33.

Lindsay, R. (1986b, July). Osteoporosis: When and how to intervene. *Drug Therapy,* 39-53.

Lingam, V.R., Lazarus, L.W., Groves, L., & Oh, S.H. (1988). Methylphenidate in treating post-stroke depression. *Journal of Clinical Psychiatry, 49,* 151-153.

Lingjaerde, O., Ahlfors, U.G., Bech, P., Dencker, S.J., & Elgen, K. (1987). The UKU side-effect rating scale: A new comprehensive rating scale for psychotropic drugs and a cross-sectional study of side effects in neuroleptic-treated patients. *Acta Psychiatrica Scandinavica, 76*(Suppl. 334), 1-99.

Linkins, R.W., & Comstock, G.W. (1990). Depressed mood and development of cancer, *American Journal of Epidemiology, 132,* 962-972.

Linn, G.S., & Stecklis, H.D. (1990). The effects of depo-medroxyprogesterone acetate (DMPA) on copulation-related and agonistic behaviors in an island colony of stumptail macaques (*Macacca arctoides*). *Physiology and Behavior, 47,* 403-408.

Linnoila, M., Mefford, I., Nutt, D., & Adinoff, B. (1987). Alcohol withdrawal and noradrenergic function. *Annals of Internal Medicine, 107,* 875-889.

Linnoila, M., Prinz, P.N., Wonsowicz, C.J., & Leppaluoto, J. (1980). Effect of moderate doses of ethanol and phenobarbital on pituitary and thyroid hormones and testosterone. *British Journal of Addiction, 75,* 207-212.

Lishman, W.A., Jacobson, R.R., & Acker, C. (1987). Brain damage in alcoholism: Current concepts. *Acta Medica Scandinavica Supplementation, 717,* 5-17.

Lissak, A., Sorokin, Y., Calderon, I., Dirnfeld, M., Lioz, H., & Abramovici, H. (1989). Treatment of hirsutism with cimetidine: A prospective randomized controlled trial. *Fertility and Sterility, 51,* 247-250.

Lobo, R.A. (1988). Endocrine therapy of hyperandrogenism. In R. Barbieri & I. Schiff (Eds.), *Re-*

productive endocrine therapeutics (pp. 101-126). New York: Alan R. Liss.

Lofstrom, A. (1979). Effect of progesterone on catecholamine content in parts of the limbic system and preoptic area. *Psychoneuroendocrinology, 4,* 75-77.

Loldrup, D., Langemark, M., Hansen, H.J., Olesen, J., & Bech, P. (1989). Clomipramine and mianserin in chronic idiopathic pain syndrome. *Psychopharmacology, 99,* 1-7.

Louvel, E., Cramer, P., Ferreri, M., Pagot, R., Regnier, F., L'Heritier, C., & Orofiamma B. (1988). Zolpidem and triazolam: Long-term multicenter studies (1-3 months) in psychiatric and general practice patients. In J.P. Sauvanet, S.Z. Langer, & P.L. Morselli (Eds.), *Imidazopyridines in sleep disorders* (pp. 327-338). New York: Raven Press.

Love, R.R. (1987). The risk of breast cancer in American women [Letter to the editor]. *Journal of the American Medical Association, 257,* 1470.

Love, R.R., Wiebe, D.A., Newcomb, P.A., Cameron, L., Leventhal, H., Jordan, V.C., Feyzi, J., & DeMets, D.L. (1991). Effects of tamoxifen on cardiovascular risk factors in postmenopausal women. *Annals of Internal Medicine, 115,* 860-864.

Lovejoy, J., & Wallen, K. (1990). Adrenal suppression and sexual initiation in group-living female rhesus monkeys. *Hormones and Behavior, 24,* 256-269.

Lowe, M.A., Schwartz, A.N., & Berger, R.E. (1989). The effects of cigarette smoking on penile function testing. *Journal of Urology, 141,* 437A.

Luck, M.R. (1989). A function for ovarian oxytocin. *Journal of Endocrinology, 121,* 203-204.

Lue, T.F. (1988). Impotence: New concepts regarding therapy. In M.I. Resnik (Ed.), *Current trends in urology. Vol. 1.* (pp. 1-9). Baltimore: Williams & Wilkins.

Lue, T.F., & Tanagho, E.A. (1987). Physiology of erection and pharmacological management of impotence. *Journal of Urology, 137,* 829-836.

Luisi, M., & Franchi, F. (1980). Double-blind group comparative study of testosterone undecanoate and mesterolone in hypogonadal male patients. *Journal of Endocrinological Investigation, 3,* 305-308.

Lukert, B.P., & Raisz, L.G. (1990). Glucocorticoid-induced osteoporosis: Pathogenesis and management. *Annals of Internal Medicine, 112,* 352-364.

Lulich, K.M., Goldie, R.G., Ryan, G., & Paterson, J.W. (1986). Adverse reactions to beta 2-agonist bronchodilators. *Medical Toxicology, 1,* 286-299.

Luttge, W.G. (1975). Stimulation of estrogen-induced copulatory behavior in castrated male rats with the serotonin biosynthesis inhibitor p-chlorophenylalanine. *Behavioral Biology, 14,* 373-378.

Lydiard, R.B., Howell, E.F., Laraia, M.T., & Balenger, J.C. (1987). Sexual side effects of alprazolam [Letter to the editor]. *American Journal of Psychiatry, 144,* 254-255.

Lynch, M.G., Whitson, J.T., Reay, H.B., Nguyen, H., & Drake, M.M. (1988). Topical beta-blocker therapy and central nervous system side effects. *Archives of Opthalmology, 106,* 908-911.

MacDonald, P.C., Dombroski, R.A., & Casey, M.L. (1991). Recurrent secretion of progesterone in large amounts: An endocrine/metabolic disorder unique to young women? *Endocrine Reviews, 12,* 372-394.

Macfarlane, C.A., Reynolds, W.J., & Rosencrantz, D.R. (1983). Yohimbine: An alternative treatment for erectile dysfunction. *Weekly Urological Clinical Letter, 27*(27), 1-2.

MacHale, S., & Phanjco, A.L. (1994). SSRIs to treat sexual dysfunction [Letter to the editor]. *British Journal of Psychiatry, 164,* 854.

MacLean, J.D., Forsythe, R.G., & Kapkin, I.A. (1983). Unusual side effects of clomipramine associated with yawning. *Canadian Journal of Psychiatry, 28,* 569-570.

MacLean, P.D. (1966). Studies of the cerebral representation of certain basic sexual functions. In R.A. Gorski & R.E. Whalen (Eds.), *Brain and behavior. Vol. 3. Brain and gonadal function* (pp. 35-79). Berkeley: University of California Press.

MacLean, P.D. (1990). *The triune brain in evolution: Role in paleocerebral functions.* New York: Plenum Press.

MacLean, P.D., Dua, S., & Deniston, O. (1963). Cerebral localization for scratching and seminal discharge. *Archives of Neurology, 9,* 485-497.

MacLean, P.D., & Ploog, D.W. (1962). Cerebral representation of penile erection. *Journal of Neurophysiology, 25,* 29-55.

MacPhee, G.J.A., Larkin, J.G., Butler, E., Beastall, G.H., & Brodie, M.J. (1988). Circulating hormones and pituitary responsiveness in young epileptic men receiving long-term antiepileptic medication. *Epilepsia, 29,* 468-475.

Maddocks, S., Hahn, P., Moller, P., & Reid, R.L. (1986). A double-blind placebo-controlled trial of progesterone vaginal suppositories in the treatment of premenstrual syndrome. *American Journal of Obstetrics and Gynecology, 154,* 573-581.

Maes, M., Jacobs, M.P., Suy, E., Minner, B., & Raus, J. (1989). Cortisol, ACTH, prolactin, and beta-endorphin responses to fenfluramine administration in major-depressed patients. *Neuropsychobiology, 21,* 192-196.

Maffla, A.F., & de Garcia, M.H. (1979). Clinical

evaluation of the symptomatic activity of a new, original psychotropic drug, minaprine. *Pharmatherapeutica, 2,* 265–270.

Magni, G. (1991). The use of antidepressants in the treatment of chronic pain. *Drugs, 42,* 730–748.

Magos, A.L., Brewster, E., Singh, R., O'Dowd, T., Brincat, M., & Studd, J.W. (1986). The effects of norethisterone in postmenopausal women on estrogen replacement therapy: A model for the premenstrual syndrome. *British Journal of Obstetrics and Gynecology, 93,* 1290–1296.

Mahajan, S.K., Abassi, A.A., Prasad, A.S., Rabbani, P., Briggs, W., & McDonald, F.D. (1982). Effect of oral zinc therapy on gonadal function in hemodialysis patients: A double-blind study. *Annals of Internal Medicine, 97,* 357–361.

Mahendra, B. (1987). *Depression: The disorder and its associations.* Lancaster, England: MTP Press.

Mahmoud, K.Z., Dakhli, M.R.E., Fahmi, I.M., & Abdel-Aziz, A.B. (1992). Comparative value of prostaglandin E1 and papaverine in treatment of erectile failure: Double-blind crossover study among Egyptian patients. *Journal of Urology, 147,* 623–626.

Maier, U., & Koinig, G. (1994). Andrological findings in young patients under long-term antidepressive therapy with clomipramine. *Psychopharmacology, 116,* 357–359.

Maj, J., Wedzony, K., & Klimek, V. (1987). Desipramine given repeatedly enhances behavioral effects of dopamine and d-amphetamine injected into the nucleus accumbens. *European Journal of Pharmacology, 140,* 179–185.

Majewska, M.D. (1987). Steroids and brain activity: Essential dialogue between body and mind. *Biochemical Pharmacology, 36,* 3781–3788.

Majewska, M.D. (1990). Steroid regulation of the $GABA_A$ receptor: Ligand binding, chloride transport, and behavior. In D. Chadwick & K. Widdows (Eds.), *Steroids and neural activity* (pp. 83–106). New York: John Wiley & Sons.

Majewska, M.D., Demirgoren, S., & London, E.D. (1990). Binding of pregnenolone sulfate to rat brain membranes suggests multiple sites of steroid action at the $GABA_A$ receptor. *European Journal of Pharmacology, 189,* 307–315.

Majewska, M.D., Mienville, J.M., & Vicini, S. (1988). Neurosteroid pregnenolone sulfate antagonizes electrophysiological responses to GABA in neurons. *Neuroscience Letters, 90,* 279–284.

Makajina, T., Post, R., Pert, A., Weiss, S., & Ketter, T. (1989). Perspectives on the mechanism of action of electro-convulsive therapy. *Anti-convulsant, Peptidergic, and C-FOS Proto-Oncogene Convulsive Therapy, 5,* 274–275.

Makhija, V.N. (1984). Maprotiline and impotence: A case report. *Delaware Medical Journal, 56,* 183–185.

Malatesta, V.J., Pollack, R.H., Crotty, T.D., & Peacock, L.J. (1982). Acute alcohol intoxication and the female orgasmic response. *Journal of Sex Research, 18,* 1–17.

Malatesta, V.J., Pollack, R.H., Wilbanks, W.A., & Adams, H.E. (1979). Alcohol effects on the orgasmic-ejaculatory response in human males. *Journal of Sex Research, 15,* 101–107.

Malcomb, R., Ballenger, J.C., Sturgis, E.T., & Anton, R. (1989). Double-blind controlled trial comparing carbamazepine to oxazepam treatment of alcoholic withdrawal. *American Journal of Psychiatry, 146,* 617–621.

Malloy, T.R., & Wein, A.J. (1988, June). Erectile dysfunction: Effects of pharmacotherapy. *Medical Aspects of Human Sexuality,* 42–48.

Malmas, C.O. (1976). The significance of dopamine versus other catecholamines, for L-dopa-induced facilitation of sexual behavior in the castrated male rat. *Pharmacology, Biochemistry, and Behavior, 4,* 521–526.

Mamelle, N., Meunier, P.J., Dusan, R., Guillaume, M., Martin, J.L., Gaucher, A., Prost, A., & Zeigler, G. (1988). Risk-benefit ratio of sodium flouride treatment in primary vertebral osteoporosis. *Lancet, 2,* 361–365.

Manberg, P.J., & Carter, R.G. (1984). Bupropion in the treatment of psychotic depression: Two case reports. *Journal of Clinical Psychiatry, 45,* 1984.

Mandenoff, A., Bertiere, M.C., Betoulle, D., & Apfelbaum, M. (1986). Action of naltrexone on the sexual impairment of obese cafeteria rats. In J.W. Haladay, D.Y. Law, & A. Herz (Eds.), *Progress in opioid research: National Institute of Drug Abuse Research Monograph 75* (pp. 489–492). Washington DC.

Maneksha, S., & Harry, T.A. (1975). Lorazepam in sexual disorders. *British Journal of Clinical Practice, 29,* 175–176.

Mann, D.R., Gould, K.G., & Collins, D.C. (1990). A potential primate model for bone loss resulting from medical oophorectomy or menopause. *Journal of Clinical Endocrinology and Metabolism, 71,* 105–110.

Mann, K.V., Abbott, E.C., Gray, J.D., Thiebaux, H.J., & Belzer, E.J. (1982). Sexual dysfunction with beta-blocker therapy: More common than we think? *Sexuality and Disability, 5,* 67–77.

Mann, T. (1968). Effects of pharmacological agents on male sexual functions. *Journal of Reproduction and Fertility, 4*(Suppl.), 101–114.

Manning, D.M., Klevens, R.M., & Flanders, W.D. (1994). Cigarette smoking: An independent risk factor for impotence? *American Journal of Epidemiology, 140,* 1003-1008.

Mansky, T., Mestres-Ventura, P., & Wuttke, W. (1982). Involvement of GABA in the feedback action of estradiol on gonadotropin and prolactin release: Hypothalamic GABA and catecholamine turnover rates. *Brain Research, 231,* 353-364.

Manso, G., Sanchez, M., Hidalgo, A., & Andres-Trelles, F. (1986). Influence of some inhibitors of arachidonic acid metabolism on oxytocin concentrations in the isolated testicular capsule of the rat. *European Journal of Pharmacology, 131,* 285-287.

Maoz, B., & Durst, N. (1980). The effects of estrogen therapy on the sex life of postmenopausal women. *Maturitas, 2,* 327-336.

March, C.M. (1979). Bromocriptine in the treatment of hypogonadism and male impotence. *Drugs, 17,* 349-358.

Marcus, M.D., Wing, R.R., Ewing, L., Kern, E., McDermott, B.S., & Gooding, W. (1990). A double-blind, placebo-controlled trial of fluoxetine plus behavior modification in the treatment of obese binge-eaters and non-binge eaters. *American Journal of Psychiatry, 147,* 876-881.

Marcus, R. (1991). Understanding osteoporosis. *Western Journal of Medicine, 155,* 53-60.

Marder, S.R., & Meibach, R.C. (1994). Risperidone in the treatment of schizophrenia. *American Journal of Psychiatry, 151,* 825-835.

Marek, G.J., Vosmer, G., & Seiden, L.S. (1990). Dopamine uptake inhibitors block long-term neurotoxic effects of methamphetamine upon dopaminergic neurons. *Brain Research, 513,* 274-279.

Margolin, A., Kosten, T., Petrakis, I., Avants, S.K., & Kosten, T. (1991). Bupropion reduces cocaine abuse in methadone-maintained patients. *Archives of General Psychiatry, 48,* 87.

Margolis, R., & Leslie, C.H. (1966). Review of studies on a mixture of nux vomica, yohimbine, and methyltestosterone in the treatment of impotence. *Current Therapeutic Research, 8,* 280-284.

Margolis, R., Prieto, P., Stein, L., & Chinn, S. (1971). Statistical summary of 10,000 male cases using aphrodex in treatment of impotence. *Current Therapeutic Research, 13,* 616-622.

Margolis, R., Sangree, J., Prieto, P., Stein, L., & Chinn, S. (1967). Clinical studies on the use of afrodex in the treatment of impotence: Statistical summary of 4,000 cases. *Current Therapeutic Research, 9,* 213-219.

Maric, D., Stojilkovic, S., Krsmanovic, L., Simonovic, Kovacevic, R., & Andjus, R. (1987). Rapid naloxone-induced alterations of androgen variables in the growing male rat. *Neuroendocrinology, 46,* 167-175.

Marks, I.M., Stern, R.S., Mawson, D., Cobb, J., & McDonald, R. (1980). Clomipramine and exposure for obsessive-compulsive rituals. *British Journal of Psychiatry, 136,* 1-25.

Marks, P., & Banks, J. (1960). Inhibition of mammalian glucose-6-phosphate dehydrogenase by steroids. *Proceedings of the National Academy of Sciences, 46,* 447-452.

Marlatt, G., Demming, B., & Reid, J. (1973). Loss of control drinking in alcoholics: An experimental analogue. *Journal of Abnormal Psychology, 81,* 233-241.

Marshall, E. (1994). Tamoxifen: Hanging in the balance. *Science, 264,* 1524-1527.

Marshall, G.A., Breza, J., & Lue, T.F. (1994). Improved hemodynamic response after long-term intracavernous injection for impotence. *Urology, 43,* 844-848.

Marshall, G.A., & Lue, T.F. (1993). Improved hemodynamic response after long-term intracavernosal injection therapy for impotence. *Journal of Urology, 149,* 320A.

Marshall, J.F., & Altar, C.A. (1986). Striatal dopamine uptake and swim performance of the aged rat. *Brain Research, 379,* 112-117.

Marson, L., & McKenna, K.E. (1990a). The identification of a brainstem site controlling spinal sexual reflexes in male rats. *Brain Research, 515,* 303-308.

Marson, L., & McKenna, K.E. (1990b). A role for 5-hydroxytryptamine in mediating spinal sexual reflexes. *Society for Neuroscience Abstracts: 20th Meeting, 16* (Pt. 2), 1066.

Martin, C.A., & Iwamoto, E.T. (1984). Diethylpropion-induced psychosis reprecipitated by an MAO inhibitor: Case report. *Journal of Clinical Psychiatry, 45,* 130-131.

Martin, P., Massol, J., Colin, J.N., Lacomblez, L., & Puech, A.J. (1990). Antidepressant profile of bupropion and three metabolites in mice. *Pharmacopsychiatry, 23,* 187-194.

Martin, R.L., Roberts, W.V., & Clayton, P.J. (1980). Psychiatric status after hysterectomy: A one-year prospective follow-up. *Journal of the American Medical Association, 244,* 350-353.

Martin, W.R., Jasinski, D.R., Haertzen, C.A., Kay, D.C., Jones, B.E., Mansky, P.A., & Carpenter, R.W. (1973). Methadone: A reevaluation. *Archives of General Psychiatry, 28,* 286-295.

Martino, V., Mas, M., & Davidson, J.M. (1987). Chlordiazepoxide facilitates erections and inhibits seminal emission in rats. *Psychopharmacology (Berlin), 91,* 85-89.

Mas, M., Gonzalez-Mora, J.L., Louilot, A., Sole, C., & Guadalupe, T. (1990). Increased dopamine release in the nucleus accumbens of copulating male rats as evidenced by in vivo voltammetry. *Neuroscience Letters, 110,* 303-308.

Mas, M., Zahradnik, M.A., Martino, V., & Davidson, J.M. (1985). Stimulation of spinal serotonergic receptors facilitates seminal emission and suppresses penile erectile reflexes. *Brain Research, 342,* 128-134.

Masand, P., & Stern, T.A. (1993). Bupropion and secondary mania: Is there a relationship? *Annals of Clinical Psychiatry, 5,* 271-274.

Mashford, M.L. (1985). Appetite suppressant drugs. *Medical Journal of Australia, 143,* 605-607.

Mashini, I.S., Devoe, L.D., McKenzie, J.S., Hadi, H.A., & Sherline, D.M. (1987). Comparison of uterine activity induced by nipple stimulation and oxytocin. *Obstetrics and Gynecology, 69,* 74-78.

Masters, W.H., & Johnson, V.E. (1966). *Human sexual response.* Boston: Little, Brown & Co.

Masters, W.H., Johnson, V.E., & Kolodny, R.C. (1988). *Human sexuality (3rd ed.).* New York: Harper Collins.

Mathes, C.W., Smith, E.R., Popa, B.R., & Davidson, J. (1990). Effects of intrathecal and systemic administration of buspirone on genital reflexes and mating behavior in male rats. *Pharmacology, Biochemistry, and Behavior, 36,* 63-68.

Mathews, A. (1983). Progress in the treatment of female sexual dysfunction. *Journal of Psychomatic Research, 27,* 165-173.

Mathews, A., Whitehead, A., & Kellett, J. (1983). Psychological and hormonal factors in the treatment of female sexual dysfunction. *Psychological Medicine, 13,* 83-92.

Mathews, K.A. Meilahn, E., Kuller, L.H., Kelsey, S.f., Caggiula, A.W., & Wing, R.R. (1989). Menopause and risk factors for coronary heart disease. *New England Journal of Medicine, 321,* 641-646.

Mattes, J.A., Boswell, L., & Oliver, H. (1984). Methylphenidate effects on symptoms of attention deficit disorder in adults. *Archives of General Psychiatry, 41,* 1059-1063.

Mattson, R.H. (1990). Selection of drugs for treatment of epilepsy. *Seminars in Neurology, 10,* 406-413.

Mattson, R.H., & Cramer, J.A. (1985). Epilepsy, sex hormones, and antiepileptic drugs. *Epilepsia, 26*(Suppl. 1), 540-551.

Mattson, R.H., Cramer, J.A., Williamson, P.D., & Novelly, R.A. (1978). Valproic acid in epilepsy: Clinical and pharmacologic effects. *Annals of Neurology, 3,* 20-25.

Max, M.B., Lynch, S.A., Muir, J., Shoaf, S.E., Smoller, B., & Dubner, R. (1992). Effects of desipramine, amitriptyline, and fluoxetine on pain in diabetic neuropathy. *New England Journal of Medicine, 326,* 1250-1256.

Mazur, A., & Lamb, T.A. (1988). Testosterone, status, and mood in human males. *Hormones and Behavior, 14,* 236-246.

Mazurek, M.F., Beal, M.F., Bird, E.D., & Martin, J.B. (1987). Oxytocin in Alzheimer's disease: Postmortem brain levels. *Neurology, 37,* 1001-1003.

McAllister, J.M., & Hornsby, P.J. (1987). TPA inhibits the synthesis of androgens and cortisol and enhances the synthesis of non-17 alpha-hydroxylated steroids in cultured human adrenocortical cells. *Endocrinology, 121,* 1908-1910.

McBride, P.A., Tierney, H., DeMeo, M., Chen, J.S., & Mann, J.J. (1990). Effect of age and gender on CNS serotonergic responsivity in normal adults. *Biological Psychiatry, 27,* 1143-1155.

McCaffrey, T.A., & Czaja, J.A. (1989). Diverse effects of estradiol-17 Beta: Concurrent suppression of appetite, blood pressure, and vascular reactivity in conscious, unrestrained animals. *Physiology and Behavior, 45,* 649-657.

McCaul, K.D., Gladue, B.A., & Joppa, M. (1992). Winning, losing, mood, and testosterone. *Hormones and Behavior, 26,* 486-504.

McClain, C., Van Thiel, D.H., Parker, S., Badzin, L.K., & Gilbert, H. (1979). Zinc, vitamin A and retinol-binding protein in chronic alcoholics: A possible mechanism for night blindness and hypogonadism. *Alcoholism: Clinical and Experimental Research, 3,* 135-141.

McClure, R.D., Oses, R., & Ernest, M.L. (1991). Hypogonadal impotence treated by transdermal testosterone. *Urology, 37,* 224-228.

McConaghy, N. (1993). *Sexual behavior: Problems and management.* New York: Plenum.

McCormick, S., Olin, J., & Brotman, A.W. (1990). Reversal of fluoxetine-induced anorgasmia by cyproheptadine in two patients. *Journal of Clinical Psychiatry, 51,* 383-384.

McCoy, N., Cutler, W., & Davidson, J.M. (1985). Relationships among sexual behavior, hot flashes, and hormone levels in premenopausal women. *Archives of Sexual Behavior, 14,* 385-394.

McDonnell, S.M., Diehl, N.K., Garcia, M.C., & Kenney, R.M. (1989). Gonadatropin releasing hormone (GnRH) affects precopulatory behavior in testosterone-treated geldings. *Physiology and Behavior, 45,* 145-149.

McDonnell, S.M., Garcia, M.C., & Kenney, R.M. (1987b). Pharmacological manipulation of sexual behavior in stallions. *Journal of Reproduction and Fertility, 35*(Suppl.), 45-49.

McDonnell, S.M., Garcia, M.C., Kenney, R.M., & Van Arsdalen, K.N. (1987a). Imipramine-induced erection, masturbation, and ejaculation in male horses. *Pharmacology, Biochemistry, and Behavior, 27,* 187-191.

McDonnell, S.M., Kenney, R.M., Meckley, P.E., & Garcia, M.C. (1986). Novel environment suppression of sexual behavior in stallions and effects of diazepam. *Physiology and Behavior, 37,* 503–505.

McElroy, J.F., Miller, J.M., & Meyer, J.S. (1984). Fenfluramine, p-chloroamphetamine, and p-fluoroamphetamine stimultion of pituitary-adrenocortical activity in rat: Evidence for differences in site and mechanism of action. *Journal of Pharmacology and Experimental Therapeutics, 228,* 593–599.

McElroy, S.L., Keck, P.E., Jr., Pope, H.J., Jr., & Hudson, J.I. (1992). Valproate in the treatment of bipolar disorder: Literature review and clinical guidelines. *Journal of Clinical Psychopharmacology, 12,* 425–525.

McEwen, J., & Meyboom, R.H.B. (1983). Testicular pain caused by mazindol. *British Medical Journal, 287,* 1763–1764.

McFarland, B.H., Miller, M.R., & Straumfjord, A.A. (1990). Valproate use in the older manic patient. *Journal of Clinical Psychiatry, 51,* 479–481.

McFarland, K.F., Boniface, M.E., Hornung, C.A., Earnhardt, W., & Humphries, J.O. (1989). Risk factors and noncontraceptive estrogen use in women with and without coronary disease. *American Heart Journal, 117,* 1209–1214.

McGregor, A., & Herbert, J. (1992a). Specific effects of beta-endorphin infused into the amygdala on sexual behavior in the male rat. *Neuroscience, 46,* 165–172.

McGregor, A., & Herbert, J. (1992b). The effects of beta-endorphin infusions into the amygdala on visual and olfactory sensory processing during sexual behavior in the male rat. *Neuroscience, 46,* 173–179.

McGuigan, J.E. (1983). Side effects of histamine H2-receptor antagonist. *Clinics in Gastroenterology, 12,* 819–839.

McHaffie, D.J., Guz, A., & Johnston, A. (1977). Impotence in patient on disopyramide. *Lancet, 1,* 859.

McIntosh, T.K., & Barfield, R.J. (1984a). Brain monoaminergic control of male reproductive behavior. I. Serotonin and the post-ejaculatory refractory period. *Behavioral Brain Research, 12,* 255–265.

McIntosh, T.K., & Barfield, R.J. (1984b). Brain monoaminergic control of reproductive behavior. II. Dopamine and the post-ejaculatory refractory period. *Behavioral Brain Research, 12,* 267–273.

McIntosh, T.K., & Barfield R.J. (1984c). Brain monoaminergic control of reproductive behavior. III. Norepinephrine and the post-ejaculatory period. *Behavioral Brain Research, 12,* 275–281.

McIntosh, T.K., Vallano, M.L., & Barfield, R.J. (1980). Effects of morphine, beta-endorphin, and naloxone on catecholamine levels and sexual behavior in the male rat. *Pharmacology, Biochemistry, and Behavior, 13,* 435–444.

McKenna, K.E., & Nadelhaft, I. (1986). The organization of the pudendal nerve in the male and female rat. *Journal of Comparative Neurology, 248*(4), 532–549.

McKenna, K.E., & Nadelhaft, I. (1989). The pudendo-pudendal reflex in male and female rats. *Journal of the Autonomic Nervous System, 27,* 67–77.

McKenna, P.J., & Bailey, P.E. (1993). The strange story of clozapine. *British Journal of Psychiatry, 162,* 32–37.

McLean, J.D., Forsythe, R.G., & Kapkin, I.A. (1983). Unusual side effects of clomipramine associated with yawning. *Canadian Journal of Psychiatry, 28,* 569–570.

McMahon, D.C., Shaffer, R.N., Hoskins, H.D., & Hetherington, J. (1979). Adverse effects experienced by patients taking timolol. *American Journal of Ophthalmology, 88,* 736–738.

McMahon, F.G. (1978). *Management of essential hypertension*. Mount Kisco, New York: Futura Publishers.

McMahon, F.G., Jain, A.K., Vargas, R., & Fillingim, J. (1990). A double-blind comparison of transdermal clonidine and oral captopril in essential hypertension. *Clinical Therapeutics, 12,* 88–100.

McNair, D.M., Goldstein, A.P., Lorr, M., et al. (1965). Some effects of chlordiazepoxide and meprobamate with psychiatric outpatients. *Psychopharmacologia, 7,* 256–265.

McNamee, B., Grant, J., Ratcliffe, W., & Oliver, J. (1979). Lack of effect of alcohol on pituitary gonadal function in women. *British Journal of Addiction, 74,* 316–317.

McNeilly, A.S., & Ducker, H.A. (1972). Blood levels of oxytocin in the female goat during coitus and in response to stimuli associated with mating. *Journal of Endocrinology, 54,* 399–406.

McSweeny, A.J., & Labuhn, K.T. (1990). Chronic obstructive pulmonary disease. In B. Spilker (Ed.), *Quality of life assessments in clinical trials* (pp. 391–410). New York: Raven Press.

Measom, M.O. (1992). Penile anesthesia and fluoxetine [Letter to the editor]. *American Journal of Psychiatry, 149,* 709.

Medical Letter. (1993). Zolpidem for insomnia. *Medical Letter on Drugs and Therapeutics, 35*(895), 35–36.

Medical Letter. (1994). Cisapride for nocturnal heartburn. *Medical Letter on Drugs and Therapeutics, 36*(915), 11–13.

Medical Letter (1995). Lamotrigine for epilepsy. *Med-*

ical Letter on Drugs and Therapeutics, 37(944), 21–22.

Meikle, A.W., Arvers, S., Dobs, A.S., Hoover, D.R., Sanders, S.W., & Mazer, N.A. (1993). Application site influences on the enhanced transdermal delivery of testosterone to hypogonadal men. *Endocrine Society 95th Annual Meeting Abstracts,* p. 146.

Melia, K.F., & Spealman, R.D. (1991). Pharmacological characterization of the discriminative stimulus effects of GBR 12909. *Journal of Pharmacology and Experimental Therapeutics, 258,* 626–632.

Melin, P., & Kihlstrom, J.E. (1963). Influence of oxytocin on sexual behavior in male rabbits. *Endocrinology, 73,* 433–438.

Melis, M.R., Argiolas, A., & Gessa, G.L. (1986). Oxytocin-induced penile erection and yawning: Site of action in the brain. *Brain Research, 398,* 259–265.

Melis, M.R., Argiolas, A., Stancampiano, R., & Gessa, G.L. (1988). Oxytocin-induced penile erection and yawning: Structure-activity relationship studies. *Pharmacological Research Communications, 20,* 1117–1118.

Melis, M.R., Argiolas, A., Stancampiano, R., & Gessa, G.L. (1990). Effect of apomorphine on oxytocin concentration of different brain areas and plasma of male rats. *European Journal of Pharmacology, 182,* 101–107.

Melis, M.R., Stancampiano, R., Gessa, G.L., & Argiolas, A. (1992). Prevention by morphine of apomorphine- and oxytocin-induced penile erection and yawning: Site of action in the brain. *Neuropsychopharmacology, 6,* 17–21.

Meliska, C.J., & Gilbert, D.G. (1991). Hormonal and subjective effects of smoking the first five cigarettes of the day: A comparison in males and females. *Pharmacology, Biochemistry, and Behavior, 40,* 229–235.

Mellgren, A. (1967). Treatment of ejaculation praecox with thioridazine. *Psychotherapy and Psychosomatics, 15,* 454–460.

Mello, N.K., Bree, M.P., Mendelson, J.H., Ellingboe, J. (1983). Alcohol self-administration disrupts reproductive function in female macacque monkeys. *Science, 221,* 677–679.

Melman, A. (1984). The effects of yohimbine upon sexual function: A double-blind study. *Journal of Urology: 79th Annual Meeting of American Urological Association Abstracts,* 302A.

Melman, A., Fersel, J., & Weinstein, P. (1984). Further studies of the effect of chronic alpha-methyldopa administration upon the central nervous system and sexual function in male rats. *Journal of Urology, 132,* 804–808.

Meltzer, H.Y., Alphs, L.D., Bastani, B., Ramirez, L.F., & Kwon, K. (1991). Clinical efficacy of clozapine in the treatment of schizophrenia. *Parmacopsychiatry, 24*(2), 44–45.

Meltzer, H.Y., Lee, M.A., & Ranjan, R. (1994). Recent advances in the pharmacotherapy of schizophrenia. *Acta Psychiatrica Scandinavica, 90*(Suppl. 384), 95–101.

Meltzer, H.Y., Wiita, B., Tricou, B.J., Simonovic, M., Fang, V., & Manov, G. (1982). Effect of serotonin precursors and serotonin agonists on plasma hormone levels. In B.T. Ho, J. Schoolar, & E. Usdin (Eds.), *Serotonin in biological psychiatry* (pp. 117–139). New York: Raven Press.

Mendelson, J.H., Ellingboe, J., Kuehnle, J.C., & Mello, N.K. (1978). Effects of chronic marijuana use on integrated plasma testosterone and luteinizing hormone levels. *Journal of Pharmacology and Experimental Therapeutics, 207,* 611–617.

Mendelson, J.H., Ellingboe, J., Keuhnle, J.C., & Mello, N.K. (1979). Effect of naltrexone on mood and neuroendocrine function in adult males. *Psychoneuroendocrinology, 3,* 231–236.

Mendelson, J.H., Kuehnle, J., Ellingboe, J., & Babor, T.F. (1974). Plasma testosterone levels before, during, and after chronic marijuana smoking. *New England Journal of Medicine, 291,* 1051–1055.

Mendelson, J.H., & Mello, N.K. (1979). Biologic concomitants of alcoholism. *New England Journal of Medicine, 301,* 912–921.

Mendelson, J.H., & Mello, N.K. (1988). Acute and chronic effects of alcohol on the hypothalamic-pituitary-gonadal axis in men and women. In R.M. Rose & J. Barrett (Eds.), *Alcoholism: Origins and outcome* (pp. 175–207). New York: Raven Press.

Mendelson, J.H., Mello, N.K., Cristofaro, P., Ellingboe, J., Skupny, A., Palmieri, S.L., Benedikt, R., & Schiff, I. (1987). Alcohol effects on naloxone-stimulated luteinizing hormone, prolactin, and estradiol in women. *Journal of Studies on Alcohol, 48,* 287–294.

Mendelson, J.H., Mello, N.K., & Ellingboe, J. (1977). Effects of acute alcohol intake on pituitary-gonadal hormones in normal human males. *Journal of Pharmacology and Experimental Therapeutics, 202,* 676–683.

Mendelson, J.H., Mello, N.K., & Ellingboe, J. (1981). Acute alcohol intake and pituitary-gonadal hormones in normal human females. *Journal of Pharmacology and Experimental Therapeutics, 218,* 23–26.

Mendelson, J.H., Mello, N.K., Teoh, S.K., Lukas, S.E., Phipps, W., Ellingboe, J., Palmieri, S.L., & Schiff, I. (1992). Human studies of the biological basis of reinforcement. In C.P. O'Brien & J.H. Jaffe (Eds.), *Addictive states* (pp. 131–155). New York: Raven Press.

Mendelson, J.H., Mendelson, J.E., & Patch, V.D. (1975). Plasma testosterone levels in heroin addiction and methadone maintenance. *Journal of Pharmacology and Experimental Therapeutics, 192,* 211-217.

Mendelson, S.D., & Gorzalka, B.B. (1986). 5-HT_{1A} receptors: Differential involvement in female and male sexual behavior in the rat. *Physiology and Behavior, 37,* 345-351.

Mendelson, W.B. (1991). Safety of short-acting benzodiazepine hypnotics in patients with impaired respiration [Letter to the editor]. *American Journal of Psychiatry, 148,* 1401.

Mendelson, W.B., Gujavarty, K., Slintak, C., Schwartz, J., & Maczaj (1990). Reported sexual dysfunction in obstructive sleep apnea patients. *Annals of Clinical Psychiatry, 2,* 93-101.

Mendoza, S.P. (1984). The psychobiology of social relationships. In P.R. Barchas & S.P. Mendoza (Eds.), *Social cohesion: Essays toward a sociophysiological perspective* (pp. 3-29). Westport, CN: Greenwood.

Mendoza, S.P., Lowe, E.L., Davidson, J., & Levine, S. (1979). The physiological response to group formation in adult male squirrel monkeys. *Psychoneuroendocrinology, 3,* 221-229.

Menkes, D.B., Thomas, M.C., & Phipps, R.F. (1994). Moclobemide for menopausal flushing. *Lancet, 344,* 691-692.

Menon, K., Okonofua, E., Agnew, J.E., Thomas, M., Bell, J., O'Brien, P.M., & Dandona, P. (1987). Endocrine and metabolic effects of simple hysterectomy. *International Journal of Gynecology and Obstetrics, 25,* 459-463.

Mersdorf, A., Goldsmith, P.C., Diederichs, W., Padula, C.A., Lue, T.F., Fishman, I.J., & Tanagho, E.A. (1991). Ultrastructural changes in impotent penile tissue: A comparison of 65 patients. *Journal of Urology, 145,* 749-758.

Meschia, M., Brincat, M., Barbacini, P., Crosignani, P.G., Albisetti, W., & Pietrogrande, V. (1988). A pilot study comparing the use of conjugated estrogens and calcitonin to calcitonin alone in the prevention and treatment of postmenopausal bone loss. *Gynecological Endocrinology, 2*(Suppl. 2), 160.

Meshorer, M., & Meshorer, J. (1986). *Ultimate pleasure: The secrets of easily orgasmic women.* New York: St. Martin's Press.

Meuwissen, I., & Over, R. (1992). Sexual arousal across phases of the human menstrual cycle. *Archives of Sexual Behavior, 21,* 101-119.

Meyerson, B.J. (1981). Comparison of the effects of beta-endorphin and morphine on exploratory and socio-sexual behavior in the male rat. *European Journal of Pharmacology, 69,* 453-463.

Meyerson, B.J., Berg, M., & Johansson, B. (1988). Neonatal naltrexone treatment: Effects on sexual and exploratory behavior in male and female rats. *Pharmacology, Biochemistry, and Behavior, 31,* 63-67.

Meyerson, B.J., & Malmnas, C.O. (1978). Brain monoamines and sexual behavior. In J.B. Hutchison (Ed.), *Biological determinants in sexual behavior* (pp. 521-554). New York: Wiley & Sons.

Meyerson, B.J., & Terenius, L. (1977). Endorphins and male sexual behavior. *European Journal of Pharmacology, 42,* 191-192.

Meyhoff, H.H., Rosenkilde, P., & Bodker, A. (1992). Non-invasive management of impotence with transcutaneous nitroglycerin. *British Journal of Urology, 69,* 88-90.

Michael, R.P., & Zumpe, D. (1990). Sexual preferences during artificial menstrual cycles in social groups of rhesus monkeys (*Macacca mulatta*). *Primates, 31,* 225-241.

Michael, R.P., Zumpe, D., & Bonsall, R.W. (1982). Behavior of rhesus monkeys during artificial menstrual cycles. *Journal of Comparative and Physiological Psychology, 96,* 875-885.

Michal, V., Kramar, R., & Pospichal, J. (1977). Arterial epigastric cavernous anastomosis for the treatment of sexual impotence. *World Journal of Surgery, 1,* 515.

Michell, G.F., Mebane, A.H., & Billings, C.K. (1989). Effect of bupropion on chocolate craving. *American Journal of Psychiatry, 146,* 119-120.

Michelson, E.L., Frishman, W.H., Lewis, J.E., Edwards, W.T., Flanigan, W.J., Bloomfield, S.S., Johnson, B.F., Lucas, C., Freis, E.D., Finnerty, F.A., Sawin, H.S., Sabol, S.A., Long, C., & Poland, M.P. (1983). Multicenter clinical evaluation of long-term efficacy and safety of labetalol in treatment of hypertension. *American Journal of Medicine, 75*(Suppl.), 68-80.

Michnovicz, J.J., & Galbraith, R.A. (1991). Cimetidine inhibits catechol estrogen metabolism in women. *Metabolism, 40,* 170-174.

Miller, L., & Griffith, J. (1983). A comparison of bupropion, dextroamphetamine and placebo in mixed-substance abusers. *Psychopharmacology, 80,* 199-205.

Miller, R.A. (1976). Propranolol and impotence. *Annals of Internal Medicine, 85,* 682-683.

Miller, W.R., & Anderson, T.J. (1988). Estrogens, progestogens, and the breast. In J.W. Studd & I.M. Whitehead (Eds.), *The menopause* (pp. 234-246). London: Blackwell Scientific.

Miller, W.W. (1968). Afrodex in the treatment of male impotence: A double-blind crossover study. *Current Therapeutic Research, 10,* 354-359.

Mills, I.H. (1979). Endocrine responses to psychotropic drugs. *British Journal of Clinical Practice, 61*(Suppl. 4), 61–64.

Mills, L.C. (1976). Sexual disorders in the diabetic patient. In W.W. Oaks, G.A. Melchiode, & I. Ficher (Eds.), *Sex and the life cycle* (pp. 163–174). New York: Grune & Stratton.

Miranda, H., Perez, E., Fernandez, E., Rosselot, F., Vergara, J.F., Wolstenholme, W.W., & Zuazo, A. (1985). Androgens and effects of opioids and catecholamines on the smooth muscle of the rat vas deferens. *Pharmacology, 30,* 168–180.

Mishell, D.R. (1991). Editorial comment on "What do physicians in practice do to prevent osteoporosis?" In D.R. Mishell, T.H. Kirschbaum, & C.P. Morrow (Eds.), *Yearbook of Obstetrics and Gynecology: 1991* (p. 391). St. Louis: Mosby.

Miskowiak, B., Janecki, A., Jakubowiak, A., & Limanowski, A. (1986). Reproductive functions in adult male rats after prolonged intraventricular administration of corticotropin-releasing factor (CRF). *Experimental and Clinical Endocrinology, 88,* 25–30.

Mitchell, J.B., & Gratton, A. (1990). Sexually relevant stimuli activate the mesolimbic dopamine system: Measurement using high-speed chronoamperommetry in freely moving animals. *Society for Neuroscience: Abstracts, 16*(1), 437.

Mitchell, J.B., & Stewart, J. (1989). Effects of castration, steroid replacement, and sexual experience on mesolimbic dopamine and sexual behaviors in the male rat. *Brain Research, 491,* 116–127.

Mitchell, J.E., Hatsukami, D., Eckert, E.D., & Pyle, R.L. (1985). Characteristics of 275 patients with bulimia. *American Journal of Psychiatry, 142,* 482–485.

Mitchell, J.E., & Popkin, M.K. (1982). Antipsychotic drug therapy and sexual dysfunction in men. *American Journal of Psychiatry, 139,* 633–637.

Mitchell, J.E., & Popkin, M.K. (1983). Antidepressant drug therapy and sexual dysfunction in men: A review. *Journal of Clinical Psychopharmacology, 3,* 76–79.

Mitchell, J.E., Pyle, R.L., & Eckert, E.D. (1991). Diet pill usage in patients with bulimia nervosa. *International Journal of Eating Disorders, 10,* 233–237.

Mitchell, W., Falconer, M., & Hill, D. (1954). Epilepsy with fetishism relieved by temporal lobectomy. *Lancet, 2,* 626–630.

Modai, I., Valevski, A., Dror, S., & Weizman, A. (1994). Serum cholesterol levels and suicidal tendencies in psychiatric inpatients. *Journal of Clinical Psychiatry, 55,* 252–254.

Modell, J.G. (1989). Repeated observations of yawning, clitoral engorgement, and orgasm associated with fluoxetine administration. *Journal of Clinical Psychopharmacology, 9,* 63–65.

Moffat, R.J., & Owens, S.G. (1991). Cessation from cigarette smoking: Changes in body weight, body composition, resting metabilism, and energy consumption. *Metabolism, 40,* 465–470.

Mogenson, G.J., Jones, D.L., & Yim, C.Y. (1980). From motivation to action: Functional interface between the limbic system and the motor system. *Progress in Neurobiology, 14,* 69–97.

Mogenson, G.J., Yang, C.R., & Yim, C.Y. (1988). Influence of dopamine on limbic imputs to the nucleus accumbens. In *Vol. 537: Annals of the New York Academy of Sciences* (pp. 86–100). New York: New York Academy of Sciences.

Moghetti, P. Castello, R., Magnani, C.M., Tosi, F., Negri, C., Armanini, B.G., & Muggeo, J. (1994). Clinical and hormonal effects of the 5α-reductase inhibitor finasteride in idiopathic hirsuitism. *Journal of Clinical Endocrinology and Metabolism, 79*(4), 1115–1118.

Mohan, P.F., & Cleary, M.P. (1989). Comparison of dehydroepiandrosterone and clofibric acid treatments in obese Zucker rats. *Journal of Nutrition, 119,* 496–501.

Moller, H., Lindvig, K., Klefter, R., Mosbech, J., & Jensen, O. (1989). Cancer occurrence in a cohort of patients treated with cimetidine. *Gut, 30,* 1558–1562.

Molloy, D.W. (1987). Hypomagnesesemia and respiratory-muscle weakness in the elderly. *Geriatric Medicine Today, 6,* 53–61.

Moltz, H. (1989). E-series prostaglandins and arginine vasopressin in the modulation of male sexual behavior. *Neuroscience and Biobehavioral Reviews, 14,* 109–115.

Money, J. (1987). Treatment guidelines: Antiandrogen and counseling of paraphilic sex offenders. *Journal of Sex and Marital Therapy, 13,* 219–223.

Money, J., & Yankowitz, R. (1967). The sympathetic-inhibiting effects of the drug Ismelin on human male eroticism, with a note on Mellaril. *Journal of Sex Research, 3,* 69–82.

Moniz, C., Savvas, M., Brincat, M., & Studd, J.W. (1989). The effects of estrogens on skin aging in the menopause. In G. Albatangelo & J.M. Davidson (Eds.), *Cutaneous development, aging, and repair* (pp. 107–111). Padova: Liviana Press (Fidia).

Monroe, R.R. (1989). Dyscontrol syndrome: Long-term follow-up. *Comprehensive Psychiatry, 30,* 490–496.

Montalto, J., Funder, J.W., Yong, A.B., Calan, A., Davies, H.E., & Connelly, J.F. (1989). Serum C-19 steroid sulphates in females with clinical hyperandrogenism. *Journal of Steroid Biochemistry, 34,* 531–534.

Monteiro, W.O., Noshirvani, H.F., Marks, I.M., & Lelliott, P.T. (1987). Anorgasmia from clomipramine in obsessive-compulsive disorder: A controlled trial. *British Journal of Psychiatry, 151,* 107–112.

Montgomery, J.C., Brincat, M., Tapp, A., Appleby, L., Versi, E., Fenwick, P.B., & Studd, J.W. (1987). Effect of estrogen and testosterone implants on psychological disorders in the climacteric. *Lancet, 1,* 297–299.

Monti, P.M., Brown, W.A., & Corriveau, D.P. (1977). Testosterone and components of aggressive and sexual behavior in man. *American Journal of Psychiatry, 134,* 692–694.

Montorsi, F., Guazzoni, G., Bergamaschi, F., Orlandini, A., Da Pozzo, L., Barbieri, L., & Rigatti, P. (1993). Intracavernous vasoactive pharmacotherapy: The impact of a new self-injection device. *Journal or Urology, 150,* 1829–1832.

Moon, T.E. (1991). Estrogens and disease prevention. *Archives of Internal Medicine, 151,* 17–18.

Moore, C. (1983). Increased sexual function with nomifensine. *Medical Journal of Australia, 2,* 538.

Moore, D.E. (1992). Management of menopause. In M.A. Stenchever (Ed.), *Office gynecology* (pp. 136–174). St. Louis: Mosby Yearbook.

Morales, A., Condra, M., Owen, J.A., Surridge, D.H., Fenemore, J., & Harris, C. (1987). Is yohimbine effective in the treatment of organic impotence? Results of a controlled trial. *Journal of Urology, 137,* 1168–1172.

Morales, A., Surridge, D.H., & Marshall, P.G. (1981). Yohimbine for treatment of impotence in diabetics. *New England Journal of Medicine, 305,* 1221.

Morales, A., Surridge, D.H.C, Marshall, P.G., & Fenemore, J. (1982). Nonhormonal pharmacological treatment of organic impotence. *Journal of Urology, 128,* 45–47.

Morales, A., Johnston, B., Heaton, J.P.W., & Clark, A. (1994). Oral androgens in the treatment of hypogonadal impotent men. *Journal of Urology, 152,* 1115–1118.

Morales, A.J., Nolan, J.J., Nelson, J.C., & Yen, S.S. (1994). Effects of replacement dose of dehydroepiandrosterone in men and women of advancing age. *Journal of Clinical Endocrinology and Metabolism, 78,* 1360–1367.

Morfin, R., & Courchay, G. (1994). Pregnenolone and dehydroepiandrosterone as precursors of native 7-hydroxylated metabolites which increase the immune response in mice. *Journal of Steroid Biochemistry and Molecular Biology, 50,* 91–100.

Morgan, J.P. (1985). Norephedrine and norpseudoephedrine: Pharmacologically and clinically distinct isomers of phenylpropanolamine. In J.P. Morgan, D.V. Kagan, & J.S. Brody (Eds.), *Phenylpropanolamine: Risks, benefits and controversies* (pp. 180–198). New York: Praeger Publishers.

Morgenstern, R., Fink, H., Ott, T., & Parvez, S.H. (1988). Interaction of serotonergic and dopaminergic transmission systems in mesolimbic structures: Target for the action of classical and atypical neuroleptics. *Biogenic Amines, 5,* 225–238.

Morrell, M.J. (1991). Sexual dysfunction in epilepsy. *Epilepsia, 32*(Suppl. 6), 538–545.

Morrell, M.J., Dixen, J.M., Carter, S., & Davidson, J.M. (1984). The influence of age and cycling status on sexual arousability in women. *American Journal of Obstetrics and Gynecology, 148,* 66–71.

Morris, N.M., Udry, J.R., Khan-Dawood, F., & Dawood, M.Y. (1987). Marital sex frequency and mid-cycle female testosterone. *Archives of Sexual Behavior, 16,* 147–157.

Morrison, A.S. (1990). Prostatic hypertrophy. In N. Wald & J. Baron (Eds.), *Smoking and hormone-related disorders* (pp. 118–134). Oxford: Oxford University Press.

Morrissette, D.L., Skinner, M.H., Hoffman, B.B., Levine, R.E., & Davidson, J.M. (1993). Effects of antihypertensive drugs atenolol and nifedipine on sexual function in older men: A placebo-controlled crossover study. *Archives of Sexual Behavior, 22,* 99–109.

Moser, M. (1989). Relative efficacy of, and some adverse reactions to, different antihypertensive regimens. *American Journal of Cardiology, 63,* 2B–7B.

Moss, H.B. (1983). More cases of anorgasmia after MAOI treatment [Letter to the editor]. *American Journal of Psychiatry, 140,* 266.

Moss, H.B., & Procci, W.R. (1981). Antihypertensive drugs and sexual dysfunction. *Psychosomatic Medicine, 43,* 473–474.

Moss, R.L., & Dudley, C.A. (1979). Sexual function and brain peptides. In A.M. Gotto Jr., E.J. Peck Jr., & E.A. Boyd (Eds.), *Brain: A new endocrinology* (pp. 329–346). New York: North Holland Biomedical Press.

Moss, R.L., & Dudley, C.A. (1984). The challenge of studying the behavioral effects of neuropeptides. In L.L. Iversen, S.D. Iversen, & S.H. Snyder (Eds.), *Handbook of Psychopharmacology, Vol. 18* (pp. 397–454). New York: Plenum Press.

Moss, R.L., Dudley, C.A., Foreman, M.M., & McCann, S.M. (1975). Synthetic LRF: A potentiator of sexual behavior in the rat. In M. Motta, P.G. Crosignani, & L. Martini (Eds.), *Hypothalamic hormones: Chemistry, physiology, and clinical use* (pp. 269–278). London: Academic Press.

Moss, R.L., Riskind, P., & Dudley, C. (1979). Effects of LH-RH on sexual activities in animal and man. In R. Collu, A. Barbeau, & J.R. Ducharme (Eds.), *Central nervous system effects of hypothalamic hormone and other peptides* (pp. 345-366). New York: Raven Press.

Moss, R.L. (1978). Effects of hypothalamic peptides on sex behavior in animal and man. In M.A. Lipton, A. DiMascio, & K.P. Killam (Eds.), *Psychopharmacology: A generation of progress* (pp. 431-440). New York: Raven Press.

MRC: Medical Research Council Working Party Trial on Mild to Moderate Hypertension (1981). Adverse reactions to bendrofluazide and propranolol for the treatment of mild hypertension. *Lancet, 2,* 539-542.

MRC: Medical Research Council Working Party Trial on Mild to Moderate Hypertension (1987). The MRC treatment trial for hypertension in the elderly: Design and progress report. In T. Strasser & D. Ganten (Eds.), *Mild hypertension: From drug trials to practice* (pp. 67-70). New York: Raven Press.

Mrozek, W.J., Leibl, B.A., & Finnerty, F.A. (1972). Comparison of clonidine and methyldopa in hypertensive patients receiving a diuretic. A double-blind crossover study. *American Journal of Cardiology, 29,* 712-717.

Mudd, J.W. (1977). Impotence responsive to glyceryl trinitrate. *American Journal of Psychiatry, 134,* 922-925.

Muir, J.W., Besser, G.M., Edwards, C.R.W., Rees, L.H., Cattell, W.R., Ackrill, P., & Baker, L.R.I. (1983). Bromocriptine improves reduced libido and potency in men receiving maintenance hemodialysis. *Clinical Nephrology, 20,* 308-314.

Muller, S., & Cleary, M.P. (1985). Glucose metabolism in isolated fat cells from lean and obese Zucker rats following treatment with dehydroepiandrosterone. *Metabolism, 34,* 278-284.

Müller, S.C., El-Damanhoury, H., Röth, J., & Lue, T.F. (1991). Hypertension and impotence. *European Urology, 19,* 29-34.

Munjack, D.J., & Crocker, B. (1986). Alprazolam-induced ejaculatory inhibition. *Journal of Clinical Psychopharmacology, 6,* 57-58.

Munjack, D.J., & Oziel, L.J. (1980). Drugs and sexual response. In D.J. Munjack & L.J. Oziel (Eds.), *Sexual medicine and counseling in office practice* (pp. 175-187). Boston: Little, Brown & Co.

Munroe, W.P., Rindone, J.P., & Kershner, R.M. (1985). Systemic side effects associated with the ophthalmic administration of timolol. *Drug Intelligence and Clinical Pharmacy, 19,* 85-89.

Muramatsu, M., Tamaki-Ohashi, J., Usuki, C. Araki, H., & Aihara, H. (1988). Serotonin-2 receptor-mediated regulation of release of acetylcholine by minaprine in cholinergic nerve terminal of hippocampus of rat. *Neuropharmacology, 27,* 603-609.

Murphy, M.J., Bowie, D.L., & Pert, C.B. (1979). Copulation elevates plasma beta-endorphin in the male hamster. *Society for Neuroscience Abstracts, 5,* P470.

Murphy, M.R., Checkley, S.A., Seckl, J.R., & Lightman, S.I. (1990). Naloxone inhibits oxytocin release at orgasm in man. *Journal of Clinical Endocrinology and Metabolism, 71,* 1056-1058.

Murphy, M.R., Seckl, J. R., Burton, S., Checkley, S.A. & Lightman, S.L. (1987). Changes in oxytocin and vasopressin secretion during sexual activity in men. *Journal of Clinical Endocrinology and Metabolism, 65,* 738-741.

Murphy, W.D., Coleman, E., Hoon, E., & Scott, S. (1980). Sexual dysfunction and treatment in alcoholic women. *Sexuality and Disability, 3,* 240-255.

Murray, F.T., Fettes, J., Wyss, H., Cameron, D., & Sciadini, M. (1988). Increased beta-endorphins and decreased penile tumescence in middle-age men. *Journal of Andrology, 9,* 20-P.

Musher, J.S. (1990). Anorgasmia with the use of fluoxetine [Letter to the editor]. *American Journal of Psychiatry, 147,* 948.

Muyard, J.P. (1972). Premiers essais cliniques de l'Agr 1240. Equipe soignante de Cour-Cheverny. *Agressologie, 13,* 337-352.

Myers, L.S., Dixen, J., Morrissette, D., Carmichael, M., & Davidson, J.M. (1990). Effects of estrogen, androgen, and progestin on sexual psychophysiology and behavior in postmenopausal women. *Journal of Clinical Endocrinology and Metabolism, 70,* 1124-1131.

Myers, L.S., & Morokoff, P.J. (1986). Physiological and subjective sexual arousal in pre- and post-menopausal women and postmenopausal women taking replacement therapy. *Psychophysiology, 23,* 283-292.

Myerson, A. (1936). The effect of benzedrine sulfate on mood and fatigue in normal and neurotic persons. *Archives of Neurology and Psychiatry, 36,* 816-822.

Nachtigal, L.E., Nachtigal, R.H., Nachtigal, R.D., & Beckman, E.M. (1979). Estrogen replacement therapy: A 10-year prospective study in the relationship to osteoporosis. *Obstetrics and Gynecology, 53,* 277-281.

Nachtigall, M.J., Smilen, S.W., Nachtigall, R.D., Nachtigall, R.H., & Nachtigall, L.E. (1992). Incidence of breast cancer in a 22-year study of women receiving estrogen-progestin replacement therapy. *Obstetrics and Gynecology, 80,* 827-830.

Nadler, R.D. (1970). A biphasic influence of progesterone on sexual receptivity of spayed female rats. *Physiology and Behavior, 5,* 95-97.

Nadler, R.D., Wallis, J., Roth-Meyer, C., Cooper,

R.W., & Baulieu, E.E. (1987). Hormones and behavior of prepubertal and peripubertal chimpanzees. *Hormones and Behavior, 21,* 118–131.

Nafziger, A.N., Herrington, D.M., & Bush, T.L. (1991). Dehydroepiandrosterone and dehydroepiandrosterone sulfate: Their relation to cardiovascular disease. *Epidemiologic Reviews, 13,* 267–293.

Nafziger, A.N., Jenkins, P.L., Bowlin, S.J., & Pearson, T.A. (1990). Dehydroepiandrosterone, lipids, and apoproteins: Associations in a free-living population [abstract]. *Circulation, 82*(Suppl. 3), 469.

Nakhla, A.M. (1987). Calcitonin induces ornithone decarboxylase in various rat tissues. *Molecular and Cellular Endocrinology, 52,* 263–265.

Napoli-Farris, L., Fratta, W., & Gessa, G.L. (1984). Stimulation of dopamine autoreceptors elicits "premature ejaculation" in rats. *Pharmacology, Biochemistry, and Behavior, 20,* 69–72.

Nappi, C., Petraglia, F., Gambardella, A., De Masellis, G., De Carlo, C., Genazzani, A.R., & Montemagno, U. (1990). Relationship between cerebrospinal fluid beta-endorphin and plasma pituitary-gonadal levels in women. *Journal of Endocrinological Investigation, 13,* 149–153.

Naranjo, C.A., Bremner, K.E., Poulos, C.X., & Lanctot, K.L. (1992). Fluoxetine decreases desire for alcohol. *Clinical Pharmacology and Therapeutics, 51*(2), 168.

Naranjo, C.A., & Sellers, E.M. (1987). Serotonin uptake inhibitors attenuate ethanal intake in problem drinkers. In M. Galanter (Ed.), *Recent developments in alcoholism. Vol. 7. Treatment research* (pp. 255–266). New York: Plenum Press.

Nathan, D.M., Singer, D.E., Godine, J.E., & Perlmutter, L.C. (1986). Noninsulin-dependent diabetes in older patients: Complications and risk factors. *American Journal of Medicine, 81*[5], 837–842. (Published erratum appears in *American Journal of Medicine,* 1988, *84*(5), 977.)

Nathan, S.G. (1986). The epidemiology of the *DSM-III* psychosexual dysfunctions. *Journal of Sex and Marital Therapy, 12,* 267–281.

Nathorst-Böös, J., Wiklund, I., Mattsson, L.A., Sandin, K., & von Schoultz, B. (1993). Is sexual life influenced by transdermal estrogen therapy? *Acta Obstetrica et Gynecologica Scandinavica, 72,* 656–660.

Naumenko, T.G., Amstislavskaja, T.G., & Osadchuk, A.V. (1991). The role of adrenoceptors in the activation of the hypothalamic-testicular complex of mice induced by the presence of a female. *Experimental and Clinical Endocrinology, 97,* 1–11.

Naylor, A.M., Ruwe, W.D., & Veale, W.L. (1986). Thermoregulatory actions of centrally-administered vasopressin in the rat. *Neuropharmacology, 25,* 787–794.

Negelev, S. (1990). Re: Topical nitrogylcerin: A potential treatment for impotence [Letter to the editor]. *Journal of Urology, 143,* 586.

Neill, J.R. (1991). Penile anesthesia associated with fluoxetine use. *American Journal of Psychiatry, 148,* 1603.

Nellans, R.E., Ellis, L.R., & Kramer-Levien, D. (1987). Pharmacological erection: Diagnosis and treatment applications in 69 patients. *Journal of Urology, 138,* 52–54.

Neppe, V.M., Tucker, G.J., & Wilensky, A.J. (1988). Introduction: Fundamentals of carbamazepine use in neuropsychiatry. *Journal of Clinical Psychiatry, 49* (Suppl. 4), 4–6.

Neri, A., Aygen, M., Zukerman, Z., & Bahary, C. (1980). Subjective assessment of sexual dysfunction of patients on long-term administration of digoxin. *Archives of Sexual Behavior, 9,* 343–347.

Nessel, M.A. (1994). Yohimbine and pentoxifylline in the treatment of erectile dysfunction [Letter to the editor]. *American Journal of Psychiatry, 151,* 453.

Nestler, J.E., Barlascini, C.O., & Clore, J.N. (1988). Dehydroepiandrosterone reduces low density lipoprotein levels and body fat but does not alter insulin sensitivity in normal men. *Journal of Clinical Endocrinology and Metabolism, 66,* 57–61.

Nestler, J.E., Beer, N.A., Jakubowicz, D.J., & Beer, R.M. (1994). Effects of a reduction in circulating insulin by metformin on serum dehydroepiandrosterone in sulfate in nondiabetic men. *Journal of Clinical Endocrinology and Metabolism, 78,* 549–554.

Nestler, J.E., McClanahan, M.A., Clore, J.N., & Blackard, W.G. (1992). Insulin inhibits adrenal 17,20-lyase activity in man. *Journal of Clinical Endocrinology and Metabolism, 74,* 362–367.

Neugarten, B.L., & Kraines, R.J. (1965). Menopausal symptoms in women at various ages. *Psychosomatic Medicine, 27,* 140–151.

Newman, R.J., & Salerno, H.R. (1974). Sexual dysfunction due to methyldopa [Letter to the editor]. *British Medical Journal, 4,* 106.

Newton, N. (1973). Interrelationships between sexual responsiveness, birth and breast feeding. In J. Zubin & J. Money (Eds.), *Contemporary sexual behavior: Critical issues in the 1970s* (pp. 77–98). Baltimore: John Hopkins University Press.

Newton, N. (1978). The role of the oxytocin reflexes in three interpersonal reproductive acts: Coitus, birth and breast-feeding. In L. Carenza, P. Pancheri, & L. Zichella (Eds.), *Clinical psychoneuroendocrinology in reproduction* (pp. 411–418). New York: Academic.

Nicholson, H.D., Swann, R.W., Burford, G.D., Wathes, D.C., Porter, D.G., & Pickering, B.T. (1984). Identification of oxytocin and vasopressin in the testis and in adrenal tissue. *Regulatory Peptides, 8,* 141-146.

Nickel, B., Schulze, G., & Szelenyi, I. (1990). Effect of enantiomers of deprenyl (selegiline) and amphetamine on physical abuse liability and cortical electrical activity in rats. *Neuropharmacology, 29,* 983-992.

Nickel, B., Szelenyi, I., & Schulze, G. (1994). Evaluation of physical dependence liability of l-deprenyl (selegiline) in animals. *Clinical Pharmacology and Therapeutics, 56,* 757-767.

Nielsen, E.B., & Scheel-Kruger, J. (1988). Central nervous system stimulants: Neuropharmacological mechanisms. In F.C. Colpaert & R. Balster (Eds.), *Transduction mechanisms of drug stimuli* (pp. 57-71). Berlin: Springer-Verlag.

Nielsen, J.A., Shannon, N.J., Berg, L., & Moore, K.E. (1986). Effects of acute and chronic bupropion on locomotor activity and dopaminergic neurons. *Pharmacology, Biochemisty, and Behavior, 24,* 795-799.

Nierenberg, A.A., Feighner, J.P., Rudolph, R., Cole, J.O., & Sullivan, J. (1994). Venlafaxine for treatment-resistant unipolar depression. *Journal of Clinical Psychopharmacology, 14,* 419-423.

Nieschlag, E., & Freischem, C.W. (1982). Androgen therapy in hypogonadism and infertility. In J. Bain, W.B. Schill, & L. Schwarzstein (Eds.), *Treatment of male infertility* (pp. 103-105). New York: Springer-Verlag.

Nieschlag, E., Waites, G.M., Paulsen, C.A., & Handelsman, D.J. (1990). Reply to: Tumorigenic effect of testosterone [Letter to the editor]. *Lancet, 2,* 1518.

Nigam, A.K., Srivastava, R.P., Saxena, S., Chavan, B.S., & Sundaram, K.R. (1994). Naloxone-induced withdrawal in patients with buprenorphine dependence. *Addiction, 89,* 317-320.

NIH Consensus Conference on Impotence. (1993). NIH consensus development panel on impotence. *Journal of the American Medical Association, 270,* 83.

Nininger, J. (1978). Inhibition of ejaculation by amitriptyline. *American Journal of Psychiatry, 135,* 750-751.

Nirenberg, T.D., Wincze, J.P., Bansal, S., Liepman, M.R., Engle-Friedman, M., & Begin, A. (1991). Volunteer bias in a study of male alcoholics' sexual behavior. *Archives of Sexual Behavior, 20,* 371-379.

Nishida, E., Akasofu, K., Hashimoto, S., Harada, T., Uchide, K., Nakagawa, T., & Tomimatsu, N. (1989). Any indication for androgen therapy? In M.L. Hermite (Ed.), *Update on hormonal treatment of the menopause* (pp. 86-94). Basel: Karger.

Noci, I., Chelo, E., Saltarelli, O., Donati Cori, G., & Scarselli, G. (1985). Tamoxifen and oligospermia. *Archives of Andrology, 15,* 83-88.

Nofzinger, E.A., Thase, M.E., Reynolds III, C.F., Frank, E., Jennings, J.R., Garamoni, G.L., Fasiczka, A.L., & Kupfer, D.J. (1993). Sexual function in depressed men. *Archives of General Psychiatry, 50,* 24-30.

Nomikos, G.G., Damsma, G., Wenkstern, D., & Fibiger, H.C. (1989). Acute effects of bupropion on extracellular dopamine concentrations in rat striatum and nucleus accumbens studied by in vivo microdialysis. *Neuropsychopharmacology, 2,* 273-279.

Noppen, M., Jacobs, A., Van Belle, S., Herregodts, P., & Somers, G. (1988). Inhibitory effects of ranitidine on flushing and serum serotonin concentrations in carcinoid syndrome. *British Medical Journal, 296,* 682-683.

Nordin, B.E. (Ed.). (1984). *Metabolic bone and stone diseases* (2nd ed.). New York: Churchill Livingston.

Nordin, B.E., Crilly, R.G., & Smith, D.A. (1984). Osteoporosis. In B.E. Nordin (Ed.), *Metabolic bone and stone disease* (pp. 1-70). London: Churchill Livingstone.

Nordin, B.E., Horsman, A., Crilly, R.G., Marshall, D.H., & Simpson, M. (1980). Treatment of spinal osteoporosis in postmenopausal women. *British Medical Journal, 280,* 451-454.

Nordin, B.E., Robertson, A., Seamark, R.F., Bridges, A., Philcox, J.C., Need, A.G., Horowitz, M., Morris, H.A., & Deam, S. (1985). The relation between calcium absorption, serum dehydroepiandrosterone and vertebral mineral density in postmenopausal women. *Journal of Clinical Endocrinology and Metabolism, 60,* 651-657.

Nordin, C., Siwers, B., & Bertilsson, L. (1981). Bromocriptine treatment of depressive disorders: Clinical and biochemical effects. *Acta Psychiatrica Scandanavica, 64,* 25-33.

Norton, R., Brown, K., & Howard, R. (1992). Smoking, nicotine dose, and the lateralization of electrocortical activity. *Psychopharmacology, 108,* 473-479.

Notelovitz, M. (1986). Postmenopausal osteoporosis: A practical approach to its prevention. *Acta Obstetrica et Gynecology Scandinavica, 134* (Suppl.), 67-80.

Notman, M.T. (1979). Midlife concerns of women: Implications of the menopause. *American Journal of Psychiatry, 136,* 1270-1274.

Notman, M.T. (1984). Psychiatric disorders of menopause. *Psychiatric Annals, 14,* 448-453.

Noyes, R., Garvey, M.J., Cook, B.L., & Samuelson, L. (1989). Problems with tricyclic antidepressant use in patients with panic disorder or agoraphobia: Results of a naturalistic follow-up study. *Journal of Clinical Psychiatry, 50,* 163–169.

Noyes, R., & Kathol, R.G. (1986). Depression and cancer. *Psychiatric Developments, 2,* 77–100.

Nurse, B., Russell, V.A., & Taljaard, J.J. (1985). Effect of chronic desipramine treatment on adrenoceptor modulation of (3H) dopamine release from rat nucleus accumbens slices. *Brain Research, 334,* 235–242.

Nyholm, H., Djursing, H., Hagen, C., Agner, T., Bennett, P., & Svenstrup, B. (1989). Androgens and estrogens in postmenopausal insulin-treated diabetic women. *Journal of Clinical Endocrinology and Metabolism, 69,* 946–949.

O'Carroll, R., & Bancroft, J. (1984). Testosterone for low sexual interest and erectile dysfunction in men: A controlled trial. *British Journal of Psychiatry, 145,* 146–151.

O'Carroll, R., Shapiro, C., & Bancroft, J. (1985). Androgens, behavior, and nocturnal erection in hypogonadal men: The effects of varying the replacement dose. *Clinical Endocrinology, 23,* 527–538.

Oesterling, J.E., Epstein, J.I., & Walsh, P.C. (1986). The inability of adrenal androgens to stimulate the adult human prostate: An autopsy evaluation of men with hypogonadotropic hypogonadism and panhypopituitarism. *Journal of Urology, 136,* 1030–1033.

O'Farrell, T.J., Choquette, K.A., & Birchler, G.R. (1991). Sexual satisfaction and dissatisfaction in the marital relationships of male alcoholics seeking marital therapy. *Journal of Studies on Alcohol, 52,* 441–447.

Ohman, K.P., & Asplund, J. (1984). Labetolol in primary hypertension: A long-term effect and tolerance study. *Current Therapeutic Research, 35,* 277–285.

Oksenberg, D., & Peroutka, S.J. (1988). Antagonism of 5-hydorxytryptamine$_{1A}$ (5-HT$_{1A}$) receptor-mediated modulation of adenylate cyclase activity by pindolol and propranolol isomers. *Biochemical Pharmacology, 37,* 3429–3433.

Olajide, D., & Lader, M. (1985). Psychotropic effects of enalapril maleate in normal volunteers. *Psychopharmacology, 86,* 374–376.

Olgiati, V.R., Guidobono, F., Netti, G., & Pecile, A. (1983). Localization of calcitonin binding sites in rat central nervous system: Evidence of its neuroactivity. *Brain Research, 265,* 209–215.

Oliveros-Palacios, M.C., Godoy-Godoy, N., & Colina-Chourio, J.A. (1991). Effects of doxazosin on blood pressure, renin-angiotensin-aldosterone, and urinary kallikrein. *American Journal of Cardiology, 76,* 157–161.

Ollat, H., Parvez, H., & Parvez, S. (1988). Alcohol and central neurotransmission. *Neurochemistry International, 13,* 275–300.

O'Meara, J., & White, W.B. (1988). Ejaculatory failure and urinary dysfunction secondary to labetolol. *Journal of Urology, 139,* 371–372.

Onaka, T., Yagi, K., & Hamamura, M. (1982). Vasopressin: Physical stress potentiates but emotional stress suppresses its secretion. In A.J. Baertschi & J.J. Dreifuss (Eds.), *Neuroendocrinology of vasopressin, corticoliberin, and opiomelanocortins* (pp. 221–225). New York: Academic Press.

Onesti, G., Bock, K.D., Heimsoth, V., Kim, K.E., & Merguet, P. (1971). Clonidine: A new antihypertensive agent. *American Journal of Cardiology, 28,* 74–83.

Ong, Y.L., Checkley, S.A., & Russell, G.F.M. (1983). Suppression of bulimic symptoms with methylamphetamine. *British Journal of Psychiatry, 143,* 288–293.

Ongini, E., & Longo, V.G. (1989). Dopamine receptor subtypes and arousal. *International Review of Neurobiology, 31,* 239–255.

Onuora, C.O., Ardoin, J.A., Dunnihoo, D.R., & Otterson, W.N. (1991). Vaginal estrogen therapy in the treatment of urinary tract symptoms in postmenopausal women. *International Urogynecology Journal, 2,* 3–7.

Orford, J., & Vellman, R. (1990). Offspring of parents with drinking problems: Drinking and drug-taking as young adults. *British Journal of Addiction, 85,* 779–794.

Ortmann, R. (1985). The conditioned place preference paradigm in rats: Effect of bupropion. *Life Sciences, 37,* 2021–2027.

Oseko, F., Morikawa, K., Nakano, A., Note, S., Endo, J., Taniguchi, A., Kono, T., & Imura, H. (1986). Effect of chronic hyperprolactemia induced by sulpiride on plasma dehydroepiandrosterone in normal men. *Andrologia, 18,* 523–528.

Oswald, I. (1974). Fenfluramine and psychosis [Letter to the editor]. *British Medical Journal, 2,* 103.

Othmer, E., & Othmer, S.C. (1987). Effect of buspirone on sexual dysfunction in patients with generalized anxiety disorder. *Journal of Clinical Psychiatry, 48,* 201–203.

Ott, S.M., & Chesnut, C.H. (1989). Calcitriol treatment is not effective in postmenopausal osteoporosis. *Annals of Internal Medicine, 110,* 267–274.

Ottesen, B. (1983). Vasoactive intestinal polypeptide as a neurotransmitter in the female genital tract. *American Journal of Obstetrics and Gynecology, 147,* 208–224.

Ottesen, B., Andersen, A.N., Gerstenberg, T. Ulrichsen, H., Manthorpe, T., & Fahrenkrug, J. (1981). VIP stimulates prolactin release in women *Lancet, 2,* 696.

Ottesen, B., Hansen, B., Fahrenkrug, J., & Fuchs, A.R. (1984). Vasoactive intestinal peptide (VIP) stimulates oxytocin and vasopressin release from the neurohypophyis. *Endocrinology, 115,* 1648-1650.

Ottesen, B., Moller, M., Willis, E., & Fahrenkrug, J. (1982). Vasoactive intestinal polypeptide (VIP) and the urogenital tract. In S.R. Bloom, J.M. Polak, & E. Lindenlaub (Eds.), *Systemic role of regulatory peptides* (pp. 365-376). New York: F.K. Schattauer Verlag.

Ottesen, B., Schierup, L., Bardrum, B., & Fahrenkrug, J. (1986). Release of vasoactive intestinal polypeptide (VIP) in breast-feeding women. *European Journal of Obstetrics, Gynecology, and Reproductive Biology, 22,* 333-336.

Ottesen, B., Wagner, G., Virag, R., & Fahrenkrug, J. (1984). Penile erection: Possible role for vasoactive intestinal polypeptide as a neurotransmitter. *British Medical Journal, 288,* 9-11.

Owen, J.A., Condra, M., Phillips, P., Surridge, D., Fenemore, J., & Morales, A. (1987). Transcutaneous nitroglycerin enhances the quality of erections in impotent men. Results of a controlled trial. *Journal of Urology, 137* (Pt. 2), 201A.

Owen, J.A., Saunders, F., Harris, C., Fenemore, J., Reid, K., Surridge, D., Condra, M., & Morales, A. (1989). Topical nitroglycerin: A potential treatment for impotence. *Journal of Urology, 141,* 546-548.

Owman, C. (1981). Pregnancy induces degenerative and regenerative changes in the autonomic innervation of the female reproductive tract. In K. Elliot & G. Lawrenson (Eds.), *Development of the autonomic nervous system* (pp. 252-279). London: Pittman Press.

Packer, M. (1992). The neurohormonal hypothesis: A theory to explain the mechanism of disease progression in heart failure. *Journal of the American College of Cardiology, 20,* 248-254.

Padma-Nathan, H., & Payton, T.R. (1986). Cigarette smoking related arterial and venous aberrations of penile erection. *Journal of Urology 135*(Suppl.), 363A.

Paganini-Hill, A., Ross, R.K., Gerkins, V.R., Henderson, B.E., Arthur, M., & Mack, T.M. (1981). Menopausal estrogen therapy and hip fractures. *Annals of Internal Medicine, 95,* 28-31.

Page, C., Benaim, S., & Lappin, F. (1987). A long-term retrospective follow-up study of patients treated with prophylactic lithium carbonate. *British Journal of Psychiatry, 150,* 175-179.

Paikoff, R.L., & Brooks-Gunn, J. (1991). Do parent-child relationships change during puberty? *Psychological Bulletin, 110,* 47-66.

Palle, C., Bredkjaer, H.E., Fahrenkrug, J., & Ottesen, B. (1991). Vasoactive intestinal polypeptide loses its ability to increase vaginal blood flow after menopause. *American Journal of Obstetrics and Gynecology, 164,* 556-558.

Palmer, A., Fletcher, A., Hamilton, G., Muriss, S., & Bulpitt, C. (1990). A comparison of verapamil and nifedipine on quality of life. *British Journal of Clinical Pharmacology, 30,* 365-370.

Palmer, R.H. (1989). Cimetidine and alcohol absorption [Letter to the editor]. *Gastroenterology, 97,* 1066-1067.

Palminteri, R., & Narbonne, G. (1988). Safety profile of zolpidem. In J.P. Sauvanet, S.Z. Langer, & P.L. Marselli (Eds.), *Imidazopyridines in sleep disorders* (pp. 351-362). New York: Raven Press.

Pani, L., Kuzmin, A., Martellotta, M.C., Gessa, G.L., & Fratta, W. (1991). The calcium antagonist PN-200-110 inhibits the reinforcing properties of cocaine. *Brain Research Bulletin, 26,* 445-447.

Papadopoulos, C. (1980). Cardiovascular drugs and sexuality. *Archives of Internal Medicine, 140,* 1341-1345.

Parada, M.A., Hernandez, L., De Parada, M.P., Paez, X., & Hoebel, B.G. (1990). Dopamine in the lateral hypothalamus may be involved in the inhibition of locomotion related to food and water seeking. *Brain Research Bulletin, 25,* 961-968.

Parker, L.N. (1989). *Adrenal androgens in clinical medicine.* New York: Academic Press.

Parker, L.N., Eugene, J., Farber, D., Lifrak, E., Lai, M., & Juler, G. (1985). Dissociation of adrenal androgen and cortisol levels in acute stress. *Hormone and Metabolism Research, 17,* 209-212.

Parker, L.N., Levin, E., & Lifrak, E. (1985). Evidence for adenocortical adaptation to severe illness. *Journal of Clinical Endocrinology and Metabolism, 60,* 947-952.

Parker, L.N., & Odell, W. (1979). Evidence for the existence of cortical androgen-stimulating hormone. *American Journal of Physiology, 236,* E616.

Parker, S., Udani, M., Gavaler, J.S., & Van Thiel, D.H. (1984). Pre- and neonatal exposure to cimetidine but not ranitidine adversely affects adult sexual functioning of male rats. *Neurobehavioral Toxicology and Teratology, 6,* 313-318.

Parmar, H., Edwards, L., Phillips, R.H., Allen, L., & Lightman, S.L. (1987). Orchidectomy versus long-acting D-Trp-6-LHRH in advanced prostatic cancer. *British Journal of Urology, 59,* 248-254.

Parry, B.L., & Rush, A.J. (1979). Oral contraceptives and depressive symptomatology: Biologic mechanisms. *Comprehensive Psychiatry, 20,* 347-358.

Patt, N. (1985). More on trazodone and priapism

[Letter to the editor]. *American Journal of Psychiatry, 142,* 783–784.

Patten, S.B. (1990). Propranolol and depression: Evidence from the antihypertensive trials. *Canadian Journal of Psychiatry, 35,* 257–259.

Patterson, J.F. (1988). Carbamazepine in the treatment of phantom limb pain. *Southern Medical Journal, 81,* 1100–1102.

Patterson, W.M. (1993). Fluoxetine-induced sexual dysfunction [Letter to the editor]. *Journal of Clinical Psychiatry, 54,* 71.

Paulsen, C.A., Enzmann, G.D., Bremner, W.J., Perrin, E.B., & Rogers, B.J. (1983). Effects of cimetidine on reproductive function in men. In S. Cohen (Ed.), *Update: H2 receptor antagonists. Proceedings of an International Symposium of the Royal Society of Medicine in London, England, 1983. Supplement to Drug Therapy* (pp. 169–178). New York: Biomedical Information Corporation.

Pearce, P., & Funder, J.W. (1980). Histamine H2-receptor antagonist radioreceptor assay for antiandrogen side effects. *Clinical and Experimental Pharmacology and Physiology, 7,* 442.

Pearson, D., & Shaw, S. (1982). *Life Extension: A practical scientific approach.* New York: Warner Books.

Peden, N.R., Cargill, N.R., Browning, M.C., Saunders, J.H., & Wormsley, K.G. (1979). Male sexual dysfunction during treatment with cimetidine. *British Medical Journal, 1,* 659.

Peden, N.R., & Wormsley, K.G. (1982). Effect of cimetidine on gonadal function in man [Letter to the editor]. *British Journal of Clinical Pharmacology, 14,* 565.

Pekkanen, J., Nissinen, A., Punsar, S., & Karvonen, M.J. (1989). Serum cholesterol and risk of accidental or violent death in a 25-year follow-up. *Archives of Internal Medicine, 149,* 1589–1591.

Penston, J.G. (1990). Medical events occurring in patients with duodenal ulcer disease during maintenance treatment with ranitidine. *Scandanavian Journal of Gastroenterology, 25 (Suppl. 177),* 87–97.

Perez, J., Zucchi, I., & Maggi, A. (1988). Estrogen modulation of the aminobutyric acid receptor complex in the central nervous system of the rat. *Journal of Pharmacology and Experimental Therapeutics, 244,* 1005–1010.

Persky, H., Charney, N., Lief, H.I., O'Brien, C.P., Miller, W.R., & Strauss, D. (1978). The relationship of plasma estradiol level to sexual behavior in young women. *Psychological Medicine, 40,* 523–535.

Persky, H., Dreisbach, L., Miller, W.R., O'Brien, C.P., Khan, M.A., Lief, H.J., Charney, N., & Strauss, D. (1982). The relation of plasma androgen levels to sexual behaviors and attitudes of women. *Psychosomatic Medicine, 44,* 305–319.

Persky, H., Lief, H.I., Strauss, D., Miller, W.R., & O'Brien, C.P. (1978). Plasma testosterone level and sexual behavior of couples. *Archives of Sexual Behavior, 7,* 157–173.

Persky, H., O'Brien, C.P., & Kahn, M.A. (1976). Reproductive hormone levels, sexual activity and moods during the menstrual cycle. *Psychosomatic Medicine, 38,* 62–63.

Persson, I., Yuen, J., Bergkvist, L., Adami, H.O., Hoover, R., & Schairer, C. (1992). Combined estrogen-progestogen replacement and breast cancer risk [Letter to the editor]. *Lancet, 340,* 1044.

Peselow, E.D., Filippi, A.M., Goodnick, R., Barouche, F., & Freve, R.R. (1989). The short- and long-term efficacy of paroxetine HCL: Data from a six-week double-blind parallel design trial versus imipramine and placebo. *Psychopharmacology Bulletin, 25,* 267–271.

Peskind, E.R., Raskind, M.A., Leake, R.D., Erwin, M.G., Ross, M.G., & Dorsa, D.M. (1987). Clonidine decreases plasma and cerebrospinal fluid arginine vasopressin but not oxytocin in humans. *Neuroendocrinology, 46,* 395–400.

Petersson, F., Fries, H., & Nillius, S.J. (1973). Epidemiology of secondary amenorrhea: Incidence and prevalence rates. *American Journal of Obstetrics and Gynecology, 117,* 80.

Petitti, D.B., Perlman, J.A., & Signey, S. (1986). Postmenopausal estrogen use and heart disease. *New England Journal of Medicine, 315,* 131–132.

Petitti, D.B., Perlman, J.A., & Sidney, S. (1987). Noncontraceptive estrogens and mortality: Long-term follow-up of women in the Walnut Creek study. *Obstetrics and Gynecology, 70,* 289–293.

Petraglia, G., DiMeo, G., D'Ambrogio, G.D., Segre, A., Ruspa, F., Facchinetti, F., Volpe, A., & Genazzani, A.R. (1985). Multiple opiatergic pathways are involved in reproductive functions. In M.J. Lewin & S. Bonfils (Eds.), *Regulatory peptides in digestive, nervous, and endocrine systems* (pp. 339–344). New York: Elsevier Science Publishers.

Petrie, W.M. (1980). Sexual effects of antidepressants and psychomotor stimulant drugs. *Modern Problems of Pharmacopsychiatry, 15,* 77–90.

Pettit, H.O., & Justice, J.B. (1991). Effect of dose on cocaine self-administration behavior and dopamine levels in the nucleus accumbens. *Brain Research, 539,* 94–102.

Petty, F., Kramer, G.L., & Speece, L.A. (1991). Diazepam and serotonin: In vivo effects of chronic treatment and withdrawal. *Biological Psychiatry, 29,* 81A.

Pfaff, D.W. (1973). Luteinizing hormone-releasing factor potentiates lordosis behavior in hypophysectomized ovariectomized female rats. *Science, 182,* 1148–1149.

Pfaff, D.W., & Schwartz-Giblin, S. (1988). Cellular mechanisms of female reproductive behaviors. In E. Knobil & J. Neill (Eds.), *The physiology of reproduction* (pp. 1487–1568). New York: Raven Press.

Pfaus, J.G., Damsma, G., Nomikos, C.G., Wenkstern, D.G., Blaha, C.D., Phillips, A.G., & Fibiger, H.C. (1990). Sexual behavior enhances central dopamine transmission in the male rat. *Brain Research, 530,* 345–348.

Pfaus, J.G., & Gorzalka, B.B. (1987). Opioids and sexual behavior. *Neuroscience and Biobehavioral Reviews, 11,* 1–34.

Pfaus, J.G., & Phillips, A.G. (1989). Differential effects of dopamine receptor antagonists on the sexual behavior of male rats. *Psychopharmacology, 98,* 363–368.

Pfaus, J.G., & Phillips, A.G. (1991). Role of dopamine in anticipatory and consummatory aspects of sexual behavior in the male rat. *Behavioral Neuroscience, 105,* 727–743.

Pfaus, J.G., & Pinel, J.P. (1989). Alcohol inhibits and disinhibits sexual behavior in the male rat. *Psychobiology, 17,* 195–201.

Phillip, M., Kohnen, R., & Benkert, O. (1994). Comparison study of moclobemide and doxepine with special reference to the effects on sexual dysfunction. *Neuropsychopharmacology, 10*(35, Part. 2), 845.

Phillips, A.G., Blaha, C.D., & Fibiger, H.C. (1988). In vivo detection of dopamine in the nucleus accumbens during self-stimulation: Effects of reuptake blockade. *Psycopharmacology: Abstracts of 2nd meeting of European Pharmacological Society, 96,* 544.

Phillips, S.M., & Sherwin, B.B. (1992). Variations in memory function and sex steroid hormones across the menstrual cycle. *Psychoneuroendocrinology, 17,* 497–506.

Phoenix, C.H., & Chambers, K.C. (1990). Sexual performance of old and young male rhesus macaques following treatment with GnRH. *Physiology and Behavior, 47,* 513–517.

Physicians Desk Reference. (1991a). *Physicians desk reference: 45th edition.* Montvale, NJ: Medical Economics Data.

Physicians Desk Reference. (1991b). *PDR drug interactions and side-effects index: 45th edition.* Montvale, NJ: Medical Economics Data.

Physicians Desk Reference. (1994). *Physicians desk reference: 48th edition.* Montvale, NJ: Medical Economics Data.

Physicians Desk Reference. (1995). *Physicians desk reference: 49th edition.* Montvale, NJ: Medical Economics Data.

Pierce, J.R. (1983). Cimetidine-associated depression and loss of libido in a woman. *American Journal of the Medical Sciences, 286,* 31–34.

Pierini, A.A., & Nusimovich, B. (1981). Male diabetic sexual impotence: Effects of dopaminergic agents. *Archives of Andrology, 6,* 347–350.

Pietrowsky, R., Dentler, M., Born, J., & Fehm, H.L. (1990). Calcitonin inhibits sensory processing. *Acta Endocrinologica, 122*(Suppl. 1), 111.

Pigott, T.A., Pato, M.T., Bernstein, S.E., Grover, G.N., Hill, J.L., Tolliver, T.J., & Murphy, D.L. (1990). Controlled comparisons of clomipramine and fluoxetine in the treatment of obsessive-compulsive disorder. *Archives of General Psychiatry, 47,* 926–932.

Pijnenburg, A.J.J., Honig, W.M.M., Van der Heyden, J.A.M., & Van Rossum, J.M. (1976). Effects of chemical stimulation of the mesolimbic dopamine system upon locomotor activity. *European Journal of Pharmacology, 35,* 45–58.

Pillay, V.K.G. (1976). Some side effects of alphamethyldopa. *South African Medical Journal, 50,* 625–626.

Pirrelli, A.M., & Nazzaro, P. (1989). Well-being during indapamide treatment: A benefit of blood pressure control. *Current Therapeutic Research, 45,* 611–620.

Pisantry, S., Rafaely, B., & Polishuk, W. (1975). The effect of steroid hormones on buccal mucosa of menopausal women. *Oral Surgery, Oral Medicine, Oral Pathology, 40,* 346–353.

Pitts, F.N., Jr. (1982b). The use of dextroamphetamine in medically ill depressed patients. *Journal of Clinical Psychiatry, 43,* 438.

Pitts, F.N., Jr. (1982a). Amphetamines, depression, and psychiatrists [editorial]. *Journal of Clinical Psychiatry, 43,* 3.

Placzek, R., Ohling, H., Waller, U., Krassnigg, F., & Schill, W.B. (1987). Calcium antagonists inhibit the motility of washed human spermatozoa. *Andrologia, 19,* 640–643.

Planitz, V. (1987). Comparison of moxonidine and clonidine HCL in treating patients with hypertension. *Journal of Clinical Pharmacology, 27,* 46–51.

Playboy (1970). Aphrodite's potions. *Playboy, 17,* 54.

Pleim, E.T., Matochik, J.A., Barfield, R.J., & Auerbach, S.B. (1990). Correlation of dopamine release in the nucleus accumbens with masculine sexual behavior in rats. *Brain Research, 524,* 160–163.

Plowman, P.N. (1993). Tamoxifen as adjuvant therapy in breast cancer: Current status. *Drugs, 46,* 819–833.

Podolsky, E. (1963). The women alcoholic and premenstrual tension. *Journal of the American Medical Women's Association, 18,* 816.

Poggioli, R., Vergoni, A.V., & Bertolini, A. (1985). Influence of yohimbine on the ACTH-induced behavioral syndrome in rats. *Pharmacological Research Communications, 17,* 671–678.

Poggioli, R., Vergoni, A.V., Santi, R., Carani, C., Baraghini, G.F., Zini, D., Marrama, P., & Bertolini, A. (1984). Sexual behavior of male rats: Influence of short- and long-term adrenalectomy. *Hormones and Behavior, 18,* 79–85.

Pogrund, H., Bloom, R.A., & Menczel, J. (1986). Preventing osteoporosis: Current practices and problems. *Geriatrics, 41,* 55–71.

Pohl, R. (1983). Anorgasmia caused by MAOIs. *American Journal of Psychiatry, 140,* 510.

Pohl, R., Yeragani, V.K., Balen, R., Lycaki, H., & McBride, R. (1992). Smoking in patients with panic disorder. *Psychiatry Research, 43,* 253–262.

Polderman, K.H., Gooren, L.J., Asscheman, H., Bakker, A., & Heine, R.J. (1994). Induction of insulin resistance by androgens and estrogens. *Journal of Clinical Endocrinology and Metabolism, 79,* 265–271.

Polivy, J., & Herman, C.P. (1976a). Clinical depression and weight change: A complex relation. *Journal of Abnormal Psychology, 85,* 338–340.

Polivy, J., & Herman, C.P. (1976b). Effects of alcohol on eating behavior: Influence of mood and perceived intoxication. *Journal of Abnormal Psychology, 85,* 601–606.

Pollack, M.H., & Rosenbaum, J.F. (1987). Management of antidepressant-induced side effects: A practical guide for the clinician. *Journal of Clinical Psychiatry, 48,* 3–8.

Poloniecki, J., & Hamilton, M. (1985). Subjective costs of antihypertensive treatment. *Human Toxicology, 4,* 287–291.

Pomerantz, S.M. (1991). Quinelorane (LY163402), a D2 dopamine receptor agonist, acts centrally to facilitate penile erections of male rhesus monkeys. *Pharmacology, Biochemistry, and Behavior, 39,* 123–128.

Pomerantz, S.M. (1992). Dopaminergic influences on male sexual behavior of rhesus monkeys: Effects of dopamine agonists. *Pharmacology, Biochemistry, and Behavior, 41,* 511–517.

Pontius, E.B. (1988). Case report of an anticholinergic crisis associated with cyproheptadine treatment of desipramine-induced anorgasmia [Letter to the editor]. *Journal of Clinical Psychopharmacology, 8,* 230–231.

Popli, S., Daugirdas, J.T., Neubauer, J.A., Hockenberry, B., Hano, J.E., & Ing, T.S. (1986). Transdermal clonidine in mild hypertension: A randomized, double-blind, placebo-controlled trial. *Archives of Internal Medicine, 146,* 2140–2144.

Popovic, A., Plecas, B., Milicevic, Z., Hristic, M., & Jovovic, D. (1990). Stereologic analysis of ventral prostate of oxytocin-treated rats. *Archives of Andrology, 24,* 247–253.

Porrino, L.J., Ritz, M.C., Goodman, N.L., Sharpe, L.G., Kuhar, M.J., & Goldberg, S.R. (1989). Differential effects of the pharmacological manipulation of serotonin systems on cocaine and amphetamine self-administration in rats. *Life Sciences, 45,* 1529–1535.

Porsolt, R.D., Pawelec, C., Roux, S., & Jalfre, M. (1984). Discrimination of the amphetamine cue: Effects of A, B, and mixed type inhibitors of monoamine oxidase. *Neuropharmacology, 23,* 569–573.

Porto, R. (1980). Double-blind study of clomipramine in premature ejaculation. In R. Forleo & W. Pasini (Eds.), *Medical sexology* (pp. 624–628). Littleton, MA: PSG Publishing Co.

Post, L.L. (1994). Sexual side effects of psychiatric medications in women. *American Journal of Psychiatry, 151,* 1246–1247.

Post, R.M., Weiss, S.R., & Chuang, D.M. (1992). Mechanisms of action of anticonvulsants in affective disorders: Comparisons with lithium. *Journal of Clinical Psychopharmacology, 12,* 235–355.

Potegal, M., Antilla, A., & Glusman, M. (1988). Alterations in aggression following GABAergic modulation of septal and raphe activity. *Psychobiology, 16,* 174–177.

Pressman, M.R., DiPillipo, M.A., Kendrick, J.I., Conroy, K., & Fry, J.M. (1986). Problems in the interpretation of nocturnal penile tumescence studies: Disruptions of sleep by occult sleep disorders. *Journal of Urology, 136,* 595–598.

Price, J., & Grunhaus, L.J. (1990). Treatment of clomipramine-induced anorgasmia with yohimbine: A case report. *Journal of Clinical Psychiatry, 51,* 32–33.

Prummel, M.F., Wiersinga, W.M., Lips, P., Sanders, G.T., & Sauerwein, H.P. (1991). The course of biochemical parameters of bone turnover during treatment with corticosteroids. *Journal of Clinical Endocrinology and Metabolism, 72,* 382–386.

Przyklenk, K., & Kloner, R.A. (1991). Angiotensin converting enzyme inhibitors improve contractile function of stunned myocardium by different mechanisms of action. *American Heart Journal, 121,* 1319–1330.

Pulvirenti, L., & Koob, G.F. (1990). Self-administration of drugs of abuse in rats: Nucleus accumbens glutamate modulates mesolimbic dopamine function. *Pharmacological Research, 22*(Suppl. 2), 418.

Pulvirenti, L., Swerdlow, N.R., & Koob, G.F. (1989).

Microinjection of a glutamate antagonist into the nucleus accumbens reduces psychostimulant locomotion in rats. *Neuroscience Letters, 103,* 213-218.

Punnonen, R. (1973). Effect of castration and peroral estrogen therapy on the skin. *Acta Obstetricia et Gynecologica Scandanavica, Suppl. 21,* 1-44.

Punnonen, R., Vilska, S., & Rauramo, L. (1984). Skinfold thickness and long-term postmenopausal hormone therapy. *Maturitas, 5,* 259-262.

Pyke, R.E., & Krause, M. (1988). Alprazolam in the treatment of panic attack patients with and without major depression. *Journal of Clinical Psychiatry, 49,* 66-68.

Pyle, R.L., Mitchell, J.E., & Eckert, E.D. (1981). Bulimia: A report of 34 cases. *Journal of Clinical Psychiatry, 42,* 60-64.

Quadraccia, A., Salvini, A., Cordani, C., & Pizzi, P. (1988). Yohimbine plus intracavernous vasodilators in mild vasculogenic impotence. *Acta Urologica Belgica, 56,* 272-278.

Quattrone, A., Tedeschi, G., Aguglia, U., Scopacasa, F., DiRenzo, G.F., & Annunziato, L. (1983). Prolactin secretion in man: A useful tool to evaluate the activity of drugs on central 5-hydroxytryptaminergic neurons. Studies with fenfluramine. *British Journal of Clinical Pharmacology, 16,* 471-475.

Quinn, N.P., Toone, B., Lang, A.E., Marsden, C.D., & Parkes, J.D. (1983). Dopa dose-dependent sexual deviation. *British Journal of Psychiatry, 142,* 296-298.

Quirk, K.C., & Einarson, T.R. (1982). Sexual dysfunction and clomipramine. *Canadian Journal of Psychiatry, 27,* 228-231.

Rabkin, J.G., Quitkin, F.M., Harrison, W., Tricarno, R., & McGrath, P. (1984). Adverse reactions to monoamine oxidase inhibitors. Part I. A comparative study. *Journal of Clinical Psychopharmacology, 4,* 270-278.

Rabkin, J.G., Quitkin, F.M., McGrath, P., Harrison, W., & Tricaro, E. (1985). Adverse reactions to monoamine oxidase inhibitors: Part II. *Clinical Psychopharmacology, 5,* 2-9.

Racke, K., Haas, U., Sperb, S., Fischbach, A., Hof, H., Sirrenberg, S., & Wammack, R. (1991). Opioid inhibition of oxytocin release, but not autoinhibition of dopamine release, may involve activation of potassium [K^+] channels. *Advances in the Biosciences, 82,* 265-267.

Radomski, S.B., Herschorn, S., & Rangaswamy, S. (1994). Topical minoxidil in the treatment of male erectile dysfunction. *Journal of Urology, 151,* 1225-1226.

Ragavan, V.V., & Frantz, A.G. (1981). Opioid regulation of prolactin secretion: Evidence for a specific role of beta-endorphin. *Endocrinology, 109,* 1769-1771.

Rajfer, J., Aronson, W.J., Bush, P.A., Dorsey, F.J., & Ignarro, L.J. (1992). Nitric oxide as a mediator of relaxation of the corpus cavernosum in response to nonadrenergic noncholinergic neurotransmission. *New England Journal of Medicine, 326,* 90-94.

Raleigh, M.J., Brammer, G.L., McGuire, M.T., Yuwiler, A., Geller, E., & Johnson, C.K. (1983). Social status related differences in the behavioral effects of drugs in vervet monkeys (*Cercopithecus aethiops sayacus*). In H.D. Steklis & A.S. Kling (Eds.), *Hormones, drugs, and social behavior in primates* (pp. 83-105). New York: Spectrum.

Raleigh, M.J., Brammer, G.L., Ritvo, E.R., Geller, E., McGuire, M.T., & Yuwiler, A. (1986). Effects of chronic fenfluramine on blood serotonin, cerebrospinal fluid metabolites, and behavior in monkeys. *Psychopharmacology, 90,* 503-508.

Raleigh, M.J., McGuire, M.T., & Brammer, G.L. (1988). Behavioral and cognitive effects of altered tryptophan and tyrosine supply. In G. Huether (Ed.), *Amino acid availability and brain function in health and disease* (pp. 299-308). New York: Springer-Verlag.

Rampling, D. (1978). Aggression: A paradoxical response to tricyclic antidepressants. *American Journal of Psychiatry, 135,* 117-118.

Rapp, M.S. (1979). Two cases of ejaculatory impairment related to phenelzine [Letter to the editor]. *American Journal of Psychiatry, 136,* 1200-1201.

Rasmussen, K., & Aghajanian, G.K. (1989). Withdrawal-induced activation of locus coeruleus neurons in opiate-dependent rats: Attenuation by lesions of the nucleus paragigantocellularis. *Brain Research, 505,* 346-350.

Rauramo, L., Lagerspetz, K., Engblom, P., & Punnonen, R. (1975). The effect of castration and peroral estrogen therapy on some psychological functions. In P.A. van Keep & C. Lauritzen (Eds.), *Estrogens in the post-menopause* (pp. 94-104). Basel: Karger.

Rausch, J.L., & Parry, B.L. (1987). Endocrinology and depression, III: The effect of gonadal steroids on affective symptomatology. In O.G. Cameron (Ed.), *Presentations of depression: Depressive symptoms in medical and other psychiatric disorders* (pp. 291-320). New York: John Wiley & Sons.

Ravn, S.H., Rosenberg, J., & Bostofte, E. (1994). Postmenopausal hormone replacement therapy: Clinical implications. *European Journal of Obstetrics, Gynecology, and Reproductive Biology, 53,* 81-93.

Ravnikar, V. (1987). Compliance with hormone therapy. *American Journal of Obstetrics and Gynecology, 156,* 1332-1334.

Raymond, C.A. (1987). Hormone replacement: Gynecologists consider the heart of the matter. *Journal of the American Medical Association, 258,* 1573-1577.

Recker, R.R., Saville, P.D., & Heaney, R.P. (1977). Effect of estrogens and calcium carbonate on bone loss in postmenopausal women. *Annals of Internal Medicine, 87,* 649-655.

Redmond, D.E. (1985). Anxiety and sexual arousal (letter to the editor). *American Journal of Psychiatry, 142,* 782-783.

Redmond, D.E., Kosten, T.R., & Treiser, M.F. (1983). Spontaneous ejaculation associated with anxiety: Psychophysiological considerations. *American Journal of Psychiatry, 140,* 1163-1166.

Regelson, W., Loria, R., & Kalimi, M. (1988). Hormonal intervention: "Buffer hormones" or "state dependency": The role of dehydroepiandrosterone (DHEA), thyroid hormone, estrogen, and hypophysectomy in aging. In W. Pierpaoli & N.H. Spector (Eds.), *Neuroimmunomodulation: Interventions in aging and cancer. Vol. 521. Annals of the New York Academy of Sciences* (pp. 260-273). New York: New York Academy of Sciences.

Regestein, Q.R., & Reich, P. (1985). Agitation observed during treatment with newer hypnotic drugs. *Journal of Clinical Psychiatry, 46,* 280-283.

Regestein, Q.R., Schiff, I., Tulchinsky, D., & Ryan, K.J. (1981). Relationships among estrogen-induced psychophysiological changes in hypogonadal women. *Psychosomatic Medicine, 43,* 147-155.

Reich, L.H., Davies, R.K., & Himmelhock, J.N. (1974). Excessive alcohol use in manic-depressive illness. *American Journal of Psychiatry, 131,* 83-86.

Reichlin, S. (1987). Basic research of hypothalamic-pituitary-adrenal neuroendocrinology: An overview. The physiological function of the stress response. In U. Halbreich (Ed.), *Hormones and depression* (pp. 21-30). New York: Raven Press.

Reid, K., Morales, A., Harris, C., Surridge, D.H.C., Condra, M., Owen, J., & Fenemore, J. (1987). Double-blind trial of yohimbine in treatment of psychogenic impotence. *Lancet, i,* 421-423.

Reid, L.D., & Hunter, G.A. (1984). Morphine and naloxone modulate intake of ethanol. *Alcohol, 1,* 35-37.

Reid, R.L., Quigley, M.E., & Yen, S.S. (1983). The disappearance of opioidergic regulation of gonadotropin secretion in postmenopausal women. *Journal of Clinical Endocrinology and Metabolism, 57,* 1107-1110.

Reimherr, F.W., Chouinard, G., Cohn, C.K., Cole, J.O., Itil, T.M., LaPierre, Y.D., Masco, H.L., & Mendels, J. (1990). Antidepressant efficacy of sertraline: A double-blind, placebo- and amitriptyline-controlled multicenter comparison study in outpatients with major depression. *Journal of Clinical Psychiatry, 51* (12, Suppl. B), 18-27.

Reinisch, J.M., Ziemba-Davis, M., & Sanders, S.A. (1991). Hormonal contributions to sexually dimorphic behavioral development in humans. *Psychoneuroendocrinology, 16,* 213-278.

Rekers, H., Drogendijk, A.C., Valkenbeurg, H.A., & Riphagen, F. (1992). The menopause, urinary incontinence, and other symptoms of the genitourinary tract. *Maturitas, 15,* 101-111.

Renaud, S., & De Lorgeril, M. (1992). Wine, alcohol, platelets, and the French paradox for coronary heart disease. *Lancet, 339,* 1523-1526.

Renri, T., Ueda, S., Anraku, T., Satoh, H., Tsujimaru, S., Nakazawa, Y., & Ueda, J. (1990). Antiepileptics and bone atrophy—three-year follow-up study. *Japanese Journal of Psychiatry and Neurology, 44,* 385-386.

Renyi, L. (1985). Ejaculations induced by p-chloroamphetamine in the rat. *Neuropharmacology, 24,* 697-704.

Renyi, L. (1986). The effect of selective 5-hydroxytryptamine uptake inhibitors on 5-methoxy-M, N-dimethyltryptamine-induced ejaculation in the rat. *British Journal of Pharmacology, 87,* 639-648.

Rex, A., Marsden, C.A., & Fink, H. (1993). Effect of diazepam on cortical 5-HT release and behavior in the guinea-pig on exposure to the elevated plus maze. *Psychopharmacology, 110,* 490-496.

Richards, D.H. (1974). A post-hysterectomy syndrome. *Lancet, 2,* 983-985.

Richelson, E. (1994). Preclinical pharmacology of antipsychotic drugs: Relationship to efficacy and side effects. *Journal of Clinical Psychiatry Monograph, 12*(2), 17-20.

Richelson, E., & Nelson, A. (1984). Antagonism by antidepressants of neurotransmitter receptors of normal human brain in vitro. *Journal of Pharmacology and Experimental Therapeutics, 230,* 94-102.

Richer, M., & Crisman, M.L. (1993). Pharmacotherapy of sexual offenders. *Annals of Pharmacotherapy, 27,* 316-320.

Rickels, K., Freeman, E.W., Sondheimer, S., & Albert, J. (1990). Fluoxetine in the treatment of premenstrual syndrome. *Current Therapeutic Research, 48,* 161-166.

Rickels, K., & Schweizer, E. (1990). Clinical overview of serotonin reuptake inhibitors. *Journal of Clinical Psychiatry, 51* (12, Suppl. B), 9-12.

Riedel, H.H., Lehman-Willenbrock, E., & Semm, K. (1988). Clinical and biochemical signs of ovarian failure after hysterectomy in young women and its treatment. In R. Lizuka & K. Semm (Eds.), *Human reproduction: Current status/future prospect* (pp. 671-679). New York: Elsevier Science Publishers.

Riggs, B.L., Hodgson, S.F., O'Fallon, W.M., Chao, E.Y., Wahner, H.W., Muhs, J.M., Cedel, S.L., & Melton, L.J. (1990). Effects of flouride treatment on the fracture rate in postmenopausal women with osteoporosis. *New England Journal of Medicine, 322,* 802-809.

Riley, A.J., Goodman, R.E., Kellett, J.M., & Orr, R. (1989). Double-blind trial of yohimbine hydrochloride in the treatment of erection inadequacy. *Sexual and Marital Therapy, 4,* 17-26.

Riley, A.J., & Riley, E.J. (1981). The effect of labetalol and propranolol on the pressor response to sexual arousal in women. *British Journal of Clinical Pharmacology, 12,* 341-344.

Riley, A.J., & Riley, E.J. (1983). Cholinergic and adrenergic control of human sexual responses. In D. Wheatley (Ed.), *Psychopharmacology and sexual disorders* (pp. 129-137). New York: Oxford University Press.

Riley, A.J., & Riley, E.J. (1986). Cyproheptadine and antidepressant-induced anorgasmia. *British Journal of Psychiatry, 148,* 217-218.

Riley, A.J., Riley, E.J., & Davies, H.J. (1982). A method for monitoring drug effects on male sexual response: The effect of single dose labetalol. *British Journal of Clinical Pharmacology, 14,* 695-700.

Rittmaster, R.S., Antonian, L., New, M.I., & Stoner, E. (1994). Effect of finasteride on adrenal steroidogenesis in men. *Journal of Andrology, 15,* 298-301.

Ritz, M.C., & Kuhar, M.J. (1989). Relationship between self-administration of amphetamine and monoamine receptors in the brain: Comparison with cocaine. *Journal of Pharmacology and Experimental Therapeutics, 248,* 1010-1017.

Ritz, M.C., Lamb, R.J., Goldberg, S.R., & Kuhar, M.J. (1987). Cocaine receptors on dopamine transporters are related to self-administration of cocaine. *Science, 237,* 1219-1223.

Rivas, F.J., & Mir, D. (1990). Effects of nucleus accumbens lesion on female rat sexual receptivity and proceptivity in a partner preference paradigm. *Behavioral Brain Research, 41,* 239-249.

Rivas, M.D.C., Barradas, E., Montiel, C., & Bianco, F.J. (1990). Pubococcygeus activity related to female orgasm. In F.J. Bianco & H. Serrano (Eds.), *Sexology: An independent field* (pp. 189-205). New York: Elsevier Science Publishers.

Robbins, M.A., Elias, M.F., & Schultz, N.R. (1990). The effects of age, blood pressure, and knowledge of hypertensive diagnosis on anxiety and depression. *Experimental Aging Research, 16,* 199-207.

Robel, P., Akwa, Y., Corpechot, C., Zhony-Yi, H., Jung-Testas, I., Kabbadj, K., Le Goascogne, C., Morfin, R., Vourc'h, C., Young, J., & Baulieu, E.E. (1991). Neurosteroids: Biosynthesis and function of pregnenolone and dehydroepiandrosterone in the brain. In M. Motta (Ed.), *Brain endocrinology* (2nd ed.) (pp. 105-130). New York: Raven Press.

Robel, P., & Baulieu, E.E. (1985). Neuro-steroids: 3 beta-hydroxy-5-derivatives in the rodent brain. *Neurochemistry International, 7,* 953-958.

Robel, P., Corpechot, C., Clarke, C., Groyer, A., Synguelakis, M., Vourhc'h, C., & Baulieu, E.E. (1986). Neurosteroids: 3 beta-hydroxy-5-derivatives in the rat brain. In G.F. Frank, A.J. Harmar, & K.W. McKerns (Eds.), *Neuroendocrine molecular biology* (pp. 367-376). New York: Plenum Press.

Robel, P., Corpechot, C., Synguelakis, M., Groyer, A., Clarke, C., Schlegel, M.L., Brazeau, P., & Baulieu, E.E. (1984). Pregnenolone, dehydroepiandrosterone, and their sulfate esters in the rat brain. In F. Celotti, L. Naftolin, & L. Martini (Eds.), *Metabolism of hormonal steroids in the neuroendocrine structures* (pp. 185-193). New York: Raven Press.

Roberts, C.D., & Sloboda, W. (1974). Afrodex versus placebo in the treatment of male impotence: Statistical analysis of two double-blind crossover studies. *Current Therapeutic Research, 16,* 96-99.

Roberts, E. (1986). Guides through the labyrinth of AD: Dehydroepiandrosterone, potassium channels, and the C4 component of complement. In T. Crook, R.T. Bartus, S. Ferris, & S. Sershon (Eds.), *Treatment development strategies for Alzheimer's disease* (pp. 173-200). Madison, Connecticut: Mark Powley Associates.

Robinson, B.W., & Mishkin, M. (1968). Penile erection evoked from forebrain structures in *Macaca mulatta. Archives of Neurology, 19,* 184-198.

Robinson, D., Friedman, L., Marcus, R., Tinklenberg, J., & Yesavage, J. (1994). Estrogen replacement therapy and memory in older women. *Journal of the American Geriatrics Society, 42,* 919-922.

Robinson, T.E., & Becker, J.B. (1986). Enduring changes in brain and behavior produced by chronic amphetamine administration: A review and evaluation of animal models of amphetamine psychosis. *Brain Research Reviews, 11,* 157-198.

Rodriguez, L.A.G., & Jicks, H. (1994). Risk of gynecomastia associated with cimetidine, omeprazole, and other antiulcer drugs. *British Medical Journal, 308,* 503-506.

Rodríguez-Manzo, G., & Fernández-Guasti, A. (1994). Reversal of sexual exhaustion by serotonergic and noradrenergic agents. *Behavioral Brain Research, 62,* 127-134.

Rolandi, E., Franceschini, R., Giberti, C., Brancadoro, T., Martorana, G., & Barreca, T. (1988). Sustained impairment of pituitary and testicular function in prostatic cancer patients treated with a depot form of a GnRH agonist. *Hormone Research, 30,* 22–25.

Rose, L.I., Underwood, R.H., Newmark, S.R., Kisch, E.S., & Williams, G.H. (1977). Pathophysiology of spironolactone-induced gynecomastia. *Annals of Internal Medicine, 87,* 398–403.

Rose, R.M., Bernstein, I.S., & Gordon, T.P. (1975). Consequences of social conflict on plasma testosterone levels in rhesus monkeys. *Psychosomatic Medicine, 37,* 50–61.

Rosen, M.P., Greenfield, A.J., Walker, T.G., Grant, P., Dubrow, J., Bettman, M.A., Fried, L.E., & Goldstein, I. (1991). Cigarette smoking: An independent risk factor for atherosclerosis in the hypogastric-cavernous arterial bed of men with arteriogenic impotence. *Journal of Urology, 145,* 759–763.

Rosen, R.C., & Beck, J.G. (1988). *Patterns of sexual arousal.* New York: Guilford Press.

Rosen, R.C., Kostis, J.B., Jekelis, A., & Taska, L.S. (1994). Sexual sequelae of antihypertensive drugs: Treatment effects on self-report and physiological measures in middle-aged male hypertensives. *Archives of Sexual Behavior, 23,* 135–151.

Rosenbaum, J.F., & Pollack, M.H. (1988). Anhedonic ejaculation with desipramine. *International Journal of Psychiatry in Medicine, 18,* 85–88.

Rosenbaum, J.F., Woods, S.W., Groves, J.E., & Klerman, G.L. (1984). Emergence of hostility during alprazolam treatment. *American Journal of Psychiatry, 141,* 792–793.

Rosenberg, L., Hennekens, C.H., Rosner, B., Belanger, C., Rothman, K.J., & Speizer, F.E. (1981). Early menopause and the risk of myocardial infarction. *American Journal of Obstetrics and Gynecology, 139,* 47–51.

Rosenvinge, H.S. (1975). Abuse of fenfluramine [Letter to the editor]. *British Medical Journal, 1,* 735.

Rosenzweig-Lipson, S., Chu, B., Delfs, J.M., & Kelley, A.E. (1990). Microinjections of cocaine, bupropion, and pipradrol into the nucleus accumbens enhance locomotor activity and potentiate responding for a conditioned reinforcer. *Society for Neuroscience: Abstracts, 164,* 749.

Ross, R.K., Paganini-Hill, A., Roy, S., Chao, A., & Henderson, B. (1988). Past and present preferred prescribing practices of hormone replacement therapy among Los Angeles gynecologists: Possible implications for public health. *American Journal of Public Health, 78,* 516–519.

Rostene, W.H. (1984). Neurobiological and neuroendocrine functions of the vasoactive intestinal polypeptide (VIP). *Progress in Neurobiology, 22,* 103–129.

Rostom, A.Y., & Gershuny, A.R. (1992). Adjuvant treatment in breast cancer [Letter to the editor]. *Lancet, 339,* 424.

Rothman, R.B. (1990). High affinity dopamine reuptake inhibitors as potential cocaine antagonists: A strategy for drug development. *Life Sciences, 46,* 17–21.

Rothschild, A.J. (1992). Disinhibition, amnestic reaction, and other adverse reactions secondary to triazolam: A review of the literature. *Journal of Clinical Psychiatry, 53*(Suppl. 12), 69–78.

Rothschild, A.J., Bessette, M.P., Carter-Campbell, J., & Murray, M. (1993). Triazolam and disinhibition [Letter to the editor]. *Lancet, 341,* 186.

Rousseau, L., Couture, M., Dupont, A., Labrie, F., & Couture, N. (1990). Effect of combined androgen blockage with an LHRH agonist and flutamide in one severe case of male exhibitionism. *Canadian Journal of Psychiatry, 35,* 338–341.

Roy, A.C., Adaikan, P.G., Sen, D.K., & Ratnam, S.S. (1989). Prostaglandin 15-hydroxydehydrogenase activity in human penile corpora cavernosa and its significance in prostaglandin-mediated penile erection. *British Journal of Urology, 64,* 180–182.

Roy, A.C., Tan, S.M., Kottegoda, S.R., & Ratnam, S.A. (1984). Ability of human corpora cavernosa muscle to generate prostaglandins and thromboxanes in vitro. *IRCS Medical Science, 12,* 608–610.

Roy, J.B., Petrone, R.L., & Said, S.I. (1990). A clinical trial of intracavernous vasoactive intestinal peptide to induce penile erection. *Journal of Urology, 143,* 302–304.

Rozenberg, S., Ham, H., Bosson, D., Peretz, A., & Robyn, C. (1990). Age, steroids, and bone mineral content. *Maturitas, 12,* 137–143.

Rozenberg, S., Ham, H., Caufriez, A., Bosson, D., Peretz, A., & Robyn, C. (1990). Sex and adrenal steroids in female in- and out-patients. In M. Flint, F. Kronenberg, & W. Utian (Eds.), *Multidisciplinary perspectives on menopause. Vol. 592. Annals of the New York Academy of Sciences* (pp. 466–468). New York: New York Academy of Sciences.

Rozenboim, I., Dgany, O., Robinzon, B., Arnon, E., & Snapir, N. (1989). The effect of tamoxifen on the reproductive traits in white leghorn cockerels. *Pharmacology, Biochemistry, and Behavior, 32,* 377–381.

Rubin, H.B., & Henson, D.E. (1976). Effects of alcohol on male sexual responding. *Psychopharmacology, 47,* 123–134.

Ruch, A., & Duhring, J.L. (1989). Postpartum myocardial infarction in a patient receiving bromocriptine. *Obstetrics and Gynecology, 74,* 448–451.

Rud, T. (1980). The effect of estrogens of gestagens on the urethral pressure profile in urinary continent and stress incontinent women. *Acta Obstetricia et Gynecologica Scandinavica, 59,* 331–335.

Rud, T., Andersson, K., Boye, N., & Ulmsten, U. (1980). Terodiline inhibition of human bladder contraction: Effects in vitro and in women with unstable bladder. *Acta Pharmacologica et Toxicologica, 46*(Suppl. 1), 31-38.

Ruggieri, S., Stocchi, F., & Agnoli, A. (1986). Lisuride infusion pump for Parkinson's disease [Letter to the editor]. *Lancet, 2,* 348-349.

Rune, S.J. (1994). Treatment strategies for symptom resolution, healing, and *Helicobacter pylori* eradication in duodenal ulcer patients. *Scandinavian Journal of Gastroenterology, 29*(Suppl. 205), 45-47.

Rupniak, N.M., Jenner, P., & Marsden, C.D. (1986). Acute dystonia induced by neuroleptic drugs. *Psychopharmacology, 88,* 403-419.

Russ, M.J., & Ackerman, S.H. (1988). Antidepressants and weight gain. *Appetite, 10,* 102-117.

Russell, J.M., MacGregor, R.J., & Watson, I. (1985). Prazosin and priapism. *Medical Journal of Australia, 143,* 321.

Russell, M., & Bigler, L. (1979). Screening for alcohol-related problems in an outpatient obstetric-gynecologic clinic. *American Journal of Obstetrics and Gynecology, 134,* 4-12.

Ryan, C. (1980). Learning and memory deficits in alcoholics. *Journal of Studies on Alcohol, 41,* 437-447.

Ryan, C., & Butters, N. (1980). Learning and memory impairments in young and old alcoholics: Evidence for the premature aging hypothesis. *Alcoholism: Clinical and Experimental Research, 4* 288-293.

Ryan, D.E., & Levin, W. (1990). Purification and characterization of hepatic microsomal cytochrome P-450. *Pharmacology and Therapeutics, 45,* 153-239.

Ryan, M.M., Dennerstein, L., & Pepperell, R. (1989). Psychological aspects of hysterectomy: A prospective study. *British Journal of Psychiatry, 154,* 516-522.

Sabelli, H.C., & Giardina, W. (1973). Amine modulation of affective behavior. In H.C. Sabelli (Ed.), *Chemical modulation of brain function* (pp. 225-259). New York: Raven Press.

Sabelli, H.C., & Moshaim, A.D. (1974). Phenylethylamine hypothesis of affective behavior. *American Journal of Psychiatry, 131,* 695-699.

Sachs, B.D., & Meisel, R.L. (1988). The physiology of male sexual behavior. In E. Knobil & J. Neill (Eds.), *The physiology of reproduction* (pp. 13893-1485). New York: Raven Press.

Sackeim, H., Decina, P., Prohownik, I., & Malitz, S. (1987). Seizure threshold in electroconvulsive therapy. *Archives of General Psychiatry, 44,* 355-360.

Sacks, O. (1973). *Awakenings.* London: Duckworth.

Saenz de Tejada, I., Ware, J.C., Blanco, R., Pittard, J.T., Nadig, P.W., Azadzoi, K.M., Krane, R.J., & Goldstein, I. (1991). Pathophysiology of prolonged penile erection associated with trazodone use. *Journal of Urology, 145,* 60-64.

Sala, M., Braida, D., Leone, M.P., Calcaterra, P., Monti, S., & Gori, E. (1990). Central effect of yohimbine on sexual behavior in the rat. *Physiology and Behavior, 47,* 165-173.

Salis, P.J., & Dewsbury, D.S. (1971). p-Chlorophenylalamine facilitates copulatory behavior in male rats. *Nature, 232,* 400-401.

Salmimies, P., Kockott, G., Pirke, K.M., Vogt, H.J., & Schill, W.B. (1982). Effects of testosterone replacement on sexual behavior in hypogonadal men. *Archives of Sexual Behavior, 11,* 345-354.

Salmon, U.J. (1941). Rationale for androgen therapy in gynecology. *Journal of Clinical Endocrinology, 1,* 162-179.

Salmon, U.J., & Geist, S.H. (1943). Effects of androgens upon libido in women. *Journal of Clinical Endocrinology, 3,* 235-238.

Salmon, U.J., Walter, R.I., & Geist, S.H. (1941). The use of estrogen in the treatment of dysuria and incontinence in postmenopausal women. *American Journal of Obstetrics and Gynecology, 42,* 845-851.

Sambhi, M.P., Gavras, H., Robertson, J.I.S., & Smith, W.M. (1993). Long-range safety and protective benefits of angiotensin-converting enzyme inhibitors for hypertension: Do we need more clinical trials? *Western Journal of Medicine, 158,* 286-294.

Sanders, D., & Bancroft, J. (1982). Hormones and the sexuality of women-the menstrual cycle. *Clinics in Endocrinology and Metabolism, 11,* 639-659.

Sanders, D., Warner, P., Backstrom, T., & Bancroft, J. (1983). Mood, sexuality, hormones, and the menstrual cycle. I. Changes in mood and physical state: Description of subjects and method. *Psychosomatic Medicine, 45,* 487-501.

Sandin, M., Jasmin, S., & Levere, T.E. (1990). Aging and cognition: Facilitation of recent memory in aged nonhuman primates by nimodipine. *Neurobiology of Aging, 11,* 573-575.

Sandler, B. (1979). Idiopathic retrograde ejaculation. *Fertility and Sterility, 32,* 474-475.

Sangal, R. (1985). Inhibited female orgasm as a side effect of alprazolam [Letter to the editor]. *American Journal of Psychiatry, 142,* 1223-1224.

Sapolsky, R.M., Krey, L.C., & McEwen, B.S. (1986). The neuroendocrinology of stress and aging: The glucocorticoid cascade hypothesis. *Endocrine Reviews, 7,* 284-301.

Sarantidis, D., & Waters, B. (1983). A review and controlled study of cutaneous conditions associated with lithium carbonate. *British Journal of Psychiatry, 143,* 42-50.

Sarosdy, M.F., Hudnall, C.H., Erickson, D.R., Hardin, T.C., & Novicki, D.E. (1989). A prospective double-blind trial of intracorporeal papaverine versus prostaglandin E1 in the treatment of impotence. *Journal of Urology, 141,* 551-553.

Sarrel, P.M. (1982). Sex problems after menopause: A study of fifty couples treated in a sex counseling programe. *Maturitas, 4,* 231-239.

Sarrel, P.M. (1986). Laser doppler measurement of peripheral blood flow. In M. Notelovitz & P.A. van Keep (Eds.), *The climacteric in perspective* (pp. 161-175). Lancaster, England: MTP Press.

Sarrel, P.M. (1987). Sexuality in the middle years. *Obstetrics and Gynecology Clinics of North America, 14,* 49-62.

Sarrel, P.M. (1988). Sexuality. In J.W. Studd & I.M. Whitehead (Eds.), *Menopause* (p. 65-75). London: Blackwell Scientific.

Sarrel, P.M. (1990). Sexuality and menopause. *Obstetrics & Gynecology, 75,* 26s-30s.

Satel, S.L., & Nelson, J.C. (1989). Stimulants in the treatment of depression: A critical overview. *Journal of Clinical Psychiatry, 50,* 241-149.

Satinoff, E. (1982). Are there similarities between thermoregulation and sexual behavior. In D.W. Pfaff (Ed), *The physiological mechanisms of motivation* (pp. 217-251). New York: Springer-Verlag.

Sauvanet, J.P., Maarek, L., Roger, M., Renaudin, J., Louvel, E., & Orofiamma, B. (1988). Open long-term trials with zolpidem in insomnia. In J.P. Sauvanet, S.Z. Langer, & P.L. Morselli (Eds.), *Imidazopyridines in sleep disorders* (pp. 339-350). New York: Raven Press.

Savion, M., Segenreich, E., Kahan, E., & Servadio, C. (1987). Pharmacologic, nonhormonal treatment of impotence. *Urology, 29,* 510-512.

Sawyer, C.H. (1966). Neural mechanisms in the steroid feedback regulation of sexual behavior and pituitary-gonad function. In R.A. Gorski & R.E. Whalen (Eds.), *Brain and behavior. Vol. 3* (pp. 221-255). Berkeley, CA: University of California Press.

Saydoff, J.A., Rittenhouse, P.A., Van de Kar, L.D., & Brownfield, M.S. (1991). Enhanced serotonergic transmission stimulates oxytocin secretion in conscious male rats. *Journal of Pharmacology and Experimental Therapeutics, 257,* 95-99.

Schaefer, C.F., Gunn, C.G., & Dubowski, K.M. (1975). Normal plasma testosterone concentrations after marijuana smoking. *New England Journal of Medicine, 292,* 867-868.

Schams, D., Baumann, G., & Leidl, W. (1982). Oxytocin determination by radioimmunoassay in cattle. II. Effect of mating and stimulation of the genital tract in bulls, cows, and heifers. *Acta Endocrinologica, 99,* 218-223.

Scharf, M.B., Fletcher, K., & Graham, J.P. (1988). Comparative amnestic effects of benzodiazepine hypnotic agents. *Journal of Clinical Psychiatry, 49,* 134-137.

Schechter, M.D. (1984). Evidence for a direct dopaminergic effect of lisuride. *Pharmacology, Biochemistry, and Behavior, 21,* 185-189.

Scher, M., Krieger, J.N., & Juergens, S. (1983). Trazodone and priapism. *American Journal of Psychiatry, 140,* 1362-1363.

Schersten, B. (1988). Effect of antihypertensive therapy on kidney function in diabetic patients. *Drugs, 35*(Suppl. 5), 59-61.

Schildkraut, J.J. (1965). The catecholamine hypothesis of affective disorders: A review of supporting evidence. *American Journal of Psychiatry, 122,* 509-522.

Schlemmer, A., Jensen, J., Riis, B.J., & Christiansen, C. (1990). Smoking induces increased androgen levels in early post-menopausal women. *Maturitas, 12,* 99-104.

Schmidt, C.W. (1983). Pharmacological methods in the treatment of sexual disorders. In J.K. Meyer, C. W. Schmidt, & T.N. Wise (Eds.), *Clinical management of sexual disorders* (2nd ed.) (pp. 161-168). Baltimore: Williams & Wilkins.

Schmidt, G.R., Schuna, A.A., & Goodfriend, T.L. (1989). Transdermal clonidine compared with hydrochlorthiazide as monotherapy in elderly hypertensive males. *Journal of Clinical Pharmacology, 29,* 133-139.

Schmidt, P.J., Lynnette, L.K., Grover, G.N., Muller, K.L., Merriam, G.R., & Rubinow, D.R. (1991). Lack of effect of induced menses on symptoms in women with premenstrual syndrome. *New England Journal of Medicine, 324,* 1174-1179.

Schneider, L.S., Tariot, P.N., & Goldstein, B. (1994). Therapy with l-deprenyl (selegiline) and relation to abuse liability. *Clinical Pharmacology and Therapeutics, 56,* 750-756.

Schneider, R.H., Mills, P.J., Schramm, W., Walton, K.G., Dillbeck, M.C., & Wallace, R.K. (1989). Dehydroepiandrosterone sulfate (DHEAS) levels in type A behavior and the transcendental meditation program. *Psychosomatic Medicine, 51,* 256.

Schnur, S.L., Smith, E.R., Lee, R.L., Mas, M., & Davidson, J.M. (1989). A component analysis of the effects of DPAT on male rat sexual behavior. *Physiology and Behavior, 45,* 897-901.

Schoeffter, P., & Hoyer, D.C. (1989). 5-Hydroxytryptamine 5-HT_{1B} and 5-HT_{1D} receptors mediating inhibition of adenylate cyclase activity. *Naunyn-Schmiedeberg's Archives of Pharmacology, 340,* 285-292.

Schon, M. (1989). Lithium prophylactics: Myths and

realities. *American Journal of Psychiatry, 146,* 573-546.

Schon, M., & Sutherland, A.M. (1960). The role of hormones in human behavior: III. Changes in female sexuality afer hypophysectomy. *Clinical Endocrinology and Metabolism, 20,* 833-841.

Schramek, P., Dorninger, R., Waldhauser, M., Konecny, P., & Porpaczy, P. (1990). Prostaglandin E1 in erectile dysfunction: Efficiency and incidence of priapism. *British Journal of Urology, 65,* 68-71.

Schreiner-Engel, P., Schiavi, R.C., Smith, H., & Shite, D. (1981). Sexual arousability and the menstrual cycle. *Psychosomatic Medicine, 43,* 199-213.

Schreiner-Engel, P., Schiavi, R.C., Smith, H., & White, D. (1982). Plasma testosterone and female sexual behavior. In Z. Hoch & H. Lief (Eds.), *Sexology* (pp. 88-92). Amsterdam: Excerpta Medica.

Schreiner-Engel, P., Shiavi, R.C., White, D., & Ghizzani, A. (1989). Low sexual desire in women: The role of reproductive hormones. *Hormone Behavior, 23*(2), 221-234.

Schreiter, F., Fuchs, P., & Stockamp, K. (1976). Estrogenic sensitivity of receptors in the urethra musculature. *Urologia Internationalis, 31,* 13-19.

Schuckit, M.A. (1983a). Alcoholic men with no alcoholic first-degree relatives. *American Journal of Psychiatry, 140,* 439-443.

Schuckit, M.A. (1983b). Alcoholic patients with secondary depression. *American Journal of Psychiatry, 140,* 711-714.

Schuckit, M.A. (1986). Genetic and clinical implications of alcoholism and affective disorders. *American Journal of Psychiatry, 143,* 140-147.

Schumacher, M., Coirini, H., Frankfurt, M., & McEwen, B.S. (1989). Localized actions of progesterone in hypothalamus involve oxytocin. *Proceedings of the National Academy of Science, USA, 86,* 6798-6801.

Schumacher, M., Coirini, H., Pfaff, D.W., & McEwen, B.S. (1990). Behavioral effects of progesterone associated with rapid modulation of oxytocin receptors. *Science, 250,* 691-694.

Schuster, C. (1988). *Alcohol and sexuality.* New York: Praeger.

Schuster, C.R., & Johanson, C.E. (1985). Efficacy, dependence potential, and neurotoxicity of anorectic drugs. In L.S. Seiden & R.L. Balster (Eds.), *Behavioral pharmacology: The current status* (pp. 263-279). New York: Alan R. Liss.

Schuster, C.R., Lewis, M., & Seiden, L.S. (1986). Fenfluramine: Neurotoxicity. *Psychopharmacology Bulletin, 22,* 148-151.

Schuurs, A.H., & Verheul, H.A. (1990). Effects of gender and sex steroids on the immune response. *Journal of Steroid Biochemistry, 35,* 157-172.

Schwartz, A.G. (1985). The effects of dehydroepiandrosterone on the rate of development of cancer and autoimmune processes in laboratory rodents. In A.D. Woodhead (Ed.), *Molecular biology of aging* (pp. 181-191). New York: Plenum Publishing.

Schwartz, A.G., Fairman, D.K., Polansky, M., Lewbart, M.L., & Pashko, L.L. (1989). Inhibition of 7, 12-Dimethyl-benz[a]anthracene-initiated and 12-0-tetradecanoylphorbol-13-acetate-promoted skin papilloma formation in mice by dehydroepiandrosterone and two synthetic analogs. *Carcinogenesis, 10,* 1809-1813.

Schwartz, A.G., Hard, G., Pashko, I., Abou-Gharbia, M., & Swern, D. (1981). DHA: An antiobesity and anticarcinogenic agent. *Nutrition and Cancer, 3,* 46-53.

Schwartz, A.G., Pashko, I.I., Henderson, E.E., Tannen, R.H., Cleary, M.P., Abou-Gharbia, M., & Swern, D. (1983). Dehydroepiandrosterone: An antiobesity and anticarcinogenic agent. In R.D. Bulbrook & D.J. Taylor (Eds.), *Commentaries on research in breast cancer* (p. 113-130). New York: Alan R. Liss.

Schwartz, A.G., Pashko, L., & Whitcome, J. (1986). Inhibition of tumor development by DHA and related steroids. *Toxicology and Pathology, 14,* 357-362.

Schweizer, E., Feighner, J., Mandos, L.A., & Rickels, K. (1994). Comparison of venlafaxine and imipramine in the acute treatment of major depression in outpatients. *Journal of Clinical Psychiatry, 55,* 104-108.

Schwinger, R.H.G., Bohm, M., & Erdmann, E. (1991). Negative inotropic activity of the calcium antagonists isradipine, nifedipine, diltiazem, and verapamil in diseased human myocardium. *American Journal of Health, 4,* 1855-1875.

Sebastian, J.L., McKinney, W.P., Kaufman, J., & Young, M.J. (1991). Angiotensin-converting enzyme inhibitors and cough: Prevalence in an outpatient medical clinic population. *Chest, 99,* 36-39.

Seckl, J.R., Haddock, J.A., Dunne, M.J., & Lightman, S.L. (1988). Opioid-mediated inhibition of oxytocin during insulin-induced hypoglycemic stimulation of vasopressin in man. *Acta Endocrinologica, 118,* 77-81.

Seeman, M.V., Denber, H.C., & Goldner, F. (1968). Paradoxical effects of phenthiazines. *Psychiatric Quarterly, 42,* 90-104.

Segal, M., & Richter, G. (1988). Involvement of serotonin in hippocampal plasticity. In H.L. Haas & G. Buzsaki (Eds.), *Synaptic plasticity in the hippocampus* Berlin: Springer-Verlag.

Segraves, R.T. (1985). Psychiatric drugs and orgasm in the human female. *Journal of Psychosomatic Obstetrics and Gynecology, 4,* 125–128.

Segraves, R.T. (1986). Reversal by bethanechol of imipramine-induced ejaculatory dysfunction. *American Journal of Psychiatry, 144,* 1243–1244.

Segraves, R.T. (1987). Treatment of premature ejaculation with lorazepam [Letter to the editor]. *American Journal of Psychiatry, 144,* 1240.

Segraves, R.T. (1988). Hormones and libido. In S.R. Leiblum & R.C. Rosen (Eds.), *Sexual desire disorders* (pp. 271–312). New York: Guilford Press.

Segraves, R.T. (1989). Effects of psychotropic drugs on human erection and ejaculation. *Archives of General Psychiatry, 46,* 275–284.

Segraves, R.T., Madsen, R., Carter, C.S., & Davis, J.M. (1985). Erectile dysfunction associated with pharmacological agents. In R.T. Segraves & H.W. Schoenberg (Eds.), *Diagnosis and treatment of erectile disturbances* (pp. 23–63). New York: Plenum Press.

Segraves, R.T., Schoenberg, H.W., & Ivanoff, J. (1983). Serum testosterone and prolactin levels in erectile dysfunction. *Journal of Sex and Marital Therapy, 9,* 19–26.

Seiden, L.S., & Ricaurte, G.A. (1987). Neurotoxicity of methamphetamine and related drugs. In H.Y. Meltzer (Ed.), *Psychopharmacology: The third generation of progress* (pp. 359–366). New York: Raven Press.

Seidmon, E.J., & Samaha, A.M. (1989). The pH analysis of papaverine-phentolamine and prostaglandin E1 for pharmacologic erection. *Journal of Urology, 141,* 1458–1459.

Semmens, T.P., Tsai, C.C., Semmens, E.C., & Loadholt, C.B. (1985). Effects of estrogen therapy on vaginal physiology during menopause. *Obstetrics and Gynecology, 66,* 15–18.

Semple, C.G., Beastall, G.H., Gray, C.E., & Thompson, J.A. (1983). Trilostane in the management of Cushing's syndrome. *Acta Endocrinologica, 102,* 107–110.

Semple, C.G., Gray, C.E., & Beastall, G.H. (1987). Adrenal androgens and illness. *Acta Endocrinologica, 116,* 155–160.

Semple, C.G., Weir, S.W., Thomson, J.A., & Beastall, G.H. (1982). Trilostane and the normal hypothalamic-pituitary-testicular axis. *Clinical Endocrinology, 17,* 99–102.

Serafini, P., & Lobo, R.A. (1985). The effects of spironolactone on adrenal steroidogenesis in hirsute women. *Fertility and Sterility, 44,* 595–599.

Serova, L.I., Kudryavtseva, N.N., Popova, N.K., & Naumenko, E.V. (1987). Relation between hormones of the hypothalamo-hypophyseal-gonadal system and peripheral blood serotonin levels. *Fiziol Zh Sssr, 73*(5), 675–679.

Serova, L.I., Kudryavtseva, N.W., Popova, N.K., Naumenko, E.V., & Parvez, S.H. (1987). Hormones of the hypothalamic-pituitary-testicular complex in the control of peripheral serotonin. *Biogenic Amines, 4,* 145–151.

Serra, G., Collu, M., & Gessa, G.L. (1988). Endorphins and sexual behavior. In R.J. Rodgers & S.J. Cooper (Eds.), *Endorphins, opiates, and behavioral processes* (pp. 237–247). New York: Wiley.

Serri, O., & Rasio, E. (1989). Temporal changes in prolactin and corticosterone response during chronic treatment with d-fenfluramine. *Hormone Research, 31,* 180–183.

Shaarawy, M., Fayad, M., Nagui, A.R., & Abdel-Azim, S. (1982). Serotonin metabolism and depression in oral contraceptive users. *Contraception, 26,* 193–204.

Shaarawy, M., & Mahmoud, K.Z. (1982). Endocrine profile and semen characteristics in male smokers. *Fertility and Sterility, 38,* 255–257.

Shabsigh, R., Fishman, I.J., Schum, C., & Dunn, J.K. (1991). Cigarette smoking and other vascular risk factors in vasculogenic impotence. *Urology, 38,* 227–231.

Shahrad, P., & Marks, R. (1977). A pharmacological effect of oestrone on human epidermis. *British Journal of Dermatology, 97,* 383–386.

Shanks, N., & Wishart, T.B. (1985). Diazepam disrupts sexual aggressive and grooming behaviors in the rat. *Society for Neuroscience, 11* (Pt. 2), 1291.

Shapiro, B.H., & Bitar, M.S. (1991). Developmental levels and androgen responsiveness of hepatic mono-oxygenases of male rats perinatally exposed to maternally administered cimetidine. *Toxicology Letters, 55,* 85–98.

Shapiro, B.H., Hirst, S.A., Babalola, G.O., & Bitar, M.S. (1988). Prospective study on the sexual development of male and female rats perinatally exposed to maternally administered cimetidine. *Toxicology Letters, 44,* 315–329.

Shapiro, E. (1986). Effect of estrogens on the weight and muscarinic cholinergic receptor density of the rabbit bladder and urethra. *Journal of Urology, 135,* 1084–1087.

Sharma, O.P., & Hays, R.L. (1976). A possible role for oxytocin in sperm transport in the male rabbit. *Journal of Endocrinology, 68,* 43–47.

Sharp, B., & Pekary, A.E. (1981). Beta-endorphin (61–69) and other beta-endorphin-immunoreactive peptides in human semen. *Journal of Clinical Endocrinology and Metabolism, 52,* 586–588.

Sheard, M.H. (1969). The effect of p-chlorophenylalanine on behavior in rats: Relation to brain serotonin and 5-hydroxy-indoleactic acid. *Brain Research, 15,* 524–528.

Sheehan, D.V., Davidson, J., Manschreck, T., & Van Wyck Fleet, J. (1983). Lack of efficacy of a new antidepressant (bupropion) in the treatment of panic disorder with phobias. *Journal of Clinical Psychopharmacology, 3,* 28–31.

Sheehy, T.W. (1992). Alcohol and the heart. *Postgraduate Medicine, 91,* 271–277.

Shen, W.W. (1982). Female orgasmic inhibition by amoxapine. *American Journal of Psychiatry, 139,* 1220–1221.

Shen, W.W., & Sata, L.S. (1983). Inhibited female orgasm resulting from psychoactive drugs. *Journal of Reproductive Medicine, 28,* 497–499.

Sherwin, B.B. (1987). Effects of hormone implants of psychological disorders in the climacteric. *Lancet, 1,* 1038–1039.

Sherwin, B.B. (1988a). Affective changes with estrogen and androgen replacement therapy in surgically menopausal women. *Journal of Affective Disorders, 14,* 177–187.

Sherwin, B.B. (1988b). A comparative analysis of the role of androgens in human male and female sexual behavior: Behavioral specificity, critical thresholds, and sensitivity. *Psychobiology, 16,* 416–425.

Sherwin, B.B. (1988c). Estrogen and/or androgen replacement therapy and cognitive functioning in surgically menopausal women. *Psychoneuroendocrinology, 13,* 345–357.

Sherwin, B.B. (1991). The impact of different doses of estrogen and progestin on mood and sexual behavior in postmenopausal women. *Journal of Clinical Endocrinology and Metabolism, 72,* 336–343.

Sherwin, B.B., & Gelfand, M.M. (1985a). Differential symptom response to parental estrogen and/or androgen administration in the surgical menopause. *American Journal of Obstetrics and Gynecology, 151,* 153–160.

Sherwin, B.B., & Gelfand, M.M. (1985b). Sex steroids and affect in the surgical menopause: A double-blind, crossover study. *Psychoneuroendocrinology, 10,* 325–335.

Sherwin, B.B., Gelfand, M.M., & Brender, W. (1985). Androgen enhances sexual motivation in females: A prospective crossover study of sex steroid administration in the surgical menopause. *Psychosomatic Medicine, 47,* 339–351.

Sherwin, B.B., & Phillips, S. (1990). Estrogen and cognitive functioning in surgically menopausal women. In M. Flint, F. Kronenberg, & W. Utian (Eds.), *Multidisciplinary perspectives on menopause. Vol. 592. Annals of the New York Academy of Sciences* (pp. 474–475). New York: New York Academy of Sciences.

Shi, Y.F., Patterson, A.P., & Sherins, R.J. (1986). Increased plasma and pituitary prolactin concentrations in adult male rats with selective elevation of FSH levels may be explained by reduced testosterone and increased estradiol production. *Journal of Andrology, 7,* 105–111.

Shillito, E.E. (1969). The effect of p-chlorophenylalanine on social interactions of male rats [abstract]. *British Journal of Pharmacology, 36,* 193P–194P.

Shillito, E.E. (1970). The effect of para-chlorophenylalanine on social interaction of male rats. *British Journal of Pharmacology, 38,* 305–315.

Shively, C.A., Manuck, S.B., Kaplan, J.R., & Koritnik, D.R. (1990). Oral contraceptive administration, interfemale relationships, and sexual behavior in *Macaca fascicularis. Archives of Sexual Behavior, 19,* 101–117.

Shopsin, B. (1983). Bupropion's prophylactic efficacy in bipolar affective illness. *Journal of Clinical Psychiatry, 44*(5), 163–169.

Shore, J.H., Fraunfelder, F.T., & Meyer, S.M. (1987). Psychiatric side effects from topical ocular timolol, a beta-adrenergic blocker. *Journal of Clinical Psychopharmacology, 7,* 264–267.

Shoupe, D., & Mishell, D.R. (1989). Norplant: Subdermal implant system for long-term contraception. *American Journal of Obstetrics and Gynecology, 160,* 1286–1292.

Sibilia, V., Netti, C., Guidobono, F., Pagani, F., & Pecile, A. (1985). Cimetidine-induced prolactin release: Possible involvement of the GABA-ergic system. *Neuroendocrinology, 40,* 189–192.

Sicuteri, F. (1974). Serotonin and sex in man. *Pharmacological Research Communications, 6,* 403–411.

Siddle, N., Sarrel, P., & Whitehead, M. (1987). The effect of hysterectomy on the age at ovarian failure: Identification of a subgroup of women with premature loss of ovarian function and a literature review. *Fertility and Sterility, 47,* 94–100.

Sideri, M., Origoni, M., Spinaci, L., & Ferrari, A. (1994). Topical testosterone in the treatment of vulvar lichen sclerosis. *International Journal of Gynecology and Obstetrics, 46,* 53–56.

Sidi, A.A. (1988). Vasoactive intracavernous pharmacotherapy. *Urologic Clinics of North America, 15*(1), 95–101.

Sidi, A.A., Cameron, J.S., Duffy, L.M., & Lange, P.H. (1986). Intracavernous drug-induced erections in the management of male erectile dysfunction: Experience with 100 patients. *Journal of Urology, 135,* 704–706.

Siegel, S., Streem, S.B., & Steinmuller, D.R. (1988). Prazosin-induced priapism: Pathogenic and therapeutic implications. *British Journal of Urology, 60,* 165.

Sifton, D.W. (Ed.). (1994). *The Physicians Desk Reference family guide to women's health and prescription drugs.* Montvale, NJ: Medical Economics.

Sillero-Arenas, M., Delgado-Rodriguez, M., Rodigues-Canteras, R., Bueno-Cavanillas, A., & Galvez-Vagas, R. (1992). Menopausal hormone replacement therapy and breast cancer: A meta-analysis. *Obstetrics and Gynecology, 79,* 286–294.

Silva, F.H.L., Witter, M.P., Boeijinga, P.H., & Lohman, A.H. (1990). Anatomic organization and physiology of the limbic cortex. *Physiological Reviews, 70,* 453–499?

Silverman, H.I. (1985). A history of therapeutic uses of phenylpropanolamine in North America. In J.P. Morgan, D.V. Kagan, & J.S. Brody (Eds.), *Phenylpropanolamine: Risks, benefits, and controversies* (pp. 11–24). New York: Praeger Publishers.

Simoons, M.L. (1994). Myocardial infarction: ACE inhibitors for all? Forever? *Lancet, 344,* 279–280.

Simpson, G.M., Blair, H.H., & Amuso, D. (1965). Effects of antidepressants on genitourinary function. *Diseases of the Nervous System, 26,* 787–789.

Simpson, W.J. (1957). A preliminary report on cigarette smoking and the incidence of prematurity. *American Journal of Obstetrics and Gynecology, 73,* 808.

Simpson, W.S., & Ramberg, J.A. (1992). Sexual dysfunction in married female patients with anorexia and bulimia nervosa. *Journal of Sex and Marital Therapy, 18,* 44–54.

Sindrup, S.H., Bjerre, U., Dejgaard, A., Brøsen, K., Aaes-Jørgensen, T., & Gram, L.F. (1992). The selective serotonin reuptake inhibitor citalopram relieves the symptoms of diabetic neuropathy. *Clinical and Pharmacology Therapy, 52,* 547–552.

Singh, H. (1963). Therapeutic use of thioridazine in premature ejaculation. *American Journal of Psychiatry, 119,* 891.

Sinha, Y.N., Gilligan, T.A., & Barkley, M.S. (1984). Inhibition of prolactin secretion by moderate and high doses of testosterone. *Proceedings of the Society for Experimental Biology and Medicine, 175,* 438–443.

Sireling, L., Freeling, P., Paykel, E.S., & Rao, B.M. (1985). Depression in general practice: Clinical features and comparison with outpatients. *British Journal of Psychiatry, 147,* 119–126.

Sirinathsinghji, D.J. (1984). Modulation of lordosis behavior of female rats by naloxone, beta-endorphin and its antiserum in the mesencephalic central grey: Possible mediation via GnRH. *Neuroendocrinology, 39,* 222–230.

Sirinathsinghji, D.J. (1985). Modulation of lordosis behavior in the female rat by corticotropin releasing factor, beta-endorphin, and gonadotropin releasing hormone in the mesencephalic central grey. *Brain Research, 336,* 45–55.

Sirinathsinghji, D.J. (1986). Regulation of lordosis behavior in the female rat by corticotropin-releasing factor, beta-endorphin/corticotropin, and luteinizing hormone-releasing hormone neuronal systems in the medial preoptic area. *Brain Research, 375,* 49–56.

Sirinathsinghji, D.J., Rees, L.H., Rivier, J., & Vale, W. (1983). Corticotropin-releasing factor is a potent inhibitor of sexual receptivity in the female rat. *Nature, 305,* 232–235.

Sitland-Marken, P.A., Wells, B.G., Froemming, J.H., Chu, C.C., & Brown, C.S. (1990). Psychiatric applications of bromocriptine therapy. *Journal of Clinical Psychaitry, 51,* 68–82.

Sitruk-Ware, R. (1989). Percutaneous and transdermal hormonal therapy. In M. L'Hermite (Ed.), *Update on hormonal treatment in the menopause* (pp. 72–85). Basel: Karger.

Sjoerdsma, A., Lovenberg, W., Engelman, K., Carpenter, W.T., Wyatt, R.J., & Gessa, G.L. (1970). Serotonin now: Clinical implications of inhibiting its synthesis with para-chlorophenylalanine. *Annals of Internal Medicine, 73,* 607–629.

Skakkebaek, N., Bancroft, J., Davidson, D., & Warren, P. (1981). Androgen replacement with oral testosterone undecanoate in hypogonadal men: A double-blind controlled study. *Clinical Endocrinology, 14,* 49–61.

Skinner, M.H., Futterman, A., Morrissette, D., Thompson, L.W., Hoffman, B.B., & Blaschke, T.F. (1992). Atenolol compared with nifedipine: Effect on cognitive function and mood in elderly hypertensive patients. *Annals of Internal Medicine, 116,* 615–623.

Slag, M.F., Morley, J.E., Elson, M.K., Trence, D.L., Nelson, C.J., Nelson, A.E., Kinlaw, W.B., Beyer, S., Nutthal, F.Q., & Shafer, R.B. (1983). Impotence in medical clinic outpatients. *Journal of the American Medical Association, 249,* 1736–1740.

Smiggan, L., & Perris, C. (1983). Memory functions and prophylactic treatment with lithium. *Psychological Medicine, 13,* 529–536.

Smith, B.D., Davidson, R.A., & Green, R.L. (1993). Effects of caffeine and gender on physiology and performance: Further tests of a biobehavioral model. *Physiology and Behavior, 54,* 415–422.

Smith, C.G., Almirez, R.G., Scher, P.M., & Asch, R.H. (1984). Tolerance to the reproductive effects of delta-9-tetrahydrocannabol: Comparison of the acute, short-term, and chronic drug effects on menstrual cycle hormones. In S. Agurell, W.L. Dewey, & R.E. Willette (Eds.), *The cannabinoids: Chemical, pharmacologic, and therapeutic aspects* (pp. 471–485). New York: Academic Press.

Smith, D.E., Moser, C., Wesson, D.R., Apter, M., Buxton, M.E., Davison, J.V., Orgel, M., & Buffum, J. (1982). A clinical guide to the diagnosis and treatment of heroin-related sexual dysfunction. *Journal of Psychoactive Drugs, 14,* 91–99.

Smith, E.R., Lee, R.L., Schnur, S.L., & Davidson, J.M. (1987a). Alpha$_2$-adrenoceptor antagonists and male sexual behavior: I. Mating behavior. *Physiology and Behavior, 41,* 7–14.

Smith, E.R., Lee, R.L., Schnur, S.L., & Davidson, J.M. (1987b). Alpha$_2$-adrenoceptor antagonists and male sexual behavior: II. Erectile and ejaculatory reflexes. *Physiology and Behavior, 41,* 15–19.

Smith, E.R., Maurice, J., Richardson, R., Walter, T., & Davidson, J.M. (1990). Effects of four beta-adrenergic receptor antagonists on male rat sex behavior. *Pharmacology, Biochemistry & Behavior, 36,* 713–717.

Smith, G.R., Conger, C., O'Rourke, D.F., Steele, R.W., Charlton, R., & Smith, S.S. (1989). Modulation of cellular immunity by meditation. *Psychosomatic Medicine, 51,* 246.

Smith, J.A., Jr. (1987). New methods of endocrine management of prostatic cancer. *Journal of Urology, 137,* 1–10.

Smith, J.A., Jr., Glode, L.M., Wettlaufer, J.N., Stein, B.S., Glass, A.G., Max, D.T., Anbar, D., Jagst, C.L., & Murphy, G.P. (1985). Clinical effects of gonadotropin-releasing hormone analogue in metastic carcinoma of prostate. *Urology, 25,* 106–114.

Smith, J.A., Jr., & Urry, R.L. (1985). Testicular histology after prolonged treatment with a gonadotrophin-releasing hormone analogue. *Journal of Urology, 133,* 612–614.

Smith, M.A., Chick, J., Kean, D.M., Douglas, R.H., Singer, A., Kendell, R.E., & Best, J.J. (1985). Brain water in chronic alcoholic patients measured by magnetic resonance imaging [Letter to the editor]. *Lancet, 1,* 1273–1274.

Smith, M.C. (1985). *Small comfort.* New York: Praeger.

Snyder, A.M., Stricker, E.M., & Zigmond, M.J. (1985). Stress-induced neurological impairments in an animal model of Parkinsonism. *Annals of Neurology, 18,* 544–551.

Snyder, S. (1989). Drug and neurotransmitter receptors: New perspectives with clinical relevance. *Journal of the American Medical Association, 261,* 3126–3129.

Snyder, S., & Karacan, I. (1981). Effects of chronic alcoholism on nocturnal penile tumescence. *Psychosomatic Medicine, 43,* 423–429.

Snyder, S., & Reynolds, I.J. (1985). Calcium-antagonist drugs: Receptor interactions that clarify therapeutic effects. *Seminars in Medicine of the Beth Israel Hospital, Boston, 313,* 995–1002.

Sobotka, J.J. (1969). An evaluation of Afrodex in the management of male impotency: A double-blind crossover study. *Current Therapeutic Research, 11,* 87–94.

Sodersten, P. (1990). Opioid peptides and sexual behavior in female rats. *Neuroendocrinology, 52* (Suppl. 1), 16.

Sodersten, P., De Vries, G.J., Buijs, R.M., & Melin, P. (1985). A daily rhythm in behavioral vasopressin sensitivity and brain vasopressin concentrations. *Neuroscience Letters, 58,* 37–41.

Sodersten, P., Forsberg, G., Bednar, I., Eneroth, P., & Wiesenfeld-Hallin, Z. (1989). Opioid peptide inhibition of sexual behavior in female rats. In R.G. Dyer & R.J. Bicknell (Eds.), *Brain opioid systems in reproduction* (pp. 203–215). Oxford: Oxford University Press.

Sodersten, P., Henning, M., Melin, P., & Ludin, S. (1983). Vasopressin alters female sexual behavior by acting on the brain independently of alterations in blood pressure. *Nature (London), 301,* 608–610.

Sodersten, P., Larsson, K., Ahlenius, S., & Engel, J. (1976). Stimulation of mounting behavior but not lordosis behavior in ovariectomized female rats by p-chlorophenylalanine. *Pharmacology, Biochemistry, and Behavior, 5,* 319–327.

Soldatos, C.R., Sakkas, P.N., Bergiannaki, P., & Stefanis, C.N. (1986). Behavioral side effects of triazolam in psychiatric inpatients: Report of five cases. *Drug Intelligence and Clinical Pharmacy, 20,* 294–297.

Solstad, K., & Garde, K. (1992). Middle-aged Danish men's ideas of a male climacteric—and of the female climacteric. *Maturitas, 15,* 7–16.

Solyom, L., Solyom, C., & Ledwidge, B. (1990). The fluoxetine treatment of low-weight, chronic bulimia nervosa. *Journal of Clinical Psychopharmacology, 10,* 421–425.

Sonda, L.P., Mazo, R., & Chancellor, M.B. (1990). The role of yohimbine for the treatment of erectile impotence. *Journal of Sex and Marital Therapy, 16,* 15–21.

Sonka, J. (1976). Dehydroepiandrosterone: Metabolic effects. *Acta Universitatis Carolinae Medica Monographia, 71,* 146–171.

Sopchak, A.L. (1957). Changes in sexual behavior, desire, and fantasy in breast cancer patients under androgen and estrogen therapy. Doctoral dissertation, Adelphi College, Garden City, New York.

Sorensen, A.S., & Bolwig, T.G. (1987). Personality and epilepsy: New evidence for a relationship? A review. *Comprehensive Psychiatry, 28,* 369–383.

Sorensen, S., Waechter, P.B., Constantinou, C.E., Kirkeby, H.J., Jonler, M., & Djurhuus, J.C. (1991). Urethral pressure and pressure variations in healthy fertile and postmenopausal women with reference to the female sex hormones. *Journal of Urology, 146,* 1434–1440.

Sorkin, E.M., & Darvey, D.L. (1983). Review of cimetidine drug interactions. *Drug Intelligence and Clinical Pharmacology, 17,* 110–120.

Soules, M.R., Cohen, N.L., Clifton, D.K., Brenner, W.J., & Steiner, R.A. (1987). Gonadotropin-releasing hormone-induced changes in testosterone secretion in normal women. *Fertility and Sterility, 48,* 423–427.

Sovner, R. (1983). Anorgasmia associated with imipramine but not desipramine: Case report. *Journal of Clinical Psychiatry, 44,* 345–346.

Sovner, R. (1984). Treatment of tricyclic antidepressant-induced orgasmic inhibition with cyproheptadine. *Journal of Clinical Psychopharmacology, 4,* 169.

Spagnoli, A., Ostino, G., Borga, A.D., D'Ambrosio, R., Maggiorotti, P., Todisco, E., Prattichizzo, N., Pia, L., & Comelli, M. (1989). Drug compliance and unreported drugs in the elderly. *Journal of the American Geriatric Society, 37,* 619–624.

Spark, R.F. (1983). Neuroendocrinolgy and impotence. *Annals of Internal Medicine, 98,* 103–105.

Spark, R.F., & Dickstein, G. (1979). Bromocriptine and endocrine disorders. *Annals of Internal Medicine, 90,* 949–956.

Spark, R.F., White, R.A., & Connolly, P.B. (1980). Impotence is not always psychogenic. *Journal of the American Medical Association, 243,* 750–755.

Spark, R.F., Wills, C.A., O'Reilly, G., Ransil, B.J., & Bergland, R. (1982). Hyperprolactemia in males with and without pituitary macroadenomas. *Lancet, 2,* 129–131.

Sparrow, D., Bosse, R., & Rowe, T.W. (1980). The influence of age, alcohol consumption, and body build on gonadal function in men. *Journal of Clinical Endocrinology and Metabolism, 51,* 508–512.

Spealman, R. (1988). Psychomotor stimulant effects of methylxanthines in squirrel monkeys: Relations to adenosine antagonism. *Psychopharmacology, 95,* 19–24.

Spedding, M. (1987). Three types of Ca^{2+} channels explain discrepancies. *Trends in Pharmacological Sciences, 8,* 115–117.

Spence, R.W., & Celestin, L.R. (1979). Gynaecomastia associated with cimetidine. *Gut, 20,* 154–157.

Sperzel, W.D., Glassman, H.N., Jordon, D.C., & Luther, R.R. (1986). Overall safety of terazosin as an antihypertensive agent. *American Journal of Medicine, 80*(Suppl. 5B), 77–81.

Stackl, W., Hasun, R., & Marberger, M. (1990). The use of prostaglandin E1 for diagnosis and treatment of erectile dysfunction. *World Journal of Urology, 8,* 84–86.

Stackl, W., Loupal, G., & Holzmann, A. (1988). Intracavernous injection of vasoactive drugs in the rabbit. *Urological Research, 16,* 455–458.

Stahl, N.I., & Decker, J. (1978). Androgenic status of males with systemic lupus erythematosus. *Arthritis and Rheumatism, 21,* 665–668.

Stamford, J.A., Kruk, Z.L., & Millar, J. (1988). Effects of uptake inhibitors on stimulated dopamine release and uptake in the nucleus accumbens studied by fast cyclic voltammetry. *British Journal of Pharmacology: Proceedings Supplement, 34,* 348P.

Stamler, J., Pick, R., & Katz, L.N. (1953). Prevention of coronary atherosclerosis by estrogen-androgen administration in the cholesterol-fed chick. *Circulation Research, 1,* 94–98.

Stampfer, M.J., Colditz, G.A., Willett, W.C., Manson, J.E., Rosner, B., Speizer, F.E., & Hennekens, C.H. (1991). Postmenopausal estrogen therapy and cardiovascular disease: Ten-year follow-up from the Nurses' Health Study. *New England Journal of Medicine, 325,* 756–762.

Stampfer, M.J., Willett, W.C., Colditz, G.A., Rosner, B., Speizer, F.E., & Hennekens, C.H. (1985). A prospective study of postmenopausal estrogen therapy and coronary heart disease. *New England Journal of Medicine, 313,* 1044–1049.

Steele, T.E., & Howell, E.F. (1986). Cyproheptadine for imipramine-induced anorgasmia [Letter to the editor]. *Journal of Clinical Psychopharmacology, 6,* 326–327.

Steers, W.D., McConnell, J., & Benson, G.S. (1984). Some pharmacologic effects of yohimbine on human and rabbit penis. *Journal of Urology, 131,* 799–802.

Steiger, A., Holsboer, F., & Benkert, O. (1988). Long-term studies on the effect of tricyclic antidepressants and selective MAO-A-inhibitors on sleep, nocturnal penile tumescence, and hormonal secretion in normal controls. In W.P. Koella, F. Obal, H. Schulz, & P. Visser (Eds.), *Sleep '86* (pp. 335–337). New York: Gustav Fischer Verlag.

Steiger, A., Von Bardeleben, U., Wiedemann, K., & Holsboer, F. (1991). Sleep EEG and nocturnal secretion of testosterone and cortisol in patients with major endogenous depression during acute phase and after remission. *Journal of Psychiatry Research, 25,* 169–177.

Steinberg, K.K., Thacker, S.B., Smith, J., Stroup, D.F., Zack, M.M., Flanders, D., & Berkelman, R.L. (1991). A meta-analysis of the effect of estrogen replacement therapy on the risk of breast cancer. *Journal of the American Medical Association, 265,* 1985–1990.

Steiner, S.S., Friedhoff, A.J., Wilson, B.L., Wecker, J.R., & Santo, J.P. (1990). Antihypertensive therapy and quality of life: A comparison of atenolol, captopril, enalapril and propranolol. *Journal of Human Hypertension, 4,* 217–225.

Steiness, I. (1957). Vibratory perception in normal

subjects. A biothesiometric study. *Acta Medica Scandinavica, 68,* 315–325.

Stenkvist, B., Bengtsson, E., Dahlquist, B. (1982). Cardiac glycosides and breast cancer revisited [Letter to the editor]. *New England Journal of Medicine, 306,* 484.

Stepan, J.J., Lachman, M., Zverina, J., Pacovsky, V., & Baylink, D.J. (1989). Castrated men exhibit bone loss: Effect of calcitonin treatment on biochemical indices of bone remodeling. *Journal of Clinical Endocrinology and Metabolism, 69,* 523–527.

Stepanski, E.J., Conway, W.A., Young, D.K., Zarick, F.J., Wittig, R.M., & Roth, T. (1988). A double-blind trial of protriptyline in the treatment of sleep apnea syndrome. *Henry Ford Hospital Medical Journal, 36,* 5–8.

Stern, K.N., Chait, L.D., & Johanson, C.E. (1989). Reinforcing and subjective effects of caffeine in normal human volunteers. *Psychopharmacology, 98,* 81–88.

Stessman, J., & Ben-Ishay, D. (1980). Chlorthalidone-induced impotence. *British Medical Journal, 281,* 714.

Stevenson, J.C., Abeyasekera, G., Hillyard, C.J., Phang, K.G., MacIntyre, I., Campbell, S., Townsent, P.T., Young, O., & Whitehead, M.I. (1981). Calcitonin and calcium-regulating hormones in postmenopausal women: Effect of estrogens. *Lancet, 1,* 693–695.

Stevenson, J.G., & Umstead, G.S. (1984). Sexual dysfunction due to antihypertensive agents. *Drug Intelligence and Clinical Pharmacy, 18,* 113–121.

Stevenson, R.W.D., & Solyom, L. (1990). The aphrodisiac effect of fenfluramine: Two case reports of a possible side effect to the use of fenfluramine in the treatment of bulimia. *Journal of Clinical Psychopharmacology, 10,* 69–71.

Stewart, B.H., & Bergant, J.A. (1974). Correction of retrograde ejaculation by sympathomimetic medication: Preliminary report. *Fertility and Sterility, 25,* 1073–1074.

Stief, C.G., & Wetterauer, U. (1988). Erectile responses to intracavernous papaverine and phentolamine: Comparison of single and combined delivery. *Journal of Urology, 140,* 1415–1416.

Stillman, R.J., Rosenberg, M.J., & Sachs, B.P. (1986). Smoking and reproduction. *Fertility and Sterility, 46,* 545–566.

Stock, S., & Uvnas-Moberg, K. (1985). Oxytocin infusions increase plasma levels of insulin and VIP but not gastrin in conscious dogs. *Acta Physiologica Scandinavica, 125,* 205–210.

Stock, S., & Uvnas-Moberg, K. (1988). Increased plasma levels of oxytocin in response to afferent electrical stimulation of the sciatic and vagal nerves and in response to touch and pinch in anesthetized rats. *Acta Physiologica Scandinavica, 132,* 29–34.

Stockamp, K., Schreiter, F., & Altwein, J. (1974). Alpha-adrenergic drugs in retrograde ejaculation. *Fertility and Sterility, 25,* 817–820.

Stoffer, S.S., Hynes, K.M., Jiany, N.S., & Ryan, R.J. (1973). Digoxin and abnormal serum hormone levels. *Journal of the American Medical Association, 225,* 1643–1644.

Stokes, G.S., Mennie, S.R., Gellatly, R., & Hill, A. (1983). On the combination of alpha- and beta-adrenoceptor blockade in hypertension. *Clinical Pharmacology and Therapeutics, 34,* 576–582.

Stoll, A.L., Mayer, P.V., Kolbrener, M., Goldstein, E., Suplit, B., Lucier, J., Cohen, B.M., & Tohen, M. (1994). Antidepressant-associated mania: A controlled comparison with spontaneous mania. *American Journal of Psychiatry, 151,* 1642–1645.

Stone, N.N., Fair, W.R., & Fishman, J. (1986). Estrogen formation in human prostatic tissue from patients with and without benign prostatic hyperplasia. *Prostate, 9,* 311–318.

Stoneham, M.D., Everitt, B.J., Hansen, S., Lightman, S.L., & Todd, K. (1985). Oxytocin and sexual behavior in the male rat and rabbit. *Journal of Endocrinology, 107,* 97–106.

Stoner, E. (1994). Three-year safety and efficacy data on the use of finasteride in the treatment of benign prostatic hyperplasia. *Urology, 43,* 284–294.

Stoner, G.R., Skirboll, L.R., Werkman, S., & Hommer, D.W. (1988). Preferential effects of caffeine on limbic and cortical dopamine systems. *Biological Psychiatry, 23,* 761–768.

Storm, T., Thamsborg, G., Steinische, T., Genant, H.K., & Sorensen, O.H. (1990). Effect of intermittent cyclical therapy on bone mass and fracture rate in women with postmenopausal osteoporosis. *New England Journal of Medicine, 322,* 1265–1271.

Strickland, D.M., Gambrell, R.D., Butzin, C.A., & Strickland, K. (1992). The relationship between breast cancer survival and prior postmenopausal estrogen use. *Obstetrics and Gynecology, 80,* 400–404.

Studd, J.W., Collins, W.P., Chakravarti, S., Newton, J.R., Oram, D., & Parsons, A. (1977). Estradiol and testosterone implants in treatment of psychosexual problems in postmenopausal women. *British Journal of Obstetrics and Gynecology, 84,* 314–316.

Studd, J.W., & Magos, A. (1987). Hormone pellet implantation for the menopause and premenstrual syndrome. *Obstetrics and Gynecology Clinics of North America, 14,* 229–247.

Stumpe, K.O., Kolloch, R., & Overlack, A. (1984). Captopril and enalapril: Evaluation of therapeutic efficacy and safety. *Therape Woche, 34,* 3290–3298.

Stunkard, A.J. (1984). New developments in the drug treatment of obesity. *Clinical Neuropharmacology, 7*(Suppl. 1), 704-705.

Sturniolo, G.C., Montino, M.C., Rossetto, L., Martin, A., D'Inca, R., & D'Odorico, A. (1991). Inhibition of gastric acid secretion reduces zinc absorption in man. *Journal of the American College of Nutrition, 10,* 372-375.

Suemaru, K., Gomita, Y., Furuno, K., & Araki, Y. (1993). Chronic nicotine treatment potentiates behavioral responses to dopaminergic drugs in rats. *Pharmacology, Biochemistry, and Behavior, 46,* 135–139.

Sullivan, G. (1987). Increased libido with trazodone. *American Journal of Psychiatry, 144,* 967.

Sullivan, G. (1988). Increased libido in three men treated with trazodone. *Journal of Clinical Psychiatry, 49,* 202–203.

Sullivan, J.M., Zwaag, R.V., Hughes, J.P., Maddock, V., Kroetz, F.W., Ramanathan, K.B., & Mirvis, D.M. (1990). Estrogen replacement and coronary artery disease: Effect on survival in postmenopausal women. *Archives of Internal Medicine, 150,* 2557-2562.

Sullivan, J.M., Zwaag, R.V., Lemp, G.F., Hughes, J.P., Maddock, V., Kroetz, F.W., Ramanthan, K.B., & Mirvis, D.M. (1988). Postmenopausal estrogen use and coronary atherosclerosis. *Annals of Internal Medicine, 108,* 358-363.

Sunderland, T., Merril, C.R., Harrington, M.G., Lawlor, B.A., Moldran, S.E., Martinez, R., & Murphy, D.L. (1989). Reduced plasma dehydroepiandrosterone concentration in Alzheimer's disease. *Lancet, 2,* 570.

Superko, H.R., Bortz, W., Jr., Williams, P.T., Albers, J.J., & Wood, P.D. (1991). Caffeinated and decaffeinated coffee effects on plasma lipoprotein, cholesterol, apolipoproteins, and lipase activity: A controlled, randomized trial. *American Journal of Clinical Nutrition, 54,* 599–605.

Surgeon-General (1990). *The health consequences of smoking.* Washington DC: United States Department of Health and Human Services.

Susset, J.G., Tessier, C.D., Wincze, J., Bansal, S., Malhotra, G., & Schwacha, M.G. (1989). Effect of yohimbine hydrochloride on erectile impotence: A double-blind study. *Journal of Urology, 141,* 1360–1363.

Sutherst, J. (1979). Sexual dysfunction and urinary incontinence. *British Journal of Obstetrics and Gynecology, 86,* 387-388.

Suzuki, H., Tominaga, T., Kumagai, H., & Saruta, T. (1988). Effects of first-line antihypertensive agents on sexual function and sex hormones. *Journal of Hypertension, 6*(Suppl. 4), S649-S651.

Suzuki, T., Suzuki, N., Daynes, R.A., & Engleman, E.G. (1991). Dehydroepiandrosterone enhances IL-2 production and cytotoxic effector function of human T-cells. *Clinical Immunology and Immunopathology, 61,* 202–211.

Swartz, C. (1986). Hormone release by electroconvulsive therapy. *Lancet, 2,* 581.

Swartz, D.A. (1994). Sertraline hydrochloride for premature ejaculation. *Journal of Urology, 151* (Suppl.), 345A.

Szele, F.G., Murphy, D.L., & Garrick, N.A. (1988). Effects of fenfluramine, m-chlorophenylpiperazine, and other serotonin-related agonists and antagonists on penile erections in nonhuman primates. *Life Sciences, 43,* 1297–1303.

Taberner, P.V. (1985). *Aphrodisiacs: The science and the myth.* Philadelphia: University of Pennsylvania Press.

Taelman, P., Kaufman, J.M., Janssens, X., & Vermeulen, A. (1989). Persistence of increased bone resorption and possible role of dehydroepiandrosterone as a bone metabolism determinant in osteoporotic women in late post-menopause. *Maturitas, 11,* 65–73.

Tagliaferro, A.R., Davis, J.R., Trachon, S., & van Hamont, N. (1986). Effects of dehydroepiandrosterone acetate on metabolism, body weight, and composition of male and female rats. *Journal of Nutrition, 116,* 1977–1983.

Tagliamonte, A., Tagliamonte, P., Gessa, G.L., & Brodie, B. (1969). Compulsive sexual activity induced by p-chlorophenylalanine in normal and pinealectomized male rats. *Science, 166,* 1433–1435.

Takahashi, Y., Ishii, N., Aboseif, S.R., Benard, F., Lue, T.F., & Tanagho, E.A. (1990). Effects of adenosine on canine penile erection. *Journal of Urology, 143,* 305A.

Talley, J.D., & Crawley, I.S. (1985). Transdermal nitrate, penile erection, and spousal headache. *Annals of Internal Medicine, 103,* 804.

Tamini, R.R., & Mavissakalian, M.R. (1991). Are effective antiobsessional drugs interchangeable? [Letter to the editor]. *Archives of General Psychiatry, 48,* 857–858.

Tanner, C.M., Goetz, C.G., & Klawans, H.L. (1986). Hypersexuality in Parkinson's disease. *Neurology, 36*(Suppl. 1), 183.

Tanner, L.A., & Bosco, L.A. (1988). Gynecomastia associated with calcium channel-blocker therapy. *Archives of Internal Medicine, 148,* 379–380.

Tappler, B., & Katz, M. (1979). Pituitary-gonadal dysfunction in low-output cardiac failure. *Clinical Endocrinology, 10,* 219–226.

Tashkin, D.P., Ashutosh, K., Bleecker, E.R., Britt, E.J., Cugell, D.W., Cummiskey, J.M., DeLorenzo, L., Gilman, M.J., Gross, G.N., Kotch, A., Lakshimarayan, S., Maguire, G., Miller, M., Plummer, A., Renzetti, A., Sackner, M.A., Skordin, M.S., Wanner, A., & Watanabe, S. (1986). Comparison of the anticholinergic bronchodilator ipratropium bromide with metaproterenol in chronic obstructive pulmonary disease. *American Journal of Medicine, 81*(Suppl. 5A), 81-89.

Tatarelli, R., Giraldi, P., & Vella, G. (1984). Symptomes-cibles des antidepresseurs. *L'Encephale, X,* 29-32.

Tattersfield, A.E. (1994). Use of $beta_2$ agonists in asthma: Much ado about nothing? Still cause for concern. *British Medical Journal, 309,* 794-795.

Teicher, M.H., Glad, C., & Cole, J.O. (1990). Emergence of intense suicidal preoccupation during fluoxetine treatment. *American Journal of Psychiatry, 147,* 207-210.

TenHouton, S. (1986). Family environment: Implications from sexual dysfunction and methaqualone dependence. *Journal of Psychoactive Drugs, 18,* 73-75.

Tennant, G., Bancroft, J., & Cass, J. (1974). The control of deviant sexual behavior by drugs: A double-blind controlled study of benperidol, chlorpromazine, and placebo. *Archives of Sexual Behavior, 3,* 261-271.

Tennes, K. (1984). Effects of marijuana on pregnancy and fetal development in the human. In M.C. Braude & J.P. Ludford (Eds.), *Marijuana effects on the endocrine and reproductive systems: National Institute of Drug Abuse Research Monographs, 44* (pp. 115-124). Rockville, MD: United States Government Printing Office.

Teoh, S.K., Mello, N.K., & Mendelson, J.H. (1994). Effects of drugs of abuse on reproductive function in women and pregnancy. In R.R. Watson (Ed.), *Drug and alcohol abuse reviews. Vol. 5. Addictive behaviors in women* (pp. 437-473). Totowa, NJ: Humana Press.

Tepper, R., Goldberger, S., May, J.Y., Luz, I.J., & Beyth, Y. (1992). Hormonal replacement therapy in postmenopausal women and cardiovascular disease: An overview. *Obstetrical and Gynecological Survey, 47,* 426-431.

Terrell, H.B. (1988). Behavioral dyscontrol with combined use of alprazolam and ethanol [Letter to the editor]. *American Journal of Psychiatry, 145,* 1313.

Tessman, I. (1979). Female sexual activity at ovulation [Letter to the editor]. *New England Journal of Medicine, 300,* 626.

Testa, M.A., Anderson, R.B., Nackley, J.F., Hollenberg, N.K., & Quality-of-Life Hypertension Study Group. (1993). Quality of life and antihypertensive therapy in men: A comparison of catopril with enalapril. *New England Journal of Medicine, 328,* 907-913.

Tetrud, J.W., & Langston, J.W. (1989). The effect of deprenyl (selegiline) on the natural history of Parkinson's disease. *Science, 245,* 519-522.

Theohar, C., Fischer-Cornelssen, K., Akesson, H.O., Ansari, J., Gerlach, J., Harper, P., Ohman, R., Ose, E., & Stegink, A.J. (1981). Bromocriptine as antidepressant: Double-blind comparative study with imipramine in psychogenic and endogenous depression. *Current Therapeutic Research, 30,* 830-842.

Thiagarajah, S., Vaughn, E.D., & Kitchin, J.D. (1978). Retrograde ejaculation: Successful pregnancy following combined sympathomimetic medication and insemination. *Fertility and Sterility, 30,* 96-97.

Thibaut, F., Cordier, B., & Kuhn, J.M. (1993). Effect of a long-lasting gonadotrophin hormone-releasing hormone agonist in six cases of severe male paraphilia. *Acta Psychiatrica Scandinavica, 87,* 445-450.

Thomas, A.J. (1983). Ejaculatory dysfunction. *Fertility and Sterility, 39,* 445-454.

Thompson, D.C., Diamond, L, & Altiere, R.J. (1990). Presynaptic alpha adrenoceptor modulation of neurally mediated cholinergic excitatory and nonadrenergic and noncholinergic responses in guinea pig trachea. *Journal of Pharmacology and Experimental Therapeutics, 254,* 306-313.

Thompson, J.W., Ware, M.R., & Blashfield, R.K. (1990). Psychotropic medication and priapism: A comprehensive review. *Journal of Clinical Psychiatry, 51,* 430-433.

Thomson, J. (1976). Double-blind study of the effect of estrogen on sleep and anxiety and depression in perimenopausal women. *Proceedings of the Royal Society of Medicine, 69,* 829-830.

Thong, K.J., & Baird, D.T. (1992). Induction of abortion with mifepristone and misoprostol in early pregnancy. *British Journal of Obstetrics and Gynecology, 99,* 1004-1007.

Thorneycroft, I.H. (1989). The role of estrogen replacement therapy in the prevention of osteoporosis. *American Journal of Obstetrics and Gynecology, 160,* 1306-1310.

Thornton, J.E., Vincent, P.A., & Feder, H.H. (1988). Facilitation of lordosis in guinea pigs by an alpha-noradrenergic agonist is independent of progestin receptor stimulation. *Hormones and Behavior, 22,* 172-177.

Tiegs, R.D., Body, J.J., Wahner, H.W., Barta, J.M., Riggs, B.L., & Heath, H. (1985). Calcitonin secretion in postmenopausal osteoporosis. *New England Journal of Medicine, 312,* 1097-1100.

Titmarsh, S., & Monk, J.P. (1987). Terazosin: A review of its pharmacodynamic and pharmokinetic properties, and therapeutic efficacy in essential hypertension. *Drugs, 33,* 461–477.

Tokuhata, G.K. (1968). Smoking in relation to infertility and fetal loss. *Archives of Environmental Health, 17,* 353–359.

Tollefson, G.D., Rampey, A.H., Potvin, J.H., Jenike, M.A., Rush, A.J., Dominguez, R.A., Koran, L.M., Shear, K., Goodman, W., & Genduso, L.A. (1994). A multicenter investigation of fixed-dose fluoxetine in the treatment of obsessive-compulsive disorder. *Archives of General Psychiatry, 51,* 559–567.

Toone, B.K. (1985). Sexual disorders in epilepsy. In T.A. Redley & B.S. Meldrum (Eds.), *Recent advances in epilepsy* (pp. 233–260). Edinburgh: Churchill Livingstone.

Toone, B.K. (1986). Hyposexuality among male epileptic patients: Clinical and hormonal correlates. In M.R. Trimble & T.G. Bolwig (Eds.), *Aspects of epilepsy and psychiatry* (pp. 61–74). New York: John Wiley & Sons.

Tordjman, G. (1982). Prolactin, sexuality, and bromocriptine. In Z. Hoch & H.I. Lief (Eds.), *Sexology: Sexual biology, behavior, and therapy* (pp. 72–76). Princeton: Excerpta Medica.

Tordjman, G. (1990). Current approach and prospect of intracavernosal injections in erectile and ejaculation disorders. In F.J. Bianco & R. Hernandez Serrano (Eds.) *Sexology: An independent field* (pp. 245–251). New York: Elsevier Science Publishers.

Tosi, R., & Cagnoli, M. (1982). Painful gynecomastia with ranitidine. *Lancet, 2,* 160.

Toth, P., & Frankenburg, F.R. (1994). Clozapine and seizures: A review. *Canadian Journal of Psychiatry, 39,* 236–238.

Tribollet, E., Audiger, S., Dubois-Dauphin, M., & Dreifuss, J.J. (1990). Gonadal steroids regulate oxytocin receptors but not vasopressin receptors in the brain of male and female rats. An autoradiographical study. *Brain Research, 511,* 129–140.

Tribollet, E., & Dubois-Dauphin, M. (1987). Castration reduces the density of oxytocin but not of vasopressin binding sites in the rat brain. *Experientia, 43,* 721.

Trichopoulos, D., MacMahon, B., & Cole, P. (1972). The menopause and breast cancer risk. *Journal of the National Cancer Institute, 48,* 605–613.

Trienekens, P., Schmidt, N., & Thijssen, J. (1986). The effect of age, weight-related parameters, and hormonal contraceptives on andrological assays. *Contraception, 33,* 503–517.

Tsai, K.S., Heath, H., Kumar, R., & Riggs, B.L. (1984). Impaired vitamin D metabolism with aging in women. *Journal of Clinical Investigation, 73,* 1668–1672.

Tsitouras, P.D., Martin, C.E., & Harman, S.M. (1982). Relationship of serum testosterone to sexual activity in healthy elderly men. *Journal of Gerontology, 37,* 288–293.

Tuomisto, J., & Mannisto, P. (1985). Neurotransmitter regulation of anterior pituitary hormones. *Pharmacological Review, 37,* 249–332.

Turkkan, J.S., & Heinz, R.D. (1991). Behavioral effects of chronic orally administered diuretics and verapamil in baboons. *Pharmacology, Biochemistry, and Behavior, 38,* 55–62.

Turner, L.A., Althof, S.E., Levine, S.B., Bodner, D.R., Kursh, E.D., & Resnik, M.I. (1992). Twelve-month comparison of two treatments for erectile dysfunction: Self-injection versus external vacuum devices. *Urology, 39,* 139–144.

Tyler, V.E., Brady, L.R., & Robbers, J.E. (1981). *Pharmacognosy* (8th ed.). Philadelphia: Lea & Febiger.

Tytgat, G.N. (1994). Long-term consequences of *Helicobacter pylori* eradication. *Scandinavian Journal of Gastroenterology, 29*(Suppl. 205), 38–44.

Udry, J.R. (1988). Biological predispositions and social control in adolescent sexual behavior. *American Sociological Reviews, 53,* 709–722.

Udry, J., & Morris, N. (1968). Distribution of coitus in the menstrual cycle. *Nature, 220,* 593–596.

Udry, J.R., & Morris, N.M. (1977). The distribution of events in the human menstrual cycle. *Journal of Reproduction and Fertility, 51,* 419–425.

Udry, J.R., & Talbert, L.M. (1988). Sex hormone effects on personality at puberty. *Journal of Personality and Social Psychology, 54,* 291, 295.

Uhde, T.W., Tancer, M.E., & Shea, C.A. (1988). Sexual dysfunction related to alprozalam treatment of social phobia [Letter to the editor]. *American Journal of Psychiatry, 145,* 531–532.

Uitti, R.J., Tanner, C.M., Rajput, A.H., Goetz, C.G., Klawans, H.L., & Thiessen, B. (1989). Hypersexuality with anti-Parkinsonian therapy. *Clinical Neuropharmacology, 12,* 375–383.

Ulmann, A., Silvestre, L., Chemana, L., Rezvani, Y., Renault, M., Aguillaume, C.J., & Baulieu, E.E. (1992). Medical termination of early pregnancy with mifepristone (RU 486) followed by a prostaglandin analogue. *Acta Obstetrica et Gynecologica Scandinavica, 71,* 278–283.

Ulmann, A., Teutsch, G., & Philibert, D. (1990). RU 486. *Scientific American, 262(6),* 42–48.

Umbricht, D.S., Pollack, S., & Kane, J.M. (1994). Clozapine and weight gain. *Journal of Clinical Psychiatry, 55*(Suppl. B), 157–160.

Upton, N. (1994). Mechanisms of action of new antiepileptic drugs: Rational design and serendipitous findings. *Trends in Pharmacological Science (TIPS), 15,* 456–463.

Utian, W.H. (1972a). The mental tonic effect of estrogens administered to oophorectomized females. *South African Medical Journal, 46,* 1079–1082.

Utian, W.H. (1972b). The true clinical features of postmenopause and oophorectomy, and their response to estrogen therapy. *South African Medical Journal, 46,* 732–737.

Utian, W.H. (1975). Definitive symptoms of postmenopause: Incorporating use of vaginal parabasal cell index. In P.A. van Keep & C. Lauritzen (Eds.), *Estrogens in the post-menopause* (pp. 74–93). Basel: Karger.

Uvnas-Moberg, K. (1990). Endocrinologic control of food intake. *Nutrition Reviews, 48,* 57–63.

VA: Veterans Administration Cooperative Study Group on Antihypertensive Agents (1972). Effects of treatment on morbidity in hypertension: III. Influence of age, diastolic pressure, and prior cardiovascular disease: Further analysis of side effects. *Circulation, 40,* 1180–1187.

VA: Veterans Administration Cooperative Study Group on Antihypertensive Agents (1977). Propranolol in the treatment of essential hypertension. *Journal of the American Medical Association, 237,* 2303–2310.

VA: Veterans Administration Cooperative Study Group for Antihypertensive Agents (1981). Comparison of prozosin with hydralazine in patients receiving hydrochlorothiazide. A randomized double-blind clinical trial. *Circulation, 64,* 772–779.

VA: Veterans Administration Cooperative Study Group on Antihypertensive Agents (1984). Low-dose captopril for the treatment of mild to moderate hypertension. I. Results of a 14-week trial. *Archives of Internal Medicine, 144,* 1947–1953.

Vaitukaitis, L., Dale, S., & Melby, J. (1969). Role of ACTH in the secretion of free DHA and its sulfate ester in man. *Journal of Clinical Endocrinology and Metabolism, 29,* 1443–1447.

Valentino, R.J., & Foote, S.L. (1986). Brain noradrenergic neurons, corticotropin-releasing factor, and stress. In T.W. Moody (Ed.), *Neural and endocrine peptides and receptors* (pp. 101–120). New York: Plenum Press.

Van Amerongen, D. (1994). Removal rates of subdermal levonorgestrel implants. *Journal of Reproductive Medicine, 39,* 873–876.

Van Amerongen, P. (1979). Double-blind controlled trials of amineptine versus trimipramine in depression. *Current Medical Research and Opinion, 6,* 101–106.

Van de Kar, L.D., Lorens, S.A., Urban, J.H., Richardson, K.D., Paris, J., & Bethea, C.L. (1985). Pharmacological studies on stress-induced renin and prolactin secretion: Effects of benzodiazepines, naloxone, propranolol, and diisopropyl fluorophosphate. *Brain Research, 345,* 257–263.

Van Den Hoof, P., & Urban, I.J.A. (1990). Vasopressin facilitates excitatory transmission in slices of the rat dorsolateral septum. *Synapse, 5,* 201–206.

Van den Pol, A.N., Wuarin, J.P., & Dudek, F.E. (1990). Glutamate, the dominant excitatory transmitter in neuroendocrine regulation. *Science, 250,* 1276–1278.

Van der Schoot, P., & Baumgarten, R. (1992). Interactions between oestradiol and the progesterone antagonist RU-486 in establishing and maintaining female rat's sex responsiveness: Central versus peripheral effects. *Behavioral Brain Research, 47,* 105–112.

Van Thiel, D. (1977). Therapy of sexual dysfunction in alcohol abusers: A Pandora's box. *Gastroenterology, 72,* 1354–1356.

Van Thiel, D.H. (1980). Alcohol and its effect on endocrine functioning. *Alcoholism, 4,* 44–49.

Van Thiel, D.H., Gavaler, J.S., Eagon, P.K., & Lester, R. (1980). Effect of alcohol on gonadal function. *Drug and Alcohol Dependence, 6,* 41–42.

Van Thiel, D.H., Gavaler, J.S. Heyl, A., & Susen, B. (1987). An evaluation of the anti-androgen effects associated with H2 antagonist therapy. *Scandanavian Journal of Gastroenterology, 22* (Suppl. 136), 24–28.

Van Thiel, D.H., Gavaler, J.S., Lester, R., Loriaux, D.L., & Braunstein, G.D. (1975). Plasma estrone, prolactin, neurophysin, and sex steroid-binding globulin in chronic alcoholic men. *Metabolism, 24,* 1015–1019.

Van Thiel, D.H., Gavaler, J.S., & Schade, R.R. (1985). Liver disease and the hypothalmic pituitary gonadal axis. *Seminars in Liver Disease, 5,* 35–45.

Van Thiel, P.H., Gavaler, B.S, Smith, W.I., & Paul, G. (1979). Hypothalmic-pituitary-gonadal dysfunction in men using cimetidine. *New England Journal of Medicine, 300,* 1012–1015.

Van Weerden, W.M., Steenbrugge, G.V., Van Kreuningen, A., Moerings, E.P., de Jong, F.H., & Schroder, F.H. (1990). Effects of low testosterone levels and of adrenal androgens on growth of prostate tumor models in nude mice. *Journal of Steroid Biochemistry and Molecular Biology, 37,* 903–907.

Van Wimersma Greidanus, T.B., & Ten Haaf, J. (1985). The effects of opiates and opioid peptides on oxytocin release. In J.A. Amico & A.G. Robinson (Eds.), *Oxytocin: Clinical and laboratory studies* (pp. 145–152). New York: Elsevier Science Publishers.

Van Zweiten, P.A. (1986). Differentiation of calcium entry blockers into calcium channel-blockers and calcium overload blockers. *European Neurology, 25*(Suppl. 1), 57–67.

Varga, E., Haher, E.J., & Simpson, G.M. (1975). Neuroleptic-induced Kluver-Bucy syndrome. *Biological Psychiatry, 10,* 65–68.

Vartiainen, E., Puska, P., Pekkanen, J., Tuomilehto, J., Lönngvist, J., & Ehnholm, C. (1994). Serum cholesterol concentration and mortality from accidents, suicide, and other violent causes. *British Medical Journal, 309,* 445–447.

Vasdev, S., Longerich, L., Johnson, E., Brent, D., & Gault, M.H. (1985). Dehydroepiandrosterone sulfate as a digitalis-like factor in plasma of healthy human adults. *Research Communications in Chemical Pathology and Pharmacology, 49,* 387–399.

Vendsborg, P.B., & Rafelson, O.J. (1976). Lithium treatment and weight gain. *Acta Psychiatrica Scandinavica, 53,* 139–147.

Vener, A.M., & Krupka, L.R. (1985). Over-the-counter anorexiants: Use and perceptions among young adults. In J.P. Morgan, D.V. Kagan, & J.S. Brody (Eds.), *Phenylpropanolamine: Risks, benefits, and controversies* (pp. 132–149). New York: Praeger Publishers.

Vereecken, R.L. (1989). Psychological and sexual aspects in different types of bladder dysfunction. *Psychotherapy and Psychosomatics, 51,* 128–134.

Vermesh, M., Fossum, G.T., & Kletzky, O.A. (1988). Vaginal bromocriptine: Pharmacology and effect on serum prolactin in normal women. *Obstetrics and Gynecology, 72,* 693–698.

Vermeulen, A. (1991). Androgens in the aging male. *Journal of Clinical Endocrinology and Metabolism, 73,* 221–224.

Vermeulen, A. (1994). Clinical problems in reproductive neuroendocrinology in men. *Neurobiology of Aging, 15,* 489–493.

Vermeulen, A., & Thiery, M. (1982). Metabolic effects of the triphasic oral contraceptive Trigynon. *Contraception, 26,* 505–512.

Versi, E., & Cardozo, L.D. (1988). Estrogens and lower urinary tract function. In J.W. Studd & I.M. Whitehead (Eds.), *The menopause* (pp. 76–84). London: Blackwell Scientific.

Versiani, M., Nardi, A.E., Mundion, F.D., Alves, A.B., Liebowitz, M.R., & Amrein, R. (1992). Pharmacotherapy of social phobia: A controlled study with moclobemide and phenelzine. *British Journal of Psychiatry, 161,* 353–360.

Vestergaard, P., Amdisen, A., & Schon, M. (1980). Clinically significant side effects of lighium treatment. *Acta Psychiatrica Scandinavica, 62,* 193–200.

Vicizian, M. (1968). Effect of cigarette smoke inhalation on spermatogenesis in rats. *Experientia, 24,* 511.

Vidal, H., & Riou, J.P. (1989). Alpha$_2$-adrenergic stimulation counteracts the metabolic effects of vasoactive intestinal peptide in isolated rat enterocytes. *Endocrinology, 124,* 3117–3121.

Vigersky, R.A., Mehlman, J., Glass, A.R., & Smith, C.E. (1980). Treatment of hirsute women with cimetidine. *New England Journal of Medicine, 303,* 1042.

Vinarova, E., Uhlir, O., Stika, L., & Vinar, O. (1972). Side effects of lithium administration. *Activitas Nervosa Superior (Praha), 14,* 105–107.

Vincent, P.A., & Feder, H.H. (1988). Alpha$_1$- and alpha$_2$-noradrenergic receptors modulate lordosis behavior in female guinea pigs. *Neuroendocrinology, 48,* 477–481.

Vine, M.F., Margolin, B.H., Morrison, H.I., & Hulka, B.S. (1994). Cigarette smoking and sperm density: A meta-analysis. *Fertility and Sterility, 61,* 35–43.

Virag, R. (1982). Intracavernous injection of papaverine for erectile failure [Letter to the editor]. *Lancet, 2,* 938.

Virag, R., & Adaikan, P.G. (1987). Effects of prostaglandin E1 on penile erection and erectile failure [Letter to the editor]. *Journal of Urology, 137,* 1010.

Virag, R., Bouilly, P., & Frydman, D. (1985). Is impotence an arterial disorder? *Lancet, 1,* 181.

Virag, R., Frydman, D., Legman, M., & Virag, H. (1984). Intracavernous injection of papaverine as a diagnostic and therapeutic method in erectile failure. *Angiology, 35,* 79–87.

Virag, R., Shoukry, K., Floresco, J., Nollet, F., & Greco, E. (1991). Intracavernous self-injection of vasoactive drugs in the treatment of impotence: 8-year experience with 615 cases. *Journal of Urology, 145,* 287–293.

Vogel, H.P., & Schiffter, R. (1983). Hypersexuality: A complication of dopaminergic therapy in Parkinson's disease. *Pharmacopsychiatry, 16,* 107–110.

Vogel, W., Klaiber, E.L., & Broverman, D.M. (1985). A comparison of the antidepressant effects of a synthetic androgen (mesterolone) and amitriptyline in depressed men. *Journal of Clinical Psychiatry, 46,* 6–8.

von Knorring, A.L., Bohman, L., von Knorring, L., & Oreland, L. (1985). Platelet MAO activity as a biological marker in subgroups of alcoholism. *Acta Psychiatrica Scandinavica, 72,* 51–58.

Wade, C.E., Lindberg, J.S., Corkrell, J.L., Lamiell, J.M., Hunt, M.M., Ducey, J., & Turney, J.H. (1988). Upon admission adrenal steroidogenesis is adapted to the degree of illness in intensive care unit patients. *Journal of Clinical Endocrinology and Metabolism, 66,* 223–227.

Waehrens, J., & Gerlach, J. (1981). Bromocriptine and imipramine in endogenous depression. *Journal of Affective Disorders, 3,* 193–202.

Wagner, G. (1985, May 28-31). *The penis: Erection and impotence.* AASECT Professional Seminar: Scandinavian Approaches to Sex Education and Therapy, Panum Institute, Copenhagen.

Wagner, G., & Brindley, G.S. (1980). The effect of atropine, alpha, and beta blockers on human penile erection: A controlled pilot study. In A.W. Zorgniotti & G. Rossi (Eds.), *Vasculogenic impotence. Proceedings of the First International Conference on corpus cavernosum revascularization* (pp. 77-81). Springfield, IL: Charles C. Thomas Publisher.

Wagner, G., & Gerstenberg, T. (1988). Vasoactive intestinal peptide facilitates normal erection. *Proceedings of the Sixth Biennial International Symposium for corpus cavernosum revascularization and the Third Biennial World Meeting on impotence.* Boston, MA: International Society for the Study of Impotence.

Wagner, G., & Levin, R.J. (1980). Effect of atropine and methylatropine on human vaginal blood flow, sexual arousal, and climax. *Acta Pharmacologica et Toxicologica, 46,* 321-325.

Wagner, J. & Clayton, T. (1995). Highlights of the 46th Institute on hospital and community psychiatry. *Psychiatric Services, 46*(1), 23-28.

Wagner, J.A., & Peroutka, S.J. (1988). Comparative neurotoxicity of fenfluramine and 3,4-methylenedioxymethamphetamine (MDMA). *Society for Neuroscience Abstracts: 18th Meeting, 14* (Pt. 1), 327.

Waldemar, G., Werdelin, L., & Boysen, G. (1987). Neurologic symptoms and hysterectomy: A retrospective survey of the prevalence of hysterectomy in neurologic patients. *Obstetrics and Gynecology, 70,* 559-563.

Waldholz, M. (1989, September 6). Federal Drug Administration asks drug makers to stop promoting lactation suppressants for new mothers. *Wall Street Journal,* A6.

Waldinger, M.D., Hengeveld, M.W., & Zwinderman, A.H. (1994). Paroxetine treatment of premature ejaculation: A double-blind, randomized, placebo-controlled study. *American Journal of Psychiatry, 151,* 1377-1379.

Waldmeier, P.C. (1987). Is there a common denominator for the antimanic effect of lithium and anticonvulsants? *Pharmacopsychiatry, 20,* 37-47.

Walker, P., Meyer, W.J., Emory, L.E., & Rubin, A.L. (1984). Antiandrogenic treatment of the paraphilias. In H. Stancer, P. Garfinkel, & V.M. Rakoff (Eds.), *Guidelines for the use of psychotropic drugs* (pp. 427-443). Toronto: Spectrum Publications.

Walker, P.W., Cole, J.O., Gardner, E.A., Hughes, A.R., Johnston, J.A., Batey, S.R., & Lineberry, C.G. (1993). Improvement in fluoxetine-associated sexual dysfunction in patients switched to bupropion. *Journal of Clinical Psychiatry, 54,* 459-465.

Walker, T.F., Bott, J.H., & Bond, B.C. (1987). Cimetidine does not demasculinize male rat offspring exposed in utero. *Fundamental and Applied Toxicology, 8,* 188-197.

Wallen, K., Mann, D.R., Davis-DaSilva, M., Gaventa, S., Lovejoy, J., & Collins, D.C. (1986). Chronic gonadotrophin-releasing hormone agonist treatment suppresses ovulation and sexual behavior in group-living female rhesus monkeys. *Physiology and Behavior, 36,* 369-375.

Wallen, K., & Winston, L.A. (1984). Social complexity and hormonal influences on sexual behavior in rhesus monkeys (*Macaca mulatta*). *Physiology and Behavior, 32,* 629-637.

Walling, M., Anderson, B.L., & Johnson, S.R. (1990). Hormonal replacement therapy for postmenopausal women: A review of sexual outcomes and related gynecological effects. *Archives of Sexual Behavior, 19,* 119-137.

Walters, M.D., Taylor, S., & Schoenfeld, L.S. (1990). Psychosexual study of women with detrusor instability. *Obstetrics and Gynecology, 75,* 22-25.

Ward, C.D. (1994). Does selegiline delay progression of Parkinson's disease? A critical re-evaluation of the DATATOP study. *Journal of Neurology, Neurosurgery, and Psychiatry, 57,* 217-220.

Warneke, L. (1990). Psychostimulants in psychiatry. *Canadian Journal of Psychiatry, 35,* 3-10.

Warner, N.J., & Rush, J.E. (1988). Safety profiles of the angiotensin-converting enzyme inhibitors. *Drugs, 35*(Suppl. 5), 89-97.

Warren, S.C, & Warren, S.G. (1977). Propranolol and sexual impotence. *Annals of Internal Medicine, 86,* 112.

Wartman, S.A. (1983). Sexual side effects of antihypertensive drugs. *Postgraduate Medicine, 73,* 133-138.

Wassertheil-Smoller, S., Blaufax, M.D., Oberman, A., Davis, B.R., Swencionis, C., Knerr, M.O., Hawkins, C.M., & Langford, H.G. (1991). Effect of antihypertensives on sexual function and quality of life: The TAIM Study. *Annals of Internal Medicine, 114,* 613-620.

Watanabe, H., & Uramoto, H. (1986). Caffeine mimics dopamine receptor agonists without stimulation of dopamine receptors. *Neuropharmacology, 25,* 577-581.

Watanabe, S. (1986). Comparison of the anticholinergic bronchodilator ipratropium bromide with metaproterenol in chronic obstructive pulmonary disease. *American Journal of Medicine, 81*(Suppl. 5A), 81-89.

Waters, C.H., Belai, Y., Gott, P.S., Shen, P., & De Giorgio, C.M. (1994). Outcomes of pregnancy associated with antiepileptic drugs. *Archives of Neurology, 51,* 250-253.

Watson, D.L., Bhatia, R.K., Norman, G.S., Brindley, B.A., & Sokol, R.J. (1989). Bromocriptine mesylate for lactation suppression: A risk for postpartum hypertension. *Obstetrics and Gynecology, 74,* 573-576.

Watson, N.V., & Gorzalka, B.B. (1994). DOI-induced inhibition of copulatory behavior in male rats: Reversal by 5-HT_2 antagonists. *Pharmacology, Biochemistry, and Behavior, 39,* 605-612.

Watters, G.R., Keough, E.J., Earle, C.M., Carati, C.J., Wisniewski, Z.S., Tulloch, A.G.S., & Lord, D.J. (1988). Experience in the management of erectile dysfunction using the intracavernosal self-injection of vasoactive drugs. *Journal of Urology, 140,* 1417-1419.

Watts, N.B., Harris, S.T., Genant, H.K., Wasnich, R.D., Miller, P.D., Jackson, R.D., Licata, A.A., Ross, P., Woodson, G.C., & Yanover, J.J. (1990). Intermittent cyclical etidronate treatment of post-menopausal osteoporosis. *New England Journal of Medicine, 323,* 73-79.

Waxenburg, S.E. (1962). Some biological correlates of sexual behavior. In G. Winoker (Ed.), *Determinants of human sexual behavior* (pp. 52-75). Springfield, IL: Charles Thomas.

Waxenberg, S.E., Drellich, M.G., & Sutherland, A.M. (1959). The role of hormones in human behavior. I. Changes in female sexuality after adrenalectomy. *Journal of Clinical Endocrinology, 19,* 193-202.

Waxenberg, S.E., Finkbeinter, J.A., Drellich, M.G., & Sutherland, A.M. (1960). Changes in sexual behavior in relation to vaginal smears of breast cancer patients after oophorectomy and adrenalectomy. *Psychosomatic Medicine, 22,* 435-442.

Wehr, T.A., & Goodwin, F.K. (1987). Can antidepressants cause mania and worsen the course of affective illness? *American Journal of Psychiatry, 144,* 1403-1411.

Weiland, S.K., Keil, U., Spelsberg, A., Hense, H.W., Hartel, U., Gefeller, O., & Dieckmann, W. (1991). Diagnosis and management of hypertension by physicians in the Federal Republic of Germany. *Journal of Hypertension, 9,* 131-134.

Wein, A.J. (1991). Practical uropharmacology. *Urologic Clinics of North America, 18,* 269-281.

Weisner, J.B., & Moss, R.L. (1984). Beta-endorphin suppression of lordosis behavior in female rats: Lack of effect of peripherally-adminisstered naloxone. *Life Sciences, 34,* 1455-1462.

Weisner, J.B., & Moss, R.L. (1986a). Behavioral specificity of beta-endorphin suppression of sexual behavior: Differential receptor antagonism. *Pharmacology Biochemistry and Behavior, 24,* 1235-1239.

Weisner, J.B., & Moss, R.L. (1986b). Suppression of receptive and proceptive behavior in ovarectomized, estrogen-progesterone-primed rats by intraventricular beta-endorphin: Studies of behavioral specificity. *Neuroendocrinology, 43,* 57-62.

Weiss, N.S., Ure, C.L., Ballard, J.H., Williams, A.R., & Daling, J.R. (1980). Decreased risk of fractures of the hip and lower forearm with post-menopausal use of estrogen. *New England Journal of Medicine, 303,* 1195-1198.

Weissman, M., & Klerman, G. (1977). Sex differences and the epidemiology of depression. *Archives of General Psychiatry, 34,* 98-111.

Weizman, R., Weizman, A., Levi, J., Gura, V., Zevin, D., Maoz, B., Wijsenbeek, H., Ben David, M. (1983). Sexual dysfunction asociated with hyperprolactinemia in males and females undergoing hemodialysis. *Psychosomatic Medicine, 45,* 259-269.

Weksler, M.E. (1993). Immune senescence and adrenal steroids: Immune dysregulation and the action of dehydroepiandrosterone (DHEA) in old animals. *European Journal of Clinical Pharmacology, 45*(Suppl. 1), 521-523.

Wender, P.H., Reimherr, F.W., Wood, D., & Ward, M. (1985). A controlled study of methylphenidate in the treatment of attention deficit disorder, residual type, in adults. *American Journal of Psychiatry, 142,* 547-552.

Wender, P.H., Wood, D.R., & Reimherr, F.W. (1985). Pharmacological treatment of attention deficit disorder, residual type (ADD, RT "minimal brain dysfunction," "hyperactivity") in adults. *Psychopharmacology Bulletin, 21,* 222-227.

Werning, C., Weitz, T., & Ludwig, B. (1988). Assessment of indapamide in elderly hypertensive patients with special emphasis on well-being. *American Journal of Medicine, 84*(Suppl. 1B), 104-108.

Wesson, D.R., & Camber, S. (1985). Phenylpropanolamine mentions in the drug abuse warning network: Numbers plus interpretations. In J.P. Morgan, D.V. Kagan, & J.S. Brody (Eds.), *Phenylpropanolamine: Risks, benefits, and controversies* (pp. 362-370). New York: Praeger Publishers.

West, C.H., & Michael, R.P. (1990). Enhanced responsiveness of nucleus accumbens units to odors associated with amphetamine administration in rats. *Society for Neuroscience, 16,* 592.

Weyerer, S., & Dilling, H. (1991). Prevalence and treatment of insomnia in the community: Results from the Upper Bavarian Field Study. *Sleep, 14,* 392-398.

Whalen, R.E. (1984). Multiple actions of steroids and their antagonists. *Archives of Sexual Behavior, 13,* 497-502.

Whalen, R.E., & Luttge, W.G. (1970). P-chlorophenylalanine methyl ester: An aphrodisiac? *Science, 169,* 1000-1001.

Whipple, B., & Komisaruk, B.R. (1985). Elevation of pain threshold by vaginal stimulation in women. *Pain, 21,* 357-367.

Whipple, B., & Komisaruk, B.R. (1988). Analgesia

produced in women by genital self-stimulation. *Journal of Sex Research, 24,* 130–140.

Whitehead, E.D. (1994). Enhancement phalloplasty: Pre-surgical information package and informed consent documentation. Paper presented at the American Urological Association Annual Meeting, May, San Francisco.

Whitehead, M.I., Lane, G., Townsend, P.T., Abeyasekera, G., Hillyard, C.J., & Stevenson, J.C. (1982). Effects in postmenopausal women of natural and synthetic estrogens on calcitonin and calcium-regulating hormone secretion. *Acta Obstetricia et Gynecologica Scandinavica Supplementum, 106,* 27–32.

Whitney, J. (1986). Effect of medial preoptic lesions on sexual behavior of female rats is determined by test situation. *Behavioral Neuroscience, 100,* 230–235.

Whyte, K.F., Gould, G.A., Airlie, A.A., Shapiro, C.M., & Douglas, N.J. (1988). Role of protriptyline and acetazolamide in the sleep apnea/hypopnea syndrome. *Sleep, 11,* 463–472.

Wiesner, J.B., Dudley, C.A., & Moss, R.L. (1986). Effect of beta-endorphin on sociosexual proclivity in a choice paradigm. *Pharmacology, Biochemistry, and Behavior, 24,* 507–511.

Wiesner, J.B. & Moss, R.L. (1984). Beta-endorphin suppression of lordosis behavior in female rats; lack of effect of peripherally-administered naloxone. *Life Sciences, 34*(15), 1455–1462.

Wiesner J.B. & Moss, R.L. (1986). Behavioral specificity of beta-endorphin suppression of sexual behavior: differential receptor antagonism. *Pharmacology, Biochemistry and Behavior, 24*(5), 1235–1239.

Wiklund, I., Karlberg, J., & Mattsson, L.A. (1993). Quality of life of postmenopausal women on a regimen of transdermal estradiol therapy: A double-blind placebo-controlled study. *American Journal of Obstetrics and Gynecology, 168,* 824–830.

Wild, R.A., Buchanan, J.R., Myers, C., & Demers, L.M. (1987). Declining adrenal androgens: An association with bone loss in aging women. *Proceedings of the Society for Experimental Biology and Medicine, 186,* 355–360.

Wild, R.A., Buchanan, J.R., Myers, C., Lloyd, T., & Demers, L.M. (1987). Adrenal androgens, sex-hormone binding globulin, and bone density in osteoporotic menopausal women: Is there a relationship? *Maturitas, 9,* 55–61.

Wildin, J.D., Pleuvry, B.J., & Mawer, G.E. (1993). Impairment of psychomotor function at modest plasma concentrations of carbamazepine after administration of the liquid suspension to naive subjects. *British Journal of Clinical Pharmacology, 35,* 14–19.

Wilens, S.L. (1947). The relationship of chronic alcoholism to atherosclerosis. *Journal of the American Medical Association, 135,* 1224–1227.

Wilhelmi, A.E., Pickford, G.E., & Sawyer, W.H. (1955). Initiation of the spawning reflex in Fundulus by the administration of fish and mammalian neurohypophyseal preparations and synthetic oxytocin. *Endocrinology, 57,* 243–254.

Willcox, S.M., Himmelstein, D.U., & Woolhandler, S. (1994). Inappropriate drug prescribing for the community-dwelling elderly. *Journal of the American Medical Association, 272,* 292–296.

Williams, C.J., Barley, V., Blackledge, G., Hutche, A., Kaye, S., Smith, D., Keen, C., Webster, D.J., Rowland, C., & Tyrrell, C. (1987). Multicenter study of trilostane: A new hormonal agent in advanced postmenopausal breast cancer. *Cancer Treatment Reports, 71,* 1197–1201.

Williams, G.H. (1988). Converting-enzyme inhibitors in the treatment of hypertension. *New England Journal of Medicine, 319,* 1517–1525.

Williamson, D.F., Madans, J., Anda, R.F., Kleinman, J.C., Giovino, G.A., & Byers, T. (1991). Smoking cessation and severity of weight gain in a national cohort. *New England Journal of Medicine, 324,* 739–745.

Wilsnack, R.W., Klassen, A.D., & Wilsnack, S.C. (1986). Retrospective analysis of lifetime changes in women's drinking behavior. *Advances in Alcohol and Substance Abuse, 5,* 9–28.

Wilsnack, R.W., Wilsnack, S.C., & Klassen, A.D. (1987). Antecedents and consequences of drinking and drinking problems in women: Patterns for a United States national survey. In P.C. Rivers (Eds.), *Nebraska Symposium on Motivation 1986* Vol. 34 (pp. 85–158). Lincoln, NB: University of Nebraska Press.

Wilsnack, S.C. (1976). The impact of sex roles on women's alcohol use and abuse. In M. Greenblatt & M.A. Schuckit (Eds.), *Alcoholism problems in women and children* (pp. 37–63). New York: Grune & Stratton.

Wilsnack, S.C. (1984). Drinking, sexuality, and sexual dysfunction in women. In S.C. Wilsnack & L.J. Beckman (Eds.), *Alcohol problems in women: Antecedents, consequences, and intervention* (pp. 189–227). New York: Guilford Press.

Wilsnack, S.C., Klassen, A.D., & Wilsnack, R.W. (1984). Drinking and reproductive dysfunction among women in a 1981 national survey. *Alcoholism: Clinical and Experimental Research, 8,* 451–458.

Wilson, C.A., Bonney, R.C., Everard, D.M., Parrott, R.F., & Wise, J. (1982). Mechanisms of action of p-chlorophylalanine in stimulating sexual receptivity in the female rat. *Pharmacology, Biochemistry and Behavior, 16,* 777–784.

Wilson, G.T. (1984). The effects of alcohol on male and female sexual function. *Sexual Medicine Today, 8*(6), 6–15.

Wilson, G.T., & Lawson, D.M. (1976a). The effects of alcohol on sexual arousal in women. *Journal of Abnormal Psychology, 85,* 489–497.

Wilson, G.T., & Lawson, D.M. (1976b). Expectancies, alcohol, and sexual arousal in male social drinkers. *Journal of Abnormal Psychology, 85,* 587–594.

Wilson, G.T., & Lawson, D.M. (1978). Expectancies, alcohol, and sexual arousal in women. *Journal of Abnormal Psychology, 87,* 358–367.

Wilson, G.T., Lawson, D.M., & Abrams, D.B. (1978). Effects of alcohol on sexual arousal in male alcoholics. *Journal of Abnormal Psychology, 87,* 609–616.

Wilson, G.T., Niaura, R.S., & Adler, T.L. (1985). Alcohol, selective attention, and sexual arousal in men. *Journal of Studies on Alcohol, 46,* 107–115.

Wilson, P.W., Garrison, R.J., & Castelli, W.P. (1985). Postmenopausal estrogen use, cigarette smoking, and cardiovascular morbidity in women over 50: The Framingham Study. *New England Journal of Medicine, 313,* 1038–1043.

Wimalawansa, S.J., Kehely, A., Banks, L.M., Stevensen, J.C., Whitehead, M.J., & MacIntyre, I. (1988). Calcitonin and estrogens in the prevention of postmenopausal bone loss. *Gynecological Endocrinology, 2*(Suppl. 2), 162.

Wincze, J., Bansal, S., & Malamud, M. (1986). Effects of medroxyprogesterone on subjective arousal, arousal to erotic stimulation, and nocturnal penile tumescence in male sex offenders. *Archives of Sexual Behavior, 15,* 293–305.

Winger, G.D., Yasar, S., Negus, S.S., & Goldberg, S.R. (1994). Intravenous self-administration studies with l-deprenyl (selegiline) in monkeys. *Clinical Pharmacology and Therapeutics, 56,* 774–780.

Winokur, G. (1973). Depression in menopause. *American Journal of Psychiatry, 130,* 92–93.

Winokur, G., & Cadoret, R. (1975). The irrelevance of the menopause to depressive disease. In E.J. Sachar (Ed.), *Topics in psychoendocrinology* (pp. 59–66). St. Louis: Mosby.

Winokur, G., Reich, T., Jimmer, J., & Pitts, F.N. (1970). Alcoholism, III: Diagnosis and familial psychiatric illness in 259 alcoholic probands. *Archives of General Psychiatry, 23,* 104–111.

Winokur, G., Rimmer, J., & Reich, T. (1971). Alcoholism, IV: Is there more than one type of alcoholism? *British Journal of Psychiatry, 118,* 525–531.

Winter, C.C., & McDonell, G. (1988). Experience with 105 patients with priapism: Update review of all aspects. *Journal of Urology, 140,* 980–983.

Winter, J.C. (1988). Generalization of the discriminative stimulus properties of 8-hydroxy-2-(di-n-propylamino) tetralin (8-OH-DPAT) and ipsapirone to yohimbine. *Pharmacology, Biochemistry, and Behavior, 29,* 193–195.

Winterer, J., Gwirtsman, H., George, D., Kaye, W., Loriaux, D., & Cutler, G. (1985). Adrenocorticotrophin-stimulated adrenal androgen secretion in anorexia nervosa: Impaired secretion at low weight with normalization after long-term weight recovery. *Journal of Clinical Endocrinology and Metabolism, 61,* 693–697.

Winters, S.J., Banks, J.L., & Loriaux, D.L. (1979). Cimetidine is an antiandrogen in the rat. *Gastroenterology, 76,* 504–508.

Wise, R.A., Fotuhi, M., & Colle, L.M. (1989). Facilitation of feeding by nucleus accumbens amphetamine injections: Latency and speed measures. *Pharmacology, Biochemistry, and Behavior, 32,* 769–772.

Wise, R.A., Murray, A., & Bozarth, M.A. (1990). Bromocriptine self-administration and bromocriptine-reinstatement of cocaine-trained and heroin-trained lever-pressing in rats. *Psychopharmacology, 100,* 355–360.

Wisneski, L.A. (1992). Review of calcitonin: Future perspectives and new opportunities in therapy. *Bone and Mineral, 16,* 213–216.

Wittels, E.H. (1985). Obesity and hormonal factors in sleep and sleep apnea. *Medical Clinics of North America, 69,* 1265–1280.

Wohrmann, S., Steiger, A., Benkert, O., & Holsboer, F. (1988). Effects of trimipramine on sleep-EEG, nocturnal penile tumescence (NPT), and nocturnal hormonal secretion in normal controls. *Psychopharmacology, 96,* 393.

Wolchik, S.A., Braver, S.L., & Jensen, K. (1985). Volunteer bias in erotica research: Effects of intrusiveness of measure and sexual background. *Archives of Sexual Behavior, 14,* 93–107.

Wolfe, M.M. (1979). Impotence on cimetidine treatment. *New England Journal of Medicine, 300,* 94.

Wolfe, S.M. (1991). *Women's health alert*: Public Citizen Health Research Group. Redding, MA: Addison-Wesley.

Wolpowitz, A., & Barnard, C.N. (1978, May 6). Impotence after heart transplantation [Letter to the editor]. *South African Mediese Tydskrif,* 693.

Wood, D.R., Reimherr, F.W., Wender, P.H., & Johnson, G.E. (1976). Diagnosis and treatment of minimal brain dysfunction in adults. *Archives of General Psychiatry, 33,* 1453–1460.

Wood, W.G., & Strong, R. (1986). Membrane changes associated with alcohol use and aging: Possibilities for nutritional intervention. In H.J. Armbrecht, J.M. Prendergast, & R.M. Coe (Eds.), *Nutritional intervention in the aging process* (pp. 159–179). New York: Springer-Verlag.

Woodhouse, C.R.J., & Tiptaft, R.C. (1983). Mazindol in the control of micturation. *British Journal of Urology, 55,* 636–638.

Woosley, R.L., & Flockhart, D.A. (1994). Evaluating drugs after their approval for clinical use [Letter to the editor]. *New England Journal of Medicine, 330,* 1394.

Wren, B.G. (1985). Estrogen replacement therapy: The management of an endocrine deficiency disorder. *Medical Journal of Australia, 142* (Suppl.), S3-S15.

Wright, G., Galloway, L., Kim, J., Dalton, M., Miller, L., & Stern, W.C. (1985). Bupropion in the long-term treatment of cyclic mood disorders: Mood stabilizing effects. *Journal of Clinical Psychiatry, 46,* 22–25.

Wright, J.M. (1994). Review of symptomatic treatment of diabetic neuropathy. *Pharmacotherapy, 14,* 689–697.

Wu, F.C.W., & Aitken, R.J. (1989). Suppression of sperm function by depot medroxyprogesterone acetate and testosterone enanthate in steroid male contraception. *Fertility and Sterility, 51,* 691–698.

Wurtman, J.J. (1983). *The carbohydrate craver's diet.* Boston: Houghton Mifflin.

Wysowski, D.K., & Baum, C. (1991). Outpatient use of prescription sedative-hypnotic drugs in the United States, 1970 through 1989. *Archives of Internal Medicine, 151,* 1779–1783.

Yager, J. (1986). Bethanechol chloride can reverse erectile and ejaculatory dysfunction induced by tricyclic antidepressants and mazindol: Case report. *Journal of Clinical Psychiatry, 47,* 210–211.

Yanagita, T., & Miyasato, K. (1976). Dependence potential of methaqualone tested in rhesus monkeys. *CIEA Preclinical Reports, 2,* 63–68.

Yasar, S., & Bergman, J. (1994). Amphetamine-like effect of l-deprenyl (selegiline) in drug discrimination studies. *Clinical Pharmacology and Therapeutics, 56,* 768 773.

Yassa, R. (1982). Sexual disorders in the course of clomipramine treatment: A report of three cases. *Canadian Journal of Psychiatry, 27,* 148–149.

Yassa, R., & Lal, S. (1985). Impaired sexual intercourse as a complication of tardive dyskinesia. *American Journal of Psychiatry, 142,* 1514–1515.

Yatham, L.N., & Mehale, P.A. (1988). Carbamazepine in the treatment of aggression: A case report and a review of the literature. *Acta Psychiatrica Scandinavica, 78,* 188–190.

Yeh, J., & Barbieri, R.L. (1989). Effects of smoking on steroid production, metabolism, and estrogen-related disease. *Seminars in Reproductive Endocrinology, 7,* 326–334.

Yen, S.S. (1977). The biology of menopause. *Journal of Reproductive Medicine, 18,* 287–296.

Yen, S.S.C., & Jaffe, R.B. (1991). *Reproductive endocrinology* (3rd ed.). Philadelphia: W.B. Saunders.

Yen, T.T., Allan, J.A., Pearson, D.V., Acton, J.M., & Greenberg, M.M. (1977). Prevention of obesity in A^{vy}/a mice by dehydroepiandrosterone. *Lipids, 12,* 409–413.

Yen, T.T., Dallo, J., & Knoll, J. (1982). The aphrodisiac effect of low doses of (-) deprenyl in male rats. *Polish Journal of Pharmacology and Pharmacy, 34,* 303–308.

Yeo, W.W., MacLean, D., Richardson, P.J., & Ramsay, L.E. (1991). Cough and enalapril: Assessment by spontaneous reporting and visual analogue scale under double-blind conditions. *British Journal of Clinical Pharmacology, 31,* 356–359.

Yeragani, V.K., & Gershon, S. (1987). Priapism related to phenelzine therapy [Letter to the editor]. *New England Journal of Medicine, 317*(2), 117–118.

Ylikahri, R.H., Huttunen, M., & Harkonen, M. (1980). Hormonal changes during alcohol intoxication and withdrawal. *Pharmacology, Biochemistry, and Behavior, 13*(Suppl. 1), 134–137.

Ylikahri, R.H., Huttunen, M., Harkonen, M., Seuderling, U., Onikki, S., Karonen, S.L., & Adlercreutz, H. (1974). Low plasma testosterone values in men during hangover. *Journal of Steroid Biochemistry, 5,* 655–658.

Ylikahri, R.H., Huttunen, M.O., Harkonen, M., Leino, T., Helenius, T., Liewendahl, K., & Karonen, S.L. (1978). Acute effects of alcohol on anterior pituitary secretion of trophic hormones. *Journal of Clinical Endocrinology and Metabolism, 46,* 715–720.

Ylikorkala, O. (1975). Clonidine in the treatment of menopausal symptoms. *Annales Chirurge & Gynaecologie. Fenn, 64,* 242–245.

Ylikorkala, O., Puolakka, J., & Vrinikka, L. (1984). Vasoconstrictory thromboxane A_2 and vasodilatory prostacylin in limacteric women: Effect of estrogen-progestogen therapy. *Maturitas, 5,* 201–205.

Ylikorkala, O., Stenman, U., & Halmesmäki, E. (1988). Testosterone, androstenedione, dehydroepiandrosterone sulfate, and sex-hormone-binding globulin in pregnant alcohol abusers. *Obstetrics and Gynecology, 71,* 731–735.

Yonezawa, A., Kawamura, S., Ando, R., Tadano, T., Nobunaga, T., & Kimura, Y. (1991). Biphasic effects of yohimbine on the ejaculatory response in the dog. *Life Sciences, 48,* PL103-PL109.

Youdim, M.B.H., & Finberg, J.P.M. (1994). Pharmacological actions of l-deprenyl (selegiline) and other selective monoamine oxidase B inhibitors. *Clinical Pharmacology and Therapeutics, 56,* 725–733.

Young, B.K. (1983). Sexual changes caused by adrenal virilizing syndromes in women. *Medical Aspects of Human Sexuality, 17*(1), 56R-56EE.

Young, R.A., & Brogden, R.N. (1988). Doxazosine: A review of its pharmacodynamic and pharmacokinetic properties and therapeutic efficacy in mild to moderate hypertension. *Drugs, 35,* 525–541.

Young, S.N., Gauthier, S., Anderson, G.M., & Purdy, W.C. (1980). Tryptophan, 5-hydroxyindoleacetic acid, and indoleacetic acid in human cerebrospinal fluid: Interrelationships and the influence of age, sex, epilepsy, and anticonvulsant drugs. *Journal of Neurology, Neurosurgery, and Psychiatry, 43,* 438–445.

Young, W. (1961). The hormones and mating behavior. In W. Young (Ed.), *Sex and internal secretions* (Vol. 2) (pp. 1173–1239). Baltimore: Williams & Wilkins.

Yu, L.C., & Han, J.S. (1990). Habenula as a relay in the descending pathway from the nucleus accumbens to periaqueductal grey subserving antinociception. *International Journal of Neuroscience, 54,* 245–251.

Yudofsky, S., Hales, R.F., & Ferguson, T. (1991). *What you need to know about psychiatric drugs.* New York: Grove Weidenfeld.

Zabik, J.E. (1987). Use of serotonin-active drugs in alcohol preference studies. In M. Galanter (Ed.), *Recent developments in alcoholism. Vol. 7. Treatment research* (pp. 211–224). New York: Plenum Press.

Zabik, J.E., Binkerd, K., & Roache, J.D. (1985). Serotonin and ethanol aversion in the rat. In C.A. Naranjo & E.M. Sellers (Ed.), *Recent advances in new psychopharmaological treatments for alcoholism* (pp. 87–105). New York: Elsevier Science Publishers.

Zahorska-Markiewicz, B., & Kucio, C. (1984). Mazindol and pain sensitivity. *Current Therapeutic Research, 36,* 445–448.

Zajecka, J., Fawcett, J., Schaff, M., Jeffries, H., & Guy, C. (1991). The role of serotonin in sexual dysfunction: Fluoxetine-associated orgasm dysfunction. *Journal of Clinical Psychiatry, 52,* 66–68.

Zanetti-Elshater, F., Pingatore, R., Beretta-Piccoli, C., Riesen, W., & Heinen, G. (1994). Calcium antagonists for treatment of diabetes-associated hypertension. *American Journal of Hypertension, 7,* 36–45.

Zenz, M., Strumpf, M., & Tryba, M. (1992). Long-term oral opioid therapy in patients with chronic nonmalignant pain. *Journal of Pain and Symptoms Management, 7,* 69–77.

Zerbe, K.J. (1992). Why eating-disordered patients resist sex therapy: A response to Simpson and Ramberg. *Journal of Sex and Marital Therapy, 18,* 55–60.

Zhang, J., Feldblum, P.J., & Fortney, J.A. (1992). Moderate physical activity and bone density among perimenopausal women. *American Journal of Public Health, 82,* 736–738.

Zhao, B., Chapman, C., & Bicknell, R.J. (1988). Opioid-noradrenergic interactions in the neurohypophysis: I. Differential opioid receptor regulation of oxytocin, vasopressin, and noradrenaline release. *Neuroendocrinology, 48,* 16–24.

Zini, D., Carani, C., Baldini, A., Cavicchioli, C., Piccinini, D., & Marrama, P. (1986). Further acquisitions on gonadal function in bromocriptine treated hyperprolactinemic male patients. *Pharmacological Research Communication, 18,* 601–609.

Zitrin, A. (1972). Changes in brain serotonin level and male sexual behavior. In J. Barchas, & E. Usdin (Eds.), *Serotonin and behavior* (pp. 365–370). New York: Academic Press.

Zitrin, A., Beach, F.A., Barchas, J.D., & Dement, W.C. (1970). Sexual behavior in male cats after administration of parachlorophenylalanine. *Science, 170,* 868–870.

Zorgniotti, A.W. (1992). "On demand" oral drug for erection in impotent men. *Journal of Urology, 147,* 308A.

Zorgniotti, A.W., & Lefleur, R.S. (1985). Autoinjection of the corpus cavernosum with a vasoactive drug combination for vasculogenic impotence. *Journal of Urology, 133,* 39–41.

Zorgniotti, A.W., & Lizza, E.F. (1991). *Diagnosis and management of impotence.* Philadelphia: B.C. Decker.

Zorgniotti, A.W., Rossman, B., & Mitchell, C. (1987). Possible role of chronic use of nasal vasoconstrictors in impotence [Letter to the editor]. *Urology, 30,* 594.

Zubenko, G.S., & Nixon, R.A. (1984). Mood-elevating effect of captopril in depressed patients. *American Journal of Psychiatry, 141,* 110–111.

Zubieta, J.K., & Demitrack, M.A. (1991). Possible bupropion precipitation of mania and a mixed affective state [Letter to the editor]. *Journal of Clinical Psychopharmacology, 11,* 327–328.

Zuckerman, B., Frank, D.A., Hingson, R., Amaro, H., Levenson, S.M., Kayne, H., Parker, S., Vinci, R., Aboagye, K., Fried, L.E., Cabral, H., Timperi, R., & Bauchner, H. (1989). Effects of maternal marijuana and cocaine use on fetal growth. *New England Journal of Medicine, 320,* 762.

Zung, N.K. (1983). Review of placebo-controlled trials with bupropion. *Journal of Clinical Psychiatry, 44,* 104–114.

Zusman, R. (1984). Renin and non-renin-mediated antihypertensive actions of converting enzyme inhibitors. *Kidney International, 25,* 969–983.

Name Index

Subject Index*

*Numbers in bold-face type indicate pages containing tables. Commercial names of drugs are indexed only when they have appeared in a heading.

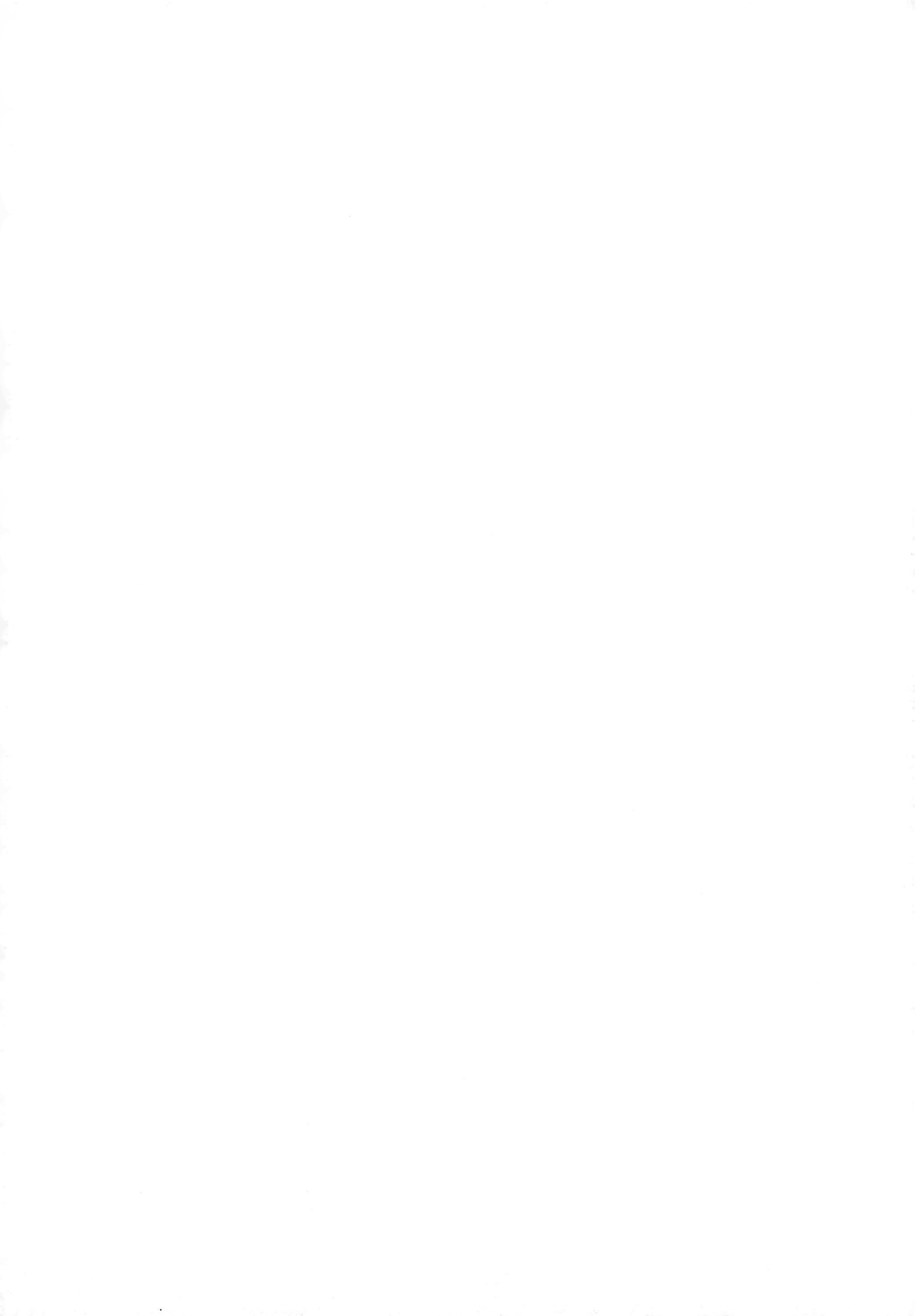

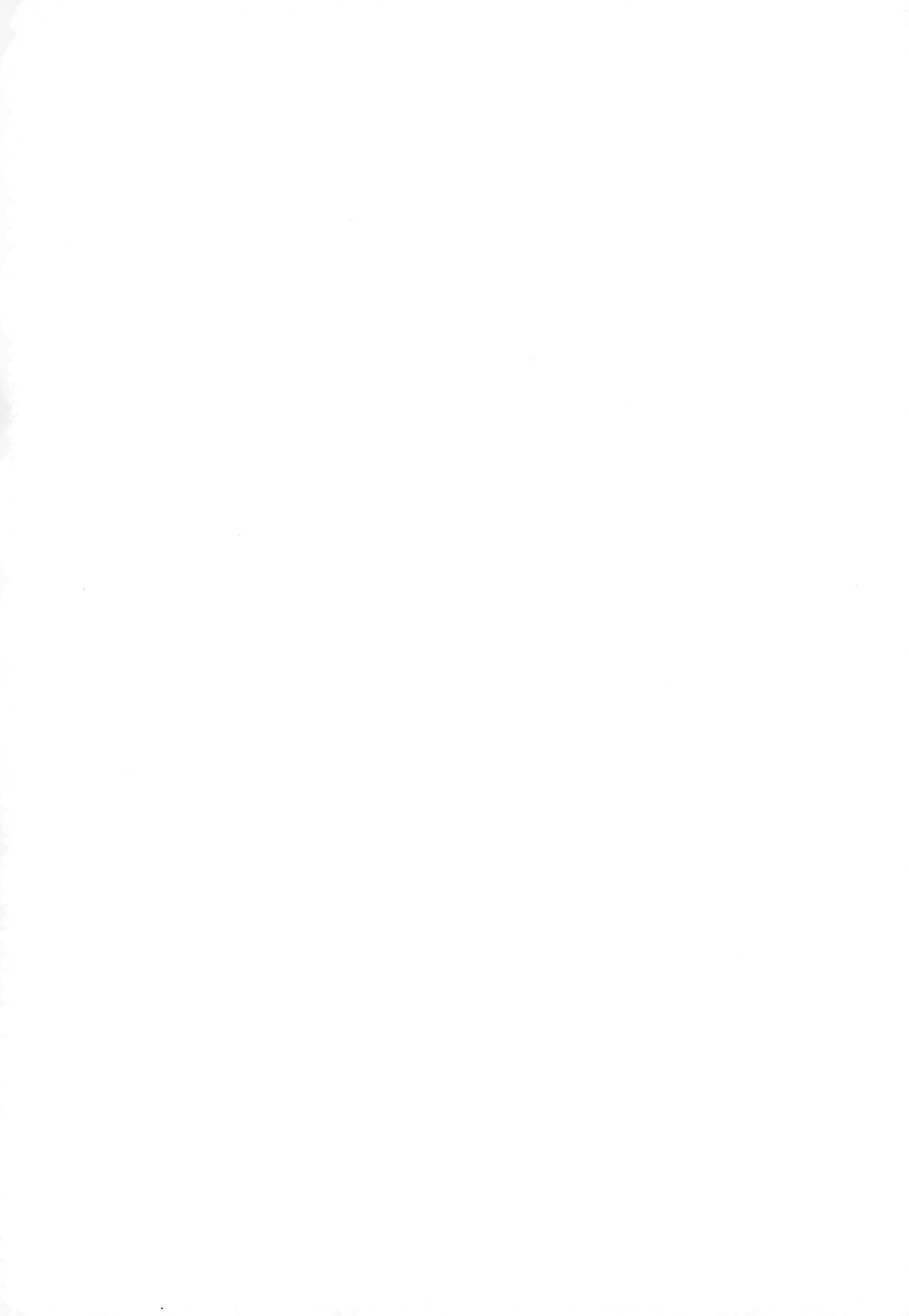